Technique
of the
Neurologic
Examination

A Programmed Text *Fourth Edition*

Technique
of the
Neurologic
Examination

A Programmed Text *Fourth Edition*

William E. DeMyer, M.D.

Professor of Neurology
Indiana University School of Medicine
Indianapolis

McGRAW-HILL, Inc.

Health Professions Division

New York St. Louis San Francisco Auckland Bogotá Hamburg
London Madrid Mexico City Montreal New Delhi Panama
Paris São Paulo Singapore Sydney Tokyo Toronto

TECHNIQUE OF THE NEUROLOGIC EXAMINATION: *A PROGRAMMED TEXT*

4567890 MALMAL 998

ISBN 0-07-016353-7

This book was set in Times Roman by University Graphics. The editor was Steven Melvin; the production supervisor was Richard C. Ruzycka; the cover designer was Marsha Cohen Parallelogram. Malloy Lithographing, Inc. was printer and binder.

Library of Congress Cataloging-in-Publication Data

DeMyer, William,
      Technique of the neurologic examination : a programmed text /
William DeMyer.—4th ed.
         p.   cm.
      Includes bibliographical references and index.
      ISBN 0-07-016353-7
      1. Neurologic examination—Programmed instruction.   I.   Title.
      [DNLM: 1.   Neurologic Examination—programmed instruction. WL 18
D389t 1993]
RC348.D44   1993
616.8′0475—dc20
DNLM/DLC
for Library of Congress   93-25996
                                                CIP

Contents

Preface to the Fourth Edition

The fourth edition adheres to the basic principles of programmed learning by eliciting active responses from the student. The text presents the real problems that the student will actually have to solve and rehearses the real responses that the student will actually have to make to master the neurologic examination.

Because programming proceeds by increments, it is the best way to learn new skills, but at the same time, it is difficult to review efficiently. This new edition adds Learning Objectives at the end of each chapter. By responding with the recitations and demonstrations specified in the Learning Objectives the student can quickly and efficiently review the contents of each chapter.

I want to thank the many students who, over the years, have made suggestions for improving the text. Let me hear from you. I am listening.

With all best wishes for a neurologic examination in which you can take pride.

William E. DeMyer

Preface to the First Edition

The purpose of this textbook is threefold: (1) to teach how to conduct a neurologic examination, (2) to review the anatomy and physiology for interpreting it, and (3) to show which laboratory tests help to clarify the clinical problem. This is not a differential diagnosis text nor a systematic description of diseases.

Anyone who sets out to write a textbook should place his manuscript on one knee and a student on the other. When the student squirms, sighs, or gives a wrong answer, the author has erred. He should correct it right then, before the ink dries. That is the way I have written this text, on the basis of feedback from the students.

The peril of student-on-the-knee teaching is that even though the student moves his lips, the words and voice remain the teacher's. To escape from ventriloquism, my text relies strongly on self-observation and induction. First, you learn to observe yourself, not as Narcissus, but as a sample of every man. Whenever possible you study living flesh, its look, its feel, and its responses. Why study a textbook picture to learn the range of ocular movements if you can hold up a hand mirror? Why memorize the laws of diplopia if you can do a simple experiment on yourself whenever you need to refresh your memory? In the best tradition of science, these techniques supplant the printed word as the source of knowledge. The text becomes a way of extending your own perceptions, of looking at the world through the eyes of experience.

Since programmed instruction is the best way for the learner himself to judge whether learning has taken place most of the text is programmed. He is not abandoned to guess whether he has learned something; the program makes him prove that he has learned. Programming, if abused or overdone, becomes incredibly dull, unmercifully slow. The reader is required to inspect a grain of sand at a time, yet he should have been shown the whole shoreline at a glance. Some programs err by bristling with objectivity, causing one to ask, "Isn't there a human being around here somewhere? Didn't someone think this, decide it, maybe even guess at it a little?" For interludes, I use quotations, anecdotes, and poetry. I even stoop to mnemonics. Sometimes I cajole, not pretending as is customary in textbooks, that the pages have been purified, relieved of an author. I am very much here, poking my head out of a paragraph now and then or peering at you through an asterisk. When I see that you are weary from filling in blanks, I offer some whimsy. When you overflow with something to say, I ask for an essay answer. Sometimes you are invited to anticipate the text, to match wits against the problem without the spoon. At all times as you practice the neurologic examination, I stand at your elbow, guiding your moves and interpretations. You should be able to do a prideful neurologic examination when you finish the book. And lastly, I include references. Only one reader in a hundred uses them? I am interested in him too, in his precious curiosity.

These then are the secrets: a lot of self-observation, a lot of programming, some irony and humor, a few editorials, and occasionally a summarizing paragraph, like this one. And as the leaven, lest they vanish from medical education, reminders of the bittersweet flowers of the mind, of tenderness, of understanding and compassion . . . like this stanza from Yeats, because it is perhaps all that should preface a text like this, into which I have poured the best teaching that I can offer, and yet the wish always exceeds the result, ah me, by far:

Had I the heavens' embroidered cloths.
Enwrought with gold and silver light,
The blue and the dim and the dark cloths
Of night and light and the half light,
I would spread the cloths under your feet;
But I, being poor, have only my dreams;
I have spread my dreams under your feet;
Tread softly because you tread on my dreams.

To the many colleagues who have shared their knowledge with me over the years, I am deeply grateful. I want especially to thank Dr. Alexander T. Ross, my own preceptor in clinical neurology, and many friends in the basic disciplines of neurology, Drs. Ralph Reitan, Charles Ferster, Sidney Ochs, Wolfgang Zeman, and Jans Muller. For their day-to-day help I thank my wife, Dr. Marian DeMyer, Dr. Mark Dyken, and the many medical students, interns, and residents who suffered through the stuttering phases of the programming. And then, Miss Irene Baird, who meticulously, maternally made the drawings; Mrs. Faith Halstead, who typed and retyped the burgeoning manuscript; medical artist James Glore; and photographer Joseph Demma.

William E. DeMyer

Preparation for the Text

I assume that you have finished at least one year of medical school and know the basic concepts of neuroanatomy and neurophysiology (but I review some of them anyway). The text will teach you the mental and manual skills needed to do the neurologic examination (NE). At the outset, I have found that students want most of all to know: just what constitutes a NE? Thus I begin my text, pages xi to xxv, (and my classes) by outlining a standard complete NE. Of course, you cannot do the NE now—that's what the rest of the text teaches—but use the outline in two ways: (1) refer back to it each time you complete a chapter, to fit what you have learned into the total examination, and (2) take it to the wards and clinics to guide you until you can do it independently.

You must have the basic examining equipment listed on pages xii to xiii, and some learning aids. As learning aids, get a hand mirror, colored pencils, and a table tennis ball. Do not start the text until you have everything. Then do the text in sequence; skipping around invites difficulty because each learning sequence locks into the preceding material and presumes its mastery. Allow approximately one hour for each nine pages you want to complete.

Since the text requires you to inspect yourself and others, study in your own living quarters, preferably with a partner. Do all of the tests on yourself or the partner as the text calls for them. The doing results in permanent learning by developing your own personal powers of observation and manipulation. Most of your education to this point has consisted of the memorization of lists and concepts compiled by someone else. Now you have to learn how to learn directly from the Pt. That requires the doing.

Abbreviations Used in This Text

AP	Anteroposterior
ARAS	Ascending reticular activating system
BE	Branchial efferent
BP	Blood pressure
C	Cervical
CT	Computerized axial tomography
cm	Centimeter
CNS	Central nervous system
cps	Cycles per second
CSF	Cerebrospinal fluid
EEG	Electroencephalogram
EMG	Electromyogram
Ex	Examiner
F	False
L	Lateral, left, or lumbar
LMN	Lower motor neuron
MLF	Medial longitudinal fasciculus
mm	Millimeters
MRI	Magnetic resonance imaging
MSR	Muscle stretch reflex
NE	Neurologic examination

OFC	Occipitofrontal circumference
PICA	Posterior inferior cerebellar artery
Pt	Patient
R	Right
RBCs	Red blood cells
S	Sacral
SA	Somatic afferent
SCA	Superior cerebellar artery
SCM	Sternocleidomastoid muscle
SE	Somatic efferent
SSSS	Solely special sensory set (cranial nerves I, II, and VIII)
SVA	Special visceral afferent
T	True or thoracic
TNR	Tonic neck reflex
UMN	Upper motor neuron
V	Vertical
VA	Visceral afferent
VE	Visceral efferent
WBCs	White blood cells

Outline of the Standard Complete Neurologic Examination (NE)

These pages outline first the NE of the conscious, responsive patient (Pt) and then of the unconscious Pt. Beginning with Chapter 1, the text explains how to do each step.

I. Introduction

A. *How the history guides the examination*

   1. The Ex completes much of the NE by observations while taking the history and assessing the Pt's mental status and the content of speech. Inspect the facial features for diagnostic abnormalities; inspect the eye movements, blinking, and the relation of the cornea to lids and the palpebral fissures; look for en- or exophthalmos; note the degree and symmetry of facial movements; observe how the Pt swallows saliva, breathes, and articulates words; inspect the posture; and look for tremors and involuntary movements.

   2. Although the Ex does a basic routine examination on every Pt, the history and preliminary observations suggest which areas need special attention: either central or neuromuscular motor systems; sensory systems; cranial nerves; or cerebral functions. For example, if the history suggests a spinal cord problem, successively test each dermatome for a sensory level and do a detailed sensory examination of the perianal region for loss or preservation of sacral sensation. But if the history suggests a cerebral lesion, emphasize tests for memory, aphasia, apraxia, astereognosis, and inattention to simultaneous stimuli.

   3. The history frequently suggests special tests tailored to the Pt's specific problems. Reproduce any conditions which the Pt reports as aggravating or triggering the symptoms, such as:

      a. Dizziness when standing up: check for orthostatic hypotension.

      b. Episodic complaints of numbness and tingling in extremities, blackouts or fainting spells, or suspected epilepsy: ask the Pt to hyperventilate for a full three minutes.

      c. Weakness in climbing stairs: watch the Pt climb stairs.

      d. Trouble swallowing: give the Pt liquids and solids to swallow.

    e. Pathologic fatigability, particularly of cranial nerve muscles: have the Pt make 100 repetitive movements, and do the edrophonium (Tensilon) test for myasthenia gravis.

The primary role of the examination becomes the testing of hypotheses derived from the history.

                                    William Landau

B. How to do an orderly, complete examination

Unless you do an orderly NE, you will forget some part of it. Neurologists may choose different orders, but they will complete the same tests. To remember the sequence I recommend, lay out your instruments in the order of use. As you finish with each one, replace it in your bag. After replacing every instrument, you will have done a complete examination without forgetting anything. Use this order:

Instruments	Use
1. Flexible steel measuring tape scored in metric system	Measurement of occipitofrontal and other body circumferences, size of skin lesions, length of extremities, etc.
2. Stethoscope	Auscultation of the neck vessels, eyes, and cranium for bruits.
3. Flashlight with rubber adapter	Pupillary reflexes, inspection of pharynx, and transillumination of the heads of infants
4. Transparent mm ruler	Measurement of pupillary size, diameter of skin lesions, distances on radiographic films.
5. Ophthalmoscope	Funduscopy, examination of ocular media and skin surface for beads of sweat.
6. Tongue blades	Three per Pt: one for depressing tongue, one for eliciting gag reflex, one broken for eliciting abdominal and plantar reflexes.
7. Opaque vial of coffee	Testing sense of smell.
8. Opaque vials of salt and sugar	Testing taste.
9. Otoscope	Examination of auditory canal and drum.
10. Tuning fork	Testing vibratory sensation and hearing (256 cps recommended).
11. 10 cc syringe	Caloric irrigation of the ear.
12. Cotton wisp	One end rolled for eliciting corneal reflex, the other loose for testing light touch.
13. Two stoppered tubes	Testing hot and cold discrimination.
14. Disposable straight pins	Testing pain sensation.

15. Reflex hammer	Eliciting muscle stretch reflexes (MSRs). Muscle percussion for myotonia.
16. Penny, nickel, dime, paper clip, and key	Testing for astereognosis.
17. Page of figure-stimuli	Screening cerebral and intellectual dysfunctions.
18. Blood pressure cuff	Routine BP and orthostatic hypotension.

II. Mental status examination

A. *General behavior and appearance.* Is the Pt normal, hyperactive, agitated, quiet, or immobile? Is the Pt neat or slovenly? Does the Pt dress in accordance with age, peers, sex, and background?

B. *Stream of talk.* Does the Pt converse normally? Is the speech rapid, incessant, under great pressure, or is it slow and lacking in spontaneity? Is the Pt discursive and unable to reach the conversational goal?

C. *Mood and affective responses.* Is the Pt euphoric, agitated, inappropriately gay, giggling, silent, weeping, or angry? Does the Pt's mood appropriately reflect the subject matter of the conversation? Is the Pt emotionally labile, histrionic, expansive, or overtly depressed?

D. *Content of thought.* Does the Pt correctly perceive reality or have illusions, hallucinations, delusions, misinterpretations, and obsessions? Is the Pt preoccupied with bodily complaints, fears of cancer or heart disease, or other phobias? Does the Pt suffer delusions of persecution, surveillance, and control by malicious persons or forces?

E. *Intellectual capacity.* Is the Pt bright, average, dull, or obviously demented or mentally retarded?

F. *Sensorium*
   1. Consciousness
   2. Attention span
   3. Orientation for time, place, and person
   4. Memory, recent and remote
   5. Calculation
   6. Fund of information
   7. Insight, judgment, and planning

III. Speech. Is it normal or does the Pt display:

A. *Dysphonia.* Difficulty in producing the voice sounds.

B. *Dysarthria.* Difficulty in articulating the individual sounds or the units (phonemes) of speech: *f*s, *r*s, *g*s, vowels, consonants, the labials (cranial nerve VII), gutterals (X), and linguals (XII).

C. *Dysprosody.* Difficulty with the melody and rhythm of speech, the accent of syllables, the inflections, pitch of voice, and intonations.

D. *Dysphasia.* Difficulty in expressing or understanding words as the symbols of communication.

IV. Head and face

A. *Inspection*
   1. What general impression does the Pt's face make? Do the features suggest a diagnostic facial *gestalt?* Does it show abnormal motility and emotional expression?
   2. Inspect the head for abnormalities in shape and asymmetry.
   3. Inspect the hair of scalp, eyebrows, and beard.
   4. Inspect the eyes for ptosis, width of palpebral fissures, relation of iris to lids, pupillary size, and interorbital distance.
   5. Inspect contours and proportions of nose, mouth, chin, and ears for malformations.

B. *Palpate* the skull of a mature Pt for lumps, depressions, or tenderness, and asymmetries and of an infant for fontanelles and sutures. Palpate the temporal arteries. Measure and record the occipitofrontal circumference of all infants.

C. *Percuss* over the sinuses and mastoid processes for tenderness if the Pt has headaches.

D. *Auscultate* for bruits over the neck vessels, eyes, temples, and mastoid processes.

E. *Transilluminate* the sinuses if the Pt has headaches. Attempt to transilluminate the head of young infants.

V. Cranial nerves

A. *Optic group:* II, III, IV, and VI
   1. Inspect width of palpebral fissures, relation of limbus to lid margins, interorbital distance, and en- or exophthalmos.
   2. *Visual functions.* Test acuity (central fields) by newsprint or Snellen chart (each eye separately), and test peripheral fields by confrontation. Test for inattention to simultaneous visual stimuli if a cerebral lesion is suspected.
   3. Test pupillary light reflexes, and record size of pupils.
   4. Do opthalmoscopy.
   5. *Ocular motility.* Test range of ocular movements by having Pt's eyes follow your finger through all fields of gaze. During convergence check for miosis. Do the cover-uncover test. Record nystagmus and any effects of eye movements on it.

B. *Branchiomotor group and tongue.* V, VII, IX, X, XI, and XII
   1. V: Inspect masseter and temporalis muscle bulk, and palpate masseters when the Pt bites.
   2. VII: Test forehead wrinkling, eyelid closure, mouth retraction, whistling or puffing out cheeks, and wrinkling of skin over neck (platysma action). Listen to labial articulations. Check for Chvostek's sign in selected cases.

3. IX and X: Listen for phonation and articulation (labial, lingual, and palatal sounds) and check swallowing, gag reflex, and palatal elevation.
4. XII: Check lingual articulations, midline and lateral tongue protrusion, and inspect tongue for atrophy, and fasciculations.
5. XI: Inspect sternocleidomastoid and trapezius contours, and test strength of head movements and shoulder shrugging.
6. If the history raises the question of pathologic fatigability, request 100 repetitive movements (eye blinks, etc.). Consider edrophonium (Tensilon) test.
7. Assess the rate, regularity, and depth of breathing.

C. *Special sensory group*
   1. *Olfaction* (I). Use aromatic, nonirritating substance and test each nostril separately.
   2. *Taste* (VII). Use salt or sugar. (Test if VIIth nerve lesion suspected.)
   3. *Hearing* (VIII).
      a. Do otoscopy.
      b. *Assess threshold and acuity* by noting the Pt's ability to hear conversational speech and to hear a tuning fork, a watch tick, or rustling of fingers.
      c. If history or preceding tests suggest a deficit, do air-bone conduction test of Rinne and vertex lateralizing test of Weber.
      d. If the history suggests a cerebral lesion, test for auditory inattention to bilateral simultaneous stimuli, using finger rustling.
      e. In infants or uncooperative Pts, try the auditopalpebral reflex as a crude screening test.
   4. *Vestibular function* (VIII). In selected Pts do caloric irrigation, and test for positional nystagmus.

D. *Somatic sensation of the face* (Testing trigeminal area sensation now obviates a return to the face after examining the Pt's anogenital area and feet.)
   1. Corneal reflex (V–VII arc).
   2. Light touch over the three divisions of the Vth nerve.
   3. Temperature discrimination over the three divisions of the Vth nerve.
   4. Pain perception over the three divisions of the Vth nerve.
   5. Test buccal mucosal sensation in selected Pts.

VI. Somatic motor systems (exclusive of cranial nerves)

A. *Inspection*
   1. *Gait testing.* Free walking, toe and heel walking, tandem walking, deep knee bend. Have a child hop on each foot and run.
   2. Inspect the Pt's posture, general activity level, and look for tremors or other involuntary movement.
   3. Undress the Pt and assess the somatotype (the build or body *gestalt*).
   4. Observe the size and contour of the muscles, looking for atrophy, hypertrophy, body asymmetry, joint malalignments, fasciculations, tremors, and involuntary movement.
   5. Search the entire skin surface for lesions, particularly neurocutaneous stigmate such as *café au lait* spots.

B. *Palpation.* Palate muscles if they seem atrophic, hypertrophic, or if the history suggests that they may be tender or in spasm.

C. *Strength testing*
  1. *Shoulder girdle.* Try to press the Pt's arms down after he or she abducts them to shoulder height. Look for scapular winging.
  2. *Upper extremities.* Test biceps, triceps, wrist dorsiflexors, and grip. Test strength of finger abduction and extension.
  3. *Abdominal muscles.* Have Pt do a sit-up. Watch for umbilical migration.
  4. *Lower extremities.* Test hip flexors, abductors and adductors, knee flexors, foot dorsiflexors, invertors, and evertors. (Knee extensors were tested by the deep knee bend and plantar flexors by toe walking.)
  5. Grade strength on a scale of 0 to 5 or describe as paralysis, severe, moderate, or minimal weakness, or normal. Discern whether any weakness follows a distributional pattern such as proximal-distal, right-left, or upper extremity-lower extremity.

D. *Muscle tone.* Make passive movements of joints to test for spasticity, clonus, rigidity, or hypotonus.

E. *Muscle stretch (deep) reflexes.* Grade 0 to 4+ and designate whether clonic:
  1. Jaw jerk (V afferent; V efferent)
  2. Biceps reflex (C5-C6)
  3. Triceps reflex (C7-C8)
  4. Finger flexion reflex (C7-T1)
  5. Quadriceps reflex (knee jerk) (L2-L4)
  6. Hamstring reflex (L5-S1)
  7. Triceps surae reflex (ankle jerk) (L5-S1-S3)
  8. Toe flexion reflex (S1-S2)

F. *Percussion.* Percuss the thenar eminence for percussion myotonia, and test for a myotonic grip if the Pt has generalized muscular weakness.

G. *Skin-muscle (superficial) reflexes*
  1. Abdominal skin-muscle reflexes (upper quadrants T8-T9); lower quadrants, (T11-T12). Do umbilical migration test (Beevor's sign) in selected cases if a thoracic cord lesion is suspected.
  2. Cremasteric reflex (afferent L1; efferent L2)
  3. Test anal pucker (S4-S5) and bulbocavernosus reflexes in Pts suspected of sacral or cauda equina lesions.

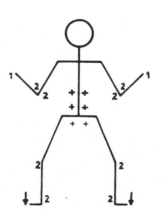

FIG. NE-1. Figure for recording muscle stretch reflexes and abdominal, cremasteric, and plantar reflexes.

    4. Extensor toe sign or Babinski sign (afferent S1; efferent L5-S1-S2).

   H. Cerebellar system. (Gait tested previously)
     1. Finger-to-nose, rebound and rapid alternating hand movements
     2. Heel-to-knee

   I. Nerve root stretching tests. Done in selected Pts.
     1. If disc or low-back disease is suspected, do leg raising tests: the straight-knee leg raising test (Laseague's sign) and the bent-knee leg raising test (Kernig's sign).
     2. If meningeal irritation is suspected, test for nuchal rigidity and concomitant leg flexion (Brudzinski's sign) and do the leg raising tests.

VII. Somatic sensory system

A. Superficial sensory modalities. (Include trigeminal area if not previously tested).
   1. Light touch over hands, trunk, and feet.
   2. Temperature discrimination over hands, trunk, and feet.
   3. Pain perception over hands, trunk, and feet.

B. Deep sensory modalities
   1. Test vibration perception at knuckles, fingernails, and malleoli of ankles and toenails.
   2. Test position sense of fingers and toes, using the fourth digits.
   3. Stereognosis
   4. Romberg (swaying) test
   5. Directional scratch test

C. Determine the distributional pattern of any sensory loss: dermatomal, peripheral nerve(s), central pathway, or nonorganic.

D. Summary of dermatomal relations (Fig. 2-10): Trigeminal nerve to interaural line where it abuts on C2 (no C1). C3-C4 over "cape" area of shoulders, 5-6-7-8-1 are pulled out on arms, C4 abuts on T2, T4 is nipple level, T10 is umbilical level, L5 to big toe, S1 to small toe, S4 and S5 to the perianal zone.

VIII. Cerebral functions

A. Do a complete Mental Status examination, emphasizing tests of the sensorium (Section II of this outline).

B. If the history or Mental Status examination suggest a cerebral lesion, test for agraphognosia, finger agnosia, poor two-point discrimination, right-left disorientation, atopognosia, and tactile, auditory, and visual inattention to bilateral simultaneous stimuli. Test for tactile inattention to simultaneous ipsilateral stimulation of face-hand and foot-hand.

C. Have the Pt do the cognitive, constructional, and performance tasks of the Halstead-Reitan screening test for cerebral dysfunction. Use Fig. NE-2 and Table NE-1.

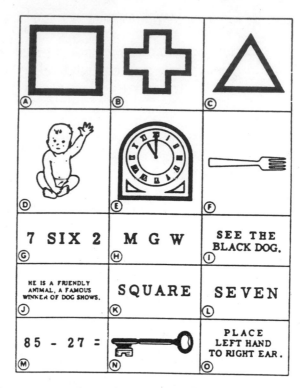

FIG. NE-2. Stimulus figures to screen for cerebral dysfunction. (From Reitan's modification of the Halstead-Wepman screening test as currently used in the Neuropsychology Laboratory at Indiana University and many other testing centers. Reitan, R. M., and Davison, L. A., *Clinical Neuropsychology: Current Status and Applications.* New York, John Wiley & Sons, 1974.)

TABLE NE-1. Instructions for the Halstead-Reitan screening test for cerebral dysfunction	
Patient's task	Examiner's instructions to the patient
1. Copy SQUARE (A) (See parts A–O, of Fig. NE-2)	FIRST, DRAW THIS ON YOUR PAPER. (Point to Square, item A). I WANT YOU TO DO IT WITHOUT LIFTING YOUR PENCIL FROM THE PAPER. MAKE IT ABOUT THIS SAME SIZE.
2. Name SQUARE	WHAT IS THAT SHAPE CALLED?
3. Spell SQUARE	WOULD YOU SPELL THAT WORD FOR ME?
4. Copy CROSS (B)	DRAW THIS ON YOUR PAPER. GO AROUND THE OUTSIDE LIKE THIS UNTIL YOU GET BACK TO WHERE YOU STARTED. MAKE IT ABOUT THIS SAME SIZE.
5. Name CROSS	WHAT IS THAT SHAPE CALLED?
6. Spell CROSS	WOULD YOU SPELL THAT WORD FOR ME?
7. Copy TRIANGLE (C)	Instruct as in 1 and 4 above.
8. Name TRIANGLE	WHAT IS THAT SHAPE CALLED?
9. Spell TRIANGLE	WOULD YOU SPELL THAT WORD FOR ME?
10. Name BABY (D)	WHAT IS THIS? (Show baby, item D)
11. Write CLOCK	NOW, I AM GOING TO SHOW YOU ANOTHER PICTURE BUT DO *NOT* TELL ME THE NAME OF IT. I DON'T WANT YOU TO SAY ANYTHING OUT LOUD. JUST WRITE THE NAME OF THE PICTURE ON YOUR PAPER. (Show clock, item E).
12. Name FORK (F)	WHAT IS THIS? (Show fork, item F)
13. Read 7 SIX 2 (G)	I WANT YOU TO READ THIS. (Show item G).
14. Read M G W (H)	READ THIS. (Show item H).
15. Reading I (I)	NOW, I WANT YOU TO READ THIS. (Show item I).
16. Reading II (J)	CAN YOU READ THIS? (Show item J).

(continued)

TABLE NE-1. **Instructions for the Halstead-Reitan screening test for cerebral dysfunction,** (continued)

Patient's task	Examiner's instructions to the patient
17. Repeat TRIANGLE	NOW, I AM GOING TO SAY SOME WORDS. I WANT YOU TO LISTEN CAREFULLY AND SAY THEM AFTER ME AS CAREFULLY AS YOU CAN. SAY THIS WORD: TRIANGLE.
18. Repeat MASSACHUSETTS	THE NEXT ONE IS A LITTLE HARDER BUT DO YOUR BEST. SAY THIS WORD: MASSACHUSETTS
19. Repeat METHODIST EPISCOPAL	NOW REPEAT THIS ONE; METHODIST EPISCOPAL.
20. Write SQUARE	DON'T SAY THIS WORD OUT LOUD. JUST WRITE IT ON YOUR PAPER. (Point to stimulus word SQUARE, item *K*.)
21. Read SEVEN (*L*)	CAN YOU READ THIS WORD OUT LOUD. (Show item *L*.)
22. Repeat SEVEN	NOW, I WANT YOU TO SAY THIS AFTER ME: SEVEN.
23. Repeat–explain.	I AM GOING TO SAY SOMETHING THAT I WANT YOU TO SAY AFTER ME. SO LISTEN CAREFULLY. HE SHOUTED THE WARNING. NOW YOU SAY IT. WOULD YOU EXPLAIN WHAT THAT MEANS?
24. Write: HE SHOUTED	NOW, I WANT YOU TO WRITE THAT SENTENCE ON THE PAPER.
25. Compute 85 − 27 = (*M*)	HERE IS AN ARITHMETIC PROBLEM. COPY IT DOWN ON YOUR PAPER ANY WAY YOU LIKE AND TRY TO WORK IT OUT. (Show item *M*.)
26. Compute 17 × 3 =	NOW, DO THIS ONE IN YOUR HEAD; 17 × 3.
27. Name KEY (*N*)	WHAT IS THIS: (Show item *N*.)
28. Demonstrate use of KEY (*N*)	IF YOU HAD ONE OF THESE IN YOUR HAND, SHOW ME HOW YOU WOULD USE IT. (Show item *N*.)
29. Draw KEY (*N*).	NOW, I WANT YOU TO DRAW A PICTURE THAT LOOKS JUST LIKE THIS. TRY TO MAKE YOUR KEY LOOK ENOUGH LIKE THIS ONE SO THAT I WOULD KNOW IT WAS THE SAME KEY FROM YOUR DRAWING. (Point to key, item *N*.)
30. Read (*O*)	WOULD YOU READ THIS? (Show item *O*.)
31. Place LEFT HAND TO RIGHT EAR	NOW, WOULD YOU DO WHAT IT SAID?
32. Place LEFT HAND TO LEFT ELBOW	NOW, I WANT YOU TO PUT YOUR LEFT HAND TO YOUR LEFT ELBOW.

Note: The average normal person with a high school education should make essentially no errors on this test and recognize immediately the impossibility of command 32. Re-test any items failed, by giving tasks similar to the failed one.

IX. Case summary

A. Write a three-line summary of the pertinent positive historical and physical findings. (If you can't put it in three lines, you don't understand the problem.)

B. Write down a provisional clinical diagnosis and outline the differential diagnosis.

C. Write out a list of the clinical problems.

D. Write down a sequential plan of management for:
   1. Diagnostic tests to discriminate between the diagnostic possibilities.
   2. Therapy: State the therapeutic goals.

3. Management of the emotional, educational, and socioeconomic problems that the illness causes the Pt.
4. Identification of and prophylaxis for other persons now known to be "at risk" because of the Pt's illness, if the illness is infectious, genetic, or environmentally induced.

Neurologic Examination of the Unconscious Patient

(Particularly the unknown Pt brought in off the street).

A. *History:* Two examiners are desirable, one for the emergency physical management of the Pt and the other to obtain a history. Contact family, friends, police, the Pt's past physicians, or anyone who witnessed the circumstances under which the Pt lost consciousness. Ask about:
   1. Possibility of head trauma.
   2. A seizure disorder.
   3. Insulin/diabetes mellitus.
   4. A recent change in mood, behavior, thinking, or neurologic condition.
   5. Depression or access to depressant drugs.
   6. Other medicines.
   7. Allergies, insect bites, and other causes of anaphylactic shock.
   8. Cardiac, hepatic, pulmonary, or lung disease.
   9. Past hospitalizations for serious health problems.
   10. Exclude red herrings. Does the Pt have preexisting neurologic or physical anomalies or dysfunctions? For example, has previous disease altered pupillary size or reactions? Has the Pt had prior strabismus, hemiplegia, etc.?

B. *Introductory note to the ABCDE ritual for the examination of the comatose Pt:* On first approaching the comatose Pt, the Ex, must have a distinct plan of priorities and procedures, summarized by the *ABCDE* mnemonic. The plan will detect any of the five *H*s that immediately threaten the brain: hypoxia, hypotension, hypoglycemia, hyperthermia, and herniation.
   1. *A and B = Airway and Breathing.* Make sure the Pt has an open airway and is breathing. Otherwise the brain, which requires a continuous supply of O_2 and glucose, will start to die within 5 min of total oxygen deprivation. If the brain dies all else is futile.
   2. *C = Circulation.* The blood must be circulating to deliver O_2 and glucose to the brain. You have only a few minutes to restore breathing and circulation.
   3. *D = Dextrose.* The dextrose level of the circulating blood must be high enough to nourish the brain.

4. *E = Examine the Eyes.* Examination of the pupillary size and reactions, optic fundi, and the position and movement of the eyes reveals more about the neurologic status of the unconscious Pt than any other steps in the examination. Fixed pupils and fixed eyes mean trouble.

C. *Physical management of the comatose patient*

1. *Check respiration.* Observe rate and rhythm of respiration. Note the Pt's color and verify air exchange by inspection, palpation, or auscultation. Look for suprasternal retraction and abdominal respiration. For inspiratory stridor, pull the mandible forward and reposition the Pt. For apnea, start mouth-to-mouth resuscitation, intubate, and assist ventilation with Ambu bag or ventilator and O_2 as needed. Note any odors such as alcohol. Before any neck maneuvers, stabilize the neck and spine if it appears that the Pt may have had trauma.

2. *Check circulation.* Palpate and auscultate the precordium. If the Pt has no heart beat, start cardiac resuscitation. Palpate the carotid and femoral pulses. Inspect for jugular distension and pedal edema. Take the blood pressure.

   a. With hypotension, treat for shock. Secure an IV line and restore blood volume: normal saline or D5W, Ringer's lactate, or whole blood or blood substitutes. See Item 17 below for processing of blood sample.

   b. With hypertension, consider a cardiac or cerebrovascular accident or hypertensive encephalopathy as the cause for the unconsciousness. Consider apresoline, but lower the blood pressure gradually over hours.

3. *Check the blood sugar level.* Prick the Pt's finger and do a glucose oxidase tape test (Dextrostix). Give 50 cc of 50% glucose IV stat for demonstrated or suspected hypoglycemia and add 500 mg of thiamine if the Pt is suspected of alcoholism.

4. *Check the eyes.* Check the pupillary light reflex. With unilaterally or bilaterally dilated pupils that are nonreactive to light, call a neurosurgeon stat. Write down the size of the pupils in millimeters. Use a ruler, do not guess.

   a. Inspect for ptosis, spontaneous blinking, and do the eyelid release test and corneal reflex.

   b. Examine ocular alignment, position, and motility:

      (1) Record alignment and the position of the eyes.

      (2) Record any spontaneous movements of the eyes.

      (3) Do doll's eye test, unless a neck/spinal cord injury is suspected. Later, do caloric irrigation if no ocular movements are elicited.

      (4) Do ophthalmoscopy.

   c. Test the faciociliary and spinociliary reflexes.

   d. Remove contact lenses to preserve the cornea.

5. *Consider naloxone:* If opiate intoxication is suspected.

6. *Inspect and palpate the Pt's head:* Look for localized edema or swelling indicative of recent trauma; look for blood behind the ear (Battle's sign) and around the eyes (racoon eyes); and for blood or CSF from the nose. Do otoscopy to look for blood behind the eardrum.

7. *Test for nuchal rigidity* but not if a neck injury is suspected. In that case splint the neck and obtain neck radiographs.

8. *Inspect the patient for persistent diagnostic postures and spontaneous patterned or repetitive movements:*

   a. Note whether the patient makes spontaneous and equal movements of face and all four extremities, or lies still, in a flaccid-compliant, dumped-in-a-heap posture indicating deep coma or flaccid quadriparesis.

    b. Look for a predominant posture:
       (1) Persistent deviation of the eyes and head
       (2) Opisthotonus
       (3) Decerebrate or decorticate posturing
       (4) Clenched jaws or immobile neck or extremities indicating tetanus
    c. Check specifically for hemiplegia by looking for paralysis of the lower part of the face on one side and of the ipsilateral extremities, with some spontaneous or pain-induced movements of the opposite side.
       (1) Acute hemiplegia in the unconscious Pt is usually flaccid. Do the eyelid release test, look for flaccidity of the cheek manifested by retraction on inspiration and puffing out during expiration, and inflict pain by supraorbital compression to check for unilateral absence of grimacing. Test muscle tone by passive manipulation of all extremities and do the wrist-, arm-, and leg-dropping tests.
       (2) The intact side of the hemiplegic patient may show the hypertonia known as *paratonia*. Record the result of tonus testing as *normal, flaccid, spastic, rigid, paratonia,* or *flexibilitas cerea* (waxy flexibility), seen in catatonic schizophrenia as well as some organic encephalopathies.
    d. Look for cyclic changes in motor activity: shivering, chewing movements, and tremors. Look for overt as well as subtle manifestations of epilepsy: eyelid fluttering, mouth twitching, myoclonic jerks, finger or toe twitching, or frank tonic-clonic generalized seizures.

9. *Strip the patient completely.* Empty all of the Pt's pockets, purse, wallet, or belongings. Look for Indentacards for diabetes or epilepsy, medications, suicide notes, or drug paraphernalia.

10. *Search the entire skin surface* for needle marks indicating subcutaneous injections of insulin or intravenous injections, bruises, petechiae, entry wounds, and turgor. Roll the Pt over and check the back.

11. *Elicit the muscle stretch reflexes:* Begin with the glabellar tap to elicit the orbicularis oculi reflexes. Next, elicit the jaw jerk, and work down through the customary stretch reflexes. Directly compare the reflexes on the two sides of the body.

12. *Try to elicit Chvostek's sign.*

13. *Elicit the superficial reflexes:* Sucking and lip-pursing reflexes and abdominal, cremasteric, anal, and plantar reflexs.

14. *Attempt to elicit grasp reflexes, forced groping, and traction responses.*

15. *Complete the physical examination,* including abdominal palpation and percussion and rectal and vaginal examinations.

16. *Initiate monitoring process and Glasgow Coma Scale (see Fig. 12-1).*
    a. Monitor pupillary size, pulse, blood pressure, respiration, and temperature continuously or at regular, frequent intervals. If increased intracranial pressure is suspected, consult a neurosurgeon about inserting an intracranial pressure monitor.
    b. Determine the Pt's level of consciousness by responsivity to voice, loud sound, light, and pain. Check the responses to pain inflicted by compression of the supraorbital ridge and nail beds of all four extremities. Record the extremity response as *none, extension, flexion, appropriate brushing,* or *movement on command.*
    c. EEG monitoring is desirable if the Pt is comatose from a postictal state or status epilepticus.

17. *Draw blood sample and anchor IV catheter.*
    a. Blood sugar (in addition to preliminary dextrose test tape)
    b. Complete blood count (CBC) and hematocrit

    c. Blood-urea nitrogen (BUN)
    d. Gases
    e. Electrolytes (Na, K, Ca, and Cl)
    f. pH
    g. Osmolality
    h. Toxicology
    i. Typing and cross match
    j. Other _____

Place a sample of the Pt's serum in the refrigerator for later chemical or toxicological testing as may be required by new information, medicolegal problems, or if the Pt dies of unknown causes.

18. *Obtain urine specimen.* Use an external bag or catheterize if the Pt is incontinent or has a distended bladder. Freeze a sample of urine for later testing as may be indicated by new information. On the routine testing of the first specimen, order these tests:
    a. Specific gravity
    b. Sugar and ketones
    c. Protein
    d. Toxicology screen
    e. Other _____

19. *Consider whether to pass a nasogastric tube.* Do so if the Pt is likely to have ingested poison, is vomiting, or is not improving and the diagnosis is obscure. Since it may induce vomiting or gagging, and cause extreme increases in intrathoracic and therefore intracranial pressure, pass it with extreme care in a Pt who may have had subarachnoid or intracranial hemorrhage, increased intracranial pressure, or is threatening brain herniation. Aspirate as often as needed to avoid fluid accumulation in the stomach and vomiting. Save a sample of any material aspirated for subsequent toxicological analysis.

20. *Make a provisional diagnosis.* At the least, assign the Pt to one of the five basic etiologic types of coma: intracranial, toxic-metabolic, anoxic, ischemic, or mental illness. See Fig. NE-3.

21. *Select the safest and most critical additional test to confirm or reject your provisional diagnosis.* The neurologic tests to consider include CT scan or MRI, echoencephalography, lumbar tap, and angiography. Generally a CT scan or MRI should precede the lumbar puncture, because the result may prove that the tap is unnecessary or dangerous. Generally Pts who are unconscious because of head trauma should have neck radiographs because of the frequency of cervical fractures.

22. During the entire examination, always assume that the Pt can hear and remember everything said or done. The pseudocomatose Pt will remember everything, while the organically comatose Pt may remember some remarks because the degree of consciousness may wax and wane. Address the Pt by name. Speak courteously. Avoid pejorative or gratuitous comments.

23. *Insure good nursing care:*
    1. Place the Pt on a comfortable surface.
    2. Cover the Pt to preserve body temperature and for modesty if the Pt regains consciousness.
    3. Keep the skin dry and avoid pressure points.
    4. Avoid compression of the peripheral nerves, particularly the ulnar nerves at the elbow and the common peroneal nerve at the head of the fibula.

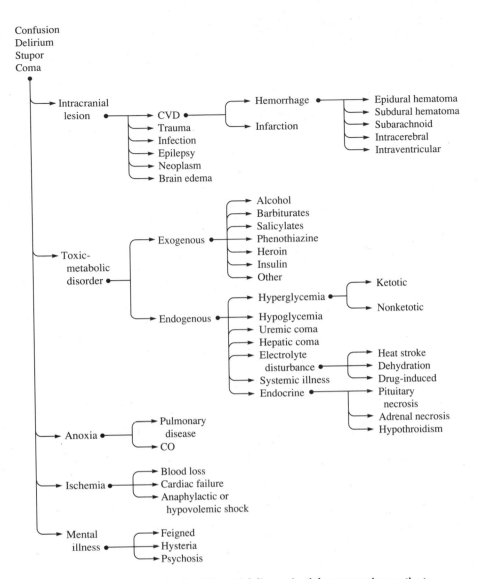

FIG. NE-3. Categories for the differential diagnosis of the unconscious patient.

Technique
of the
Neurologic
Examination

A Programmed Text   *Fourth Edition*

Chapter One

Examination of the Face and Head

Disease is of antiquity and nothing about it changes. It is we who change as we learn to recognize what was formerly imperceptible.

Jean-Martin Charcot (1825–1893)

I. Introduction to the neurologic examination

A. *Symptoms and signs of neurologic disease*
   1. All neurologic disease manifests clinically by *mental, motor,* or *sensory* symptoms and signs, and by abnormal body contours.
   2. The examiner (Ex) discovers the symptoms and signs of neurologic disease by the neurologic history and the neurologic examination (NE). The NE consists of a series of standardized operations of four types: *inspections, questions, requests,* and *maneuvers.*
      a. *Inspections* disclose the patient's (Pt's) body contours and spontaneous and elicited behaviors.
      b. *Questions* determine the Pt's mental status and perceptions.
      c. *Requests* test the Pt's volitional actions.
      d. *Maneuvers* impose stimuli to elicit sensations and reflexes.
   3. In each step of these operations, the Ex assesses some designated endpoint. The chosen endpoint may be some specific feature of the Pt's body configuration, or an isolated behavior, such as a pupil constricting in response to light or a muscle contracting in response to stretch, or the Ex may assess complex behaviors, such as walking and talking.

B. *The neurologic examination as a standardized way to assess designated behaviors*
   1. For purposes of the NE, we may define behavior as *any detectable change produced by neural activation of an effector.*
   2. Because we have only two types of effectors, namely glands and muscles, our neural circuits can produce behaviors by only two actions: by secreting something and by adjusting the length of our muscle fibers.
      a. Thus, our neural circuits can cause the secretion of sweat, tears, saliva, mucus, hormones, and digestive juices.

*The light vertical rule on the left side of the text sets off an answer column. Cover the answers with a card until you have responded to the text. Then after each response, slide the card down to check your answer.

The heavy vertical rule denotes optional material.

  b. Or our neural circuits can adjust the length of our muscle fibers. The result of changing the length of muscle fibers is:

   (1) *To operate our skeletal levers* (to move ourselves, and objects around)

   (2) *To open and close or vibrate our apertures* (eyelids, mouth, vocal cords, and other sphincters)

   (3) *To move gases and liquids through our tubes* (air, blood, secretions, food, feces, and urine)

3. The purpose of reducing behavior to its stark biological elements is not to deny the Pt's humanity and sentiency. The conception of the Pt as an organism consisting of a set of levers, apertures, tubes, and glands operated by neural circuits emphasizes that our elemental needs and natures are all alike. We all arrive, live, and die by the same biological processes, and we all exult and suffer alike. "Because I was flesh and a breath that passeth away. . . ." Appreciation of our common biological bonds supersedes liking or disliking the Pt and obviates any pejorative ruminations about the Pt's personality, life style, or perceived transgressions. Undistracted and unimpeded by such judgmental intrusions, the physician accepts all Pts with equal humility and grace. Because of your carefully fostered accessibility, each particular nervous system before you, operating its levers, apertures, tubes, and glands, can disclose itself and its sentiency as a whole person, whether saint or sinner, without fear of retribution, reprisal, or condemnation. Only when Pts can disclose themselves freely can the physician discover and effectively respond to the Pt's real medical needs.

II. Inspection of the patient

"You can see an awful lot just by looking."   **Attributed to Yogi Berra**

  If permitted to do only one part of the examination, you should choose to look at the Pt. Inspection, the most efficient method of physical diagnosis, begins the moment you approach your Pt. Immediately you might notice pinpoint pupils and numerous needle scars over the antecubital veins. In two glances you have recognized a drug addict. This is the diagnostic power of inspection. But hold on a minute. Eyedrops used to treat glaucoma may have constricted the pupils, and repeated blood transfusions may have scarred the antecubital veins. Every sign or combination of signs requires a differential diagnosis. The diagnostic value of a sign emerges only after integration with a complete history and a general physical examination. No single diagnostic technique suffices by itself.

  After a lifetime of looking, you may think you are already a keen observer. To test how well you have observed something, try to draw it. What you have seen well, you can draw well. Complete the requested drawings faithfully. They are tremendous teachers.

  A. Inspection of the eyes

   1. *Anatomy of the eye (as learned by self-inspection)*

    a. Observing your eyes in a hand mirror, draw the contours of your eyelid margins on a piece of paper. Heed the configuration at the medial and lateral angles. Compare your drawing with Fig. 1-1, and learn the names in the figure.

    b. Look into your mirror to identify the parts of your eye as listed in Fig. 1-1*A*. (If you don't have a mirror, get one. Come on now, be fair. Give these tactics a chance.)

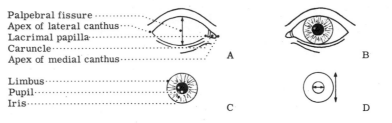

FIG. 1-1. Nomenclature of the eye.

    c. In your mirror study your own limbus, iris, and pupil.
      (1) The *external* circumference of the iris, at the junction of the cornea and sclera, forms the limbus.
      (2) The *internal* circumference of the iris forms the pupil, the opening that admits light into the eye (horizontal arrow, Fig. 1-1*D*).
    d. Notice the caruncle, the tiny meaty mound of tissue occupying the medial canthus.
    e. In your mirror study the relation of the upper and lower lid margins to the limbus when you look straight ahead. Does one lid margin cover more of the iris than the other?

Ans: The upper lid partially covers the upper margin of the limbic iris while the lower lid is tangential to the limbus.

Check against Fig. 1-1. If you erred, redraw the iris in the right eye of Fig. 1-2.

    f. Set aside your mirror and from memory draw the iris of the left eye in Fig. 1-2, showing its exact relation to the lid margins.

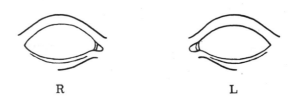

FIG. 1-2. Blank for drawing the relation of the limbus, iris, and pupil to the lid margins when the patient looks straight ahead.

    g. From memory, label Fig. 1-2 with names learned in Fig. 1-1, and check your results against Fig. 1-1.
  2. *Relation of canthi to caruncles*
    a. Look in your mirror and also study another person to learn the relationship of the limbus to the canthi and caruncles when the eyes are turned as far as possible to the *right* or *left* sides. If the person wears glasses, remove them.
    b. With the eyes turned to one side as far as possible, how much scleral white shows between the limbus and the *apex* of the lateral canthus of the *abducted* eye? _____

None or virtually none

_____.

    c. The limbus cannot reach the apex of the medial canthus because the caruncle occupies it. Instead the limbus reaches to, or nearly to, the lateral margin of the caruncle. Thus, with the eyes to one side, the limbus of the *abducted* eye reaches to, or nearly to, the _____ of the lateral canthus, and the limbus of the *adducted* eye reaches to, or nearly to, the margin of the _____.

Apex

Caruncle

d. In Fig. 1-3 draw the relation of the limbus, iris, and pupils to the lids when the patient looks to the left.

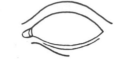

FIG. 1-3. Blank for drawing the relation of the limbus, iris, and pupil to the lid margins when the patient looks to the left as far as possible.

e. A line drawn through the apex of the medial and lateral canthi of one eye defines the *angle* of the palpebral fissure (Fig. 1-4).

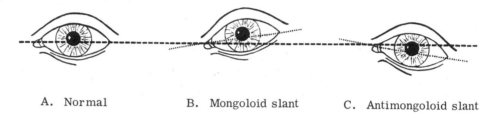

A. Normal   B. Mongoloid slant   C. Antimongoloid slant

FIG. 1-4. Left eye, showing angulations of the palpebral fissure.

3. *Anatomic variations of the medial canthus*
    a. Normally the iris is just about centered between the medial and lateral angles of the eyelids. See Fig. 1-5*A*.
    b. If you have an infant or young child, notice that the medial canthus covers more of the conjunctiva than in adults. When the medial canthus is displaced laterally relative to the limbus, as in many young children, the Pt *appears* to have inward deviation of the eyes, although the eyes are perfectly straight, as in Fig. 1-5*B*.

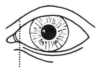 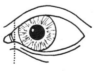

A. Normal adult   B. Young child   C. Canthus dystopia

FIG. 1-5. Left eye, showing variations in the relation of the medial canthus and lacrimal papilla (vertical line) to the corneal limbus. Notice the decreasing distance between the caruncle and the limbus in *A*, *B*, and *C*.

c. Lateral displacement of the medial canthus, which moves the lacrimal punctum out toward the limbus, is termed *canthus dystopia* (dys = bad; topos = place; hence, badly placed canthus).
d. Sometimes a skin fold covers the medial canthus. Since the fold is *upon* the canthus, it is called an *epicanthal* fold. In spaces *A*, *B*, and *C* in Fig. 1-6, write down your diagnosis, whether *epicanthal fold, normal,* or *canthus dystopia.*

A. Normal

B. Canthus dystopia

C. Epicanthal fold

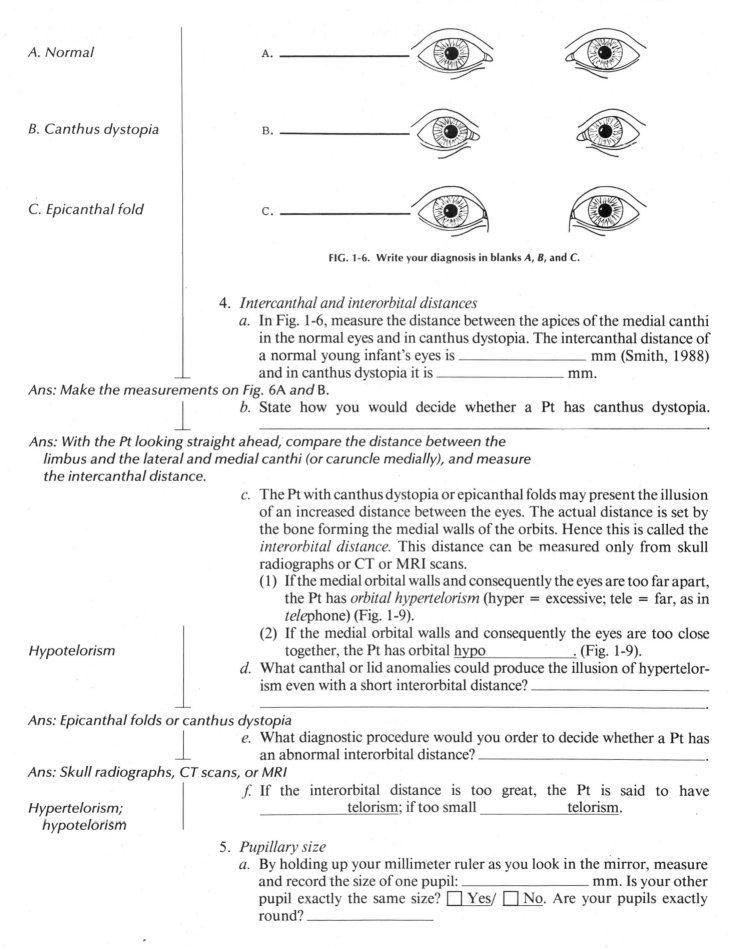

A. _____

B. _____

C. _____

FIG. 1-6. Write your diagnosis in blanks *A*, *B*, and *C*.

4. *Intercanthal and interorbital distances*
   a. In Fig. 1-6, measure the distance between the apices of the medial canthi in the normal eyes and in canthus dystopia. The intercanthal distance of a normal young infant's eyes is _____ mm (Smith, 1988) and in canthus dystopia it is _____ mm.

Ans: Make the measurements on Fig. 6A and B.

   b. State how you would decide whether a Pt has canthus dystopia. _____

Ans: With the Pt looking straight ahead, compare the distance between the limbus and the lateral and medial canthi (or caruncle medially), and measure the intercanthal distance.

   c. The Pt with canthus dystopia or epicanthal folds may present the illusion of an increased distance between the eyes. The actual distance is set by the bone forming the medial walls of the orbits. Hence this is called the *interorbital distance.* This distance can be measured only from skull radiographs or CT or MRI scans.
      (1) If the medial orbital walls and consequently the eyes are too far apart, the Pt has *orbital hypertelorism* (hyper = excessive; tele = far, as in *tele*phone) (Fig. 1-9).
      (2) If the medial orbital walls and consequently the eyes are too close together, the Pt has orbital hypo_____. (Fig. 1-9).

Hypotelorism

   d. What canthal or lid anomalies could produce the illusion of hypertelorism even with a short interorbital distance? _____
   _____

Ans: Epicanthal folds or canthus dystopia

   e. What diagnostic procedure would you order to decide whether a Pt has an abnormal interorbital distance? _____.

Ans: Skull radiographs, CT scans, or MRI

   f. If the interorbital distance is too great, the Pt is said to have _____ telorism; if too small _____ telorism.

Hypertelorism;
  hypotelorism

5. *Pupillary size*
   a. By holding up your millimeter ruler as you look in the mirror, measure and record the size of one pupil: _____ mm. Is your other pupil exactly the same size? ☐ Yes/ ☐ No. Are your pupils exactly round? _____

Anisocoria

Corectasia

Corectopia

b. Most people have exactly round, equal pupils, or *isocoria* (iso = equal, cor = pupil)—the core is the center of anything. The prefix *a-* or *an-* negates the term that follows. Thus, any congenital or acquired difference in pupillary size is called an _____ , which means *not equal pupils*.

c. An enlarged pupil can be called *pupillodilation,* but since *cor* means pupil, pupillodilation can be called _____ ectasia. (Similarly, an enlarged bronchial diameter is called *bronchiectasia.*)

d. An abnormally small pupil is called *cormiosis* or simply *miosis*.

e. Study the width of your iris and its concentricity with the pupils. An eccentric pupil is called _____ ectopia.

f. Although the pupils normally are exactly equal, the height of the palpebral fissures may differ slightly in normal subjects, because of slight drooping of an eyelid. Pathologic or excessive drooping of the upper lid is called *ptosis.* Check in your mirror to see whether one of your lids droops more than the other.

6. *Height of the palpebral fissure*

a. As you move your mirror up and down, observe the surface area of your upper lid. Hold your head still and follow the mirror only with your eyes. In which direction do you see most of the surface area of the lid? ☐ eyes up/ ☐ eyes straight ahead/ ☐ eyes down.

☑ *Eyes down*

Ptosis

b. If an eyelid droops too much when the Pt looks straight ahead, the condition is called _____.

c. A palpebral fissure that is too wide may result from protrusion of the eye, *exophthalmos* (proptosis). If the fissure is too narrow, it may be the result of a sunken eye, called en_____.

Enophthalmos

Ptosis
Enophthalmos

d. Two conditions which might reduce the height of the palpebral fissure are drooping of an eyelid, called _____, or a sunken eyeball, called _____.

e. A pathologically small eyeball is called *micro*phthalmos, an overlarge eyeball, *macro*phthalmos. Correspondingly, the eyeball may have a *micro*cornea or *macro*cornea. What term would describe complete absence of an eyeball? (What prefex negates?) _____

Anophthalmos

f. Write the correct diagnosis in Fig. 1-7. Be sure to compare the two eyes *systematically*—pupils, iris, and lids.

A. *Ptosis and cormiosis on L (anisocoria)*

B. *Exophthalmos on R*

C. *Normal*

D. *Canthus dystopia*

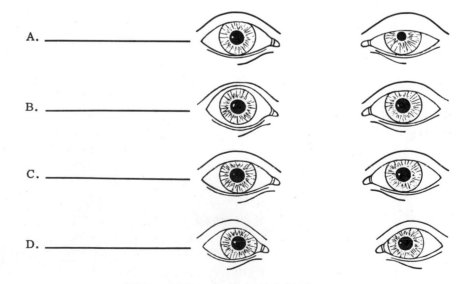

A. _____

B. _____

C. _____

D. _____

FIG. 1-7. Write your diagnosis in blanks *A* to *F*.

E. Macrocornea and corectasia

F. Cormiosis on L (anisocoria)

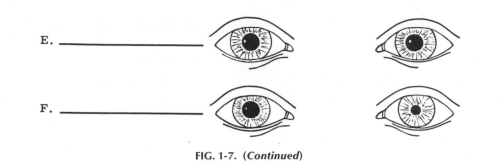

E. _____

F. _____

FIG. 1-7. (*Continued*)

    g. All of the ocular anomalies described are frequent features of facial malformation syndromes. Intercanthal, interpupillary, and interorbital distance measurements frequently aid in diagnosis of these syndromes (Smith, 1988).

  B. *Inspection of the remainder of the face and hair*
    1. *Inspection of the nose, mouth, chin, and ears*
      a. After inspecting the eyes, look systematically at the nose, mouth, chin, and ears.
      b. Nose. Consider the bridge, the nostrils, and the relation of the nose to other facial proportions.
      c. Mouth. Consider the vermillion border of the lips, the philtrum, median labial tubercle of the upper lip, and the line formed by lip closure. Do the lips make a horizontal closure line? Are the lips closed when the Pt's face is at rest? Does the Pt have microstomia or macrostomia?
      d. Chin. Look for a small chin, *micrognathia,* or a large protuberant chin, *macrognathia,* as in pituitary gigantism (acromegaly).
      e. Ears. Check for contour, shape, and asymmetry. Learn to draw a normal ear and label its parts as shown in Fig. 1-8.

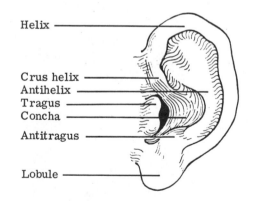

Helix —————
Crus helix —————
Antihelix —————
Tragus —————
Concha —————
Antitragus —————
Lobule —————

FIG. 1-8. Anatomy of the normal ear, lateral view. Compare your own ear with the drawing and identify the parts.

    2. *Inspection of the hair of the scalp, eyebrows, and beard*
      a. Notice the border of the hairline of the scalp. How does it relate to the forehead and to the nape of the neck? Is the hairline too high or too low? What is the texture of the scalp hair?
      b. Observe whether the eyebrows are full, scanty, absent, or joined in the midline. For example, absence of the lateral part of the eyebrows is common in hypothyroidism. Midline union of the eyebrows (synophrys) occurs in some malformation syndromes (Fig. 1-9*G*).

  c. Inspect the hair of the beard and face for its distribution and texture. Ask a male Pt how often he has to shave. Alterations in the distribution and texture of the hair occur in diverse disorders, in infections, congenital malformations, endocrine, and intersex syndromes.

3. *Inspection of the skin of the face and general body surface*

  a. Various neurocutaneous stigmata are virtually pathognomonic of the underlying disease.

   (1) Multiple flat brown spots (café au lait spots): Von Recklinghausen's multiple neurofibromatosis (Fig 1-9*B*).

   (2) Irregular linear blotches of brown pigmentation of the infant's skin: incontinenti pigmenti.

   (3) Ash leaf–shaped white spots (naevus anemicus) or facial angiofibromata in the butterfly area and chin: tuberous sclerosis.

   (4) Facial hemangiomas in the trigeminal nerve area: Sturge-Weber syndrome (Fig. 1-9).

  b. Corneal rings

   (1) Brownish corneal ring near the limbus: Wilson's hepatolenticular degeneration.

   (2) Grayish-white ring near the corneal limbus: arcus senilis of aging.

4. *A note on facial diagnosis*

  a. When the Pt's face looks a little odd, that is to say the gestalt or expression seems unusual, pay heed to it. From abnormalities in the face alone, the perceptive Ex can diagnose literally hundreds of disorders, ranging from infectious diseases such as leprosy, to endocrinopathies, mental and neurologic disorders, and especially malformation syndromes. In many malformation syndromes with abnormal facies, the brain also suffers, causing mental retardation. Diagnosing the face of such a Pt, the physician often can predict with a fair degree of certainty the Pt's intellectual potential. Thus, in these instances the face predicts the brain (DeMyer, 1975).

  b. Begin by observing the Pt's facial gestalt. Then dissect the face into parts for individual inspection. Imagine the face as a pair of eyes. Are they too close together or too far apart? Are the pupils equal? Simply ask each question for which your observations will provide an answer. Then visualize the Pt's forehead, nose, mouth, chin, and a pair of ears. Even if you cannot recite all of the possible pathologic deviations of these structures, by knowing what is normal you can detect the abnormal. Then you can consult one of the following references to make the diagnosis. Review the facial abnormalities in Fig. 1-9.

FIG. 1-9. Montage of diagnostic facial and body abnormalities detected by inspection. (A) Infant with rounded face, slight mongoloid obliquity of the palpebral fissures, open mouth, and short upper extremities. The frog-legged position of the lower extremities reflects hypotonia: Down's syndrome, trisomy 21. **(B)** Infant with antimongoloid obliquity of the palpebral fissures, orbital hypertelorism, broad forehead, and one incidental café au lait spot on the left side of the forehead: agenesis of the corpus callosum with mild macrocephaly and mild mental retardation. **(C)** Boy with hypertelorism, canthus dystopia, and flat nasal bridge with slight vertical groove: median cleft face syndrome (DeMyer, 1967 and 1975). Also called frontonasal dysplasia. Such patients generally have normal mentality. **(D)** Infant with microcephaly, orbital hypotelorism, flat nasal bridge, and median cleft of the upper lip: holoprosencephaly. Fig. 1-15 shows this type of brain. This face predicts a brain malformation of holoprosencephalic type and severe retardation (DeMyer, 1975).

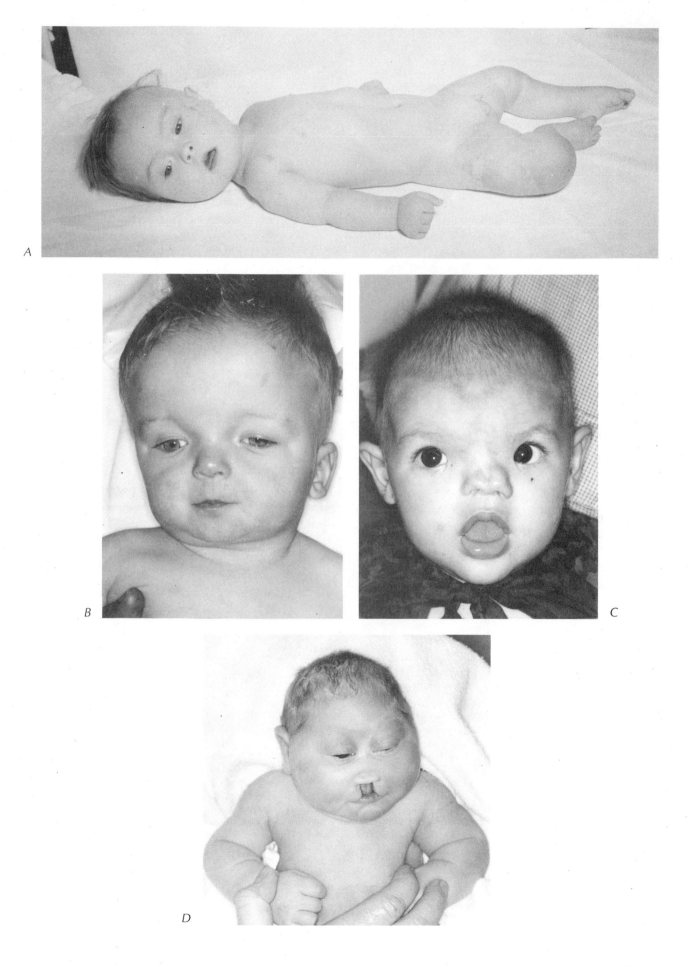

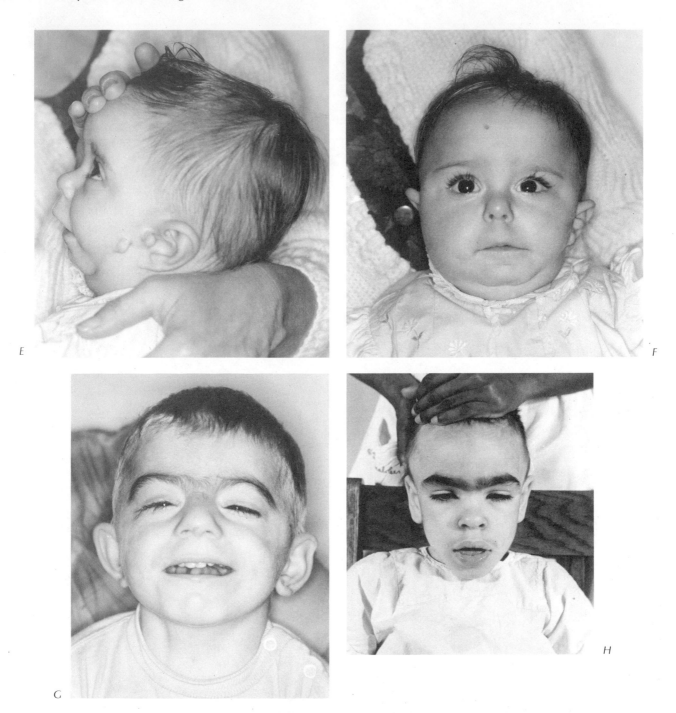

FIG. 1-9. (*Continued*) (*E*) Infant girl with dysplasia of the ear, extra tag of tissue and unilateral micrognathia: unilateral first branchial arch syndrome. The dysmorphia affects the parts of the face derived from the first branchial arch (mandibular and maxillary process) on the left (Figs. 2-19 and 2-20). (*F*) Infant girl pictured in *E* showing small palebral fissure. Hypoplastic zygoma and mandible, and slight macrostomia on the left: unilateral first branchial arch syndrome. Notice the symmetrical corneal light reflections, indicating intact ocular muscles, which derive from somites, not branchial arches. (*G*) Boy with midline eyebrows (synophrys), small midfacial segment, mild micrognathia, and severe mental retardation: Cornelia de Lange's syndrome. The patient also had a lumbar hair patch and hypoplasia of the radius and thumb, typical of this syndrome. (*H*) Boy with megalocephaly, coarse facial features, midline eyebrows, slight hypertelorism, concave nasal bridge, thick lips, and an open mouth with thick tongue: Hurler's syndrome, mucopolysaccharidosis I-H, with megalocephaly secondary to metabolic megalencephaly (DeMyer, 1993).

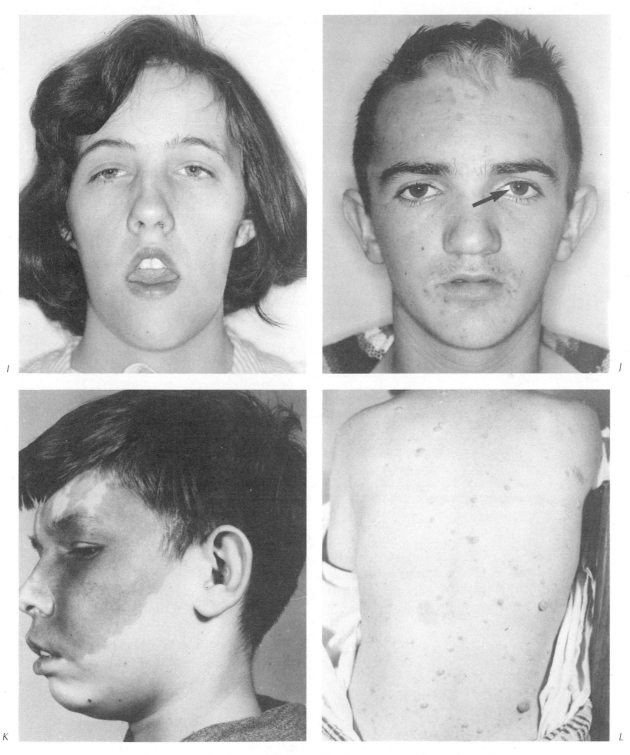

FIG. 1-9. (Continued) (I) Young woman with temporal and masseter muscle atrophy (hollowing of the temples and posterior cheeks), expressionless face, and sagging jaw with inverted-U upper lip: myotonic dystrophy. **(J)** Young man with white forelock, slight synophrys, slight hypertelorism and heterochromia of the iris *(arrow)*, slightly broadened nose, and mild deafness: Waardenburg's syndrome, Type II. Type I patients have dystopia canthorum. **(K)** Boy with port wine stain, mainly affecting the maxillary division of the trigeminal nerve and to a lesser extent, the ophthalmic division: Sturge-Weber syndrome of angiomatosis. The patient had epileptic seizures due to meningeal and cortical involvement by the angiomatosis. **(L)** Boy with multiple neurofibromas and café au lait spots: neurofibromatosis, type I. This disorder, like Sturge-Weber syndrome, belongs to the neurocutaneous syndromes, a group of congenital diseases which affect the brain and the skin.

REFERENCES FOR CRANIOFACIAL MEASUREMENTS AND MALFORMATIONS

Farkas LG: *Anthropometry of the Head and Face in Medicine.* Amsterdam, Elsevier/North Holland, 1981

Jones KL: *Smith's Recognizable Patterns of Human Malformation* (4th ed). Philadelphia, Saunders, 1988

Suggested reading for craniofacial malformations

Bysse ML (ed): *Birth Defects Encyclopedia.* Cambridge, Mass., Blackwell Scientific Publications, 1990

DeMyer W: The median cleft face syndrome: Differential diagnosis of cranium bifidum, hypertelorism, and median cleft nose, lip, and palate. *Neurology* 1967;17:961–971

DeMyer W: Median facial malformations and their implications for brain malformations *Birth Defects* 1975; 11(7):155–181

Gorlin RJ, Pindborg JJ, Cohen MM: *Syndromes of the Head and Neck* (3d ed). New York, Oxford University Press, 1990

Stricher M, Van Der Meulen J, Raphael B, Mazzola R: *Craniofacial Malformations.* Edinburgh, Churchill Livingstone, 1990

C. *Palpation, percussion, and auscultation of the head*
  1. *Palpation*
     a. *Skull.* It is perfectly natural to touch what you see. The laying on of hands, an ancient habit of healers, serves at once as a source of information to the physician and of comfort to the Pt. Therefore, after inspection, grasp the Pt's head between your fingertips (or your own head in lieu of a Pt's) and, using fairly firm pressure, search for soft spots, lumps, depressions, and areas of tenderness. Notice your own frontal and parietal eminences. By feeling along the midline and then out laterally, locate the depression between the prominences of the frontal and parietal bones, the depression marking the site of the coronal suture. Is the frontal or parietal region the widest region of the head? Feel in the midline posteriorly, where the nape of the neck meets the skull, and find your external occipital protuberance.
     b. *Arteries.* Palpate the temporal arteries. Lay your index finger lightly just in front of your tragus, and follow the pulsating temporal artery as far distally as possible. It is generally not wise to palpate or compress the carotid arteries in Pts suspected of atherosclerosis because of the danger of dislodging embolic material from ulcerated plaques.
  2. *Percussion* over the sinuses or mastoid processes may disclose tenderness in these regions when their cavities are infected, but the percussion note from the skull itself has little value.
  3. *Auscultation of the head and neck*
     a. Aneurysms, arteriovenous malformations or fistulae, and occlusive vascular disease may cause bruits over the carotid arteries or head. Loud cardiac sounds transmit along the neck vessels. In normal infants and children to five years of age, benign bruits heard over the head are common. A continuous venous hum is generally innocuous.
        (1) Sometimes benign bruits are heard over the carotid arteries of normal adults, but a strong, localized bruit suggests stenosis. Such bruits indicate a significant risk of a subsequent stroke, particularly if the Pt has hypertension, diabetes, or coronary artery disease.
        (2) Pathologic bruits become audible over the carotids when the vessel is about 50 percent occluded. The loudness may increase as the ste-

nosis increases. At about 90 percent occlusion the most ominous bruit appears, which has a soft, high pitched sound that continues throughout systole into diastole. At about 95 percent or more occlusion, the bruit disappears.

b. To survey for bruits of the neck vessels, place a rubber-edged stethoscope bell gently at various sites along the carotid and vertebral arteries. Carotid bruits ordinarily are heard along the anterior border of the sternocleidomastoid muscle, vertebral artery bruits along the posterior edge. Then place the bell over the mastoid processes, frontal and parietal regions, and over each eye after the Pt gently closes the eyelid. In Fig. 1-10*A,* notice the course of the carotid and vertebral arteries. In Fig. 1-10*B,* draw lines showing where to place the stethoscope bell to listen for carotid or vertebral artery bruits, and then make an X at the other sites showing where to place the bell to listen for a cranial bruit.

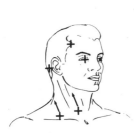

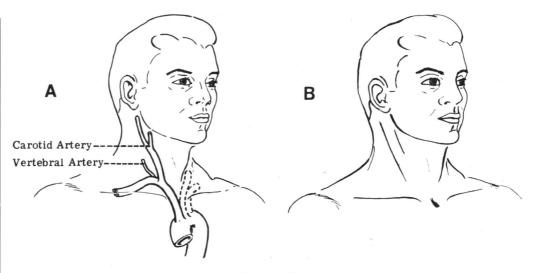

Carotid Artery - - - - - - -
Vertebral Artery - - - - - -

FIG. 1-10. Auscultation of the neck vessels for bruits. (*A*) Phantom view of carotid and vertebral arteries in the neck. (*B*) Blank to mark sites of auscultation for bruits.

c. Using your stethoscope, listen to what (I hope) will be the silence over your own head. Can you hear sounds when you auscultate your carotid arteries?

d. When you place the bell over the eye, what do you have to ask the Pt to do to eliminate noise caused by contraction of the orbicularis oculi muscle? _____.

Ans: Relax the eyelid. The light pressure of the bell will keep the lid closed to protect the cornea.

e. Further investigation of a bruit may require Doppler ultrasonography, phonocardiography, angiography, and MRI or CT scan.

SUGGESTED READING FOR AUSCULTATION OF THE HEAD AND NECK

Sandock BA, Whisnant JP, Furlan AJ, Mickell JL: Carotid artery bruits: prevalence survey and differential diagnosis. *Mayo Clinic Proc* 1982;57:227–230
Toole JF, Patel AN: *Cerebrovascular Disorders* (4th ed). New York, Raven, 1990
Whisnant JP, Basford JR, Bernstein EF, et al: Classification of cerebrovascular disease III. *Stroke* 1990;21:637–676

D. *Abnormalities in the size and shape of the head*

    1. *Origin of the skull bones.* The cephalic mesoderm produces skull bones by two different histogenetic sequences. The *endochondral* bone of the cranial base develops from preformed cartilage. The *membranous* bone of the cranial vault and facial skeleton develops directly from osteoid. Learn the four endochondral bones of the cranial base in Fig. 1-11. Then you can easily remember the membranous origin of all of the other bones.

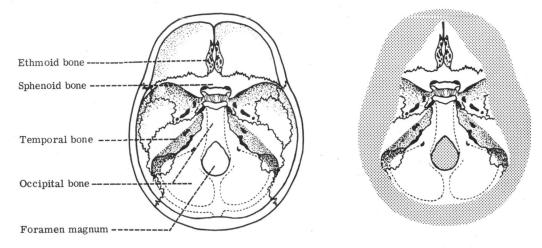

Ethmoid bone

Sphenoid bone

Temporal bone

Occipital bone

Foramen magnum

FIG. 1-11. Interior view of skull base on the left. On the right, only the endochondral bone is shown.

    2. *Functional arthrology of the skull*

        a. When a joint cavity separates the two bones at a joint, the joint is called a *diarthrosis.* If connective tissue occupies the space between the bones, leaving no joint cavity, the joint is a *synarthrosis.*

        b. The temporomandibular joints and joints of the ear ossicles are diarthroses. All other skull joints are synarthroses.

        c. During morphogenesis, *cartilaginous* connective tissue unites the joints of the endochondral bones at the cranial base. Such synarthroses are called *synchondroses.* Similarly, *fibrous* connective tissue unites the membranous bones of the cranial vault and face to each other and to endochondral bones. Such synarthroses are called *sutures.*

Sutures

Synchondroses

        d. Wherever membranous bones contact each other or endochondral bones, the joints are called _____, but wherever endochondral bones contact other endochondral bones, the joints are called

_____.

        e. In fetuses, the fibrous connective tissue at the sutures is broad and loose. It forms large, nonossified membranes between the margins of some skull bones. These sites are called *fontanels.* Learn the *sutures, fontanels,* and *bones* in Fig. 1-12*A* and *B*.

Frontal; parietal

        f. The largest fontanel, the anterior, is formed at the junction of four bones, the two _____ bones and the two _____ bones.

    3. *Pliancy of the synarthroses in the infant's skull*

        a. At the fontanels, the broad sheet of connective tissue allows an up and down, diaphragm-like action, whereas the narrower connective tissue strip at the sutures permits only a limited, hinging action. Thus the

☑ *Fontanels*

infant skull is most pliant at the ☐ sutures/ ☐ fontanels.

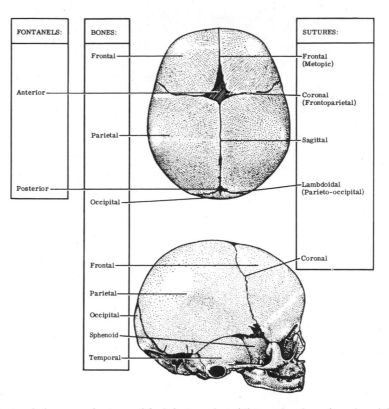

FIG. 1-12. Fontanels, bones, and sutures of the infant cranium. (*A*) Superior view of cranium. (*B*) Lateral view of cranium.

Fontanels; sutures; synchondroses

b. The cartilage uniting the synchondroses of the cranial base is less pliant than fibrous connective tissue. Rank the three skull synarthroses, the synchondroses, fontanels, and sutures, in order from most to least pliant _____, _____, and _____.

c. *Ossification of skull synarthroses*

(1) During morphogenesis, the skull serves the contradictory functions of plasticity and rigidity. The plastic fetal calvarium yields to accommodate the expanding brain. The skull's plasticity permits deformation during passage through the birth canal, when the sutures and fontanels permit a hinge-like action and may allow one cranial bone margin to overlap another. The deformation of the skull may damage the brain by compression or by rupture of veins and venous sinuses. The rigidity of the synchondroses prevents buckling of the skull base against the brainstem during birth, which would imperil the passenger even more than deformation of the calvarium.

(2) With maturation, the cranium becomes relatively rigid. The synchondroses, sutures, and fontanels progressively unite and finally ossify completely. Before the synarthroses ossify, we say they are "open." Afterwards, they are "closed." The time of closure varies considerably, as summarized in Table 1-1.

d. *Response of the skull to increased intracranial pressure before closure of the synarthroses*

(1) To the palpating finger, the anterior fontanel is resilient, as every mother knows, for she calls it the "soft spot." Normally with the infant supported upright, and not struggling or crying, the anterior

TABLE 1-1 Time of ossification of some cranial synarthroses. (Reference only, do not memorize.)	
Synarthrosis	Ossification
Frontal (metopic) suture	2 years
Coronal suture	30 years
Basilar synchrondroses	2–20 years
Anterior fontanel	1.5 years (range 3–27 months)
Posterior fontanel	Birth to 2 months

fontanel is slightly concave, as demonstrated by running a finger across it, or as shown by shining a flashlight beam obliquely across it. If the infant is held upside down, gravity distends the intracranial veins with blood and forces the brain against the roof of the skull. The anterior fontanel, the soft spot, bulges. When the infant is held upright, the opposite shift in intracranial contents occurs and the fontanel assumes its normal ☐ concave/ ☐ flat/ ☐ convex contour.

☑ *Concave*

(2) When crying, the infant expires against a partially closed glottis. Contraction of the expiratory muscles increases intrathoracic pressure, which is transmitted intracranially by the venous system. As the intracranial pressure increases, the anterior fontanel ☐ becomes sunken/ ☐ bulges.

☑ *Bulges*

(3) Dehydration reduces the blood and tissue volume, reducing intracranial pressure. The anterior fontanel ☐ becomes more sunken/ ☐ bulges more.

☑ *Becomes more sunken*

(4) Write a statement relating the contour of the anterior fontanel to the intracranial pressure. _____

_____

_____

Ans: When the intracranial pressure is increased, the anterior fontanel becomes more and more convex; when the intracranial pressure is normal or low, the fontanel becomes more and more concave.

4. *Causes of head enlargement*

   a. Normally the head increases in size as the skull yields to the growth pressure of the brain. A pathologic increase in head size may result from two basic classes of conditions:

     (1) Presence of abnormal substances within the cranium, such as neoplasms, hematomas, edema, or abnormal accumulation of metabolic substances.

     (2) Presence of increased amounts of cerebrospinal fluid, either from obstruction to its absorption or from its excessive production.

   b. If the intracranial pressure increases, what part of the fetal or infant skull would yield most rapidly and obviously to the increased intracranial pressure? ☐ anterior fontanel/ ☐ sutures/ ☐ synchrondroses.

Ans: The soft spot. Bulging of the anterior fontanel is the first sign of increased intracranial pressure.

   c. In what position would you place an infant to inspect whether the fontanel is bulging from a pathologic increase in intracranial pressure? ☐ inverted/ ☐ reclining/ ☐ upright.

Explain: _____

_____

_____.

Ans: ☑ *Upright to allow the fontanel to assume its normal concavity as gravity pulls down on the brain.*

    d. Should you try to estimate pathologic increased pressure from examination of the fontanel if the infant is struggling or crying vigorously? ☐ Yes/ ☐ No/ ☐ Makes no difference. Explain: _____

_____.

Ans: ☑ *No. When the intrathoracic pressure increases, the intracranial pressure also increases. You may err in considering physiologic bulging as pathologic.*

    5. *Closure of the sutures and fontanels*

        a. The anterior fontanel usually closes by 18 months. Suppose increased intracranial pressure began after that time. Which synarthrosis would yield next to the pressure, the synchondroses of the cranial base, or the sutures of the cranial vault? _____.

Sutures

        b. Wide separation or "splitting" of the sutures can be detected by palpation. Otherwise, skull radiographs or CT scans are essential. If the sutures split what happens to the head size? _____.

Increases

        c. Although suture closure by ossification continues into adulthood, *functional* closure occurs earlier. By 10 to 12 years of age the sutures usually adhere so firmly, although nonossified, that they no longer yield to increased intracranial pressure. Suppose you have examined a 16-year-old boy with a big head and spreading of his sutures, as shown by a skull radiograph. What is the *minimum* time the patient could have had increased intracranial pressure? _____.

4 to 6 years

        d. List three physical signs of pathologic increased intracranial pressure in a young infant: _____

_____

_____.

Ans: Bulging anterior fontanel, split sutures (as shown by palpation or radiography), and increased head size.

    6. *Head Size: the occipitofrontal circumference (OFC)*

        a. Record every infant's OFC at every examination. Place a steel tape measure around the maximum occipitofrontal circumference, from the external occipital protuberance (inion) to the glabella. Compare with the normal values given in Fig. 1-13. Any OFC value ±2.5 cm from the mean is suspicious, while any value ±3.0 cm is virtually certain to be pathologic, if the body weight, chest circumference, length, and other proportions are normal. Record the OFC of parents and siblings to make allowance for normal variations of somatotype.

        b. Too large a head is called *megalocephaly* or *macrocephaly,* too small, *microcephaly.* An infant's head may be too large or too small at birth, or the head may become abnormal in size later. To best recognize an abnormal trend in head size as the infant develops, plot successive OFC measurements on a chart (Fig. 1-14). In Fig. 1-14, trend line A displays an abnormally enlarging head, while trend line B shows a lagging head size.

Megalencephaly or macrencephaly

        c. If the brain or encephalon is too small and weighs too little the condition is called *micrencephaly.* If the brain is too large and heavy, it is called _____ *encephaly.*

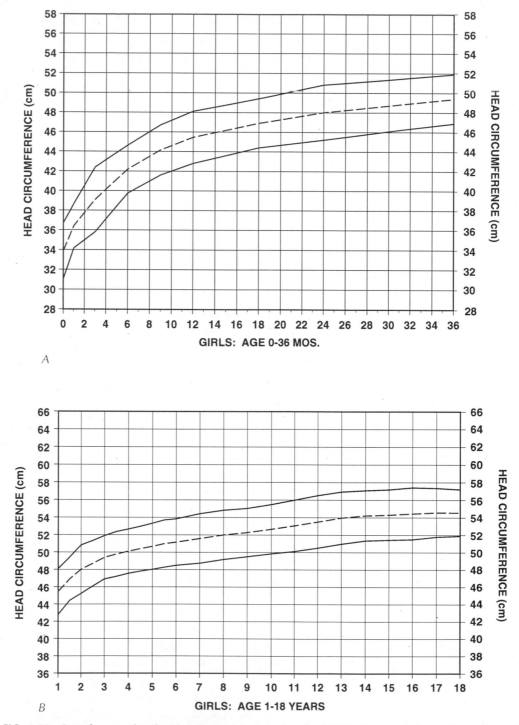

A

B

FIG. 1-13. Growth curve for the occipitofrontal circumference (OFC). The areas shown for males and females include two standard deviations above and below the mean. Ninety-five percent of normal children fall within these limits.

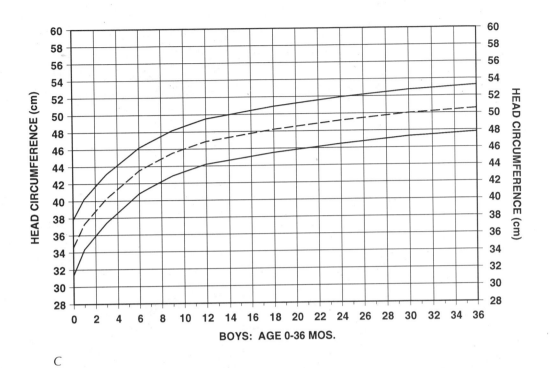

C

BOYS: AGE 0-36 MOS.

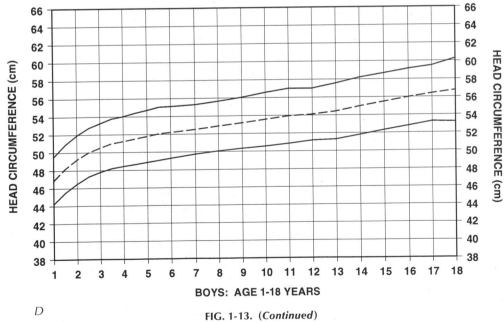

D

BOYS: AGE 1-18 YEARS

FIG. 1-13. (*Continued*)

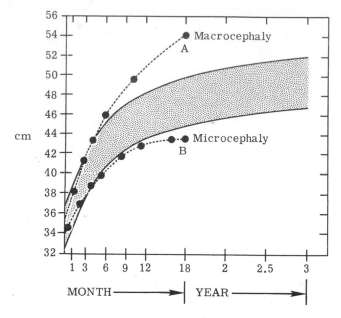

FIG. 1-14. Successive plots of abnormal head sizes.

☑ *Micrencephaly*

d. Of necessity, a Pt with microcephaly has ☐ megalencephaly/ ☐ micrencephaly/ ☐ a normal brain size.

e. Of necessity, a Pt with a big brain must have a big head, but it is not true that a Pt with a big head must have a big brain. In megalocephaly, the brain may be normal in weight, too large or too small. In fact, Pts with little or no cerebrum may have microcephaly, normocephaly, or megalocephaly. If the brain does not fully fill the skull, fluid occupies the extra space. Study Fig. 1-15.

f. Thus we can conclude which of the following:
   ☐ *(1)* The OFC and brain weight have a strict, linear correlation in normal and pathologic conditions.
   ☐ *(2)* While the OFC and brain weight generally correlate, the OFC predicts the maximum weight the brain may have, but not the minimum.
   ☐ *(3)* While the OFC and brain weight correlate roughly, the OFC predicts the minimum weight the brain may have, but not the maximum.

☑ *2*

   ☐ *(4)* None of these answers apply.

g. If the brain volume is small relative to skull volume, as in Fig. 1-15, the space unoccupied by brain contains cerebrospinal fluid (CSF). Whenever the volume of CSF is significantly increased, the condition is called *hydrocephaly,* irrespective of brain size or head size; irrespective of the location of the CSF, whether within the ventricles or the subarachnoid space; and irrespective of the intracranial pressure. Thus, the one condition necessary to justify the term *hydrocephaly* is an excessive volume of _____ within the intracranial cavity.

CSF (fluid)

h. It happened that the Pt in Fig. 1-15 had *microcephaly* and *micrencephaly.* The disproportionately small brain left a large space to be filled with fluid. Thus, this Pt had hydrocephaly as well as microcephaly and micrencephaly.

i. Thus far the combining terms *micro-, megalo-,* and *hydro-* have been used in a purely quantitative sense to mean too much or too little of something. Thus, they are descriptive terms like *gigantism* or *dwarfism,* not diagnoses. *Hydrocephaly* is used in a second sense to mean a

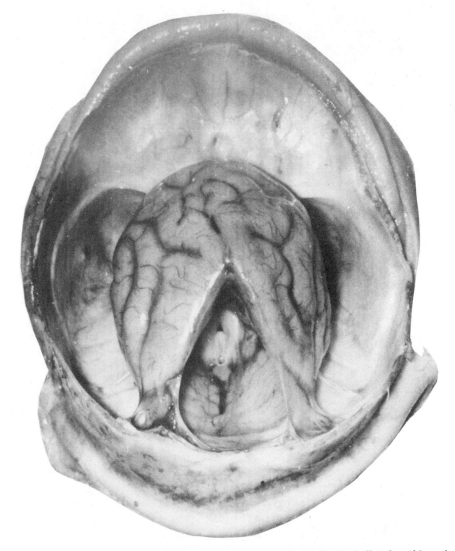

FIG. 1-15. Postmortem photograph of a microencephalon in a microcephalic skull. When this patient died at the age of 4 months, the OFC was only 32 cm (normal 41 cm). In spite of the tiny head, the disproportionately small brain failed to fill the intracranial space. (From DeMyer W, White P: EEG in holoprosencephaly (arhinencephaly). *Arch Neurol* 1964;11:507.

triad of increased head size (if the process occurs before suture closure), increased volume of CSF, and increased intracranial pressure. If the excessive CSF is under pressure in the ventricles, the cerebral wall thins and the ventricles dilate (Fig. 1-16).

j. When the brain is too small, as from atrophy, hypoplasia, or destructive lesions, and the excessive CSF merely fills in the unoccupied space (hydrocephalus ex vacuo), the intracranial pressure may be normal. Is the term *hydrocephaly* admissible in this context? ☐ Yes/ ☐ No Explain:

_____

Ans: ☑ *Yes, the first definition, the purely quantitative one of frame 6g applies, but the Pt does not have increased intracranial pressure.*

k. Suspicion of an abnormal head size requires the Ex to visualize the size and shape of the brain and its ventricles and subarachnoid spaces. You can do this by one of several imaging methods, using ultrasound in young infants, or CT or MRI scan at any age, as explained in Chap. 13. See Figs. 1-16 and 1-17.

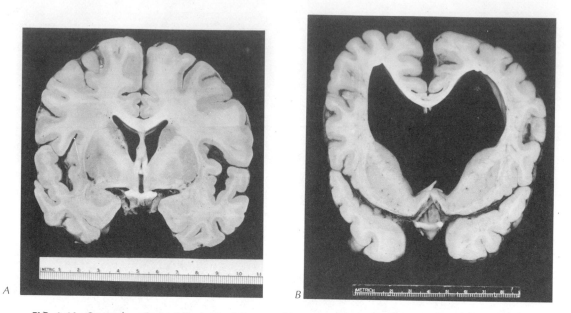

FIG. 1-16. Coronal sections of the brain. (*A*) Normal brain to show the configuration of the anterior horns of the lateral ventricles. (*B*) Hydrocephalic brain to show the enormous symmetrical dilation of the lateral ventricles. The septum pellucidum, which is shown intact in *A*, has stretched thin and ruptured in *B*. Compare with Fig. 1-17*A* and *B*.

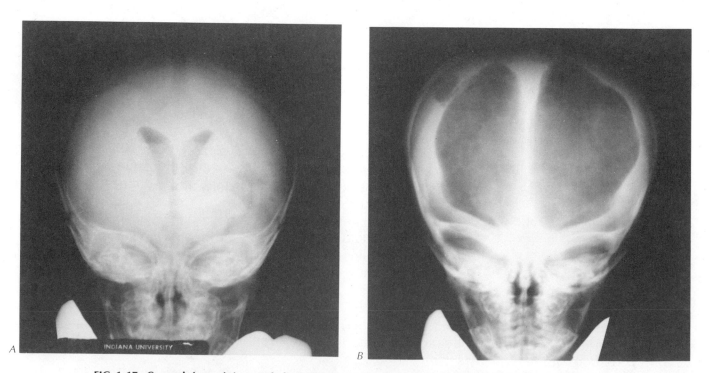

FIG. 1-17. Coronal views of air encephalograms. Compare with Fig. 1-16*A* and *B*. Although CT and MRI scans have supplanted it, the older procedure of air encephalography showed the ventricular cavities equally well. Compare with MRI scans in Figs. 13-8 and 13-9. (*A*) Normal sized lateral ventricles (paired, dark, comma-shaped areas). (*B*) Greatly enlarged lateral ventricles in infant with severe obstructive hydrocephalus. Notice the extreme thinness of the cerebral wall caused by ventricular distension.

SUGGESTED READING FOR ABNORMAL HEAD SIZE

Baum J, Searls D: Head shape and size of newborn infants. *Dev Med Child Neurol* 1971;13:572–575

Baum J, Searls D: Head shape and size of pre-term low-birthweight infants. *Dev Med Child Neurol* 1971;13:576–581

Davies P, Davis J: Very low birthweight and subsequent head growth. *Lancet* 1970;2:1216–1219

Dekaban AS: Tables of cranial and orbital measurements, cranial volume and derived indexes in males and females from 7 days to 20 years of age. *Ann Neurol* 1977;2:485–491

DeMyer W: Microcephaly, micrencephaly, megalocephaly, and megalencephaly. In Swaiman K (ed.): *Pediatric Neurology* (3d ed). St. Louis, Mosby-Year Book, 1993

Finnstrom O: Studies on maturity in newborn infants. I: Birthweight, crown-heel length, head circumference, and skull diameters in relation to gestational age. *Acta Paediat Scand* 1971;60:685–694

Nellhaus G: Head circumference from birth to eighteen years. *Pediatrics* 1968;41:106–114

Nelson K, Deutschberger J: Head size at one year as a predictor of 4-year I.Q. *Dev Med Child Neurol* 1970;12:487–495

O'Neal E: Minimal rates of head growth in the first four months of life. *Arch Dis Child* 1962;37:363–365

Sher PK, Brown SB: A longitudinal study of head growth in pre-term infants. II: Differentiation between "catch-up" head growth and early infantile hydrocephalus. *Dev Med Child Neurol* 1975;17:711–718

Weaver D, Christian J: Familial variation of head size and adjustment for parental head circumference. *J Pediatr* 1980;96:990–994

7. *Transillumination of the infant's head*
   a. Transillumination of an infant's head is clinically useful to screen for excessive quantities of intracranial fluid and to confirm the need for further study by imaging of the brain by ultrasound or radiography (Fig. 1-18).
      (1) *Procedure.* Take the infant into a completely dark closet and allow several minutes for dark-adaptation of your eyes. Press an ordinary flashlight fitted with a rubber adaptor against the infant's head, and move it over the various regions of the cranial vault.
      (2) *Results.* Normally, a small halo of transillumination, less than a centimeter in diameter, will appear around the adaptor margin. Under four conditions, the halo will be large or even the entire head will light up.
         (a) Increased fluid or edema in the scalp or in the subgaleal space between the galea aponeurotica and cranium (Fig. 1-19*A*).
         (b) Increased fluid in the subdural space (subdural hygroma), between the dura mater and the brain or in the subarachnoid space (Fig. 1-19*B*).
         (c) Increased fluid within the brain because of thinning by stretching, destruction, atrophy, or hypoplasia (Fig. 1-19*C* and *D*).
         (d) Premature infants with huge fontanels and very thin cranial bones.
   b. *Systemic analysis of the cause of transillumination*
      (1) First decide whether the fluid which causes the transillumination is outside or inside the skull. If outside the skull, the fluid must be in the scalp or subgaleal space.

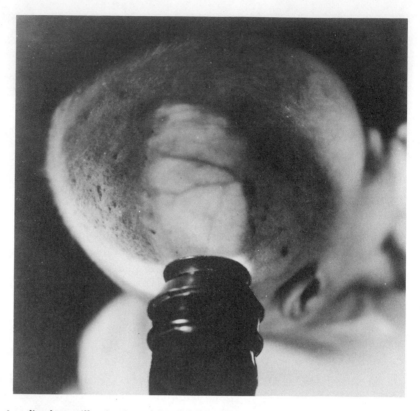

FIG. 1-18. Localized transillumination of the parietal region. A parietal craniotomy was done to relieve a combined intracerebral and subdural hematoma caused by a head injury. Clear fluid then accumulated between the dura and cerebrum (subdural gygroma) and gradually bulged through the surgical defect in the parietal bone. Observe the scalp vessels coursing over the bulge.

(2) *Detection of scalp edema.* The commonest causes of scalp edema are head injuries and infiltration of intravenous fluid given through a scalp vein. The pitting test discloses scalp edema. Press the ball of your finger firmly against the scalp in the area of transillumination. Hold it firmly and it will sink through the edema fluid, allowing the finger to press the scalp against the bone. After removal of your finger, a pit remains.

(3) *Detection of subgaleal fluid.* Subgaleal fluid elevates the scalp from the skull. The skull can be more or less ballotted. Finger pres-

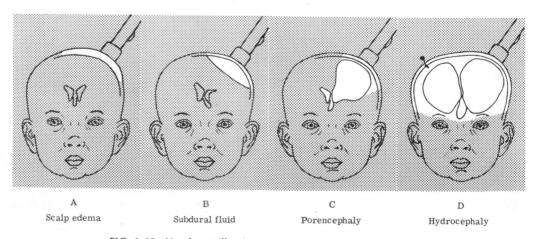

A	B	C	D
Scalp edema	Subdural fluid	Porencephaly	Hydrocephaly

FIG. 1-19. Head transillumination with lesions of different types.

sure readily discloses the distance between the scalp and skull, but the scalp does not pit.

(4) *Fluid inside the skull* is in the subdural or subarachnoid spaces or is intracerebral. If intracerebral, the fluid is in the ventricles or a cystic lesion (Fig. 1-19*C* and *D*). After a head injury, the epidural space may contain blood, but epidural blood is too opaque to transilluminate. Exact localization of intracerebral fluid requires imaging (Chap. 13). In some instances subdural fluid may be diagnosed by inserting a needle through the lateral angle of the anterior fontanel or a burr hole drilled through the skull.

(5) To prove that you can systematically analyze transillumination, place your hand on top of your head and recite the possible extracranial and intracranial locations of the fluid. Then complete Table 1-2.

Scalp; fingertip pressure for pitting edema

Subgaleal space; fingertip pressure for elevation of scalp

Subdural space; imaging or taps

Within the brain; imaging

TABLE 1-2 Tests for location of excess fluid when the head transilluminates

Location of fluid	Test procedure to verify
Extracranial {	
Intracranial {	

c. Rarely, the cerebellum is absent or is displaced by a large cyst. The posterior fossa (inferior occipital region) will then transilluminate. This fact demonstrates that you should move the flashlight over the entire cranial vault, including the inferior occipital region, to do a thorough examination.

d. In general, transillumination is useless in Pts more than 2 years of age. The skull is usually too thick and well ossified to transmit light. If you find transillumination in an older Pt, almost the only explanation would be that the fluid is located _____.

Ans: Outside of the skull in the scalp or subgaleal space.

e. Review Fig. 1-15. Would you expect the head of this young infant to transilluminate? ☐ Yes/ ☐ No.

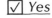 *Yes*

2

f. Review Figs. 1-16-*B* and 1-17*B*. You would expect these infants' heads to transilluminate only if they are less than _____ years old.

g. One of the ironies of a people like us, who worship technology, is that the law requires biochemical screening of every infant for phenylketonuria, but the law does not require a thorough physical examination. By measuring and transilluminating the head of every infant, you will discover more lesions, many of them life-threatening yet treatable, such as subdural fluid and hydrocephaly, than by screening for phenylketonuria. Dazzled by laboratory tests, are we demeaned if we have to candle an infant's head? Harvey Cushing (1869–1939) put it well when he remarked that we have increasing numbers of laboratory tests: . . . "the vast majority of which are but supplementary to, and *as nothing* compared with, the careful study of the Pt by a keen observer using his eyes and ears and fingers and a few simple aids."

SUGGESTED READING FOR TRANSILLUMINATION

Sjogren I, Engsner G: Transillumination of the skull in infants and children. *Acta Paediat Scand* 1972;61:426–428

8. *Differential analysis of megalocephaly (macrocephaly)*
   a. The discovery that a Pt has an enlarged head, megalocephaly, is merely a statistical description, not a diagnosis. Basically, one of five conditions causes megalocephaly. Be able to recite them. DeMyer (1986) gives a full list of differential diagnoses for megalocephaly.

   MEGALOCEPHALY

   → Obstruction hydrocephalus

   → Brain edema

   → Subdural hematoma/hygroma

   → Thickened skull

   → Megalencephaly

   b. *Essential steps in the NE of a megalocephalic Pt are:*
   (1) In infants palpate the fontanel and sutures and attempt to transilluminate the skull.
   (2) In megalocephaly as in microcephaly compare the somatotype and OFC of the Pt with siblings, and parents. Does the Pt match or differ from the family pattern?
   (3) Obtain MRI or CT scans if the OFC is abnormal, or if the history or examination discloses slow development.

SUGGESTED READING FOR MEGALENCEPHALY

DeMyer W: Megalencephaly: Types, clinical syndromes, and management. *Ped Neurol* 1986;2:321–328

9. *Mechanism of skull growth*
   a. In response to the normal pressure of the gently growing brain, bone is deposited along the suture margins, keeping the suture margins in con-

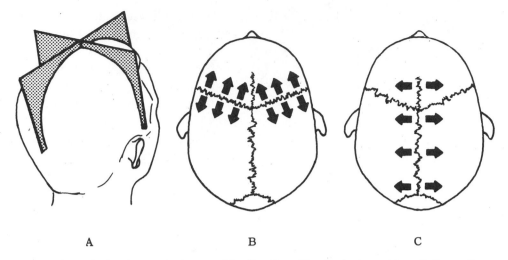

FIG. 1-20. The sagittal and coronal sutures and the direction of head enlargement from their growth zones. (*A*) Schematic projection of the planes of the sagittal and coronal sutures. (*B*) Growth along the coronal suture increases the anteroposterior diameter of the head. (*C*) Growth along the sagittal suture increases the lateral diameter of the head.

tact. Excessive intracranial pressure forces the skull sutures apart. Clinically, the most important growth occurs along the sagittal and coronal sutures. Study Fig. 1-20.

☑ A-P

b. Bone deposition along the *coronal* suture increases the head diameter which is perpendicular to it, the ☐ antero-posterior (A-P)/ ☐ lateral diameter.

Lateral

c. Bone deposition along the *sagittal* suture increases the head diameter which is perpendicular to it, the _____ diameter.

Perpendicular

d. As a general law, we can state that growth along a suture margin increases the head diameter which is _____ to the plane of the suture.

e. Look at the heads of your classmates. Some heads will be unusually short and wide and others long and thin. The OFC in the two groups will be approximately the same. Therefore, a head that is relatively small in one diameter will, in compensation, be relatively large in another diameter. Anthropologists call short-headedness *brachycephaly* (brachy = short) and long-headedness *dolichocephaly* (dolicho = long). Which head type would have the greatest lateral diameter? _____.

Brachycephaly
Sagittal
Coronal
Coronal
Sagittal

f. In brachycephaly, growth from the _____ suture proceeds rapidly relative to that from the _____ suture.

g. In dolichocephaly, growth from the _____ suture proceeds rapidly relative to that from the _____ suture.

10. *Abnormalities in skull shape: the craniosynostoses*

a. The terms *dolichocephaly* and *brachycephaly* express normal variations in the ratio of width and length of the skull. The sutures are basically normal. Sometimes one or more sutures and fontanels do not form or, if formed, close (ossify) prematurely. Such a disorder is called *craniosynostosis.*

Increases

b. What would happen to the intracranial pressure if the sutures close while the brain is still growing? _____

c. You must recognize craniosynostosis in young infants, for whom surgical treatment is most effective. Removal of strips of bone creates artificial sutures. Early surgery produces the best cosmetic results and prevents later complications (increased intracranial pressure, brain damage, and blindness) which may result when severe craniosynostosis prevents normal expansion of the brain.

d. *Clinical detection of craniosynostosis*

(1) In craniosynostosis, the overgrowth and fusion of bone at the sutures results in a palpable ridge. The bony overgrowth and absence of the sutures can be confirmed by skull radiographs or CT scans.

Coronal

(2) If the examination of a 3-month-old baby shows that its head is too short, you would suspect a deficiency of growth from the _____ suture.

e. You would have to decide whether the child's head shape was simple brachycephaly and therefore a normal variant, or whether he had craniosynostosis of the coronal suture. What do you do to determine the state of the sutures? _____

_____

_____.

Ans: *Palpate for a bony ridge and order skull radiographs or a CT scan (CT scans show bone, whereas MRI scans do not).*

f. *Terminology for craniosynostosis*

(1) Clinicians use special terms to describe the abnormal head shapes caused by craniosynostosis, in contrast to the anthropologic terms for normal variations. The terms here follow Ford's usage, but there are many synonyms which vary from author to author.

Coronal

(2) The pathologic condition of short-headedness due to craniosynostosis is called *acrobrachycephaly* (Fig. 1-21*A*). In such a patient, the closed suture is the _____ suture.

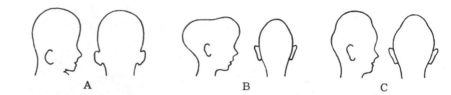

FIG. 1-21. **Silhouettes of abnormal head shapes caused by craniosynostosis. (***A***) Acrobrachycephaly. (***B***) Scaphocephaly. (***C***) Oxycephaly.**

(3) In acrobrachycephaly, the head is too short because coronal suture closure restricts its A-P diameter. The head becomes too wide because it expands perpendicular to the less affected suture, the _____ suture.

Sagittal

(4) The pathologic condition of long-headedness from craniosynostosis is called *scaphocephaly* (scapho = skiff or boat). The head looks like an inverted boat (Fig. 1-21*B*). The closed suture is the _____ suture.

Sagittal

(5) In scaphocephaly, the head becomes long because it expands perpendicular to the less affected suture, the _____ suture.

Coronal

(6) The pathologic head shape in Fig. 1-21*C* is called *oxycephaly* (oxy = keen or sharp). The head is reduced in both the lateral and A-P diameters. What does this head shape imply about the cranial sutures? _____

Ans: *Coronal and sagittal sutures are both synostosed.*

(7) Complete Table 1-3.

TABLE 1-3 Comparison of terms for head shapes		
Skull shape	Term for extreme variation of normal skull	Pathologic term for craniosynostosis
Skull too short and wide		
Skull too long		
Skull too short and narrow	None	

Brachycephaly; acrobrachycephaly

Dolichocephaly; scaphocephaly

Oxycephaly

(8) Would acrobrachycephaly, scaphocephaly, or oxycephaly most likely cause microcephaly and increased intracranial pressure? _____. Explain: _____

_____

Ans: Oxycephaly. Neither major suture allows skull expansion, thus limiting head size and brain growth.

g. The increased intracranial pressure in craniosynostosis causes the weakest part of the skull to yield. The thin orbital plates bulge downwards, causing the eyes to protrude. The general term for eyeball protrusion is _____.

Exophthalmos (proptosis)

h. Although usually bilateral, craniosynostosis may obliterate the sutures only on one side of the head. The affected hemicranium is small, and the skull and face are asymmetrical, a condition termed *plagiocephaly* (plagio = oblique). However, the term plagiocephaly crops up indiscriminately for any asymmetrical skull.

i. Craniosynostosis causes only a portion of misshapen, asymmetrical skulls. Intrinsic diseases such as rickets and syphilis deform the skull as does extrinsic pressure. Striking examples occurred in certain societies which in pursuit of beauty shaped the heads of infant girls, by tight bandages. If an infant has a neurologic deficit which causes it to rest on one part of its head, the head deforms to become flat on the "down" side. If the infant reclines on its back, the occiput becomes flattened. If the infant reclines on one parieto-occipital region, it flattens and the head becomes skewed. Sometimes no cause for skull asymmetry can be identified. In any event, an abnormal size or shape of the skull warns of an abnormal brain, often requiring further investigation by MRI or CT scan.

j. Complete Table 1-4 to fix the diagnostic terms for head shapes firmly in mind.

Acrobrachycephaly
Plagiocephaly

Scaphocephaly
Dolichocephaly
Oxycephaly
Brachycephaly

TABLE 1-4 Terms for abnormal skull shapes	
_____cephaly:	too short a skull because of lack of a coronal suture.
_____cephaly:	an asymmetrical skull because of lack of sutures on one side.
_____cephaly:	too long a skull because of lack of a sagittal suture.
_____cephaly:	too long a skull without craniosynostosis.
_____cephaly:	a short, narrow skull because of craniosynostosis.
_____cephaly:	a short skull without craniosynostosis.

k. What do you do to decide whether an infant with an abnormal head shape has craniosynostosis? _____

_____

Ans: Palpate for suture ridging and premature fontanel closure, and order plain skull radiographs or CT scans with bone windows.

SUGGESTED READING FOR CRANIOSYNOSTOSIS

Cohen MM (ed): *Craniosynostosis: Diagnosis, Evaluation, and Management,* New York, Raven, 1986

Ford F: *Diseases of the Nervous System in Infancy, Childhood and Adolescence* (6th ed). Springfield, IL, Charles C. Thomas, 1973

Shillito J Jr, Matson D: Craniosynostosis: A review of 519 surgical patients. *Pediatrics* 1968;41:829–853

III. General rules for the neurologic examination

Having learned some of the operations of the NE, you can now appreciate the general *operational, analytic,* and *attitudinal* rules that govern the success of the NE.

A. *Operational (technical) rules for the neurologic examination*
  1. *Follow the prescribed technique for each step of the NE.* Among the countless ways to do anything, whether phrasing questions or inspecting the eyes, only one is likely to be correct.
  2. *Systematize the NE.* The actual order is less important than the fact that you follow an order.
      a. Anatomic order. Work from top-to-bottom (rostro-caudal order).
      b. Instrument order. Lay out your instruments in the order that you will use them (again the rostro-caudal principle, see pages xii–xiii).
      c. Functional order. Test for mental, motor, and sensory dysfunctions in packages. The outlined NE, pages xi–xx, follows this rule.
  3. *Quantify the NE.* Measure the measurable and grade or scale the rest (number is the language of science).
      a. Measure pupillary size, occipitofrontal and limb circumferences, weight, etc., when relevant to the clinical problem.
      b. Grade strength as 0 to 5, muscle stretch reflexes as 0 to 4+, or other functions as *minimally, mildly, moderately,* or *severely* abnormal.
      c. Match or titrate the Pt's functions against your own: visual acuity, extent of visual fields, sensory thresholds, and strength.
      d. In deciding whether a body part deviates from normality, compare it against three standards:
        (1) Compare each part with the established norm for a person of like age and sex.
        (2) Compare each part with its mate on the opposite side.
        (3) Compare the Pt with the other family members. Does the Pt deviate from or repeat the appearances expected from the genetic background?
  4. *Do a complete examination on every Pt.* Since you must assume that everything is abnormal until proven otherwise, you must examine everything, or at least you must examine everything that is pertinent to the history and clinical problem:

      a. Take in the *gestalt* of the Pt: What is the total impact of the Pt's personality, facial appearance, and somatotype?

      b. *Look* over every square centimeter of skin and mucous membrane; look into every orifice, aperture, or opening.

      c. *Feel* every part.

      d. *Listen* to every sound over the chest, abdomen, head, and blood vessels.

      e. *Smell* every odor.

5. *Adapt the basic routine examination to the clinical problem.* Although each Pt must receive a basic routine examination, dismiss immediately the idea that one invariant, mindless examination protocol serves every Pt. The NE of a Pt with acute pain radiating down a leg differs considerably from the neurodevelopmental examination of an infant, or of the unconscious Pt. The Pt's mental status, the age, the symptoms that require investigation, and the diseases suspected require intelligent extensions of the routine examination.

B. *Analytic rules for the neurologic examination*

1. *Record all endpoint results objectively.* Write down objectively what actually occurred as the result of each operation of the NE, not an interpretation.

2. *After recording the findings objectively, interpret their neurophysiological and neuropathological implications and convert to technical terminology,* e.g., the observed weakness and hyperreflexia on one side becomes *hemiplegia* from pyramidal tract interruption. The *interpretation* locates the lesion in the CNS. Thus far the text in Chap. 1 has presented the observational examination for deviations in body contour. All subsequent chapters will be concerned with circuitry.

3. *Think circuitry.*

      a. As corollaries of the definition of behavior (see p. 1) we can state that:

        (1) *All* behavior depends on neuroanatomic connections.

        (2) *Every* behavior, spontaneous or induced, which the Pt can or cannot produce conveys valuable information as to whether the underlying neuroanatomic connections are intact.

      b. By "thinking through" the neuroanatomic circuits responsible for each end action, the Ex plugs into and can determine which circuits or pathways of the nervous system are intact and which are impaired; for example:

        (1) If the pupil of the eye constricts in response to light, the neural pathway from the retina to the midbrain and back to the pupilloconstrictor muscle is intact. If the pupil does not react, the neuroanatomic circuit is blocked at some point.

        (2) If the large toe flexes in response to plantar stimulation, the pyramidal tract and the afferent and efferent nerve fibers of the foot are intact, but if the toe extends (Babinski sign) the pyramidal tract is interrupted. Thus, blockage of the circuits at various sites alters the effector actions in characteristic ways.

4. *Localize the lesion. Postulate an anatomic site where the lesion has interrupted a nerve, pathway, or circuit.*

      a. Because the clinical signs of lesions at different levels of a motor, sensory, or mental circuit vary, the NE discloses which level of the circuit is interrupted. If the Pt is weak or paralyzed, the NE localizes the lesion to the pyramidal tract, ventral horn neuron, nerve root, peripheral nerve, neuromyal junction, or the muscle itself. If the Pt is blind, the NE localizes the lesion to the retina, optic nerve, chiasm or optic tract, the geniculo-calcarine tract, or the calcarine (visual) cortex itself.

b. By knowing the anatomical conjunctions of the various neural circuits, the Ex localizes the lesion to a specific anatomic site. If the Pt has a VIth nerve palsy and a contralateral hemiplegia, the lesion is in the basis pontis, near the pontomedullary junction, at the conjunction of the VIth cranial nerve and the pyramidal tract. If the Pt has expressive dysphasia and weakness of the right lower half of the face, the lesion is in the left posterior inferior frontal region, in the motor areas for speech and face movements, which are adjacent.

5. *Propose an etiologic diagnosis.*

a. By integrating the history, the anatomic localization, the pathophysiology, and the probability of various diseases, the Ex achieves a presumptive *etiologic diagnosis,* which in turn determines any required laboratory workup to reach a *final etiologic diagnosis.* The final etiologic diagnosis sets the prognosis and therapy.

b. The following catechism summarizes the analytic process applied to every Pt: Is there a lesion? Where is the lesion? What is the lesion or disease present? What do I need to do to confirm the diagnosis? What is the management?

C. *Attitudinal rules for success in the NE:* the mindset for success. First and foremost, the success of the NE depends on the attitude, the mindset, with which you approach the Pt.

1. *React professionally.* Whether the Pt is a murderer, street person, pedophile, or saint, the physician accepts every Pt with equal dignity, humility, and grace. Remain nonjudgmental and emotionally neutral to whatever behavior the Pt presents, whether compliant or hostile, or to whatever clinical problem, whether a hangnail or AIDS. Accept all of the Pt's behavior objectively as clinical phenomena, as the activation of glands and muscles by nerve impulses shuttling through neuroanatomic circuits. The Ex cannot complete a competent, analytical, and thorough NE while plagued with emotions of attraction or repulsion, or while making moral judgments about the Pt's lifestyle and worthiness.

2. *Expect the abnormal.* Maintain a paranoid suspicion that every finding will be abnormal. The trained mind discovers what it is trained to discover. Since the physician's training is to discover disease, not to deny it, assume that everything is abnormal until proven otherwise. The mindset that a finding will be normal results in loss of vigilance and a sloppy or incomplete examination. If you assume that the ear drums or rectum are normal, you won't examine them carefully. The design, the very purpose of medical investigations, is to discover whether the Pt deviates from mental and physical norms. If the patient does deviate from the norm, determine in what way (qualitatively) and to what degree (quantitatively).

3. *Enjoy the neurologic examination.*

a. Convert parts of the NE into a friendly contest or game.

(1) Visual fields. Ask the Pt, "Let's see whether you can see out as far to the side as I can."

(2) Strength testing. "Don't let me win."

(3) Sensory testing. "Let's see how light a touch you can feel."

b. Such challenges elicit the Pt's interest and best performance and maintain your own interest. Then both you and the Pt will enjoy the NE. If you do something 20 times a day for the rest of your career, you might as well learn how to enjoy it.

c. The NE gives you the privilege of entering the Pt's neural circuitry to discover the way lesions alter mental, motor, and sensory functions. If you are curious and inquisitive, and take pride in your knowledge, technique, and competence, the whole process of the NE and its derivative conclusions becomes immensely gratifying—in fact, downright fun. Viewed this way each NE becomes an opportunity for enjoyment. That is what I want this text to offer you: the competence to do an enjoyable NE in which you can take pride and derive satisfaction.

D. *Summary of the neurologic examination* The NE is a systematic series of inspections, questions, commands, and maneuvers, designed to disclose mental, motor, or sensory dysfunction or deviations in bodily configuration. Each step assesses some specific endpoint, usually a behavioral endpoint. The behavioral endpoint may be a spontaneous or elicited, verbal or nonverbal behavior. The behavior may be simple, such as a pupil constricting, or complex, such as having the Pt walk or talk. The Ex records the endpoint result objectively, quantifies it where possible, and judges it as normal, borderline, or abnormal. The Ex then interprets each behavior in terms of the integrity of the neuroanatomic circuits that mediate it. From knowledge of the course and conjunctions of neuroanatomic circuits, the Ex makes an *anatomic diagnosis* of the lesion site. By integrating the results of the NE with the history, the Ex arrives at the presumptive *etiologic diagnosis.* The presumptive etiologic diagnosis serves as the basis for ordering confirmatory laboratory tests to reach the final diagnosis, which determines the prognosis and therapy. When completed, the whole process, with its beauty, power, and intellectual symmetry, leads to immense gratification.

IV. Summary of the initial examination of the head and face

How do we insure that you can apply these general principles and the specific data of this chapter to the actual examination of a Pt? We do it by instituting a ritual of review and rehearsal of just what it is the chapter teaches you to do, until you do it automatically. Although you may prefer to call it simply practicing, behavioral psychologists would say that they want you to emit the terminal behavior of the learning sequence. By terminal behavior, the psychologist means those recitations and performances which provide evidence to yourself and anyone watching that you have learned what you should have. First, review the Learning Objectives in the section that follows. Then get a partner and practice the terminal behavior outlined in Section IV, A–E of the Summarized Neurologic Examination (page xiv). As you do so, notice how the four techniques of *inspection, palpation, percussion,* and *auscultation* impose their order on the examination and how the anatomic arrangement of the body parts imposes its order.

Learning Objectives for Chapter One

I. Introduction to the neurologic examination

1. Name the four types of operations that the Ex performs during the NE.

2. The endpoint of each operation of the NE is the observation of some bodily contour or of some spontaneous or elicited behavior. Define behavior as applied to the NE.

II. Inspection of the Pt

A. Inspection of the eyes

1. Make a drawing of the eye labeling the following structures and point them out on another person or in your mirror: medial and lateral canthi, corneal limbus, iris, pupil, caruncle, and lacrimal papilla (Fig. 1-17).
2. Make drawings which show the relation of the limbus to the upper and lower eyelids when the Pt looks straight ahead and of the relation of the limbus to the canthi and caruncle when the Pt moves the eyes as far as possible to the side (Fig. 1-3).
3. Describe and name the abnormal angulations of the palpebral fissures (Fig. 1-4).
4. Define these eye abnormalities: canthus dystopia, epicanthal folds, hypertelorism, hypotelorism, isocoria, anisocoria, cormiosis, corectasia, corectopia, ptosis, enopthalmos and exophthalmos, anopthalmia, microphthalmia, and macrophthalmia (Fig. 1-7).
5. Describe the effect of exophthalmos and enophthalmos on the height of the palpebral fissure.
6. Name the diagnostic procedure necessary to establish true bony ocular hypertelorism and hypotelorism.
7. What is the size of the normal pupil in millimeters and what terms describe very large or very small pupils?

B. Inspection of the remainder of the face and hair

1. Draw and label the parts of the external ear (pinna) (Fig. 1-8).
2. Describe how to systematically inspect the face and hair for anatomical deviations.

C. Palapation, percussion, and auscultation of the head

1. Describe the normal bumps and depressions felt on palpation of the skull.
2. Locate the carotid and temporal artery pulses (Fig. 1-9).
3. Describe and demonstrate auscultation of the neck and head for bruits.
4. Describe the type of carotid bruit associated with an increased risk of stroke?

D. Abnormalities in the size and shape of the head

1. Name the endochondral bones of the skull (Fig. 1-11).
2. Distinguish between a synarthrosis and a diarthrosis and state which joints of the skull are diarthroses.
3. Rank the skull synarthroses (synchondroses, fontanels, and sutures) in order of pliancy.
4. Name the bones that border on the anterior fontanel.
5. Describe the proper conditions for examining the contour of the anterior fontanel of an infant. Explain why you would not attempt to judge the contour of the fontanel with the infant struggling or crying.

6. Describe the contour of the normal anterior fontanel in a neonate or young infant.
7. Explain what is meant by closure of the sutures and describe when functional closure of the sutures occurs.
8. Draw the shape of the normal curve for increase in the OFC from birth, and show trend lines indicating evolving macrocephaly (megalocephaly) and microcephaly (Fig. 1-15).
9. List three physical findings on examination of the head of an infant that indicate increased intracranial pressure.
10. Distinguish between megalocephaly (macrocephaly), hydrocephaly, and megalencephaly (macrencephaly).
11. Discuss the use and limitations of the OFC in predicting the actual size and weight of the brain.
12. Define hydrocephaly (hydrocephalus) and explain why some Pts have normal pressure with hydrocephalus and others have increased pressure.
13. Describe the bedside tests and reasoning used to analyze abnormal transillumination of an infant's head (Table 1-2).
14. Name five general categories of causes for megalocephaly (macrocephaly).
15. State the law relating the direction of head growth to the plane of the sutures.
16. State the physical findings that indicate some type of craniosynostosis.
17. Give the terms for normal variations in the length and breadth of the head and for the various abnormal head shapes caused by craniosynostosis (Tables 1-3 and 1-4).

III. The philosophy of physical diagnosis

1. Describe some techniques or principles that insure a systematic basic minimum NE.
2. What factors might require the Ex to extend the basic minimum NE?
3. Describe the types of comparisons made to determine whether any particular finding on the NE is normal or abnormal.
4. Describe the differences in reacting professionally to the Pt and in the usual social and attitudinal reactions. Explain why professional responses are required of the physician.
5. Explain whether to approach each operation of the NE with the attitude that the finding will be normal or abnormal.
6. As the overall learning objective of Chap. 1, describe and demonstrate how to examine the face and head by inspection, palpation, percussion, transillumination, and auscultation.

Chapter Two

A Brief Review of Clinical Neuroanatomy

But chieflye the anatomye
Ye oughte to understande:
If ye will cure well anye thinge,
That ye doe take in hande.
  John Halle (1529–1566)

I. Gross subdivisions of the neuraxis

Introductory note: To interpret the neurologic examination requires a firm grasp of basic neuroanatomy. If the audience just groaned, let me distinguish two types of neuroanatomy: *tonguetip* neuroanatomy that you can recite on the spot, for immediate clinical use, and *fingertip* neuroanatomy that you refer to in a book as the need arises. This chapter clearly separates the two.

A. *Two main parts of the nervous system:* The *nervous system* consists of two main parts, the *central* nervous system (CNS) and the *peripheral* nervous system (PNS).
  1. The *CNS* or *neuraxis* consists of the *brain* and *spinal cord* (Fig. 2-1).
  2. The *PNS* consists of *cranial nerves, spinal nerves,* and associated *ganglia* and *plexuses.*
  3. To separate the CNS from the PNS, simply snip all cranial and spinal nerves at their attachment sites to the brain and spinal cord.

B. *How to cut out the basic subdivision of the neuraxis that you want*
  1. To separate the *brain* from the *spinal cord,* sweep your scalpel transversely across the neuraxis at the plane of the foramen magnum. The *spinal cord* is *caudal* to the transection; the *brain* is rostral (Fig. 2-1). Locate the foramen magnum in Fig. 2-1.
    a. The *brain* consists of the *brainstem, cerebellum, diencephalon,* and the *cerebral hemispheres.*
    b. In Fig. 2-1, differentiate the *cerebrum, brain,* and *brainstem.* [These definitions of the cerebrum and brainstem follow the current *Nomina Ana-*

---

*The light vertical rule on the left side of the text sets off an answer column. Cover the answers with a card until you have responded to the text. Then after each response, slide the card down to check your answer.
The heavy vertical rule or asterisk denotes optional material.

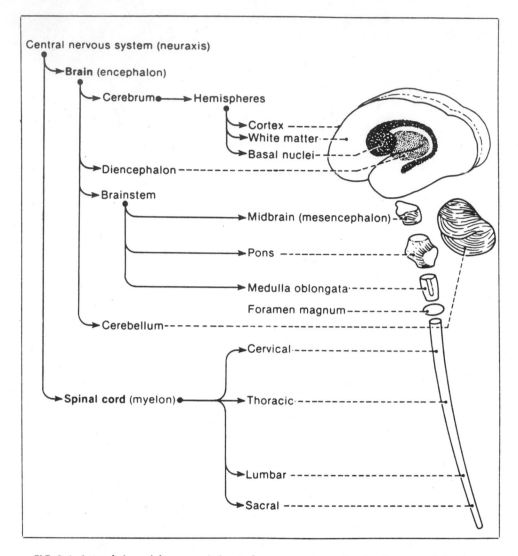

FIG. 2-1. Lateral view of the neuraxis (central nervous system), showing its gross subdivisions.

tomica (1980) and differ from the original BNA of 1895 and the definitions given in the last edition (1980) of this text].

2. *Dissecting out the brainstem:* The previous cut across the foramen magnum severed the brain from the spinal cord at the medullocervical junction. To separate the *brainstem* from the rest of the brain, make these cuts:

   a. Transect the mesencephalon just as it emerges from its attachment to the diencephalon and deep white matter at the base of the cerebrum (Figs. 2-1 and 2-22).

   b. Then remove the cerebellum by slicing through the peduncles, which attach it to the pons (Figs. 2-1 and 8-3). The brainstem remains.

   c. To subdivide the brainstem into the *midbrain, pons,* and *medulla,* make transverse cuts at the mesencephalopontine junction and at the pontomedullary junction (Fig. 2-1).

3. *Dissecting out the diencephalon:* Having removed the brainstem and cerebellum from the brain, separate the *diencephalon* from the cerebrum, by coring it out with a paring knife. Commence at the base of the brain, where the diencephalon presents on the surface as the hypothalamus and optic chiasm (Fig. 2-22). Internally, the basal ganglia and deep cerebral white matter (internal capsule) surround the diencephalon (Fig. 13-8*A* and *B*). Caudally the diencephalon abuts on the midbrain.

4. *Composition of the cerebrum:* After disposal of all of the foregoing parts of the brain, the *cerebrum* remains, consisting of two cerebral hemispheres. Sections of each hemisphere disclose:
   a. A superficial lamina of cortical gray matter containing layers of neurons.
   b. Deep white matter containing axonal pathways.
   c. Deep nuclear gray matter called *basal ganglia,* periventricular in location.
   d. Ventricular cavities. Review all of these structures in Fig. 13-8*A* and *B*.

C. *Fissures, lobes, and sulci of the cerebrum*
   1. The cerebral surface displays two types of crevices: *fissures* and *sulci.*
      a. Important fissures include:
         (1) The *interhemispheric* (longitudinal) *fissure,* which separates the *medial* faces of the two cerebral hemispheres (Fig. 13-8*A* and *B*).
         (2) The *sylvian* or *lateral fissure,* which separates the temporal lobe from the frontal lobe anteriorly and from the parietal lobe posteriorly (Fig. 2-2*A*).
      b. Important *sulci* include the *central sulcus* which separates the frontal and parietal lobes, the *parieto-occipital sulcus,* which separates the parietal and occipital lobes medially, and the *calcarine sulcus.* The posterior part of the calcarine sulcus divides the occipital lobe into dorsal and ventral halves (Fig. 2-2*B* and *C*).
   2. Each hemisphere has four traditional lobes, named because of the overlying bones of the skull: the *frontal, parietal, temporal,* and *occipital.* Learn and be able to draw the named features of Fig. 2-2. Then test your mastery in frames D.1 to D.10 that follow.

D. *Boundaries of the cerebral lobes:* Some of the lobar boundaries are natural landmarks while others are purely arbitrary lines.

Central

1. The boundary between the *posterior* margin of the frontal lobe and the *anterior* margin of the parietal lobe is marked by the plane of the _____ sulcus.
2. The sylvian fissure extends *anterior* and *posterior* to the plane of the central sulcus (Fig. 2-2*A*). The *anterior* part of the sylvian fissure divides the

Frontal; temporal
Parietal
Temporal

_____ lobe above from the _____ lobe below.
3. The *posterior* part of the sylvian fissure divides the _____ lobe above from the _____ below.
4. *Laterally,* the anterior boundary of the occipital lobe is an arbitrary line drawn from the _____ _____.

Superior to the inferior pre- occipital notch

5. *Laterally,* given the pre-occipital notch line, describe the boundary between the posterior part of the parietal lobe and the temporal lobe.

_____
_____.

Ans: Draw a perpendicular line from the half-way point of the pre-occipital notch line until it meets the Sylvian fissure.

Parietal; temporal

6. *Laterally,* the superior part of the occipital lobe abuts anteriorly on the _____ lobe, and inferiorly on the _____ lobe.

Parieto-occipital

7. *Medially,* the natural boundary that divides the occipital and parietal lobes is the _____ sulcus.
8. *Medially,* the occipital lobe is separated from the temporal lobe by an arbitrary line drawn from _____ _____.

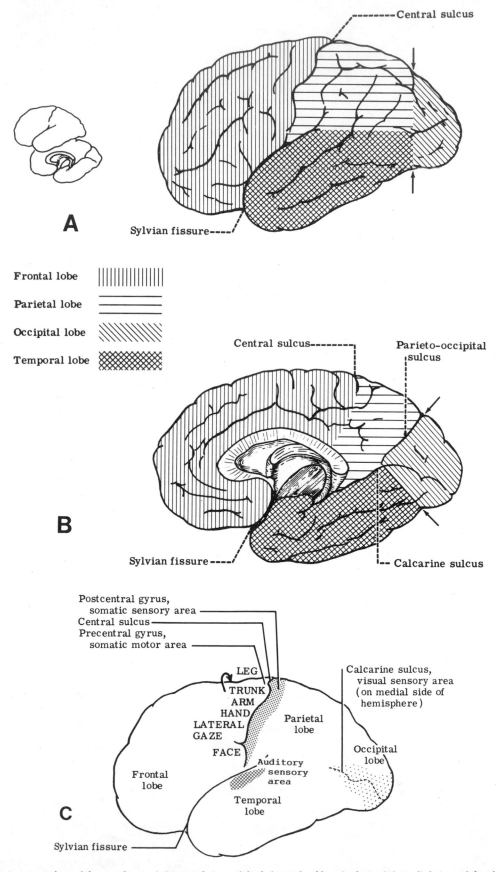

FIG. 2-2. **Lobes of the cerebrum.** (*A*) Lateral view of the left cerebral hemisphere. (*B*) Medial view of the right cerebral hemisphere. (*C*) Lateral view of the left cerebral hemisphere showing the location of somatomotor, somatosensory, visual, and auditory regions. The leg area of the sensorimotor cortex extends over onto the medial aspect of the hemisphere.

Ans: The inferior pre-occipital notch to the junction of the calcarine and parieto-occipital sulci (Fig. 2-2B).

Parietal

9. By knowing all of the boundaries of just *one* lobe, you can fairly well define the boundaries of *all* four major lobes. The keystone lobe is the _____ lobe.

10. Draw medial and lateral views of the cerebrum, and demarcate and label the major fissures, sulci, and lobes. Compare your effort with Fig. 2-2 *A* and *B*.

E. *The fifth and sixth cerebral lobes*
1. To the traditional four lobes, Paul Broca (1824–1880) added the *limbic lobe* (Fig. 2-3).

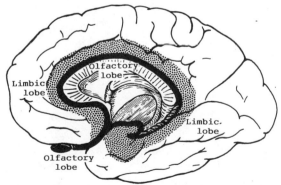

FIG. 2-3. Medial view of left cerebral hemisphere showing the limbic lobe (entire stippled ring) and the olfactory lobe (entire black ring inside limbic lobe and the olfactory bulb and tract extending anteriorly and inferiorly from the ring).

2. Notice that the limbic lobe encircles the junction of the hemispheric wall with the midline structures that connect the two hemispheres at their hilus. The general term for such a junction zone, as of the cornea with the sclera at the periphery of the iris, is *limbus.*

3. Finally we may recognize a sixth lobe, the *olfactory lobe.*

F. *Localization of function in the cerebral cortex*

1. The *somatomotor cortex* occupies the *pre*central gyrus, located just in front of the central sulcus, and to a lesser extent the postcentral gyrus (Fig. 2-2*C*). The motor cortex originates the *pyramidal tract,* the single most important pathway for volitional movement. The motor cortex represents the body parts inversely, with the leg area superomedial and the face area inferolateral (Fig. 2-2*C*).

2. The *somatosensory cortex* occupies the *post*central gyrus, just behind the central sulcus (Fig. 2-2*C*). It receives the somatosensory pathways from the thalamus of the diencephalon that mediate skin sensations and the discriminative senses, such as position sense and stereognosis (form recognition). The somatosensory cortex, like the somatomotor cortex, represents the body parts inversely.

3. The *auditory receptive cortex* occupies the transverse temporal gyri, which are tucked in the sylvian fissure, just under the parietal lobe (Fig. 2-2*C*). This cortex receives the auditory pathway from the *medial* geniculate body of the thalamus.

4. The *visual receptive cortex* occupies the superior and inferior banks of the occipital part of the calcarine sulcus (Fig. 2-2*C*). It receives the visual pathway from the *lateral* geniculate body of the thalamus.

5. Make an outline of Fig. 2-2*C* and shade or color the somatomotor, somatosensory, visual, and auditory areas.

6. The *association cortex,* the large cortical areas surrounding the primary sensory receptive cortices, receive and send association pathways to and from them, associating the primary sensory information with its meaning and with motor responses. The association cortex performs the so-called *gnostic* functions of recognizing the general meaning or import of the primary sensory information.

7. The *olfactory lobe* mediates smell. Phylogenetically the *limbic lobe* derived from the olfactory system, and retains close anatomic connections with the olfactory lobe, amygdala, hippocampal formation, and hypothalamus. Limbic lobe pathways with the hypothalamus and thalamus mediate the experience of emotions and the behavioral expression of emotions in autonomic and endocrine activity and in overall motor activity. Hippocampal, thalamic, and limbic circuits also mediate recent memory. Some diseases, such as herpes simplex encephalitis, selectively attack the temporal lobe and limbic connections. These Pts display emotionality and loss of recent memory but so do Pts with diffuse cerebral disease. The rabies virus strongly attacks the hippocampus, and emotionality, such as hydrophobia, is prominent in association with the throat spasms of the disease. Deep midline neoplasms, such as gliomas of the septum pellucidum, hippocampus-fornix, corpus callosum, and adjacent limbic lobe also cause behavioral changes, loss of emotional control, and loss of recent memory. The complicated clinical correlations between brain lesions and behavior go beyond this resumé of cerebral localization.

II. The neuron and the neuron doctrine

A. *Definition of a neuron.* The neuron is the parenchymal cell of the CNS and PNS. All *neurons* have a *nucleus* (karyon), *cell body* (perikaryon), and one or more *branches.*

1. The vast *majority* of neurons typically display two types of branches, *dendritic* and *axonal* (Fig. 2-4).

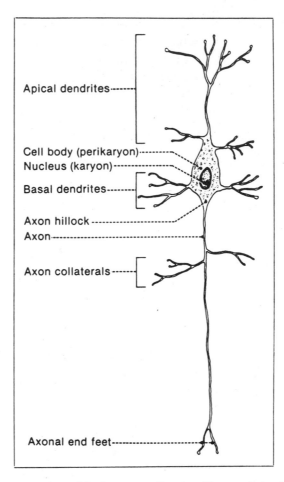

Apical dendrites

Cell body (perikaryon)
Nucleus (karyon)
Basal dendrites

Axon hillock
Axon

Axon collaterals

Axonal end feet

FIG. 2-4. Typical components of a multipolar neuron *(Reprinted by permission from W. DeMyer: Neuroanatomy, Baltimore, Williams & Wilkins, 1988.)*

   2. A small *minority* of neurons (amacrine neurons) produce branches that are difficult to classify as axons and dendrites.

B. *Function of neurons*
   1. The basic function of neurons is *communication.* When stimulated, neurons produce *nerve impulses* that influence other neurons or effector cells (gland cells or muscle cells) by activating or inhibiting them.
   2. The *nerve impulse,* when electronically recorded and measured, consists of a wave of electrical depolarization called an *action potential.* The action potential propagates along the surface of the neuronal membrane to the axonal tips, the *end feet.* The end feet form *synapses* on a dendrite, perikaryon, or axon of one or more neurons or on an effector cell. A synapse consists of:
      a. A presynaptic membrane provided by an axonal end foot.
      b. A synaptic cleft.
      c. A postsynaptic membrane of a neuron or effector cell.
   3. The branching of axons increases the number of synapses a given neuron can provide to subsequent neurons or to effector cells. The branching of dendrites increases the surface area of any given neuron to receive greater numbers of synapses.
   4. At a synapse the axon terminal releases a chemical called a *neurotransmitter.* The neurotransmitter crosses the synaptic cleft to attach to receptor sites on the postsynaptic membrane thus altering its electrical polarization. *Excitatory* neurotransmitters *depolarize* the postsynaptic cell, promoting

impulse generation, while *inhibitory* transmitters *hyperpolarize* the post-synaptic cell, opposing impulse generation.

5. In vertebrates, the simplest communication loop, called a *reflex arc,* involves an *afferent* neuron which responds to a stimulus, and a single central synapse which fires an *efferent* neuron which then activates an effector (Fig. 2-5).

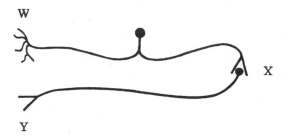

FIG. 2-5. Conventional representation of a synapse at X. A receptor (W) is any sensory nerve ending. An effector (Y) is any motor nerve ending on a gland cell or a muscle fiber.

☑ *WXY*

6. A synapse is a one-way valve. The flow of nerve impulses at a synapse is *from* the incoming axon *to* the next neuron. In Fig. 2-5, the flow of impulses is ☐ WXY/ ☐ YXW.

C. *The neuron doctrine* consists of six tenets, asserting that the neuron is the *genetic, anatomic, functional, directional, pathologic,* and *regenerative* unit of the nervous system.

1. Each neuron is an *anatomic* unit: Each neuron has a continuous surface membrane that separates it from all other cells.

2. Each neuron is a *functional* unit: The neuron is the smallest unit capable of receiving, generating, and transmitting nerve impulses.

3. Each neuron is a *directional* unit: In general a neuron in situ conducts impulses only in one direction, from dendrite to axonal tip (amacrine cells excepted).

4. Each neuron is a *genetic* unit: Each neuroblast develops by mitosis as an independent cell. Its nucleus contains a genetic code unique for each species of neuron, which gives that species its own anatomic and biochemical characteristics.

5. Each neuron is a *pathologic* unit: If the perikaryon dies, all branches die. Any part of a neuron separated from its perikaryon dies, although the rest of the cell may live.

   a. The genetic code produces numerous species of neurons, which differ in biochemistry and structure. Such differences determine the susceptibility of that neuron species. A given pathogen such as a genetic defect, a virus, or a toxin, may affect only one system of susceptible neurons, causing that neuronal species to degenerate, while completely sparing neighboring groups. Thus the poliomyelitis virus is relatively selective in attacking motoneurons; the herpes zoster virus has an affinity for dorsal root ganglia; and methanol attacks the optic nerves.

   b. This *differential susceptibility* leads to an almost endless number of genetic, viral, or toxic diseases that cause *systematized degeneration* of specific tracts or neuronal groups, while all other neurons survive. If the susceptible neurons are in the retina, the Pt becomes blind, if in the auditory ganglion, the Pt becomes deaf.

6. Each neuron is a *regenerative* unit: Mature neurons cannot multiply, but some can regenerate axons.

    a. After transection of an axon, the distal part, severed from its perikaryon dies, a process called *wallerian degeneration* (Fig. 7-23).

    b. The surviving neuronal perikaryon of a peripheral axon may regenerate its severed axon (Ochs, 1977), but effective axonal regeneration of severed tracts of CNS axons in humans has never been convincingly demonstrated. The promotion of axonal regeneration is now one of the most important areas of research (Carlson, 1990; Seil, 1988).

REFERENCES FOR AXONAL REGENERATION

Carlson BM (ed): *Regeneration and Transplantation.* Canton, Mass., Science History Publishing, 1990

Ochs S: The early history of nerve regeneration beginning with Chuckshank's observations in 1776. *Med Hist* 1977;21:261–274

Seil F (ed): *Neural Regeneration and Transplantation.* New York, Alan R Liss, 1988

Shepherd GM: Foundation of the Neuron Doctrine. New York, Oxford University Press, 1991.

III. The spinal cord, somites, and spinal nerves

How to get to the neurology clinic through the muck and slime of phylogenesis, the maelstroms of embryogenesis, and a little help from set theory.

A. Somites and the segmental level of the neuraxis

  1. During ontogeny and phylogeny, paired tissue masses called *segments* or *somites* develop along each side of the neuraxis (Fig. 2-6*A*).

  2. The parts of the neuraxis opposite the somites, the *brainstem* and *spinal cord,* constitute the *segmental* level of the nervous system. The *diencephalon* and *cerebrum* are the *suprasegmental* levels of the neuraxis.

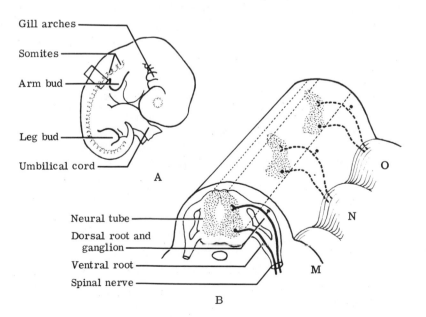

FIG. 2-6. Somites in a 5-week-old human embryo. (*A*) Serial arrangement of the somites lateral to the neuraxis. (*B*) Enlargement of neuraxis and the somites blocked off in *A*. Notice that each somite (M, N, and O) receives only one nerve.

3. The primitive cells of each somite differentiate into a *dermatome, myotome,* and *sclerotome.* The dermatome spreads out under the epidermis to form the dermis, the myotome differentiates into muscle, and the sclerotome into bone. These tissues form the skeletal muscles, neck, extremities, and parietes.

4. Each member of the somite pair receives one spinal nerve (Fig. 2-6*B*), and one spinal artery, which thus are also paired. The spinal nerves also innervate the underlying viscera.

B. *Spinal nerves and the theory of nerve components*
   1. The spinal cord has approximately 30 pairs of somites and 30 pairs of spinal nerves: 8 cervical, 12 thoracic, 5 lumbar, and 5 sacral.
   2. Each spinal nerve is formed by the union of *dorsal* and *ventral roots* (Fig. 2-7).

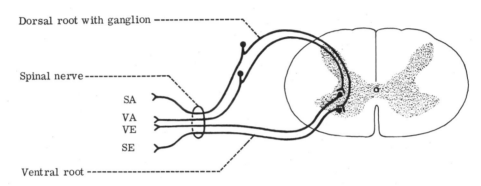

FIG. 2-7.   Cross section of spinal cord to show the typical four functional types of axons in a spinal nerve: SA, somatic afferent; VA, visceral afferent; VE, visceral efferent; and SE, somatic efferent.

3. *The theory of nerve components* states that the spinal and cranial nerves and nerve roots convey axons of specific functional types.
   a. The law of Bell and Magendie states that the *dorsal* roots convey *sensory* axons and the *ventral, motor.* The internal plan of the gray matter of the segmental nervous system reflects this sensorimotor dichotomy because the dorsal horns are mainly sensory and the ventral mainly motor.
   b. Notice that perikarya in *dorsal root ganglia* provide the axons of the somatosensory afferents (SA) from the dermatome, myotome, and sclerotome, and viscerosensory afferents (VA) from the viscera (Fig. 2-7).
   c. Notice that perikarya in the *ventral horns* of the spinal gray matter provide somatic efferent (SE) axons to the striated muscle derived from the myotomes. Perikarya in the *intermediate horn* provide visceral efferent (VE) axons to innervate glands and the smooth muscle of the viscera (via a synapse in an outlying ganglion). *Virtually all spinal nerves contain all four components: SA, VA, VE, and SE.*
   d. Fig. 2-7 shows that the SA or VA axons may synapse directly or *monosynaptically* on their respective SE or VE motor neuron. *Read all circuit diagrams by tracing along the course of the nerve impulses.* In Fig. 2-7, start at a receptor ending, let us say the SA receptor. Trace the impulse centrally past the dorsal root ganglion to the motoneuron. Excitation of the motoneuron then causes contraction of the skeletal muscle fibers innervated by the SE axon.

4. Draw and label a cross section of the spinal cord showing the dorsal and ventral horns and roots and their functional nerve components. Check your drawing against Fig. 2-7.

C. *Three functional types of neurons:* afferent (sensory), efferent (motor), and internuncial
1. The theory of nerve components recognizes distinct *afferent* and *efferent* pools of neurons. *Afferent* neurons consist of dorsal root ganglia of the spinal cord and their counterparts on the cranial nerves, including the trigeminal ganglion, cochleovestibular ganglia, geniculate ganglion, olfactory ganglion, and the analogous retinal neurons. *The perikarya of virtually all afferent neurons, except for the retina, are in ganglia outside of the CNS, but their proximal axons enter the CNS.*
2. *Efferent* neurons consist of somatic and autonomic (visceral) motoneurons in the gray matter of the spinal cord and brainstem, including an added group of branchial motoneurons at the brainstem level. *The perikarya of all of these efferent motoneurons are always within the CNS but their axons exit into the PNS to reach their effectors.*
3. A third type of neuron, *internuncial* or *intercalary* neurons, interpose themselves between the afferent and efferent pools. The perikarya of internuncials, their processes, and their connections are all *inside* of the CNS. These neurons, comprising the vast majority of all neurons, provide for alternative, polysynaptic circuits of greater complexity and plasticity than the direct monosynaptic afferent-efferent reflex arcs that can only cause simple muscular twitches (Fig. 2-8).
4. *Dispersion of afferent axons:* On entering the CNS, afferent axons could synapse at the level of entry, ascend or descend, or cross to the opposite side. The entering axon may synapse on efferent neurons or internuncial neurons at the same or different levels. In fact axons choose all of these options, ending monosynaptically (Fig. 2-7) or on internuncial neurons (Fig. 2-8).

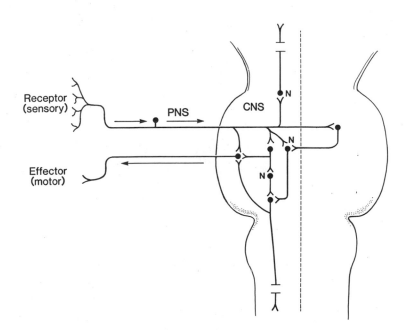

FIG. 2-8. Polysynaptic reflex arc consisting of a primary sensory neuron in a dorsal root ganglion, any number of internuncial neurons (N) in the CNS, and a motoneuron that innervates an effector. Contrast with the monosynaptic arc shown in Fig. 2-7.

The number of internuncial neurons in the circuit between afferent axon and effectors varies from none to countless (Fig. 2-8).

D. *Somite migrations and the law of original innervation*
1. The phylogenetic specializations leading to limb and head development obscure the simple serial arrangement of the somites. The proximal portions of the dermatomes attenuate as they extend out into the limbs. Finally the limbs stretch the somites so thin that C4 abuts on T2 (Figs. 2-9 and 2-10).

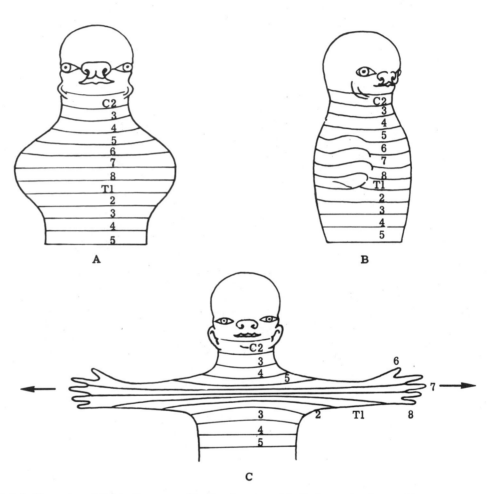

FIG. 2-9. Dermatomal dislocations caused by development of the limbs. Notice that no dermatomes are represented rostral to C-2. Cranial nerve V innervates facial sensation.

2. The myotomes and sclerotomes also undergo migrations. For example, the myotomes of cervical somites 3, 4, and 5 produce the diaphragm. The diaphragm then migrates to the level of T-12. It drags its somite nerves, united into the phrenic nerves, along with it from the cervical region. Many of the extremity muscles contain contributions from more than one myotome. Table 2-1 lists the segmental composition of the muscles, and Table 2-2, the segmental innervation of reflexes tested clinically. Do not memorize these figures and tables. They are fingertip neuroanatomy that you look up as needed.
3. *The law of original innervation: wherever a somite derivative migrates, it retains its original somite nerve.* Even when various muscles and bones receive contributions from several somites, the spinal nerve of each somite

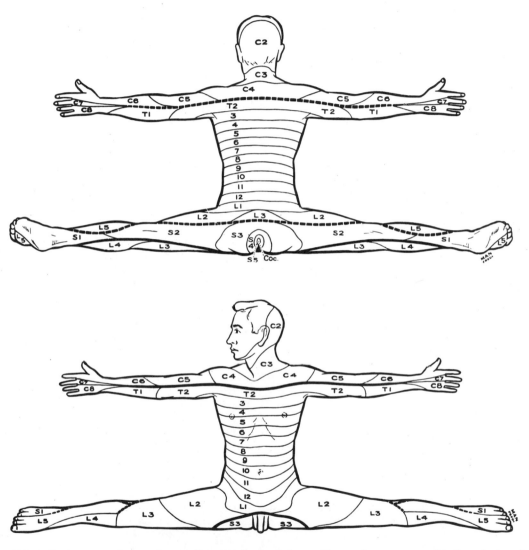

FIG. 2-10. Sensory cutaneous innervation areas by dermatomes. The numbers correspond to the spinal cord level of the dermatome. C = cervical, T = thoracic, L = lumbar, S = sacral. (*From W. Haymaker and B. Woodhall: Peripheral Nerve Injuries, 2d ed, Philadelphia, W. B. Saunders, 1962.*)

TABLE 2-1 Segmental innervation of muscles

Action tested	Roots*	Nerves	Muscles
CRANIAL			
Closure of eyes, pursing of lips, exposure of teeth	Cranial VII	Facial	Orbicularis oculi Orbicularis oris, etc.
Elevation of eyelids, movement of eyes	Cranial III, IV, VI	Oculomotor, trochlear, abducens	Extraocular
Closing and opening of jaw	Cranial V	Motor trigeminal	Masseters Pterygoids
Protrusion of tongue	Cranial XII	Hypoglossal	Lingual
Phonation and swallowing	Cranial IX, X	Glossopharyngeal, vagus	Palatal, laryngeal, and pharyngeal
Elevation of shoulders, anteroflexion and turning of head	Cranial XI	Spinal accessory	Trapezius, sternomastoid
BRACHIAL			
Adduction of extended arm	C-5, C-6	Brachial plexus	Pectoralis major
Fixation of scapula	C-5, C-6, C-7	Brachial plexus	Serratus anterior
Initiation of abduction of arm	C-5, C-6	Brachial plexus	Supraspinatus
External rotation of flexed arm	C-5, C-6	Brachial plexus	Infraspinatus
Abduction and elevation of arm up to 90°	C-5, C-6	Axillary nerve	Deltoid
Flexion of supinated forearm	C-5, C-6	Musculocutaneous	Biceps, brachialis
Extension of forearm	C-6, C-7, C-8	Radial	Triceps
Extension (radial) of wrist	C-6	Radial	Extensor carpi radialis longus
Flexion of semipronated arm	C-5, *C-6*	Radial	Brachioradialis
Adduction of flexed arm	C-6, *C-7*, C-8	Brachial plexus	Latissimus dorsi
Supination of forearm	C-6, C-7	Posterior interosseous	Supinator
Extension of proximal phalanges	*C-7*, C-8	Posterior interosseous	Extensor digitorum
Extension of wrist (ulnar side)	C-7, C-8	Posterior interosseous	Extensor carpi ulnaris
Extension of proximal phalanx of index finger	*C-7*, C-8	Posterior interosseous	Extensor indicis
Abduction of thumb	C-7, C-8	Posterior interosseous	Abductor pollicis longus and brevis
Extension of thumb	*C-7*, C-8	Posterior interosseous	Extensor pollicis longus and brevis
Pronation of forearm	C-6, C-7	Median nerve	Pronator teres
Radial flexion of wrist	C-6, C-7	Median nerve	Flexor carpi radialis
Flexion of middle phalanges	C-7, *C-8*, T-1	Median nerve	Flexor digitorum superficialis
Flexion of proximal phalanx of thumb	C-8, *T-1*	Median nerve	Flexor pollicis brevis
Opposition of thumb against fifth finger	C-8, *T-1*	Median nerve	Opponens pollicis
Extension of middle phalanges of index and middle fingers	C-8, *T-1*	Median nerve	First, second lumbricals
Flexion of terminal phalanx of thumb	*C-8*, T-1	Anterior interosseous nerve	Flexor pollicis longus
Flexion of terminal phalanx of second and third fingers	*C-8*, T-1	Anterior interosseous nerve	Flexor digitorum profundus
Flexion of distal phalanges of ring and little fingers	C-7, *C-8*	Ulnar	Flexor digitorum profundus
Adduction and opposition of fifth finger	C-8, *T-1*	Ulnar	Hypothenar
Extension of middle phalanges of ring and little fingers	C-8, *T-1*	Ulnar	Third, fourth lumbricals
Adduction of thumb against second finger	C-8, *T-1*	Ulnar	Adductor pollicis
Flexion of proximal phalanx of thumb	*C-8*, T-1	Ulnar	Flexor pollicis brevis
Abduction and adduction of fingers	C-8, *T-1*	Ulnar	Interossei

TABLE 2-1 Segmental innervation of muscles (*Continued*)

Action tested	Roots*	Nerves	Muscles
CRURAL			
Hip flexion from semiflexed position	*L-1*, *L-2*, L-3	Femoral	Iliopsoas
Hip flexion from externally rotated position	L-2, L-3	Femoral	Sartorius
Extension of knee	L-2, *L-3*, *L-4*	Femoral	Quadriceps femoris
Adduction of thigh	*L-2*, *L-3*, L-4	Obturator	Adductor longus, magnus, brevis
Abduction and int. rotation of thigh	*L-4*, *L-5*, S-1	Superior gluteal	Gluteus medius
Extension of thigh	*L-5*, *S-1*, S-2	Inferior gluteal	Gluteus maximus
Flexion of knee	L-5, *S-1*, S-2	Sciatic	Biceps femoris Semitendinosus Semimembranosus
Dorsiflexion of foot (medial)	*L-4*, L-5	Peroneal (deep)	Anterior tibial
Dorsiflexion of toes (proximal and distal phalanges)	*L-5*, S-1		Extensor digitorum longus and brevis
Dorsiflexion of great toe	*L-5*, S-1		Extensor hallucis longus
Eversion of foot	L-5, S-1	Peroneal (superficial)	Peroneus longus and brevis
Plantar flexion of foot	*S-1*, S-2	Tibial	Gastrocnemius, soleus
Inversion of foot	L-4, *L-5*	Tibial	Tibialis posterior
Flexion of toes (distal phalanges)	L-5, *S-1*, S-2	Tibial	Flexor digitorum longus
Flexion of toes (middle phalanges)	*S-1*, S-2	Tibial	Flexor digitorum brevis
Flexion of great toe (proximal phalanx)	S-1, S-2	Tibial	Flexor hallucis brevis
Flexion of great toe (distal phalanx)	L-5, *S-1*, S-2	Tibial	Flexor hallucis longus
Contraction of anal sphincter	S-2, S-3, S-4	Pudendal	Perineal muscles

*Italics indicate major nerve root involved.

SOURCE: Reprinted by permission from Adams RA and Victor M: *Principles of Neurology* (4th ed). New York, McGraw-Hill, 1989.

continues to innervate its original tissue. Only the thoracicoabdominal wall retains somites in their original or primordial segmental order. Since no limbs disturb this region, the nerves, muscles, ribs, and intercostal vessels preserve the simple segmental pattern (Figs. 2-9 and 2-10).

4. *Plexuses and peripheral nerves.* To reach their original somites, the axons of the spinal nerves may redistribute themselves in the *cervical, brachial,* and *lumbosacral* plexuses to share peripheral nerves. Thus the peripheral nerves distal to the plexus may contain dorsal and ventral root axons from more than one spinal cord segment. A lesion in or distal to a plexus thus causes deficits that may exceed the boundary of one somite. By mapping the patterns of sensory or motor loss and comparing them to Figs. 2-10 and 2-11, the Ex can decide whether the Pt suffers from a *root, plexus,* or a *peripheral nerve* lesion.

E. *Segmental composition and motor distribution of the major peripheral nerves from the spinal plexuses.*

NOTE: Study section E.1 to 3 to learn only the principal movements served by the major peripheral nerves.

1. *Motor distribution of the cervical plexus:* The cervical plexus (roots C-1 to C-4) mainly supplies the neck muscles which turn the head and open the jaw and shares the trapezius muscle with cranial nerve XI. C-4 usually is

TABLE 2-2 Segmental innervation of spinal reflexes

Deep muscle reflexes	Superficial reflexes	Methods of elicitation	Normal results	Segment(s) traversed
Biceps		Tap biceps tendon	Flexion of the forearm at the elbow	C-5 to C-6
Triceps		Tap triceps tendon	Extension of the forearm at the elbow	C-6 to C-7
Brachioradial		Tap styloid process of the radius, with forearm held in semipronation	Flexion of the forearm at the elbow	C-7 to C-8
Finger flexion		Flick palmar surface of the tip of the finger	Flexion of the fingers	C-7 to T-1
Abdominal muscle stretch reflexes		Tap lowermost portion of the thorax or abdominal wall; or tap symphysis pubis	Contraction of the abdominal wall or, when the symphysis is tapped, adduction of the legs	T-8 to T-12
	Abdominal skin-muscle reflexes	Stroke skin of the upper and lower abdominal quadrants	Contraction of the abdominal muscles and retraction of the umbilicus to the stimulated side	T-8 to T-12
	Cremasteric	Stroke skin of the upper and inner thigh	Upward movement of the testicle	L-1 to L-2
Adductor		Tap medial condyle of the tibia	Adduction of the leg	L-2 to L-4
Quadriceps		Tap tendon of the quadriceps femoris	Extension of the lower leg	L-2 to L-4
Triceps surae		Tap Achilles tendon	Plantar flexion of the foot	L-5 to S-2
	Plantar	Stroke sole of the foot	Plantar flexion of the toes	S-1 to S-2
	Anal	Prick skin of the perianal region	Constriction of the anal sphincter—"anal wink"	S-4 to Co-1
	Bulbocavernous	Prick skin of the glans penis	Contraction of the bulbocavernosus muscle and constrictor urethrae	S-3 to S-4

the main source of the phrenic nerve, with contributions from C-3 and C-5.

2. *Motor distribution of the brachial plexus:* The brachial plexus (roots C-5 to T-1) innervates a number of proximal muscles of the shoulder girdle. From it issues five major terminal nerves as follows:
   a. The *circumflex* nerve (C-5 to C-6) innervates the deltoid muscle which elevates the arm.
   b. The *musculocutaneous* nerve (C-5 to C-7) is the flexor nerve of the brachium on the shoulder and of the forearm on the brachium (with the exception of the brachioradialis muscle).
   c. The *radial* nerve (C-5 to C-8) is the extensor nerve of the arm, the elbow, the wrist, and the fingers, except that the intrinsic hand muscles extend the distal phalanges. In addition it supplies the brachioradialis, a flexor muscle of the elbow.
   d. The *median* nerve (C-6 to C-8) innervates the long forearm muscles that flex the wrist and the fingers, the opponens pollicis, the two lateral lumbricals, the abductor pollicis brevis, and part of the flexor pollicis brevis.
   e. The *ulnar* (C-7 to C-8) nerve in the forearm innervates the flexor carpi ulnaris exclusively, and collaborates with the median nerve in supplying the long flexor muscles of the wrist. In the hand, the ulnar nerve innervates all hypothenar muscles, all of the interossei, lumbricals to digits 4 and 5, the adductor pollicis, and part of the flexor pollicis brevis.

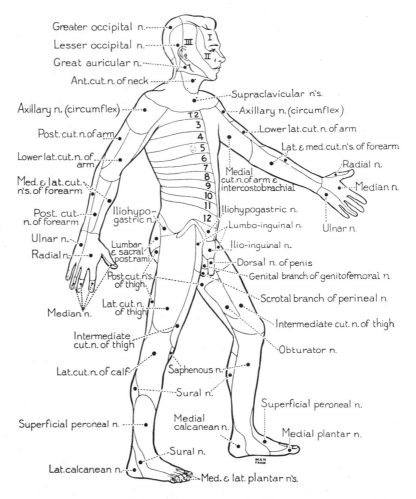

FIG. 2-11. Sensory innervation areas by peripheral nerves. Peripheral nerves may contain axons from one or more somite nerves. By using Figs. 2-10 and 2-11, the clinician determines whether the patient's sensory loss matches a dermatomal or peripheral nerve distribution. (*From K. Poeck: Einführung in die Klinische Neurologie, Berlin, Springer-Verlag, 1966.*)

  f. *Actions of the fingers*
    (1) The lumbricals, supplied by median and ulnar nerves, flex the metacarpophalangeal joints and extend the two distal phalanges. The interossei, innervated by the ulnar nerve, waggle the fingers laterally as well as helping the lumbricals flex the proximal phalanges.
    (2) *Learn this:* The thumb action tests all three motor nerves to the hand—*extension* of the thumb, *radial; abduction* of the thumb and *opposition* of the thumb to the little finger, *median; adduction* of the thumb, *ulnar.*
 3. *Motor distribution of the lumbosacral plexus* (L-1 to S-4). This plexus provides proximal branches to the glutei and hip abductors. Major terminal nerves are:
  a. The *femoral* nerve (L-2 to L-4), the *extensor* nerve of the knee (quadriceps femoris).
  b. The *obturator* nerve (L-2 to L-4), the *adductor* nerve of the thigh.
  c. The *sciatic* nerve (L-4 to S-3), the extensor nerve of the hip (glutei) and the *flexor* nerve of the knee (hamstrings). The sciatic nerve divides in the popliteal space into the *tibial* and *peroneal* nerves, the flexor and extensor nerves of the ankle and toes.
    (1) The *tibial* nerve (L-4 to S-3) innervates the plantar flexors of the foot and toes and the muscle that *inverts* the foot when the foot is plantar flexed.

(2) The *peroneal* nerve (L-4 to S-1) innervates the dorsiflexors of the ankle and toes, and the muscle that *everts* the foot when the foot is dorsiflexed.

   d. The *pudendal* nerve (S-2 to -4) innervates the urogenital diaphragm, voluntary bowel and bladder sphincters, and sexual organs.

   e. The *pelvic splanchnic* nerve (S-2 to -4) innervates the bladder wall and involuntary sphincter.

F. The axonal pathways in the spinal cord: Learn the location of the major descending internuncial tracts from the brain, essentially the pyramidal and reticulospinal tracts, and the ascending afferent pathways (Fig. 2-12*A*).

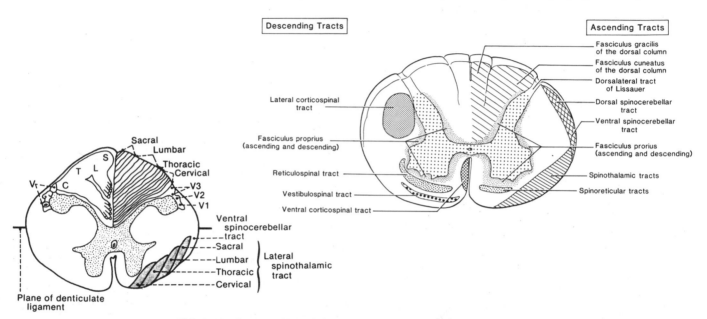

FIG. 2-12. Cross sections of the spinal cord. (*A*) Location of the major descending and ascending tracts of the white matter. (*B*) Topographic lamination of axons in the dorsal columns and the lateral spinothalamic tract for pain and temperature.

IV. Anatomic organization of the brainstem

A. For clinical neurology you must know:
1. The three *transverse* and the three *longitudinal* subdivisions of the brainstem.
2. The location of major tracts on cross section of the brainstem and their decussations.
3. The location of the cranial nerve nuclei.
4. The name, number, and fiber components of the cranial nerves.
5. The point where each cranial nerve attaches to the neuraxis and exits from the skull.

B. Three transverse and three longitudinal subdivisions of the brainstem
1. The three transverse subdivisions of the brainstem, the *mesencephalon* (midbrain), *pons,* and *medulla* (Fig. 2-1), consist of three *longitudinal* units, the *tectum, tegmentum,* and *basis* (Fig. 2-13).
2. *The tectum (= roof, the roof of the brainstem).* The tectum consists of the quadrigeminal plate that roofs the midbrain aqueduct and the anterior and posterior medullary vela that roof the 4th ventricle of the pons and medulla. The cerebellum does not belong to the tectum. Tectal lesions produce no specific neurologic syndromes.
3. *The tegmentum (= covering, the covering of the basis).* The tegmentum,

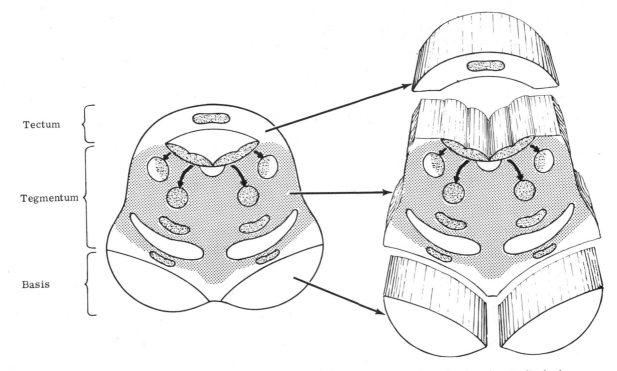

FIG. 2-13. Exploded view of a generalized cross section of the brainstem to show the three longitudinal subdivisions into tectum, tegmentum, and basis.

the block of tissue sandwiched between the tectum and basis, consists of vitally important *gray matter* and *tracts.*

4. *The basis (= the bottom, the bottom of the brainstem)*
   a. The basis mesencephali, basis pontis, and basis medulli (the medullary pyramids) convey the longitudinally coursing corticofugal motor pathways, consisting of the pyramidal tract and the corticopontine tracts.
   b. In addition the basis of the pons contains nuclei which swell it enormously. These nuclei receive the corticopontine tracts and relay to the cerebellum.

C. *Cross-sectional organization of the brainstem*
   1. Learn one cross section of the brainstem which shows the common plan for the arrangement of gray and white matter in midbrain, pons, and medulla (Fig. 2-14). Use Figs. 2-15 to 2-18 and Table 2-3 for reference.
   2. The tegmental gray matter consists of:
      a. The motor and sensory nuclei of cranial nerves. The *cranial nerve nuclei*

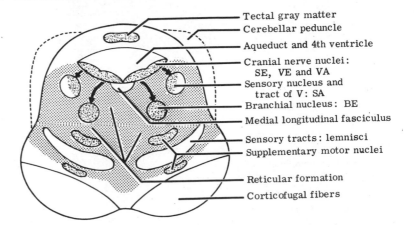

FIG. 2-14. Generalized cross section of the brainstem. Nuclei are heavily stippled, the reticular formation is lightly stippled, and white matter is white. Learn this figure.

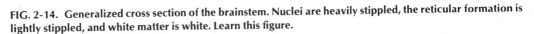

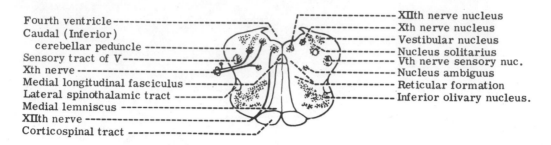

Fourth ventricle
Caudal (Inferior) cerebellar peduncle
Sensory tract of V
Xth nerve
Medial longitudinal fasciculus
Lateral spinothalamic tract
Medial lemniscus
XIIth nerve
Corticospinal tract

XIIth nerve nucleus
Xth nerve nucleus
Vestibular nucleus
Nucleus solitarius
Vth nerve sensory nuc.
Nucleus ambiguus
Reticular formation
Inferior olivary nucleus.

FIG. 2-15. Transverse section of medulla oblongata.

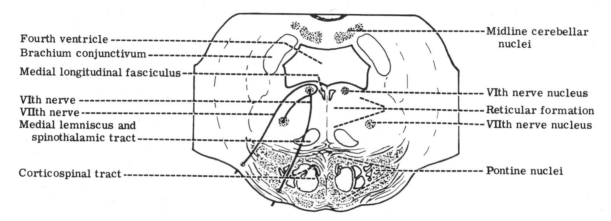

Fourth ventricle
Brachium conjunctivum
Medial longitudinal fasciculus
VIth nerve
VIIth nerve
Medial lemniscus and spinothalamic tract
Corticospinal tract

Midline cerebellar nuclei
VIth nerve nucleus
Reticular formation
VIIth nerve nucleus
Pontine nuclei

FIG. 2-16. Transverse section of pons, VIIth nerve (caudal) level.

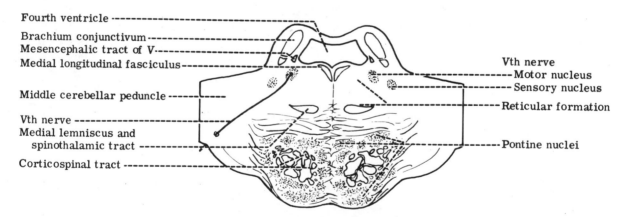

Fourth ventricle
Brachium conjunctivum
Mesencephalic tract of V
Medial longitudinal fasciculus
Middle cerebellar peduncle
Vth nerve
Medial lemniscus and spinothalamic tract
Corticospinal tract

Vth nerve
Motor nucleus
Sensory nucleus
Reticular formation
Pontine nuclei

FIG. 2-17. Transverse section of pons, Vth nerve (rostral) level.

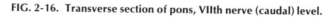

Superior colliculus
Cerebral aqueduct
Mesencephalic tract of V
Medial longitudinal fasciculus
Medial lemniscus and spinothalamic tract
IIIrd nerve
Corticospinal tract

IIIrd nerve nucleus
Reticular formation
Red nucleus
Substantia nigra

FIG. 2-18. Transverse section of mesencephalon, IIId nerve level.

TABLE 2-3 Summary of cranial nerve nuclei and tracts of the brainstem

Cranial nucleus	Upper cervical cord	Medulla	Pons	Mesencephalon
SE	Ventral motoneurons	Hypoglossal n. (XII)	Abducens n. (VI)	Oculomotor n. (III) Trochlear n. (IV)
BE	Spinal access accessory n.	Ambiguus n. (IX, X, XI)	Facial n. (VII) Trigeminal n. (V)	—
VE	—	Dorsal motor n. of vagus (X)	Salivatory n. of VII	Pupilloconstrictor n. (III)
VA	—	N. solitarius (IX, X)	—	—
SVA (Taste)	—	N. solitarius (VII, IX, X)	—	—
SA	Dorsal column n. Spinal root of V	External cuneate n. Spinal root of V	Main sensory n. of V	Mesencephalic root of V
SSA	—	Vestibular and cochlear n. (VIII)		—
Supplemental motor n.	—	Reticular formation Inf. olivary n.	Reticular formation N. of basis pontis	Reticular formation Substantia nigra, red n.
Tracts	Corticospinal, MLF Spinocerebellar tracts	Corticobulbar Corticospinal, MLF Caudal cerebellar peduncle	Corticobulbar Corticospinal, MLF Middle cerebellar peduncle	Corticobulbar Corticospinal, MLF Rostral cerebellar peduncle
Lemnisci	Spinothalamic tracts Dorsal columns Spinal root of V	Spinal lemniscus Medial lemniscus Spinal root of V Trigeminal lemniscus	Spinal lemniscus Medial lemniscus Trigeminal lemniscus Lat. lemniscus (auditory)	Spinal lemniscus Medial lemniscus Trigeminal lemniscus Lat. lemniscus

MLF = medial longitudinal fasciculus, n. = nucleus, SE = somatic efferent, BE = branchial efferent, VE = visceral efferent, VA = visceral afferent, SA = somatic afferent, SVA = special visceral afferent, SSA = special somatic afferent

in the brainstem consist of III to XII, XI excepted. They tend to cluster in the dorsal half of the tegmentum, in proximity to the aqueduct or fourth ventricle. However, the branchial efferent (BE) nuclei are always located lateral (ventrolateral) to the somatic efferent nuclei (Fig. 2-14).

b. Supplementary motor nuclei. The *supplementary motor nuclei* cluster in the ventral half of the tegmentum, or occupy the basis in the special case of the pons. The midbrain contains the substantia nigra and red nucleus, the medulla contains the inferior olivary nuclei, and the basis pontis contains the pontine nuclei (Figs. 2-14 to 2-18 and Table 2-3).

c. Reticular formation. The *reticular formation,* a mixture of neuronal perikarya, axons and dendrites, fills in the tegmental space not occupied by nuclei or long tracts.

3. The brainstem *white matter* contains the following tracts (Fig. 2-14 and Table 2-3):

a. Many *short*- and *medium*-length ascending and descending pathways of the reticular formation and supplementary motor nuclei. The *central tegmental tract* conveys descending pathways to the olivary nuclei of the medulla and conveys some of the catecholaminergic pathways and other diffuse pathways which ascend from the reticular formation to the fore-brain. Because the central tegmental tract spreads rather diffusely in the tegmentum, Figs. 2-14 to 2-18 do not show it.

  b. Long *ascending sensory tracts,* the *lemnisci,* which ascend through the brainstem from the body and face. By definition a lemniscus is a tract of axons from the secondary neuron of a sensory pathway, destined to terminate in a thalamic sensory nucleus of the diencephalon that relays to the cerebral cortex. The lemnisci migrate to the lateroventral part of the tegmentum (Figs. 2-14 to 2-18, Fig. 2-27, and Table 2-3).

  c. Long *descending motor tracts,* the corticofugal tracts, consisting of the pyramidal and corticopontine tracts, run in the basis.

  d. The afferent *cerebellar tracts* cluster along the dorsolateral aspect of the pontomedullary tegmentum.

  e. The *medial longitudinal fasciculus* interconnects the vestibular nuclei with cranial nerves III, IV, and VI, and the spinal cord. It runs just ventral to the floor of the aqueduct and fourth ventricle (Figs. 2-14 to 2-18).

  f. The figures showing the brainstem omit many known tracts, such as the *rubrospinal* and *tectospinal* tracts, because their interruption causes no known or specific clinical deficits.

 4. Learn Fig. 2-14 by drawing the perimeter and filling in the gray matter on one drawing, the white on another, and both on a third. Compare each drawing with the original.

 D. Functional significance of the additional neuronal pools of the brainstem

  1. Like the spinal cord, the cranial nerve nuclei mediate monosynaptic reflexes, but the additional neurons in reticular formation, supplementary motor nuclei, quadrigeminal plate, and cerebellum provide polysynaptic internuncial circuits for the complicated brainstem reflexes controlling posture, eye movements, breathing, feeding, and homeostasis.

  2. For additional internuncial sensory circuits, the vestibular nuclei and the cerebellum in particular evolved with the proprioceptive system in general. The cochlear nuclei and the superior olivary nuclear complex similarly serve the auditory pathway.

V. Anatomic review of the twelve pairs of cranial nerves

So the present classification of the cranial nerves into 12 numbered pairs was devised by a German medical student (Samuel Soemmering, 1755– 1830) nearly two centuries ago. Its basis is the holes in the floor of the skull through which nerves extend out from the cranial cavity to organs as diverse as the eyes and the bowels. Only in part does it sort the nerves according to their function or ultimate distribution. Although rather arbitrary and awkward, it seems likely to be with us for some time.

             —C. Wilbur Rucker

 A. Number and name of the cranial nerves

  1. By definition, a cranial nerve is any major nerve trunk that traverses one of the major foramina in the base of the skull. Learn Table 2-4.

  2. The *number* conveys the rostrocaudal sequence in which the nerve exits from the base of the skull, and this nearly duplicates the sequence of attachment of the nerves along the rostrocaudal axis of the brain.

  3. The *name* conveys at least something about the components, function, or distribution of the nerve. Learn Table 2-5.

 B. Functions of the cranial nerves. In order to express the function of each cranial nerve in the fewest words, learn Table 2-6. It is the ultimate simplification.

TABLE 2-4 Exit foramina for the cranial nerves in the base of the skull

Anterior fossa	I	Perforations in cribriform plate
Middle fossa	II	Optic foramen
	III, IV, VI, and ophthalmic division of V	Superior orbital fissure
	Maxillary division of V	Foramen rotundum
	Mandibular division of V	Foramen ovale
Posterior fossa	VII and VIII	Internal auditory meatus
	IX, X, and XI	Jugular foramen
	XII	Hypoglossal foramen

TABLE 2-5 Relation of cranial nerve name to anatomy or function

Number and name of nerve	Functional or anatomic significance of name
I Olfactory	It smells
II Optic	It sees
III Oculomotor	Its muscles move the eyeball
IV Trochlear	Its muscle moves the eyeball after running through a trochlea or pulley
V Trigeminal	It has three large sensory branches to the face
VI Abducens	It abducts the eye
VII Facial	It moves the muscles of all facial orifices
VIII Vestibulocochlear	It equilibrates, hears
IX Glossopharyngeal	It supplies taste fibers to the tongue and activates the pharynx during swallowing
X Vagus	It is a vagrant, wandering from the pharynx to the splenic flexure of the colon
XI Spinal accessory	It arises in the cervical spinal cord, runs into the skull, out again, and conveys accessory fibers to the vagus
XII Hypoglossal	It runs under the tongue

TABLE 2-6 Function of cranial nerves

Number: function
I: Smells
II: Sees
III, IV, and VI: Move eyes: III constricts pupils
V: Chews and feels front of head
VII: Moves the face, tears, tastes, salivate
VIII: Hears, equilibrates
IX: Tastes, salivates, swallows, monitors carotid body and sinus
X: Tastes, swallows, lifts palate, phonates, afferent and parasympathetic efferent to thoracico-abdominal viscera
XI: Turns head, shrugs shoulders
XII: Moves tongue

C. *Three functional sets of cranial nerves: solely special sensory, somitic, and branchial*

1. The brainstem evolves sensory and motor nuclei that provide for special nerve components, in addition to those present in the spinal cord.
   a. *Branchial efferent* (BE) nuclei are added to innervate the skeletal muscle derived from the gill arches, also called *special visceral efferent nuclei* (SVE).
   b. A *special visceral afferent* (SVA) nucleus is added for taste, and *special somatic afferent* (SSA) nuclei for auditory and vestibular functions. Any given cranial nerve may contain one or more but never all of the seven possible components (Table 2-7).

TABLE 2-7   Functional types of axons in the spinal nerves and the three sets of cranial nerves

Nerve	Functional type of axon						
	SE	BE	VE	VA	SVA	SA	SSA
A. Spinal Nerves	+		+	+		+	
B. Cranial nerves							
1. Solely special sensory set							
I					+		
II							+
VIII							+
2. Somatomotor set							
III	+		+			+*	
IV	+					+*	
VI	+					+*	
XII	+					+*	
3. Branchial set							
V		+				+	
VII		+	+	+	+	+	
IX		+	+	+	+	+	
X		+	+	+	+	+	
XI		+				+*	

*Cranial nerve V may mediate some or all of the SA component, which is proprioceptive.

2. From the theory of nerve components, and from phylogenetic and embryologic data, we can divide the 12 cranial nerves into three sets: *solely special sensory, somitic,* and *branchial.*
3. Set one, the *solely special sensory set* (SSSS), contains *three* nerves, *I, II,* and *VIII,* which have no motor fibers. Nerves VII, IX, and X mediate the only other special sense, taste.
4. Set two, the *somitic set,* contains *four* cranial nerves—*III, IV, VI,* and *XII.* Being direct homologs of the spinal nerves, these nerves innervate cranial somite derivatives, i.e., the extraocular muscles and the tongue.
5. Set three, the *branchial* set, contains *five* cranial nerves—*V, VII, IX, X,* and *XI*—that serially innervate branchial (gill) arches in analogy with the serial innervation of somites by somite nerves. Since the branchial arches are limited to the head region, only cranial nerves contain branchial efferent (BE) components (Fig. 2-20).

D. *The somitic set of cranial nerves: III, IV, VI, and XII*
   1. *Fate of the cranial somites*
      a. Of the dozen somites opposite the brainstem, only a few survive the travail of evolution. All cranial dermatomes retrogress, but some myotomes remain. The first cervical dermatome (C-1) also disappears. Hence, the most rostral dermatome, the one adjacent to the face, is _____.

Ans: C-2. Review Fig. 2-10 if you missed.

      b. Of the rostral myotomes, three survive, wondrously transformed into extraocular skeletal muscles. Pursuant to the law of original innervation, these three myotomes must retain their three original nerves. Thus, three somite nerves run to the eye muscles: nerves _____, _____, and _____.

Ans: III, IV, and VI. (If you had trouble recalling, sort through the cranial nerves one by one, I to XII. That's a good habit. See Table 2-6.)

☑ *SE*

      c. Supplying skeletal muscle derived from somites, these nerves must all have a ☐ VA/ ☐ SE/ ☐ VE component.
      d. We will assume that any nerve supplying SE fibers to a *skeletal* muscle also returns proprioceptive SA fibers from it. We will further assume that since these nerves have lost their individual dorsal root ganglia, their proprioceptive afferents (SA) derive from anastomotic branches from cranial nerve V.
      e. Only nerve III of the somitic group conveys VE axons. They innervate the *pupilloconstrictor* muscle which adjusts pupillary size, and the *ciliary* muscle, which adjusts lens thickness. No VA fibers return to the neuraxis in nerve III.
   2. The *middle* cranial somites disappear as do their nerves. The *caudal* cranial somites lose their *dermatomes,* but their *sclerotomes* merge into the base of the skull, and their *myotomes* merge into the tongue muscle. Although XII courses to the tongue muscles as a single trunk, it conveys axons from several somites. Not innervating any viscera, XII has only two components,

☑ *SE*; ☑ *SA*
  (proprioception)

      ☐ SE/ ☐ VE/ ☐ VA/ ☐ SA.
   3. Learn B-2 in Table 2-7 and test yourself in Table 2-8.

III IV VI XII

III IV VI XII

SA	☑	☑	☑	☑
VA				
VE	☑			
SE	☑	☑	☑	☑

TABLE 2-8 Nerve components of the somitic cranial nerves				
	III	IV	VI	XII
SA				
VA				
VE				
SE				

E. *The branchial set of cranial nerves . . . "or human face divine"*
   1. To the poet, Milton, it was the human face divine, created in final form by a deity, in one stroke, and then passed along from generation to generation without a history. But to the biologist, William Gregory, the face evolved gradually from the branchial arches. He stated "that the real ancestral face belonged not to a precreated man but to a poor mudsucking protochordate of pre-Silurian times; that when in some far-off dismal swamp a putrid prize was snatched by scaly forms, their facial masks already bore our eyes and nose and mouth" (Gregory, 1929).

2. The branchial arches create the face by usurping the task of the retrogressive cranial somites and forming the cheeks, jaw and ears (Fig. 2-19). Thus, the embryologic or ontogenetic elaboration of the branchial arches recapitulates the phylogenetic history of the face, from fish to man, illustrating the law of Ernest Haeckel (1834–1919) that ontogeny recapitulates phylogeny.

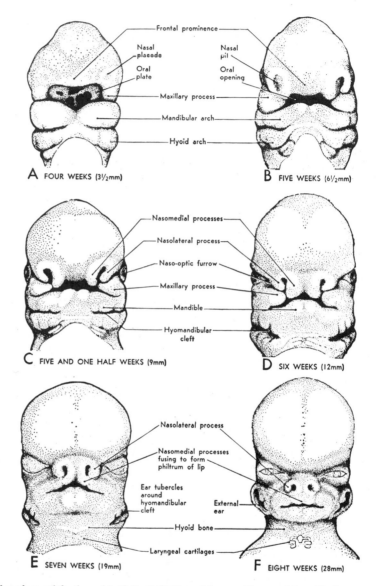

FIG. 2-19. **Embryology of the face. (*A–F*) Contribution of the maxillary and mandibular processes of the first branchial arch to the development of the face (cheeks, jaws, and ears). (*Reproduced by permission from B. M. Patton: Human Embryology, 2d ed, New York, Blakiston, 1953.*)**

3. On comparison, the branchial arches remarkably resemble somites in fundamental plan.
   a. Thus, the branchial arches are arranged serially and each receives only one nerve and only one artery (Fig. 2-20).
   b. The branchial arches produce the dermis, muscles, and bones of the cheeks, jaw, and ears (Fig. 2-19).
   c. Throughout their transformations, the branchial arch derivatives retain their original branchial nerve. The cranial nerve distributions are dia-

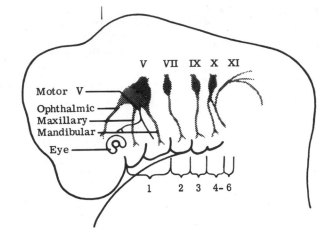

FIG. 2-20. Phantom view of a 6-week-old human embryo to show the innervation of the branchial arches (Roman numerals) by the branchial set of cranial nerves (Arabic numerals). The first arch divides into two processes, the maxillary and the mandibular.

grammed in the context of clinical testing. For now test your knowledge of their names, numbers, and general functions by completing Table 2-9.

TABLE 2-9 Summary of the branchial set of cranial nerves

Arch number	Cranial nerve number	Name	General function
1			
2			
3			
4			
5–6			

V trigeminal

VII facial

IX glossopharyngeal

X vagus

XI spinal accessory
For function,
check Table 2-6

F. The solely special sensory set of cranial nerves: I, II, and VIII

    1. In contrast to the *transverse* segmentation of the solid body wall and face into somites and branchial arches, the hollow viscera, including the neuraxis itself, are *longitudinal* tubes. After pinching off from their ectodermal or entodermal surfaces, both the neural and alimentary tubes elaborate by a single morphogenetic mechanism, *evagination* (Fig. 2-21).

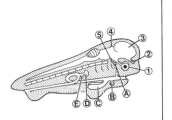

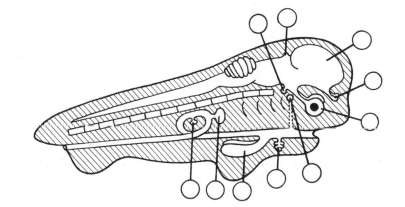

FIG. 2-21. Phantom view of a generalized vertebrate to show how the neural and alimentary tubes undergo evagination, their common mode of elaboration of accessory parts.

    a. In Fig. 2-21, place letters in rostrocaudal sequence along the *alimentary tube* to label the *evaginations* that form the: (A) adenohypophysis (Rathke's pouch), (B) thyroid gland, (C) lungs, (D) gallbladder, and (E) pancreatic duct.

    b. In Fig. 2-21, place numbers in sequence along the *neural tube* to label the evaginations that form the: (1) optic bulbs, (2) olfactory bulbs, (3) cerebral hemispheres, (4) pineal body, and (5) neurohypophysis.

    c. The mechanisms of body wall and facial elaboration are *migration, proplasia,* or *atrophy* of somites and branchial arches. In contrast, the mechanism of elaboration of the visceral tubes is the outpouching of evaginations (DeMyer, 1988).

2. *Cranial nerve I* consists only of axons from olfactory ganglion neurons located in the nasal mucosa (Fig. 9-1). These axons penetrate the cribriform plate of the skull to synapse on the olfactory evagination. These fragile axons tear away from the olfactory bulb upon removal of the brain. Hence they do not remain with the other cranial nerves on the base of the brain when the brain is removed.

3. So-called *cranial nerve II* is neither developmentally nor histologically a peripheral nerve. Instead it is the retained stalk of the optic evagination that extended the retina out to the facial surface from the diencephalon to receive light rays (Figs. 2-21 and 2-24). Demyelinating diseases like multiple sclerosis that affect oligodendroglial myelin of the CNS attack the optic nerves, whereas a different set of diseases attack the Schwann cell myelin of true peripheral nerves.

4. *Cranial nerve VIII* differentiates with the cochlear apparatus for detecting sound and the vestibular apparatus for detecting motion and position. Of the three solely special sensory cranial nerves, VIII is the only true peripheral nerve histologically. The cochleovestibular ganglia, that correspond to dorsal root ganglia, produce the axons of VIII (Fig. 9-7). It attaches to the brainstem at the *pontomedullary* sulcus, a crevice between the pons and the medulla (nerve VIII, Fig. 2-22).

5. *Fill in Table 2-10 to recapitulate the three sets of cranial nerves:*

Somitic; III, IV, VI, XIII
Branchial; V, VII, IX, X, XI
Solely special sensory; I, II, VIII

TABLE 2-10 Summary of the nerves in each of the three sets of cranial nerves		
Name of set	Characterized by	Nerves in set
1.	(1 per body segment)	
2.	(1 per gill arch)	
3.	(no motor axons)	

  G. *The points of attachment of the cranial nerves to the brain*

    1. Learn now, once and for all, that nerves *VI, VII,* and *VIII*—thus a *somite,* a *branchial,* and a *special sensory nerve*—attach, in *ventrodorsal* order, at the pontomedullary sulcus (see Fig. 2-22). By knowing this one fact and the special embryology of the olfactory and optic bulbs, you can fairly well deduce where all cranial nerves attach. Nerves III to V must be *caudal* to II, yet *rostral* to the pontomedullary sulcus. Color each of the three sets of cranial nerves with a different color and in so doing, learn Fig. 2-22. Then do the test frames G.2 to G.13.

I (Fig. 9-1)
II

    2. The only cranial nerve with an extracranial ganglion synapsing directly on a bulb that evaginated from the cerebrum is number _____.

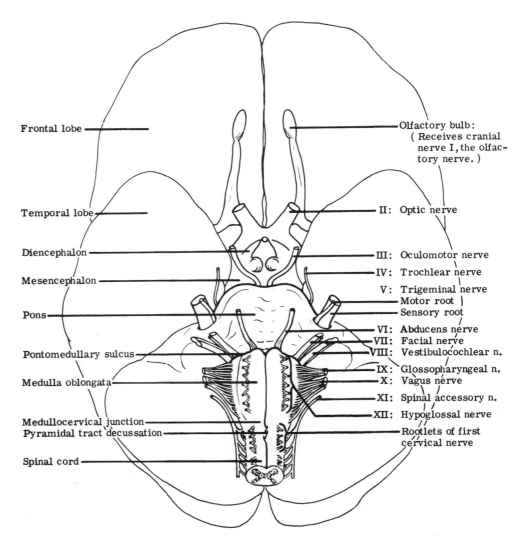

FIG. 2-22. Ventral aspect of the brain to show where the cranial nerves attach. The origin of cranial nerve IV, which attaches to the dorsal surface of the mesencephalon, does not show in this view.

VIII
Pontomedullary

III; ☑ mesencephalon

I, II

III, IV

V

VI, VII, VIII

IX, X, XII
XI

3. The stalk of a diencephalic evagination forms cranial nerve _____.
4. The only special sensory cranial nerve that is a true peripheral nerve histologically is _____. It attaches to the brainstem at the _____ sulcus.
5. The most rostral somite nerve and the most rostral *motor* cranial nerve is _____. It attaches to the ☐ diencephalon/ ☐ mesencephalon.
6. The only cranial nerves attaching to the brain rostral to the mesencephalon are _____.
7. The attachment of IV to the tectum (dorsum) of mesencephalon does not show in Fig. 2-22. It is the only cranial nerve to attach to the dorsal aspect of the brainstem. The two cranial nerves attached to the mesencephalon are _____ and _____.
8. The only cranial nerve attached to the lateral sides of the bulging belly of the pons is _____.
9. The three cranial nerves attaching at the pontomedullary sulcus in ventrodorsal order are _____, _____, and _____.
10. Three additional cranial nerves that attach to the medulla are _____, _____, and _____.
11. The only cranial nerve originating from the spinal cord is _____.

It enters the skull through the foramen magnum and exits from the jugular foramen.

12. In Fig. 2-22, notice that cranial nerves III, VI, and XII and the first cervical nerves attach in a *parasagittal* line along the brainstem.

   a. To remember this fact, use the same color as for the somite set of nerves and draw a line connecting C-1 with cranial nerve III.

   b. Discounting the anomalous dorsal attachment of IV, we find that the somite cranial nerves line up anatomically with the somite spinal nerves, just as they are phylogenetic homologs. The nerves of the branchial set then all attach ☐ lateral to/ ☐ medial to/ ☐ in line with the somitic set.

☑ *lateral to*

13. Draw Fig. 2-22 from memory.
14. Review the exit foramina of the cranial nerves (Table 2-4).

H. *Location of the cranial nerve nuclei*

   1. Color the sets of cranial nerve nuclei, using the same colors as for Fig. 2-22, and connect them longitudinally with colored lines. Then learn Fig. 2-23 and complete frames I.1 to I.10 to prove that you know it. Remember to sort through the cranial nerves one by one, I to XII, for each frame.

   2. The cranial nerve nuclei limited to the mesencephalon are numbered _____.

III, IV

   3. The cranial nerve *motor* nuclei limited to the pons are for numbers _____.

V, VI, VII

   4. The two cranial nerve *sensory* nuclei which straddle the pontomedullary junction and serve VIII are the _____ and _____ nuclei.

Cochlear; vestibular

   5. The cranial nerve *motor* nuclei limited to the medulla are for nerves numbered _____.

IX, X, XII

   6. The sensory nucleus limited solitarily to the medulla is called nucleus _____. It serves the visceral sensory functions of the medullary branchial nerves numbered _____.

Solitarius
IX, X

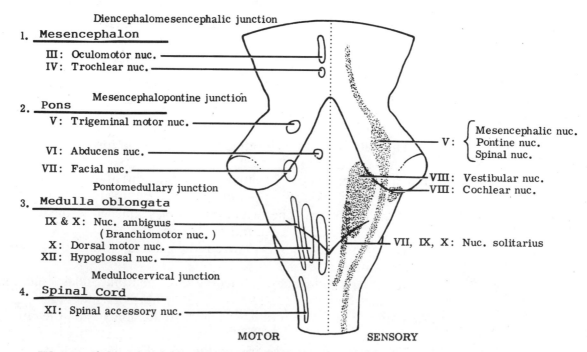

FIG. 2-23. **Phantom dorsal view of the cranial nerve nuclei in the brainstem and rostral portion of the cervical cord; motor nuclei on the left, sensory nuclei on the right.**

7. The one cranial nerve nucleus extending from the spinal cord to the mesencephalon belongs to cranial nerve _____.

8. The two cranial nerve nuclei found in the rostral part of the cervical cord are _____ (sensory) and _____ (motor).

9. In column 1 of Table 2-11, list, in rostrocaudal sequence, the numbers of the *branchial* cranial nerves. Then complete the rest of the table.

V (sensory)

V; XI

TABLE 2-11 Number, name, and location of branchial efferent nuclei (rostrocaudal order)		
Number of cranial nerve	Name of branchial motor nucleus	Anatomic subdivision of neuraxis containing the nucleus

V; trigeminal; pons

VII; facial; pons

IX; ambiguus; medulla

X; ambiguus; medulla

XI; spinal accessory; spinal cord

10. State how the nuclei and sites of brainstem attachment of the two sets of motor cranial nerves are located with respect to the midsagittal plane.

_____

_____

_____

Ans: The somitic nuclei are all paramedian, that is, adjacent to the midsagittal plane, and the nerves attach in a paramedian line along the brainstem. The branchial nuclei align more laterally and their nerves attach more laterally. (The actual location of the branchial nuclei with respect to the somitic nuclei is ventrolateral. See Fig. 2-14.)

I. *The distributional plan of the branchial nerves:* V, VII, IX, X, and XI

1. *Elimination of V and XI*

   a. Nerves V and XI are relatively simple in composition and distribution. Both are sensorimotor nerves and have only BE and SA components. Neither conveys special senses (Table 2-7).

   b. Nerve V has a huge SA component for sensation of the skin of the entire face and related mucous membranes. Its relatively modest number of BE axons innervates the chewing muscles and returns proprioceptive SA fibers from them.

   c. Nerve XI is the reciprocal of V in consisting mostly of BE axons to laryngeal, sternocleidomastoid, and trapezius muscles, while its tiny sensory component consists only of a small contingent of proprioceptive SA fibers from these muscles.

2. *Common plan of cranial nerves VII, IX, and X*

   a. These, the most complicated of the cranial nerves, pursue radically different peripheral courses, but they all have the same components and adhere to a common plan. Hence, to learn a great deal about one of them is to learn a great deal about all of them. As a prototype, refer to Fig. 9-6, the VIIth cranial nerve, as you study these common features of VII, IX, and X in Table 2-12:

	Branchiomotor (BE)	Visceromotor (VE) (all parasympathetic)	VA	Taste (SVA)	SA
TABLE 2-12 Nerve components of cranial nerves VII, IX, and X and their peripheral distribution					
VII	To all muscles of face and facial orifices and to stapedius muscles	To lacrimal, submandibular, and sublingual glands: all large exocrine glands of head except parotid. To nasal mucosa	From posterior nasopharynx and soft palate	Anterior two-thirds of tongue	Cutaneous twig to ear
IX	To pharyngeal plexus for swallowing	Parotid gland and pharyngeal mucosa	Soft palate and upper pharynx, carotid body and sinus	Posterior one-third of tongue	Cutaneous twig to ear
X	To pharyngeal plexus and laryngeal muscles (via accessory branch of XI)	To glands of pharyngeal and laryngeal mucosa and to glands and smooth muscle of thoracico-abdominal viscera. Inhibitory axons to the heart	Pharynx and larynx and thoracico-abdominal viscera	From region of epiglottis	Cutaneous twig to ear

   b. Each conveys BE axons to striated muscle derived from a gill arch.
   c. Each conveys VE (preganglionic parasympathetic) axons to a peripheral ganglion located in or near one of the large exocrine glands of the head or to glands in mucous membranes or viscera.
      (1) Nerve VII sends VE axons to the lacrimal glands and to the mucous glands of the nasal mucosa via the sphenopalatine ganglia, and to the submandibular and sublingual glands via the submandibular ganglia. VII passes through the parotid gland, but does not innervate it.
      (2) Nerve IX sends VE axons to the parotid gland via the otic ganglion and to the glands of the pharyngeal mucosa.
      (3) Nerve X sends VE axons to the glands of the pharyngeal and laryngeal mucosa and to the smooth muscle and glands of the thoracico-abdominal viscera, as far as the splenic flexure of the colon.
   d. Each conveys VA fibers from the palatopharyngeal mucosa. The Xth nerve also carries afferents from the thoracicoabdominal viscera.
   e. Each conveys SVA fibers for taste: VII from the anterior two-thirds of the tongue, IX from the posterior third, and X from the palatal orifice (rostrocaudal sequence). Clinically taste is tested only via VII.
   f. Each conveys SA fibers from the skin of the external auditory canal but not auditory fibers. The ear twigs from these nerves underscore the complex origin of the ear from several branchial arches. The skin area of V on the face, and the skin twigs of VII, IX, and X, demonstrate that the dermis of the branchial arches is retained while the dermis of the cephalic somites retrogresses.

BE, VE, VA, SVA, SA
(Table 2-7)

   g. List the nerve components of VII, IX, and X. _____

3. Review Table 2-12 to visualize the peripheral distributions of nerves VII, IX, and X in rostrocaudal sequence of face, VII; upper constrictors of pharynx, IX; and lower constrictors of pharynx and larynx, X; and so on through the table.

VI. The reticular formation

A. *Anatomic composition.* Anatomically, the reticular formation consists of a vast pool of neurons, more or less loosely arranged into nuclei. It extends throughout the brainstem tegmentum from the rostral end of the spinal cord into the caudal end of the diencephalon. The reticular formation receives collaterals from the sensory, motor, and limbic pathways. Endless polysynaptic pathways interconnect the various regions of the reticular formation.

B. *Function.* The reticular formation mediates functions as diverse as consciousness and breathing. Transection of the tegmentum at the midpontine level divides the reticular formation into *rostral* and *caudal* halves which have different functions.
  1. The *rostral* or *ponto-mesencephalic* half of the reticular formation sends ascending pathways to the thalamus and cerebral cortex. This *ascending reticular activating system* activates consciousness and the waking state (Section II, D of Chapter 12).
  2. The *caudal* or *ponto-medullary* half of the reticular formation mediates a variety of complicated brainstem reflexes related to eye movements, posture, feeding, breathing, homeostasis, and the control of BP and P. This part of the reticular formation in collaboration with cranial nerves V, VII, IX, X, and XII controls the oro-naso-pharyngeal apertures and conduits for feeding and breathing.
    a. Feeding-related reflexes include sucking, chewing, salivating, and swallowing.
    b. Breathing-related actions or reflexes include phonation, sneezing, coughing, sighing, and hiccoughing. (See Chapter 6, Section VIII and Fig. 6-13 for the neuroanatomy of breathing and its clinical testing.)

VII. The diencephalon

A. *The four nuclear subdivisions of the diencephalon.* The diencephalon consists of the four nuclear subdivisions, the *epithalamus, thalamus dorsalis, thalamus ventralis* (subthalamus), and *hypothalamus*. These nuclei form the walls and floor of the third ventricle (Figs. 2-24 and 13-8*B*).

B. The *epithalamus* consists of the pineal body, habenula, and membranous roof of the third ventricle.

C. The *thalamus (thalamus dorsalis)* consists of a group of nuclei with diverse connections that modulate all sensory, motor, and mental functions, including cognition, memory, speech, and affective experience. The thalamus receives all ascending sensory pathways (except smell); all ascending motor impulses originating in the reticular formation, cerebellum, and basal motor nuclei; the ascending reticular activating system; and limbic pathways. By means of thalamocortical and corticothalamic feedback circuits the thalamus links its nuclei with appropriate cortical motor, sensory, association, and limbic areas. By these extensive connections, the thalamus controls and modulates all cerebral functions. Virtually nothing gets into or out of the cortex without submitting to thalamic modulation. Conversely thalamic lesions can impair mental, motor, and sensory functions. Thus thalamic lesions can cause coma, dementia, thalamic dysphasia, thalamic hemispatial neglect, and a variety of sensory

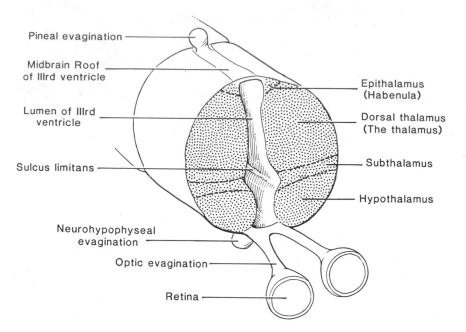

FIG. 2-24. Transverse (coronal) section of the embryonic diencephalon, showing its four nuclear zones bordering the IIId ventricle. (1) Epithalamus. (2) Thalamus dorsalis. (3) Thalamus ventralis (subthalamus). (4) Hypothalamus.

and motor syndromes. If you would know the brain you must know the thalamus. Five groups of thalamic nuclei can be recognized:

1. *Specific sensory nuclei* receive impulses from the optic tract and all lemnisci (the medial, lateral, spinal, and trigeminal) (Table 2-3) and relay them to the respective sensory areas of the cerebral cortex. Of all of the senses, only olfaction lacks a specific thalamic sensory relay nucleus and a lemniscus.
2. *Somatomotor* nuclei relay impulses from the cerebellum and basal motor nuclei to the cerebral motor cortex that modulate pyramidal tract function.
3. *Association nuclei* relate to the association cortex of the frontal, parietal, temporal, and occipital lobes. The association cortex does not receive direct sensory pathways nor does it originate specific motor pathways.
4. *Limbic nuclei* relate to the limbic lobe.
5. *Midline and intralaminar nuclei* relay ascending reticular activating impulses to the cortex at large for alerting responses and consciousness, and connect, by reciprocal short chain pathways, with the hypothalamus, reticular formation, and periaqueductal gray matter to mediate vegetative functions.

D. *The subthalamus (thalamus ventralis)* consists of the subthalamic nucleus of Luys and the zona incerta, which modulate somatomotor activity as components of the basal motor nuclei and relay to the motor cortex through the somatomotor nuclei of the thalamus (Fig. 2-30 and Table 2-15).

E. *The hypothalamus* is an integrative center for homeostatic, hormonal, and autonomic functions, strongly connected with the limbic lobe, hippocampus, amygdala, thalamus, periaqueductal gray matter, reticular formation, and pituitary gland.

VIII. The contralaterality of the central nervous system

A. The contralateral representation of the visual fields

1. The most important single fact about the course of the CNS pathways is that they decussate. The decussations determine whether lesions cause ipsilateral or contralateral clinical signs. By understanding *one* decussation, involving the optic pathway, you will understand *all* decussations, sensory and motor, because these decussations derive from the optic decussation. In asking about the biological necessity, the utility, or survival value, of decussations we will discover a profound fact: the very wiring diagram of our own nervous system derives from the physical properties of light (Rucker, 1958). The way the physical optics of the eye form a retinal image determines the wiring diagram for processing that image by the CNS. Santiago Ramon y Cajal stated the theory this way:

> Perhaps, I thought, the fundamental crossing of the optic tracts is necessarily bound up with the physical mechanism of vision. Let us seek then in this Mechanism for the logical reason of such an organization. Once it is ascertained, nothing will be easier than to explain as compensatory and corrective arrangements, the primordial decussations of the motor and sensory pathways.

> Rejecting other conjectures, I became possessed obsessively by the following thought: Everything will have a simple explanation if it is admitted that the correct perception of an object implies the congruence of the cerebral surfaces of projection, that is those representing each point in space. Hence, in order that the mental perception may be unified and may agree exactly with the external reality, or, in other words, in order that the image conveyed through the right eye may be continuous with that conveyed through the left eye, the intercrossing of the optic paths from side to side is quite necessary; a total crossing in animals with panoramic vision, a partial crossing in animals endowed with a common visual field [binocular stereoscopic vision].

> The accompanying diagrams explain the foregoing theory clearly.

> The first diagram [Fig. 2-25A] shows the form and direction which the mental visual image would have had on the supposition that the optic nerves had not crossed.

> The incongruity of the two images is evident: that projected through the right eye does not fit with that from the left eye, and it would be impossible for the animal to synthesize the two images into a continuous representation. The horizon would be presented as a panoramic view formed from two photographs, the right and left ones being laterally inverted.

> Let us now examine the mental image resulting from the intercrossing of the optic nerves, an intercrossing adopted by nature in the case of lenticular eyes. [Fig. 2-25B] shows with the greatest clearness that, thanks to the crossing, the two images, right and left, correspond and make a continuous panorama, the lateral inversion disappearing.

> Things take place somewhat differently in the mammals, in which the double visual projection reproduces the same region of space. In these animals there exists the uncrossed tract [Fig. 2-26], through which the duplication of visual images is ingeniously avoided, while the advantages of the crossing are retained.

> [Fig. 2-25B] shows also that the visual decussation has brought about the decussations of the principal voluntary motor and of the sensory paths.

> **Santiago Ramon y Cajal** (1852–1934)

2. In mammalia, which have a cortex, the pathway from the retina runs to the calcarine area of the occipital lobe. The pathway conveys the image of each

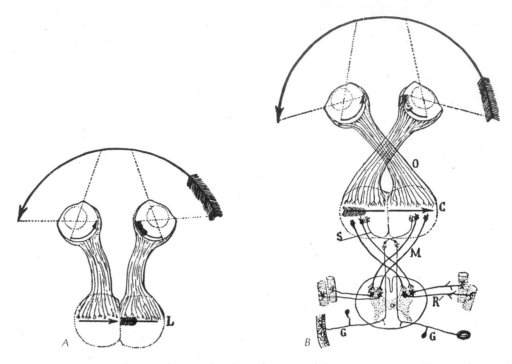

FIG. 2-25. Formation of the retinal images by physical optics and the representation of the visual image in the CNS without and with an optic nerve decussation. *(From S. Ramon y Cajal: Recollections of my life, New York, Garland, 1988). (A)* The *discontinuous* representation of the visual image from the two eyes in lower animals with panoramic vision presuming that the optic nerves do not decussate. *(B)* The *continuous* representation of the visual images from the two eyes in lower animals with panoramic vision when the optic nerves do decussate. Compare with Fig. 2-26 to see how partial decussation of optic axons in higher animals with binocular stereoscopic vision results in continuous central representation of the visual image.

right or left half of the visual field in uninterrupted fashion because of the semidecussation of axons at the optic chiasm (Fig. 2-26). The crucial fact is that each hemisphere receives the image from the opposite half of space.

B. *Contralaterality of the somatosensory pathways*
  1. Since one cerebral hemisphere receives its visual information from the contralateral half of space, logically it should also receive the somatosensory information from that contralateral half of the body. Then that hemisphere can readily associate the afferent data from the somatosensory and visual sensory areas and thus relate the proprioceptive and tactile stimuli from the limbs to visual space.
  2. *Pathways for somatic sensation.* For somatic sensation, start with a *primary neuron* in a dorsal root ganglion (Fig. 2-27).
     a. The *peripheral branch* of the dorsal root neuron receives a stimulus mediating the superficial modalities of touch, pain, and temperature or the deep modalities of form, texture, vibration, position sense (proprioception) stereognosis, and barognosis.
     b. The *central branch* synapses on a *secondary neuron* in the gray matter of the spinal cord. *The axon of the secondary neuron then decussates* and ascends to the thalamus. The critical factor in tracing sensory pathways is the level of the secondary neuron, which determines the level of the decussation.
        (1) The primary axons for *pain* and *temperature* synapse on their secondary neurons at or near the level at which the dorsal root enters the CNS, thus near the segment of origin of the dermatome served by the dorsal root. The axons of the secondary neurons then decus-

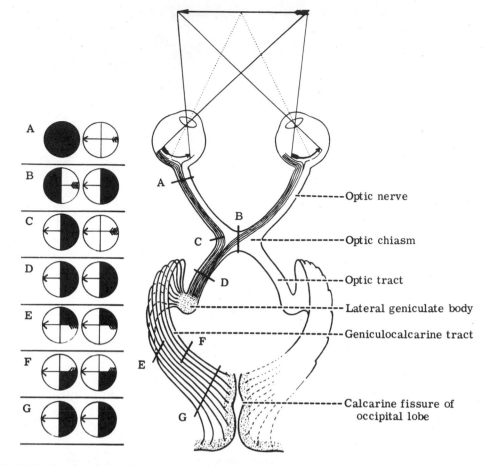

FIG. 2-26. Visual pathway from retina to occipital cortex in higher animals with binocular stereoscopic vision. The small scale of the drawing precludes showing the synapse of the retinogeniculate axons at the lateral geniculate body. A to F indicate lesion sites and the corresponding defects produced in the visual field.

TABLE 2-13 Summary of the clinically important decussations of the central nervous system	
Pathway	Site of decussation
Optic decussation	Optic chiasm (Fig. 2-26)
Somatic sensory decussations	
Pain and temperature	Near or at levels of entry of the dorsal root (Fig. 2-27)
Light touch	Two routes: near or at levels of entry and cervicomedullary junction (Fig. 2-27)
Vibration and position sense (deep modalities)	Cervicomedullary junction (Fig. 6-27)
Descending reticulospinal respiratory pathways	Cervicomedullary junction dorsal to other decussations (Fig. 6-13)
Pyramidal tract	
Corticobulbar component	Various sites along the brainstem (Fig. 2-28)
Corticospinal component	Cervicomedullary junction (Fig. 2-28)
Horizontal eye movement pathway	
Corticobulbar component	Decussates broadly from the midbrain level to the rostral pons (Fig. 2-31)
Medial longitudinal fasciculus component	Decussates near the VIth nerve level to make the medial rectus act equal to the lateral rectus, fulfilling Hering's law (Fig. 2-31)
Cerebro-ponto-cerebello-thalamo-cerebral pathway	Decussates at the pons on the way down from the motor cortex and the midbrain on the way back up to the thalamus and motor cortex (Fig. 2-29)

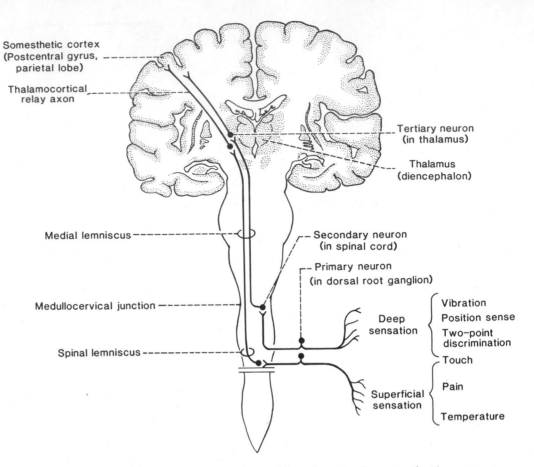

FIG. 2-27. **Decussations of the somatosensory pathways. The pathway for deep sensation decussates at one level, the cervicomedullary junction. The pathway for pain and temperature synapses at or near the level of entry of the primary axon, thus all up and down the cord. The impulses that mediate light touch travel in both pathways.**

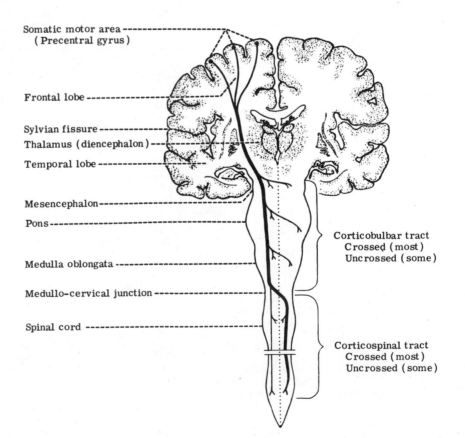

FIG. 2-28. **Coronal section of the neuraxis to show the pyramidal tract pathway from the cerebral motor cortex to the brainstem and spinal cord.**

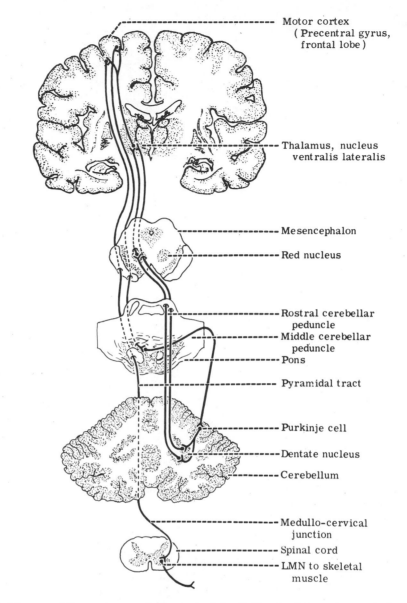

Motor cortex
(Precentral gyrus,
frontal lobe)

Thalamus, nucleus
ventralis lateralis

Mesencephalon

Red nucleus

Rostral cerebellar
peduncle
Middle cerebellar
peduncle
Pons

Pyramidal tract

Purkinje cell

Dentate nucleus

Cerebellum

Medullo-cervical
junction
Spinal cord
LMN to skeletal
muscle

FIG. 2-29. Diagram of the cerebro-cerebello-cerebral circuit. The circuit from one cerebral motor area to a cerebellar hemisphere and back crosses the midline twice. Thus one cerebellar hemisphere coordinates the muscular contractions projected by the pyramidal tract of the opposite cerebral motor cortex. Because it decussates, the pyramidal tract then produces coordinated movements on the side of the body *ipsilateral* to the cerebellar hemisphere.

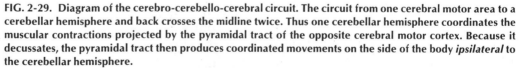

sate and turn rostrally in the *contralateral* ventrolateral quadrant of the spinal cord white matter as part of the spinal lemniscus which joins the medial lemniscus (Figs. 2-12 and 2-27).

(2) The primary axon for the *deep sensory modalities* enters the spinal cord white matter and ascends in the *ipsilateral* dorsal column to synapse on the nuclei gracilis and cuneatus located at the cervico-medullary junction (Fig. 2-27). The axons from the *secondary neurons* in these nuclei then decussate at that level. The axons turn rostrally in the *contralateral* half of the brainstem tegmentum, where they ascend as the *medial lemniscus* to the thalamus (Fig. 2-27).

(3) Both dorsal and ventral column pathways mediate touch (Fig. 2-27).

3. The *third order neuron* for all of the somatosensory pathways resides in a sensory relay nucleus of the thalamus. The thalamic neurons relay to the ipsilateral somatosensory cortex in the postcentral gyrus of the parietal lobe.

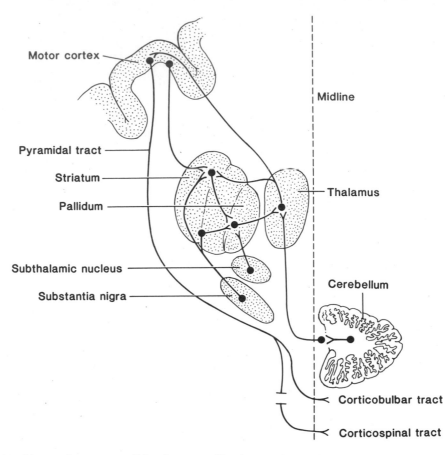

FIG. 2-30. Diagram for conceptualizing the maze of basal motor circuits that feed back through the thalamus into the ipsilateral cerebral motor cortex. The decussation of the pyramidal tract then projects the influence of the basal motor nuclei on movement to the contralateral side.

Association fibers then connect the visual and somatosensory areas with association cortex, with each other, and with the motor cortex.

4. The systems of two special senses, the olfactory and auditory, partially violate the contralaterality law. Their stimuli, odors and sounds, go around corners, in contrast to light. Auditory impulses, via commissures and decussations through the trapezoid body and superior olivary nuclei, travel to the thalamus via bilateral pathways (Fig. 9-7). Thus a unilateral lesion of the central auditory pathways does not cause a strongly lateralized deficit, as with lesions of the somatosensory and visual pathways.

C. *The lemnisci and the role of the thalamus in sensation*

1. All somatic sensations and all special sensations, except smell, relay through a lemniscus to a specific thalamic nucleus. With the exception of the special senses of taste and equilibrium, the relay nucleus is known with certainty. Thus as one of its main functions the thalamus relays sensory information to the somesthetic cortex located in the _____ gyrus of the _____ lobe.

Postcentral
Parietal

2. Since pathways for all somatic modalities cross and then relay in the thalamus, a severe destructive lesion of the thalamus would cause loss of somatic sensation on the ☐ ipsilateral/ ☐ contralateral side of the body.

☑ *Contralateral*

3. Learn Table 2-14 and test yourself with the frames C.4 to C.12.

TABLE 2-14 Origin of the lemnisci, thalamic termination, and cortical projection

Lemniscus and origin	Thalamic nucleus of termination	Cortical area of projection
Spinal, spinal gray matter	N. ventralis posterior (lateralis)	Somesthetic cortex of the postcentral gyrus
Medial, n. gracilis & cuneatus	N. ventralis posterior (lateralis)	Somesthetic cortex of the postcentral gyrus
Trigeminal, trigeminal n.	N. ventralis posterior (medialis)	Somesthetic cortex of the postcentral gyrus
Lateral, cochlear n.	Medial geniculate body	Auditory receptive area, transverse gyri of the temporal lobe
Optic tract, retina	Lateral geniculate body	Visual receptive area, calcarine cortex of the occipital lobe

Trigeminal

☑ *Medial (or combined spinal and medial) (Fig. 2-27).*
☑ *Lateral*

4. The trigeminal sensory nuclei that mediate facial sensation send axons to the thalamus by the _____ lemniscus.
5. Somatic sensory impulses from the remainder of the body, exclusive of the face, connect with the thalamus via the ☐ lateral/ ☐ medial/ ☐ trigeminal lemniscus.

6. The cochlear pathway runs to the thalamus via the ☐ medial ☐ lateral lemniscus.

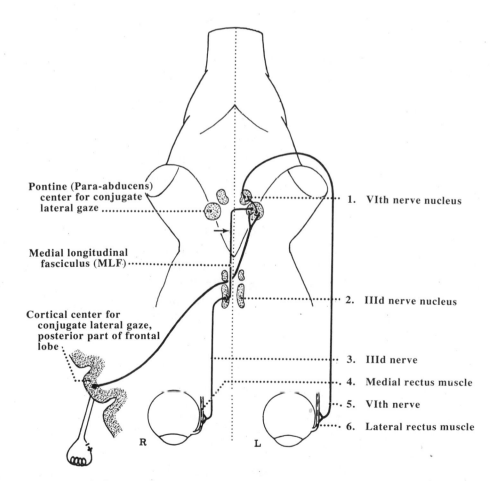

Pontine (Para-abducens) center for conjugate lateral gaze

Medial longitudinal fasciculus (MLF)

Cortical center for conjugate lateral gaze, posterior part of frontal lobe

R   L

1. VIth nerve nucleus
2. IIId nerve nucleus
3. IIId nerve
4. Medial rectus muscle
5. VIth nerve
6. Lateral rectus muscle

FIG. 2-31. Corticobulbar pathway for contralateral horizontal conjugate eye movements.

☑ *Secondary*
Crossed

Lateral
Lateral geniculate

Medial geniculate

Ventralis posterior
Ganglia
Thalamus

7. In general the lemnisci contain axons from ☐ primary/ ☐ secondary/ ☐ tertiary neurons which have _____ the midline. A partial exception to this rule, since it has many uncrossed axons, is the _____ lemniscus.

8. The thalamic relay nucleus for sight is called the _____ body.

9. For hearing, a special somatic sensation, it is the _____ _____ body.

10. For general somatic sensation it is nucleus _____.

11. All *primary* neurons for somatic sensation are located in _____. The *tertiary* neurons are located in the _____.

12. Therefore, to learn a sensory pathway, you only have to memorize the location of the secondary neuron. From knowing that fact, you get this bonus: the axons from the secondary neurons decussate. Hence by knowing the location of the second-order neuron, you know where the lemnisci begin.

D. *Union of the lemnisci in the brainstem*
1. All lemnisci unite in the brainstem to travel to the thalamus as one with the medial lemniscus.

    a. The medial lemniscus proper, at medullary levels, carries axons derived from _____.

Ans: Dorsal column nuclei (nuclei gracilis and cuneatus)

    b. As the medial lemniscus travels rostrally into the pons, the spinal and trigeminal lemnisci unite with it and then the lateral lemniscus.

    c. After the spinal, trigeminal, and medial lemnisci unite, at pontine and mesencephalic levels, the single name *medial* lemniscus is still used. Thus the medial lemniscus has different components, depending on the level of the brainstem.

2. *The domain of the lemnisci on transverse section of the brainstem*

    a. The *tectum* contains no long pathways, only a cerebellar pathway cutting through.

    b. The *basis* transmits only corticofugal tracts.

    c. The lemnisci, therefore, must run through the ☐ tectum/ ☐ tegmentum/ ☐ basis of the brainstem.

☑ *Tegmentum*

    d. Trace the medial lemniscus through Figs. 2-15 to 2-18, noting its crescentric shape.

E. *Thalamocortical connections.* From the thalamus, the tertiary neurons in the thalamic sensory nuclei relay to various areas of the cerebral cortex.

1. Touch, pain and temperature, and dorsal column modalities relay to the somesthetic cortex in the _____ gyrus of the _____ lobe.

Postcentral; parietal

2. Visual impulses relay to the _____ lobe, and auditory impulses relay to the _____ lobe.

Occipital
Temporal

IX. The contralaterality of motor innervation by the pyramidal tract

A. *The relation of sensory pathways to movement.* In reaching your hand out to pick up an item located by vision, the sequence of muscles you activate and the rate and strength of their contractions depend on where your hand starts from and the obstacles it might encounter on the way. The sensory information by which one cerebral hemisphere guides movement comes mainly from two great afferent systems, the *visual* and *proprioceptive* systems. By appropriate decussations, the visual and somatosensory pathways bring the information from one half of visual space or one half of the body mainly to the ☐ ipsilateral/ ☐ contralateral cerebral hemisphere.

☑ *Contralateral*

1. The calcarine receptive cortex of the *left* occipital lobe represents the ☐ left/ ☐ right half of the visual field.

☑ *Right*

2. The somatosensory cortex of the postcentral gyrus of the left parietal lobe represents sensation from the ☐ left/ ☐ right half of the body.

☑ *Right*

3. If the sensory information required for movement comes to one cerebral hemisphere from the contralateral side, nothing could be simpler or more efficient than for that hemisphere to control movement on the contralateral side. One cerebral hemisphere directs movement on the contralateral side via a tract of paramount importance, the pyramidal tract.

B. *The pyramidal tract: the pathway for volitional movement*

> *It would seem, therefore, that we may look upon the pyramidal system as an internuncial, a common, pathway by which the sensory system initiates and continuously directs, in willed movements, the activities of the nervous motor mechanisms. This sensory afflux is a condition of willed movements, and unless we consider both in association we cannot hope to see the purpose of either.*
>
> **F.M.R. Walshe** (1885–1973)

1. The pyramidal tract, which mediates willed movements, begins in the motor cortex, located in the precentral and, to a lesser extent, the postcentral gyri (Russell and DeMyer, 1961) (Fig. 2-28).
2. The pyramidal tract projects through the deep white matter of the cerebrum to synapse on internuncial or efferent neurons in the brainstem and spinal cord. It divides into two components, the *corticobulbar* and the *corticospinal.*
   a. The *corticobulbar* component decussates at various levels to synapse on neurons of the brainstem.
   b. The *corticospinal* component mainly decussates at the cervicomedullary junction, where the dorsal column sensory pathway also decussates (Figs. 2-27 and 2-28).
3. *Paresis and paralysis after pyramidal tract interruption*
   a. Interruption of the pyramidal tract in the cerebrum or brainstem paralyzes volitional movement on the *contralateral* side of the body. Complete or near complete paralysis on one side is called *hemiparalysis* or *hemiplegia.* Paresis or incomplete paralysis on one side is called *hemiparesis.*

☑ *Contralateral*

   b. Interruption of a pyramidal tract *rostral* to its decussation causes hemiplegia ☐ ipsilateral/ ☐ contralateral to the lesion.

☑ *Ipsilateral*

   c. Interruption of a pyramidal tract just *caudal* to its decussation causes hemiplegia ☐ ipsilateral/ ☐ contralateral to the lesion.

C. *The law of contralateral hemispheric sensorimotor innervation.*
1. Using a colored pencil, superimpose the pyramidal pathway of Fig. 2-28 onto Fig. 2-27. Then, mentally trace a nerve impulse from a somatic sensory receptor to the cerebral cortex and back to the lower motoneurons via the pyramidal tract, noting the decussations.
2. You should now appreciate this most fundamental neuroanatomic law, the *law of contralateral hemispheric sensorimotor innervation:* one cerebral

hemisphere receives the visual information from the contralateral half of space and the somatosensory information from the contralateral half of the body and in turn controls the motor activity of the contralateral half of the body.

D. *The concept of upper motor neuron (UMN) paralysis and lower motor neuron (LMN) paralysis.*
   1. Clinicians describe paralysis due to interruption of the pyramidal tract as UMN paralysis.
   2. *LMNs* are all neurons of the spinal ventral horns and brainstem tegmentum that send motor axons to skeletal muscles (branchial and somitic). No UMN axons leave the neuraxis. All motor axons in peripheral nerves come from LMNs.
   3. Paralysis due to disease of the motoneurons, either of their perikarya or their axons in ventral roots and peripheral nerves, is called LMN paralysis.
   4. *Upper motor neuron versus lower motor neuron paralysis*
      a. The hallmark of pyramidal tract interruption is paresis or paralysis of volitional *movements* of the parts, not the individual muscles. Volitional movements, even if ostensibly simple, involve the action of more than one muscle. Flex your finger, smile, or lift your arm—in every case more than one muscle springs into action. Movements, then, are compounded of the actions of several muscles.
      b. The hallmark of LMN or motor nerve interruption is paralysis of *all* and *only* the individual muscle(s) supplied by particular groups of LMNs or their peripheral nerve.
      c. If the Pt has paresis or paralysis of one muscle or a restricted set of muscles, while other movements of the limbs remain normal, the lesion must of necessity involve the ☐ UMNs/ ☐ LMNs.
      d. If the Pt has paresis or paralysis of all movements of one side of the body the lesion most likely affects the ☐ UMNs/ ☐ LMNs.
      e. Taking some poetic license, we may summarize this conclusion by saying that UMN lesions paralyze ☐ movements/ ☐ muscles while LMN lesions paralyze ☐ movements/ ☐ muscles.

☑ *LMNs*

☑ *UMNs*

☑ *Movements*
☑ *Muscles*

X. The connections of the cerebellum

A. *Sensorimotor modulation of the motor cortex.* Just as sensation modulates motor activity, the cerebellum, basal motor nuclei, and motor cortex function by modulating each other. The cerebellum and basal motor nuclei feed into motor nuclei of the thalamus, which feed to the cerebral motor cortex. Feedback loops link all of these regions. The next sections show how the motor pathways of the cerebellum and basal motor nuclei respect the law of contralateral innervation.

B. *Anatomy and functions of the cerebellum*
   1. *The gray matter of the cerebellum* consists of cortex and nuclei buried deep in its white matter.
   2. *Motor afferents* to the cerebellum come from the motor cortex via the cortico-ponto-cerebellar system, and proprioceptive afferents come from the vestibular system and trigemino- and spino-cerebellar tracts, and from the inferior olivary nuclei.

3. *Efferents* from the cerebellum project via deep cerebellar nuclei, particularly the dentate nucleus, to the thalamus and thence to the cerebral motor cortex. By these connections, the cerebellum modulates the output of the cerebral motor cortex to produce coordinated volitional movements via the pyramidal tract. Without cerebellar modulation, the pyramidal tract cannot coordinate the muscles that contract under its command.
4. *Cerebellar signs* consist of *hypotonia* and *ataxia* (Chapter 8).

C. *Decussations of the cerebellar pathways*
   1. In Fig. 2-29 start at one motor cortex and trace the three decussations in the cerebro-cerebello-cerebro-pyramidal-LMN pathway. These three decussations are:
      a. The decussation of the cerebro-ponto-cerebellar pathway in the basis pontis.
      b. The decussation of the dentatothalamic pathway in the midbrain.
      c. The decussation of the pyramidal tract at the medullocervical junction.
   2. The foregoing three decussations explain why the signs of cerebellar dysfunction appear *ipsilateral* to a lesion of a cerebellar hemisphere: The cerebellar pathway with its two decussations (Fig. 2-29) and the pyramidal decussation leads to a clinical law that paralysis is *contra*lateral to a *cerebral* hemisphere lesion, but ataxia is *ipsi*lateral to a *cerebellar* hemisphere lesion.

XI. The connections of the basal motor nuclei

A. *Components of the basal ganglia.* The basal ganglia consist of the caudate nucleus and putamen (the striatum), globus pallidus (the pallidum), claustrum, and amygdala (Fig. 13-8).
   1. The amygdala belongs to the limbic system, and the function of the claustrum is unknown.
   2. The striatum and pallidum can be considered components of the *basal motor nuclei,* also called the *extrapyramidal motor system.* The basal motor nuclei also include the subthalamic nuclei, red nuclei, substantia nigra, and parts of the reticular formation. These nuclei, in more or less close anatomic proximity at the base of the brain, modulate somatomotor activity by means of numerous feedback circuits that ultimately relay through the somatomotor nuclei of the thalamus to the motor cortex (Table 2-15 and Fig. 2-30).

TABLE 2-15 Outline of the basal motor nuclei of the extrapyramidal system

A. *Cerebrum*
   1. Caudate-putamen, the "striatum"
   2. Globus pallidus, the "pallidum"
B. *Diencephalon*
   1. Somatomotor relay nuclei of the thalamus (nucleus ventralis anterior and nucleus ventralis lateralis)
   2. Subthalamus: subthalamic nucleus and zona incerta
C. *Midbrain*
   1. Reticular formation
   2. Red nucleus
   3. Substantia nigra

B. *Signs of lesions of the basal motor nuclei*

Whereas cerebellar lesions lead to a dysmodulation of the motor cortex resulting in ataxia, lesions of the basal motor nuclei result in motor dysmodulation manifested by:

1. Muscular rigidity
2. Bradykinesia/akinesia (slowness or difficulty in initiating and executing volitional movements).
3. Hyperkinesias (involuntary movements) consisting of:
   a. Tremor, frequently a tremor of the part at rest.
   b. Patterned involuntary movements called chorea, athetosis, and dystonia. The type and distribution of the movements predict the nuclei or connections affected by the lesion, as described in Chap. 7.

C. *Connections of the basal motor nuclei*

1. The basal motor nuclei project to the cerebral motor cortex through the ipsilateral somatomotor nuclei of the thalamus (Review Fig. 2-30).
2. Thus, a unilateral lesion of the basal motor connections results in motor signs expressed *contra*laterally through dysmodulation of output via the motor cortex and the crossing of the pyramidal tract.
3. A key difference between basal motor nuclei signs and ataxia is that ataxia only appears when the Pt makes some type of volitional muscular contraction. Ataxia does not occur with the muscles at rest. To the contrary, the rigidity, and most involuntary movements, may appear both at rest and during volitional movements. The signs of basal motor nuclei lesions represent, in large part, dysmodulation of the motor cortex. The proof comes from the fact that the involuntary movements and rigidity disappear after destruction of the motor cortex or of the pyramidal tract. Thus if a Pt has hemichorea, transection of the pyramidal tract serving that side abolishes or reduces the chorea. Of course the Pt loses voluntary movement of the parts also. *We come to the anomalous almost heretical conclusion that pyramidal tract interruption paralyzes both voluntary and involuntary movements.* (This statement applies to acquired lesions in previously normal brains. Infants born with no pyramidal tracts do move, but this is another issue.)

XII. The connections of the cerebral cortex

A. *Ontogeny of cortical connections.* To best understand cerebral pathways, we had best start with their ontogeny. Simply ask what *possible* connections can any axon make when growing out from its cortical perikaryon.

1. *Association pathways.* An outgrowing axon may connect with an *ipsilateral* cortical neuron to *associate* the functions of the two neurons. Numerous long and short *association* pathways course through the cerebral white matter to connect the various cortical areas of one hemisphere. The longest such association fibers drive rectilinearly or in sweeping arcs through the white matter to connect the frontal, occipital, and temporal poles and the areas in between (Fig. 2-32).
2. *Commissural pathways.* Any outgrowing axon may cross to the *contralateral* cerebral hemisphere, to end in a mirror-image site, forming *commissural* fibers. A commissure, by definition, conveys axons that cross the mid-

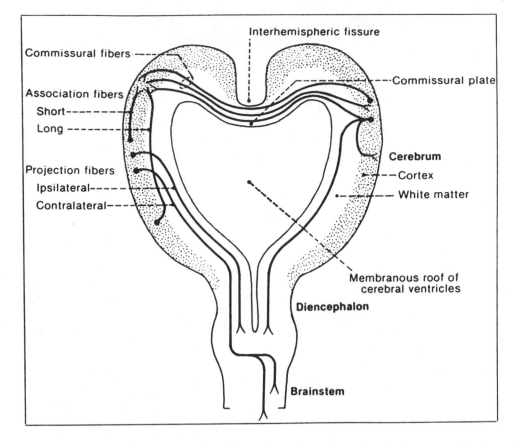

FIG. 2-32. Dorsal view of horizontal section of the embryonic cerebrum, showing the outgrowth of association, projection, and commissural axons. (*Reprinted by permission from W. DeMyer; Neuroanatomy, Baltimore, Williams & Wilkins, 1988.*)

line to connect mirror-image sites of the cortex or nuclear gray matter of the two sides. Commissures enable each right or left half of the neuraxis to inform the other half of what is going on. The cerebrum contains the largest commissures of all, the corpus callosum and anterior commissure. Similar commissures exist at all levels of the neuraxis.

3. *Projection pathways.* Any outgrowing cortical axon may end on *infracortical* internuncial neurons or on efferent neurons that are either *ipsilateral* or *contralateral* (Fig. 2-32). Such axons *project* the cortical influence to the next neuron in line. Those axons that cross the midline to end on non-mirror image sites are called *decussations,* to distinguish them from commissures. Like commissures, decussations arise from cortical and nuclear gray matter at all levels of the neuraxis. The corpus callosum and anterior commissure convey decussating as well as commissural fibers.

4. Hence the outgrowing axons of the cerebral neurons establish *associational, commissural,* and *projectional* connections.

5. The common denominator of commissures and decussations is that they _____ the midline.

6. The essential difference between commissures and decussations is that

Cross

_____

Ans: Commissures connect mirror-image points of the cortical and nuclear gray matter of the two sides, whereas decussations connect non–mirror-image points of the cortex or infracortical gray matter.

B. *Recapitulation of the pathways of the cerebral white matter.* You will now appreciate that the cerebral white matter consists of the following pathways:
1. *Association pathways,* long and short, connect ipsilateral cortical areas.
2. *Commissural pathways* connect mirror image areas of the two hemispheres: corpus callosum and anterior commissure.
3. *Projection pathways* connect the cerebral cortex with ipsilateral and contralateral infracortical gray matter. The projections run through pyramidal, corticopontine, corticostriatal, corticothalamic, and optomotor pathways.
4. *Thalamocortical-corticothalamic pathways* connect thalamic nuclei to sensory, somatomotor, association, and limbic cortex.
5. Most of the incoming and outgoing cortical pathways, including the massive thalamocortical and corticothalamic circuits, fan out from or funnel down into the *internal capsule* (Fig. 13-8*B*).
6. Lesions of the white matter, in addition to interrupting sensorimotor pathways, disconnect various cortical areas from each other or from the thalamus, giving rise to various cerebral disconnection syndromes of dysphasia, dyspraxia, dementia, amnesia, hemispatial neglect, and altered emotionality.

XIII. Summary

A. *A tabular summary of decussations.* Review Table 2-13, page 71, in conjunction with Figs. 2-26 to 2-31.

B. *Brief summary of clinical signs of motor system lesions.* Recite in principle the effects of lesions at the various components of the motor system (Table 2-16).

TABLE 2-16 Brief summary of clinical syndromes of lesions at various levels of the motor system	
Motor disability	Pathway affected
Paralysis of individual muscles	Lower motoneurons
Paralysis of movements	Upper motoneurons

Rigidity
Hypokinesia
Involuntary movements
  Tremor
  Patterned hyperkinesias
	Basal motor nuclei

Ataxia/hypotonia	Cerebellum

BIBLIOGRAPHY

Barr ML, Kiernan JA: *The Human Nervous System: An Anatomical Viewpoint,* (4th ed). Philadelphia, Harper & Row, 1983

Carpenter MB: *Core Text of Neuroanatomy* (4th ed). Baltimore, Williams & Wilkins, 1991

Crosby EC, Humphrey T, Lauer EW: *Correlative Anatomy of the Nervous System.* New York, MacMillan, 1962

DeMyer W: *Neuroanatomy.* Baltimore, Williams & Wilkins, 1988

Fix JD: *Atlas of the Human Brain and Spinal Cord.* Rockville, MD, Aspen Publishers, 1987

Gregory W: *Our Face from Fish to Man.* New York, Putnam's, 1929

Jones EG: *The Thalamus.* New York, Plenum, 1985

Paxinos G: *The Human Nervous System.* San Diego, Academic, 1990

Peters A, Jones EG (eds): *Cerebral Cortex.* (vol 1: *Cellular Components of the Cerebral Cortex).* New York, Plenum, 1984

Ramon y Cajal S: *Recollections of My Life (Genes, Cells, and Organisms).* New York, Garland, 1988

Rucker CW: The concept of a semidecussation of the optic nerves. *Arch Opthal* 1958;59:159–171

Rucker CW: History of the numbering of the cranial nerves. *Mayo Clin Proc* 1966;41:453–461

Russell J, DeMyer W: The quantitative cortical origin of pyramidal axons in *Macaca rhesus. Neurology* 1961;11:96–108

Schaltenbrand G, Walker AE: *Stereotaxy of the Human Brain.* Stuttgart, G Thieme, 1982

Learning Objectives for Chapter Two

I. Gross subdivisions of the neuraxis

1. Make a lateral view diagram which shows the major subdivisions of the central nervous system (neuraxis) (Fig. 2-1).
2. Define *brain, cerebrum,* and *brainstem* (Fig. 2-1).
3. Name, in rostrocaudal order, the three transverse subdivisions of the brainstem (Fig. 2-1).
4. Describe how to separate the brainstem from the cerebrum and spinal cord.
5. Name the four levels of the spinal cord in rostrocaudal sequence (Fig. 2-1).
6. On lateral and medial drawings of the cerebrum, label and describe the boundaries of the four traditional lobes of the cerebrum (Fig. 2-2).
7. On a medial drawing of a cerebral hemisphere, shade the olfactory lobe and the limbic lobe of Broca (Fig. 2-3).
8. Describe and draw the location of the somatosensory, auditory, visual, and motor cortices.
9. State, in principle, the functional significance of the association cortex.
10. State, in principle, the functional significance of the limbic lobe.

II. The neuron and the neuron doctrine

1. Draw and label a typical neuron (Fig. 2-4).
2. Define a synapse and explain how it functions.
3. Explain the six tenets of the neuron doctrine summarized by the statement that the neuron is the anatomic, functional, directional, genetic, pathologic, and regenerative unit of the nervous system.
4. Explain why so many genetic, toxic, and viral diseases cause degeneration of only one specific group of neurons while sparing other neuronal groups.
5. Describe the difference in regeneration of central versus peripheral axons.

III. The spinal cord, somites, and spinal nerves

1. Define a somite and describe the types of tissue derived from it.
2. Draw a cross section of the spinal cord showing the composition of a spinal nerve. Label the functional type of axons (nerve components) in the dorsal and ventral roots of the typical spinal nerve (Fig. 2-7).
3. Describe the location of the perikarya of the three functional types of neurons, *afferent* (primary sensory), *internuncial,* and *efferent* (motor neurons), and the relation of their axons to the central and peripheral nervous systems.
4. Explain, in principle, the functional importance of internuncial neurons (Table 2-8).
5. Explain why dermatome C4 abuts on T2 (Figs. 2-9 and 2-10).
6. Explain why the diaphragm receives its innervation from cervical segments 3, 4, and 5 (the law of retained original innervation).
7. Explain why the distribution of the dermatomes and peripheral nerves differs in the extremities but conforms in the thoracic region (Figs. 2-9, 2-10, and 2-11).
8. Describe, in principle, the movements (e.g., flexes the elbow) mediated by the major terminal peripheral nerves of the spinal plexuses: circumflex, musculocutaneous, radial, ulnar, median, femoral, obturator, sciatic, tibial, peroneal, pudendal, and pelvic splanchnic.
9. Describe how to test the integrity of the radial, ulnar, and median nerves in a Pt whose entire forearm and hand are encased in a cast, except for the thumb, which is free to move.
10. Make a cross section of the spinal cord to show the location of the clinically important tracts (Fig. 2-12).

IV. Anatomic organization of the brainstem

1. Name in rostrocaudal order the three *transverse* subdivisions of the brainstem (Fig. 2-1).
2. Name in dorsoventral order the three *longitudinal* plates or subdivisions of the brainstem (Fig. 2-13).
3. Draw a generalized cross section of the brainstem and label the clinically important regions of gray and white matter (Fig. 2-14 and Table 2-3).
4. Name the supplementary large motor nuclei in the ventral part of the midbrain tegmentum, basis pontis, and the ventral part of the medullary tegmentum.
5. Describe the location of the major tracts of clinical significance seen on cross section of the brainstem.
6. Explain, in principle, and by giving examples, why the brainstem has more elaborate pools of internuncial neurons (reticular formation) than the spinal cord.

V. Anatomic review of the twelve pairs of cranial nerves

1. Define a cranial nerve.
2. Give the number, name, and foramen of exit of the cranial nerves (Tables 2-4 and 2-5).
3. Describe, in the fewest possible words, the function of each of the cranial nerves (Table 2-6).
4. Divide the cranial nerves into three functional sets, and list the number of the cranial nerves belonging to each set (Table 2-7).
5. Describe, in principle, the fate of the rostral, intermediate, and caudal cranial somites.
6. Make a table of the nerve components of the somite set of cranial nerves (Table 2-8).
7. Describe which part of the face derives from branchial arches (Fig. 2-19).
8. Describe the fundamental morphologic similarities of branchial arches and somites.
9. Describe the embryologic origin of the olfactory and optic bulbs.
10. Explain why demyelinating diseases of the CNS would attack the optic nerve but not the other two special sensory nerves, I and VIII.
11. Name in ventrodorsal sequence the cranial nerves that attach to the pontomedullary sulcus. Explain why knowledge of this one fact helps you to remember where all of the remaining cranial nerves attach.
12. Draw a ventral view of the brain to show where the cranial nerves attach (Fig. 2-22).
13. Draw a dorsal phantom view of the brainstem showing the location of the motor and sensory cranial nerve nuclei. Draw the motor nuclei on one side and the sensory on the other (Fig. 2-23).
14. Describe, in principle, the similarities in the peripheral distribution of cranial nerves VII, IX, and X (Table 2-12).
15. Describe how the peripheral distribution of the cranial nerves relates in more or less rostrocaudal sequence to the rostrocaudal sequence of the nuclei of VII, IX, and X in the brainstem (Table 2-12).

16. Make a table of the nerve components of the 12 cranial nerves (Table 2-7).

VI. The reticular formation

1. Give an anatomic definition of the reticular formation.
2. State, in principle, the major functional differences between the rostral half (ponto-mesencephalic) of the reticular formation and the caudal half (pontomedullary).

VII. The diencephalon

1. State, in dorsoventral order, the four nuclear zones that comprise the diencephalon (Fig. 2-24).
2. Describe, in principle, the relation of the thalamus (thalamus dorsalis) to the cerebral cortex.
3. Describe, in principle, the functions of the five nuclear subdivisions of the thalamus.
4. State the system to which the subthalamus belongs.
5. State, in principle, the role of the hypothalamus.

VIII. The contralaterality of the central nervous system

1. Draw the visual pathway from the retina to the cerebral cortex in the human brain (Fig. 2-26).
2. Explain and show by drawings how the physical properties of light have determined the visual pathways, led to the law of contralateral cerebral sensorimotor innervation, and thus have, in effect, determined the wiring diagram of the CNS (Figs. 2-25 and 2-26).
3. Draw the pathway for pain and temperature sensation from the periphery to the cerebral cortex (Fig. 2-27).
4. Draw the pathway for deep sensation from the periphery to the cerebral cortex (Fig. 2-27).
5. Describe the pathways for touch from periphery to cerebral cortex (Fig. 2-27).
6. Recite the lemnisci and their origin and termination, naming the nucleus and its cortical projection area (Table 2-14).
7. Describe the difference between the medial lemniscus at its origin at the medullocervical junction and its course through the rostral part of the brainstem.
8. Locate the lemniscal crescent on cross sections of the brainstem (Figs. 2-14 to 2-18).

IX. The contralaterality of motor innervation by the pyramidal tract

1. Draw the pyramidal pathway from origin to termination (Fig. 2-28).
2. Recite and explain the law of contralateral hemispheric sensorimotor innervation.
3. Explain the difference in the laterality of paralysis from interruption of the pyramidal tract in the brain or spinal cord.
4. Define upper motor neurons (UMNs) and lower motor neurons (LMNs).
5. Contrast the effect of UMN and LMN lesions on movements and muscles.

X. The connections of the cerebellum
1. Describe, in principle, the afferent and efferent connections of the cerebellum.
2. State the effect of cerebellar lesions on coordination and muscle tone.
3. Diagram the circuit that explains the laterality of signs due to a lesion of the right cerebellar hemisphere (Fig. 2-29).

XI. The connections of the basal motor nuclei
1. List the nuclei ordinarily included in the basal ganglia (excluding the claustrum and amygdala) and the additional basal motor nuclei of the extrapyramidal system (Table 2-15).
2. State the categories of clinical motor deficits caused by lesions of the basal motor nuclei (Table 2-16).
3. Diagram, in principle, the circuit that explains the laterality of choreiform movements of the left extremities secondary to a lesion of the right caudate-putamen (Fig. 2-30).

4. Explain the effect on voluntary and involuntary movements of interruption of the pyramidal tract.

XII. The connections of the cerebral cortex
1. Distinguish between association, commissural, and projection fibers of cortical neurons (Fig. 2-32).
2. Distinguish between commissures and decussations.
3. Describe, in principle, the pathways of the cerebral white matter.

XIII. Chapter review
1. Recite the clinically important decussations of the CNS, beginning with the optic system (Table 2-13 and Figs. 2-26 to 2-31).
2. Recite in principle the major clinical signs that are caused by lesions of the LMNs, UMNs (pyramidal), cerebellum, and basal motor nuclei (extrapyramidal system) (Table 2-16).

Chapter Three

Examination of Vision

Seasons return; but not to me returns Day,
Or the sweet approach of even or morn,
Or sight of verbal bloom or Summer's rose,
Or flocks, or herds, or human face divine.
  John Milton (on his own blindness, at age 43)

I. Introduction to the optic system

A. *Anatomy of the eyeball.* Learn Fig. 3-1. Yes, prove that you have learned it by drawing it.

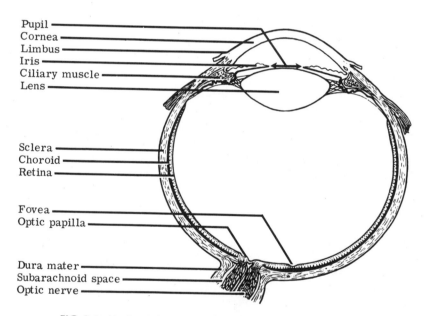

Pupil
Cornea
Limbus
Iris
Ciliary muscle
Lens

Sclera
Choroid
Retina

Fovea
Optic papilla

Dura mater
Subarachnoid space
Optic nerve

FIG. 3-1. Horizontal section of the right eye. Learn this figure.

B. *Duality of the optic system. The optic system is a dual system, consisting of a sensory (afferent) component and a motor (efferent) component.*
  1. The *sensory* component is itself dual, consisting of *visual* and *somatosensory* afferent axons.
      a. The optic nerve, II, conveys afferents for vision and pupilloconstriction.

*The light vertical rule on the left side of the text sets off an answer column. Cover the answers with a card until you have responded to the text. Then after each response, slide the card down to check your answer.
The heavy vertical rule denotes optional material.

b. The trigeminal nerve, V, conveys afferents for proprioception from the extraocular muscles, and for ocular pain, the corneal reflex, and tearing.

2. The *motor* component *finds, fixates, focuses, aligns* on, and *follows* visual targets. III, IV, and VI convey the efferent axons for these actions.

C. *Afferent pathway for vision and the pupillary light reflex.* Light initiates afferent impulses for vision and pupilloconstriction by exciting the rod and cone receptor neurons of the retina.

1. The *unipolar* rod and cone neurons synapse on the *bipolar* neurons of the adjacent layer of the retina.

2. The *bipolar* neurons synapse on *multipolar neurons* of the ganglion cell layer. The axons from the multipolar neurons exit from the eyeball at the *optic disc* to form the *optic nerve.* The optic nerve runs through the *optic chiasm* to the *optic* tract. The optic tract terminates by dividing into two further tracts:

   a. The *retinopretectal tract* synapses in the pretectum and midbrain for pupillary light reflexes (Fig. 4-30).

   b. The *retinogeniculate tract* synapses on the lateral geniculate body of the thalamus. The *geniculocalcarine* tract then synapses on the primary occipital (calcarine) cortex. The association cortex surrounding the calcarine cortex then interprets and gives value and meaning to the visual image. Trace the entire retinogeniculocalcarine tract to the cortex in Fig. 3-5

D. *Formation of the retinal and visual images*

1. *To understand vision, we commence with an arrow as the visual target.* The physical optics of the eye produce an inverted real *retinal image* of the visual target (Fig. 3-2).

   a. Neurophysiological processing from retina to cortex then converts the real retinal image into a mental abstraction called a *visual image.*

   b. The actual image formed on the retina by the physical optics of the eye is called the _____ image, whereas the image formed by the mind is called the _____ image.

Retinal; visual

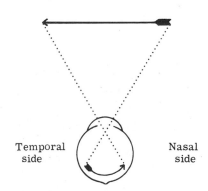

Temporal side   Nasal side

FIG. 3-2. Retinal image formed during monocular fixation with the left eye.

2. *Projection of the visual image by the mind*

   a. As Fig. 3-2 shows, the light rays which form the *nasal* half of the retinal image come from the ☐ temporal/ ☐ nasal half of the object viewed.

   b. By a process of learning, we associate the point of retinal stimulation with the reverse half of space. Hence, if light rays fall on the *temporal*

☑ *Temporal*

☑ *Nasal*

Lower

☑ *Opposite*

half of the retina, the mind perceives the object as in the ☐ temporal/ ☐ nasal half of space.

c. If the image of an object falls on the *nasal* side of the retina, we would reach for the object in the *temporal* half of space. Similarly, if the image falls on the *upper* half of the retina, we would reach for the object in the _____ half of space.

d. Thus the law regarding projection of the visual image states that *the mind projects the visual image derived from one half of the retina to the* ☐ same/ ☐ opposite half of space.

e. This particular law exemplifies a general law of sensation: *the mind projects afferent impulses to their usual site of origin in all sensory systems.* If an electrode stimulated your right auditory nerve, you would experience a sound as if it came from the right side of space. If you bump your ulnar nerve at the elbow, you would feel a shock-like sensation down your forearm into your little finger, even though no afferent impulses arose from the finger itself. In each case, we say that the afferent impulses have initiated a sensation which the mind *projects* or *refers* to the usual site of origin of the stimuli.

II. The visual fields

The visual field is . . . "an island of vision surrounded by a sea of blindness."

Harry Traquair

A. *Definition of the visual field:* Cover one eye and stare fixedly straight ahead. The entire area of vision is called the *visual field* of that eye.

B. *Duality of the visual field*
1. The entire visual field consists of a *central* field and a *peripheral* field, based on the duality of the *cone* and *rod* receptors of the retina.
   a. *Cone* neurons occupy the *macula*, which forms a disc centered on the fovea centralis (Figs. 3-1 and 3-15*A*).
   b. *Rod* neurons occupy the remaining retina, concentrically surrounding the macular disc.
2. The *cones* mediate the *central* field of vision and its two functions:
   a. Visual acuity (20/20).
   b. Color vision. (The mnemonic of the 4 *c*s: the *c*ones in the *c*enter are for a*c*uity and *c*olor.)
3. The *rods* mediate the *peripheral* field of vision and its two functions:
   a. Night vision.
   b. Motion detection.
4. If a Pt complained of decreasing visual acuity and had no opacities such as a cataract, the lesion would most likely affect the ☐ cones/ ☐ rods in the retina or their axonal pathway to the cerebrum.
5. If a Pt complained of inability to see in dim light but acuity was preserved, the lesion would most likely affect the ☐ central/ ☐ peripheral part of the retina which contains the ☐ rods/ ☐ cones.

☑ *Cones*

☑ *Peripheral*
☑ *Rods*

C. *Self-demonstration of the central field of vision*
1. Although the total field of vision when you look straight ahead is nearly 180 degrees wide, the limited central field of visual acuity may surprise you.

2. *Do this experiment to demonstrate visual acuity*
   a. Position yourself one meter from a long row of books or get close to a short row, so that the books extend beyond the limit of your peripheral vision. Stare fixedly at one book title, without moving your eyes at all. Can you read more than one book title? ☐ Yes/ ☐ No.

Ans: ☑ *No. If you could read more than one, you shifted fixation. Do the*
  experiment again.

   b. The central area of sharpest visual acuity is the *central* field. The experiment showed how small it is.
3. *Do this experiment to demonstrate color vision*
   a. Fixate on the same book. Make sure you position yourself so that the row of books extends to the peripheral limit of your field. While staring at a book directly in front of you, try to determine the color of the most distant book that you can see in the periphery. After trying to determine the color, shift your gaze to look straight at the book. How does the color of the book differ when seen in your central field of vision as contrasted to its color when seen in the peripheral field? _____

Ans: Peripherally, the book is drab, nearly colorless. With central vision it
  immediately becomes bright and vivid.

   b. Now do this experiment:
      (1) Hold a colored pen, preferably red, or any other small colored item out at the periphery of your temporal field.
      (2) Stare fixedly straight ahead and move the colored item until it is in line with your central vision. What is the difference in the color as the item moves from peripheral to central vision? _____

Ans: The more peripheral the item, the drabber the color.

D. *Self-demonstration of the perimeter of the peripheral fields*
   1. Close or cover one eye and fixate straight ahead with the other. Extend the arm ipsilateral to the fixating eye straight out to the side, and point your index finger up. Now, keeping the elbow extended, rotate the arm forward. The point at which you first see the finger defines the *temporal* perimeter of your visual field.
   2. Repeat the foregoing experiment, fixating with the same eye and closing the other. This time use the arm *contralateral* to the fixating eye, and rotate the finger forward until it just becomes visible. Did you have to move it farther forward than the ipsilateral arm? ☐ Yes/ ☐ No.

☑ Yes

   3. Ostensibly the nose would seem to limit the nasal part of the visual field. Developmentally and phylogenetically this may be true, but the extent of the retina itself limits the extent of the nasal field (Tate and Lynn, 1977).
   4. To locate the *vertical* perimeter of the visual field, fixate straight ahead with one eye, while bringing your index finger down from above and, next, up from below. What structure limits the height of the visual field? _____

Ans: The eyebrow or the eyelid if it is ptotic.

   5. If the lid is ptotic, it should be held up when you test the Pt's visual fields.

E. *Nomenclature for the visual fields and visual field defects*
   1. Learn the nomenclature of the visual fields in Fig. 3-3.
   2. Visual field defects tend to fall into patterns of one-quarter or one-half of the visual fields (Fig. 3-4). Blindness in one-quarter of a field is called *quad-*

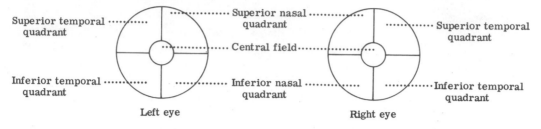

FIG. 3-3. Nomenclature of the normal visual fields.

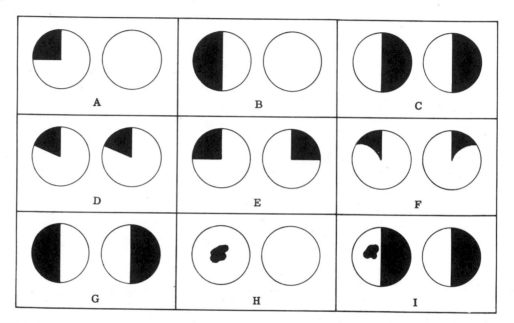

FIG. 3-4. Patterns of visual field defects (A–I). The darkened area is the area of blindness. The Pt's left eye is to the reader's left. Imagine that you are looking through the Pt's eyes.

Quadrantanopia

2. Visual field defects tend to fall into patterns of one-quarter or one-half of the visual fields (Fig. 3-4). Blindness in one-quarter of a field is called *quadrantanopia* (literally: quadrans = ¼; an = without; opic = vision). Since the superior temporal quadrant in Fig. 3-4A is completely blind, the full name is *complete left superior temporal* _____.

3. Blindness in one-half of a field, or a *hemi* defect, as in Fig. 3-4B, would be called *hemianopia*. The complete name for the field defect is complete temporal hemianopia of the left eye.

4. When corresponding quadrants or halves of the fields, e.g., the right halves, are affected, the defect is termed *homonymous,* and it is described as *right* or *left*. What is the complete name for the field defect in Fig. 30-4C? _____

Ans: Complete right homonymous hemianopia.

5. The terms *homonymous* or *corresponding,* as applied to visual field defects, thus mean that the defect corresponds to the way the visual cortex represents the retinal and visual images of the right and left visual fields during binocular vision. Refer to Fig. 3-4C. When the Pt with a complete right homonymous hemianopia looks straight ahead, he would be blind in the ☐ right/ ☐ left half of space and see in the ☐ right/ ☐ left half.

☑ *Right;* ☑ *left*

6. Name the defect in Fig. 3-4D. _____

Ans: Incomplete left superior homonymous quadrantanopia.

Quadrantanopia

7. *Noncorresponding* field defects are sometimes called *heteronymous* to contrast them with homonymous (Fig. 3-4*E*). It is simpler to describe them directly. Thus the defect in Fig. 3-4*E* would be called complete superior bitemporal _____.

8. Fig. 3-4*F* is called _____

_____

Ans: Incomplete superior bitemporal quadrantanopia.

Complete bitemporal
  hemipanopia

9. Fig. 3-4*G* the defect is called _____

_____.

10. The field defects of Figs. 3-4*E*, *F*, and *G* would not be homonymous because _____

_____

_____.

Ans: The defect is not in corresponding parts of the fields according to the way the visual cortex represents the right and left halves of space (as in Fig. 3-4C).

Central

11. An irregular field defect, not approximating a quadrantic defect, is called a *scotoma*. A scotoma may be *central, paracentral,* or *peripheral.* The defect in Fig. 3-7*H* would be called a _____ scotoma of the left eye.

F. *Anatomic basis of visual field defects.* Use these instructions to learn Fig. 3-5.
  1. Learn the names down the right side.
  2. Notice that light rays from the *right half* of space fall on the *nasal* side of the *right* retina, and on the *temporal* side of the *left* retina.

A Complete
  blindness, L eye
B Complete
  bitemporal
  hemianopia
C Complete nasal
  hemianopia, L eye
D Complete R
  homonymous
  hemianopia
E Complete R
  superior
  homonymous
  quandrantanopia
F Complete R
  inferior
  homonymous
  quadrantanopia
G Complete R
  homonymous
  hemianopia

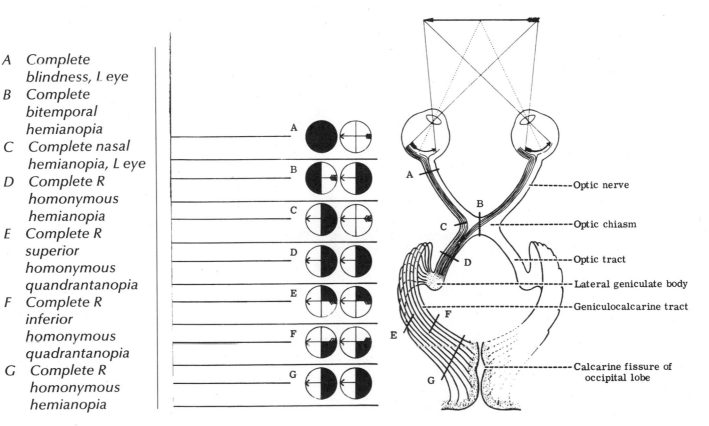

FIG. 3-5. Visual pathway from retina to occipital cortex. The small scale of the drawing precludes showing the synapse of the retinal axons at the lateral geniculate body. Fill in the blanks with the correct names for the field defects produced by the lesions represented at A to G.

3. At the chiasm, axons from the *nasal* half of the right retina decussate to travel through the optic tract with the axons from the *temporal* half of the left retina.
4. The retinal axons synapse on neurons of the lateral geniculate body, a thalamic nucleus which relays sensory impulses to the cerebral cortex. The thalamus is part of the diencephalon. The tract of axons formed by geniculate body neurons is called the *optic radiation* or *geniculocalcarine tract.*
5. Using a colored pencil, draw in the retinal pathway from the *nasal* half of

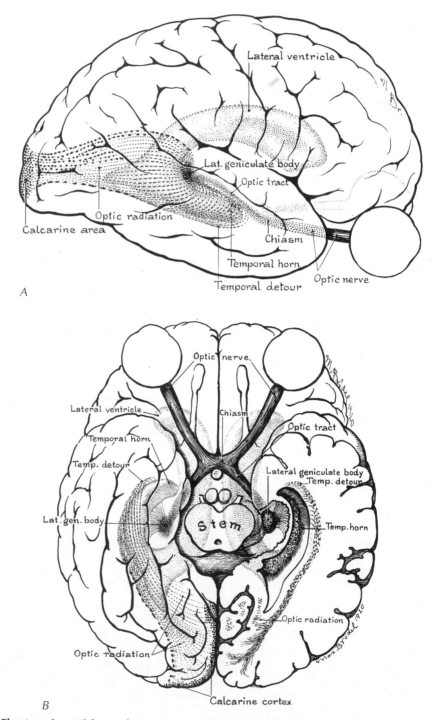

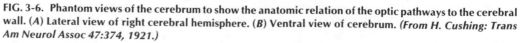

FIG. 3-6. Phantom views of the cerebrum to show the anatomic relation of the optic pathways to the cerebral wall. (*A*) Lateral view of right cerebral hemisphere. (*B*) Ventral view of cerebrum. (*From H. Cushing: Trans Am Neurol Assoc 47:374, 1921.*)

the left retina and *temporal* half of the right. Include the geniculate body synapse. Make sure you draw a mirror image of the corresponding axons already in the drawing.

6. Bars are drawn across the optic pathways at A to G to simulate lesions at various sites. At the left, label the field defects resulting from the lesions.

7. Note that lesions of the *superior* fibers, F, of the geniculocalcarine tract cause contralateral *inferior* homonymous quadrantanopia.

8. Practice drawing the entire optic pathway from the retina to the occipital cortex.

9. Figure 3-6 shows the actual course of the optic pathways through the cerebrum. Note that visual field testing assays the integrity of large parts of the temporal and occipital lobes, and the inferior margin of the parietal lobe.

III. Clinical testing of central vision

A. Bedside testing of visual acuity

1. Screen visual acuity at the bedside by having the Pt read fine print held at a distance. Test each eye separately. The Pt keeps his glasses on. Although glasses improve acuity by correcting for a refractive error, they do not improve acuity impaired by retinal or optic nerve lesions.

   a. If the history or screening test suggests a visual complaint, use a Snellen, Jaeger, or Rosenbaum chart for a numerical evaluation of acuity, and consider referring the Pt to an ophthalmologist for tangent screen testing as explained below.

   b. For a small child or mentally defective Pt, use a large E printed on a card and have the Pt point in the direction of the bars as you rotate the card.

2. Test the acuity of partially blind Pts by having them count the number of fingers held up at various distances. If the visual loss is so severe that the Pt cannot see fingers, find out whether light perception remains. That is to say, push the analysis to the limit.

3. Color vision is not tested in the basic neurologic exam (NE). If necessary, use Ishihara color vision cards.

B. Tangent screen testing of central vision

If a defect in central vision is detected or suspected, test the Pt by means of a *tangent screen*. The Pt sits 1 or 2 meters away from a black screen 1 or 2 meters square, fixating on its center (with one eye covered). The Ex moves a 1- to 5-mm white spot through the field of vision. After mapping the physiologic blind spot, the Ex systematically searches the central field for pathologic blind spots, called *scotomas*. The chart becomes part of the medical record (Fig. 3-7).

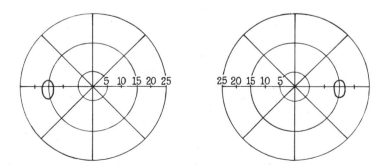

FIG. 3-7. Chart for recording the central portion of the visual fields, as determined by tangent screen examination.

C. *Mapping the physiologic blind spot and central scotomas*
   1. Do this experiment with Fig. 3-8.
      a. Hold the page about 30 cm away.
      b. Cover your left eye.
      c. Fixate on the left cross. Make sure you do not break fixation from the left cross at any time, but you should be able to make out the right cross also.
      d. Move your face slowly toward the page. As you maintain fixation on the left cross, attend to the image of the right cross.
      e. At some point the right cross disappears. As you continue to move closer, it reappears. If this does not happen you broke your fixation on the left cross—try again.
      f. Again cover your left eye, fixate on the left cross, and position your head so that the right cross disappears. Put your pencil point in the blind spot (i.e., at a position on the paper where you cannot see it) and move it very slowly toward the left cross. Make a mark on the paper when the point just becomes visible. By working around the blind spot, you can map out its perimeter. Be careful: if your fixation wavers, your blind spot will have irregular borders. The blind spot or other scotomas are mapped more accurately on a distant tangent screen than with the short target distance of this experiment.

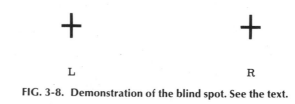

L   R

FIG. 3-8. Demonstration of the blind spot. See the text.

   2. Get a partner. Draw an *x* on a piece of paper to fixate on, and fasten the paper to a wall, making your own tangent screen. Seat the partner 100 cm away and map out the blind spot. Move a test object (a 5-mm circle of white paper stuck on the end of a wire) from the far right through the blind spot, toward the fixation point. Then work from the center of the blind spot to its periphery to outline it.
   3. We do not ordinarily recognize our own blind spots. We attend to the fixation point of the visual axes and ignore the blind spot.
   4. *Anatomic basis of the blind spot*
      The blind spot is caused by the absence of receptor neurons at the optic papilla or optic nerve head. Normally the diameter of the blind spot depends on the diameter of the optic papilla (Fig. 3-9).

D. *Pathologic blind spot enlargement and scotomas*
   1. Retinal lesions such as hemorrhages or exudates may prevent light from penetrating to the receptor neurons or may destroy them. The pathologic enlargement of the blind spot or scotoma produced depends on the size and location of the lesion. Although in theory quadrantic or hemianopic field defects could result from retinal or optic nerve lesions, in practice this virtually never occurs. These patterned field defects generally mean that the lesion affects the chiasm, optic tract, geniculocalcarine tract, or occipital lobe (Fig. 3-5*B* to *G*). Thus lesions of the pathways from the chiasm to the occipital lobe usually cause *patterned* defects, while lesions of the retina or

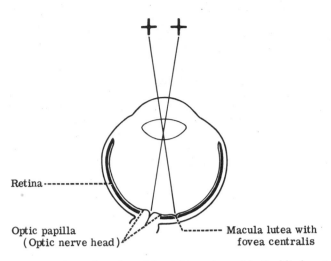

FIG. 3-9. Horizontal section of the right eye to explain the blind spot.

Retina --------------

Optic papilla
(Optic nerve head)

Macula lutea with
fovea centralis

optic nerve, if not so severe as to cause blindness, cause scotomas, *irregular* field defects.

2. A Pt who had sudden loss of visual acuity without blindness would be expected to have a macular lesion, if the lesion is in the retina. If the scotoma is large, the Ex can detect it by carefully moving a pencil tip or small white object the size of a small pearl *very slowly* through the central field. Ophthalmoscopic examination, of course, will disclose a retinal lesion. If the lesion is in the optic nerve, the retina may look normal. Supportive evidence of an organic cause of the loss of acuity will be the demonstration of a central scotoma by tangent screen examination.

3. *The blind spot in papilledema.* When the optic papilla swells the normal blind spot increases in size (section VI, Ophthalmoscopy).

4. Fig. 3-4*I* shows the visual fields of a 53-year-old hypertensive Pt who complained of headaches, sudden loss of vision on the right side and blurring of vision in the left eye. Write out the name of the defects. _____

_____

_____

Ans: Complete right homonymous hemianopia with left superior quadrant paracentral scotoma. The Pt had an infarct of the left occipital lobe, causing the right hemianopia, and a recent hypertensive hemorrhage in the left retina, causing the scotoma.

IV. Technique for confrontation testing of the peripheral visual fields
(Fig. 3-10)

A. *Positioning*

1. Confront the Pt by stationing yourself directly in front. Start with your *left* eye directly in line with the Pt's *right* eye, at a distance of about 50 cm, thus eye to eye, but not breath to breath. The Pt covers his left eye with his hand.

2. Hold up your left index finger just outside your own peripheral field, in the inferior temporal quadrant. Hold the finger about equidistant between your eye and the Pt's. (As shown in Fig. 3-6, A = A'.) Wiggle the finger slowly and move it very slowly toward the central field. Request the Pt to say "Now" as soon as the wiggling finger is seen. *The point is to match the*

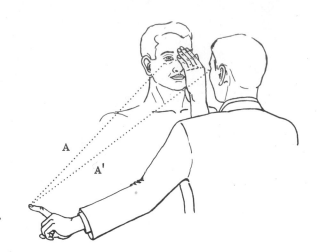

FIG. 3-10. Position of doctor and Pt for testing the visual fields by confrontation.

perimeter of the Pt's visual field against your own. Test all quadrants of each eye separately, starting at the limit of your own vision.

B. *Technical pointers*
1. Position both yourself and the Pt comfortably.
2. State clearly what you want the Pt to do. The best instructions are: "I want you to look directly into my eye. Don't look away. Now I want to find out what you can see out of the corner of your eye. Say, 'Now' as soon as you see my finger wiggle." Do not ask the Pt to look at your nose. The Pt's eyes will converge and your fields will not match the Pt's. Try to fit or titrate your island of vision against the Pt's.
3. Test the midpoint of the quadrants, at about 45, 135, 225, and 315 degrees (Fig. 3-11), rather than at 0, 90, 180, and 270 degrees. If you test along the vertical or horizontal axes, you may miss a full quadrant defect, because of the intact fields on the border of the defect. See the left eye in Fig. 3-4*A*.
4. Confrontation is suitable for detecting large erosions of the island of vision by the sea of blindness. Practice confrontation testing of the visual fields, using a normal person.

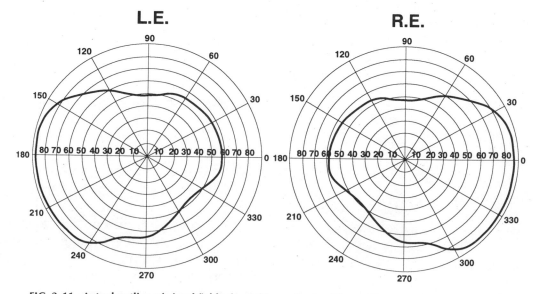

FIG. 3-11. Actual outline of visual fields charted by perimetry. The numbers are readings in degrees.

C. Quantitative mapping of the visual fields and blind spot
Detailed mapping of the *peripheral fields* requires *perimetry* by an ophthalmologist or neurologist. Accurate plotting of the fields discloses the somewhat irregular outline in Fig. 3-11, rather than the exactly round shape we have depicted. The tangent screen and perimeter, while valuable in themselves, only supplement, but do not supplant, confrontation testing by the attending physician.

V. Suppression of vision

A. Physiologic suppression of vision. Try this experiment:
1. Fixate on a distant point straight ahead. Place your palm on your forehead with your wrist directly between your eyes, while maintaining fixation on a distant point. Close one eye and then open it. Under which condition do you see more of your wrist? ☐ one eye open/ ☐ both eyes open

☑ *One eye open*

2. By closing one eye, you prove that the light rays from the wrist are striking photosensitive areas of the retina, yet the wrist is visible to one eye but nearly vanishes when both eyes are open. We interpret the experiment to mean that the medial, overlapping portions of the visual fields undergo suppression during binocular vision (Fig. 3-12). This is an example of *physiologic suppression* to rid the visual image of confusing elements.

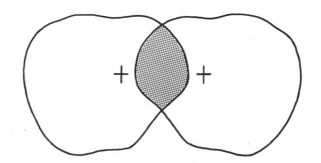

FIG. 3-12. The overlapping, shaded area of the visual fields that undergoes physiologic suppression.

B. Pathologic suppression of vision
1. *Suppression amblyopia (amblyopia ex anopsia).* If one of an infant's eye turns in or out, the infant learns to suppress the image from the errant eye. If suppression continues for the first few years of life, the Pt ultimately becomes completely blind in the deviating eye, even though the retina and visual pathways are structurally intact. Chapter 4 discusses this type of *suppression amblyopia.*
2. *Visual inattention or visual extinction to double simultaneous stimulation*
   a. Fixate straight ahead.
   b. Hold your arms out to the sides, in the upper or lower quadrant, with your index finger pointing up.
   c. Rotate your arms forward until your index fingers just come into view in each eye. Notice that you can make out both fingertips at the periphery of your fields, even though you look straight ahead. The presentation of two stimuli, such as the two fingers, on opposite sides, is called *double* or *simultaneous stimulation.*
   d. Technique for simultaneous stimulation of visual fields. Assume the same position as for regular confrontation, but the Pt keeps both eyes open. Extend your fingers into your inferior temporal quadrants, near,

but not beyond, the periphery of your own visual fields. Wiggle one finger and request the Pt to point to *the* finger that moves. Then wiggle both fingers simultaneously and ask the Pt to point to *any* finger that moves. The normal person, perceiving both stimuli, points to both fingers. Repeat the test in the upper temporal quadrants and then simultaneously stimulate upper and lower nasal and temporal quadrants of one eye at a time.

e. *Results and interpretation of inattention to simultaneous stimulation*

(1) Pts with parietal or parieto-occipital lobe lesions, particularly on the right side of the cerebrum, when presented with simultaneous stimuli, will not attend to the stimulus from the *contralateral* side. If, as in the usual case, the Pt does not attend to stimuli from the *left* half of space, the lesion is in the ☐ right/ ☐ left parietal lobe.

☑ *Right*

(2) However, when the Pt is tested by confrontation, using a single finger in the left visual field, no defect is demonstrated. The Pt is then said to have *visual inattention* for the left side of space.

Simultaneous or double

f. Hemianopia is detected by using a single stimulus, while visual inattention is detected by using _____ stimuli.

Hemianopia

g. If the Pt is blind in one-half of the visual field, it is called _____. If the Pt fails to recognize a stimulus in one-half of a visual field when both halves are stimulated, it is called _____.

Ans: Visual inattention or visual suppression.

h. Explain the difference between hemianopia and visual inattention. ___
_____
_____

Ans: Hemianopia means that the Pt is blind for single and double stimuli in one visual field. Visual inattention means that the Pt does not perceive one of simultaneous right- and left-sided stimuli, but has no hemianopia when tested with a single stimulus.

i. Pts with right parietal lobe lesions also may fail to attend to auditory or tactile stimuli from the left side (Chap. 10).

C. *Neuro-ophthalmologic findings in cortical blindness with double hemianopsia.*

1. Bilateral destruction of the visual cortex, as from infarction, hypoxia, or trauma, results in *cortical blindness,* characterized by:

a. Complete blindness, with no light perception and no response to visual stimuli.

b. Loss of smooth pursuit of the Ex's moving finger in testing the range of eye movements, while volitional movements are preserved; no optokinetic nystagmus.

c. Normal pupillary reactions and funduscopic examination; no nystagmus.

d. Not uncommonly the Pt will deny the blindness and will claim that vision is present.

2. MRI scan will confirm the bioccipital lesions.

FURTHER READING FOR VISION AND VISUAL FIELDS

Bajandas FJ, Cline LB: *Neuro-ophthalmology Review Manual* (3d ed). Slack, New Jersey, 1988.

Bedwell CH: *Visual fields: A Basis for Efficient Investigation.* London, Heineman, 1982.

Bender MB, Bodis-Wollner I: Visual dysfunctions in optic tract lesions. *Ann Neurol,* 1978; 3:187–193.

Bender MB, Rudolph SH, Stacy CB: The neurology of the visual and oculomotor systems, in Joynt RJ (ed): *Clinical Neurology.* Philadelphia, Lippincott, 1990.

Frisen L: *Clinical Tests of Vision.* New York, Raven, 1990.

Gassel M, Williams D: Visual function in patients with homonymous hemianopia. Part II: Oculomotor mechanisms, *Brain,* 1963; 86:1–36.

Glaser JS: *Neuro-ophthalmology* (2d ed). Philadelphia, Lippincott, 1990.

Harrington D: *The Visual Fields: A Textbook and Atlas of Clinical Perimetry* (4th ed). St. Louis, C.V. Mosby, 1976.

Leicester J, Sidman M, Stoddard L, et al: Some determinants of visual neglect, *J Neurol Neurosurg Psychiatr,* 1969; 32:580–587.

Miller NR (ed): *Walsh and Hoyt's Clinical Neuro-ophthalmology* (4th ed). Baltimore, Williams & Wilkins, 1982.

Tate GW, Lynn JR: *Principles of Quantitative Perimetry: Testing and Interpreting the Visual Field.* New York, Grune and Stratton, 1977.

VI. Ophthalmoscopy

A. Introduction

1. By now, you know what I would have you do to learn ophthalmoscopy. Sit down with a normal person and, using colored pencils, draw the optic fundus and draw it faithfully, precisely, and in exquisite detail. Listen—you will never, *never,* do competent opthalmoscopy unless you can draw the fundus. Moreover, you should often use drawings in your clinical notes rather than laborious written descriptions.

2. Making a drawing forces you to search the fundus systematically. Do it systematically the first time and every time for the rest of your career.

B. Technique of ophthalmoscopy

1. Remove your and your partner's or the Pt's glasses, unless one or both of you have a severe refractive error. The closer you can get your eye to the ophthalmoscope and the closer you can get the scope to the Pt's eye, the larger the area of fundus visible.

2. Darken the room leaving only a little background illumination.

3. Ask the Pt to gaze fixedly on a specific object straight ahead. Hold the ophthalmoscope in your right hand and use your right eye to examine the Pt's right eye; hold the scope in your left hand and use your left eye to examine the Pt's left eye. Otherwise you are nose to nose. When looking through the scope, keep both eyes open, attending only to the image from the eye behind the scope. Learn this art. It well repays the time required.

4. Instruct the Pt to breathe, but the Ex should generally not breathe in the Pt's face. Both Pt and Ex should be in a comfortable position. Establish a "proprioceptive circuit" to steady the Pt's head and your hand and head. (Fig. 3-13).

5. Turn the rheostat on the ophthalmoscope down a little to avoid too strong a beam of light. Start with the ophthalmoscope 10 to 15 cm from your partner's eye and, with a strong positive lens, focus on the media in succession from cornea to lens to vitreous, using successively weaker lenses. Inspect the cornea both with and without the scope for opacities, and for a circular ring near the limbus. If grayish-white the ring is an arcus senilis; if greenish-

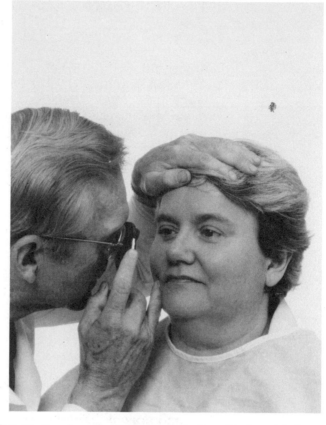

FIG. 3-13. **Proprioceptive link to steady the Pt and Ex for ophthalmoscopy.**

brown, a Kayser-Fleischer ring pathognomonic of Wilson's hepatolenticular degeneration.

6. Next focus on a retinal vessel using whatever lens setting from zero to a strong plus or minus that is necessary to overcome refractive errors. After locating a retinal vessel, follow it along until you find the optic disc (optic papilla). Now study Figs. 3-14 and 3-15*A* before continuing.

7. Next, identify the pigment ring around the disc, note the disc color, and the presence or absence of a physiologic cup. If present, the physiologic cup is white as compared to the rest of the disc. Identify the arteries, the thin, brighter-appearing vessels and the thicker, duller-appearing veins. Look for

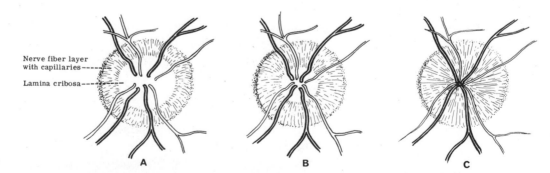

Nerve fiber layer
with capillaries

Lamina cribosa

A   B   C

FIG. 3-14. **Normal variation in the size of physiologic cup of the optic papilla. The size of the cup depends on whether the nerve fibers perforate the lamina cribrosa only at its periphery or all over its surface. (*A*) Large cup. Notice the large white ring of lamina cribrosa showing between the nerve fibers and the rim of nerve fibers. Notice the spread of the vessels where they perforate the lamina cribrosa. (*B*) Medium-sized cup. Notice the small white ring and the more compact relation of the vessels. (*C*) Absence of a physiologic cup in an otherwise normal disc. The vessels originate as from a point.**

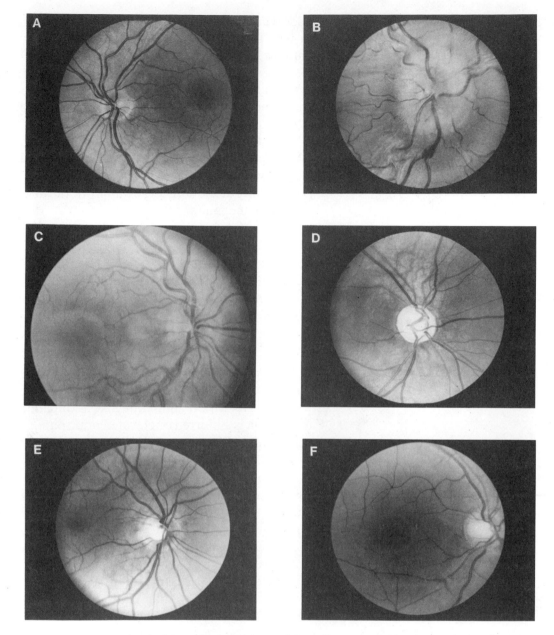

FIG. 3-15. Photographs of optic papilla in various conditions. *(Courtesy of Dr. Eugene Helveston.)* (*A*) Normal. (*B*) Papilledema. Notice how the edematous swelling engulfs and obscures the proximal segments of many vessels. Also notice the hemorrhage along the course of the vessel just inferior to the disc. (*C*) Pseudopapilledema. (*D*) Primary optic atrophy. Notice the chalk-white disc with cookie-cutter sharp edges. (*E*) Secondary optic atrophy. Notice the pale, gray-white color laterally (to the reader's left) and the shaggy margins. (*F*) Large physiologic cup, a normal variation.

venous pulsations where the veins bend over the edge of the physiologic cup. Press on the sclera through the Pt's eyelid and watch the veins collapse. Follow each artery out as far as possible. Locate the macula, a darker, avascular area two disc diameters *lateral* to the disc. Note the pearl of light reflecting from its center, the fovea centralis. Study the texture of the retina.

8. Now make your drawing of your partner's fundus, and to check how observant you have been, answer questions 8a to l. Write your answers in the left-hand margin, and you will have created your own program.

   a. What is the normal ratio of arterial diameter to venous (A-V ratio)?

   b. What is the width of the stripe of light reflected from the arteries?

   c. Do the arteries nick or indent the veins where they cross?

    d. Between the superior and inferior temporal branches of the retinal artery, how many blood vessels can you count coursing over the disc? Be sure to have the disc sharply in focus.

    e. Which margin of the disc shows the most pigment?

    f. Which borders of the disc—the superior, inferior, nasal, or temporal—normally look more blurred than the other borders?

    g. What is the normal color of the disc?

    h. Which half of the disc, the nasal or temporal, is the palest?

    i. What is the range of normal variability in the diameter of the physiologic cup? (Answer only after you have looked at several eyes.)

    j. How many disc diameters away from the disc is the macula?

    k. Describe the macula.

    l. Does the fundus appear perfectly smooth or does it have a leathery texture?

9. Now, after trying to answer the questions, decide whether you should repeat the drawing. The questions cannot be bluffed. Either you know the answers or you don't. Should you try again? While wrestling with your conscience, listen to Walt Whitman:

> *Failing to fetch me at first keep encouraged,*
> *Missing me one place, search another,*
> *I stop somewhere waiting for you.*

C. *Papilledema.* Definition and pathogenesis of papilledema.

    1. Papilledema is a blurred or elevated optic papilla (optic nerve head or optic disc), resulting from edema fluid in the nerve fibers as they cross the disc to perforate the lamina cribrosa and enter the optic nerve.

    2. Most often, papilledema results from transmission of increased intracranial pressure into the eye via the subarachnoid space, which extends out along the optic nerve (Fig. 3-16). The retinal veins converge on the optic papilla to form the ophthalmic vein, which enters the retinal end of the optic nerve. If the pressure around it increases, the ophthalmic vein, being thin-walled, collapses, obstructing the retinal veins. The retinal veins and papillary capillaries distend, leaking fluid into the nerve fibers on the optic papilla and into the surrounding retina. The veins may rupture, causing visible hemorrhages on or around the papilla.

    3. *Ophthalmoscopic features of progressive papilledema*

        a. Blurring of the nerve fibers as they converge on the disc.

        b. Hyperemia of the disc and venous engorgement with loss of venous pulsations.

        c. Obliteration of the physiologic cup, and later disc elevation and hem-

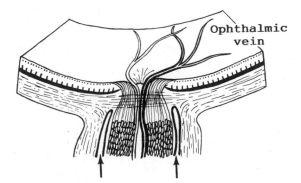

FIG. 3-16. Section of optic papilla and optic nerve. The arrows show how the subarachnoid space extends out around the optic nerve.

TABLE 3-1 Optic disc anomalies confused with papilledema (reference only)
Medullated nerve fibers: a whitish-yellow patch of fibers which radiates into the retina from the disc
Congenital vascular anomalies of the vessels with glial overgrowth
Small scleral aperature: the disc appears protruded; usually seen in a hyperopic eye with a short sagittal axis
Drusen (waxy appearing bodies which push up beneath and may protrude through the disc)
Pseudopapilledema: see next section
Papillitis: see later section

orrhages. Peripapillary rugae or folds may also occur in papilledema. From Fig. 3-15, pick out the retina which shows papilledema (and one hemorrhage). ☐ A/ ☐ B/ ☐ C/ ☐ D/ ☐ E/ ☐ F/.

Ans: ☑ *B. The hemorrhage is at the vein bifurcation, just inferior to the optic disc.*

D. *Differential diagnosis of papilledema, disc anomalies, and pseudopapilledema*

1. Although true papilledema is always pathologic, not all that looks like papilledema is papilledema (Table 3-1).
2. *Differential diagnosis of true papilledema and pseudopapilledema*
   a. Perhaps 5 percent of normal individuals have some blurring and even elevation of the optic papilla, a condition called *pseudopapilledema*. Pseudopapilledema often unduly alarms the clinician and leads to unnecessary, painful, and even harmful diagnostic investigations, when in most instances careful clinical observations, based on drawings and periodic assessment of the disc, would lead to the correct, benign diagnosis of pseudopapilledema. The difficulty arises in distinguishing early papilledema from pseudopapilledema. The experienced Ex has little difficulty recognizing advanced papilledema, which shows extreme papillary swelling, venous congestion, and hemorrhages.
   b. In pseudopapilledema, the disc margins look blurred, but the central portion of the disc protrudes rather than the peripheral part, as in true papilledema, and the vessels show preretinal branching (Fig. 3-17).
   c. The elevated disc of pseudopapilledema in some Pts may come from drusen (hyaloid bodies) pressing up from beneath the nerve fiber layer.
   d. Drusen and pseudopapilledema occur most frequently in blond Cau-

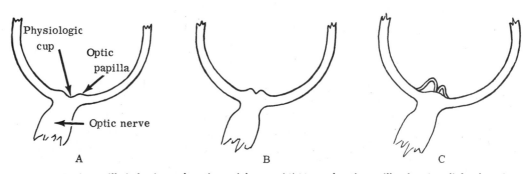

FIG. 3-17. Optic papilla in horizontal sections of the eye. (*A*) Normal optic papilla, showing slight elevation of the papillary margins and normal depth of the physiologic cup. (*B*) Early true papilledema, showing elevation of the papillary margins and beginning obliteration of the physiologic cup. (*C*) Pseudopapilledema, showing preretinal branching of the vessels, central elevation of the optic papilla, and absence of a physiologic cup.

casians. Also, pseudopapilledema most often occurs in hyperopic rather than myopic Pts. If you suspect pseudopapilledema in a blond Caucasian or hyperopic Pt, inspect the fundi of family members. Since these conditions often are hereditary, the answer becomes clear if other family members also have blurred discs. From Fig. 3-15, select the disc which shows pseudopapilledema: ☐ A/ ☐ B/ ☐ C/ ☐ D/ ☐ E/ ☐ F.

☑ *C*

  e. Two further tests help identify papilledema in doubtful cases: measurement of the blind spot's size and the fluorescein dye test.

  (1) *Measurement of the blind spot.* The optic papilla causes a blind spot in the visual field because it contains no light-receptive neurons. As edema from the optic disc infiltrates the surrounding retina, it impairs receptor function, causing the blind spot to increase in size. Serial measurements of the diameter of the blind spot aid in differentiating papilledema and pseudopapilledema. In pseudopapilledema, the blind spot is normal in size and remains so, while in papilledema, the blind spot increases in size. What type of visual field examination would you order to measure the blind spot? _____.

Ans: Tangent screen examination of the central field.

  (2) *The fluorescein dye test.* After injection of fluorescein into an arm vein, the fundus is photographed. Fluorescein can be visualized in the papilla and the surrounding retina after it passes through the leaky walls of the distended retinal vessels.

  f. Thus the two tests in addition to ophthalmoscopic examination to diagnose papilledema are _____.

Ans: Measure the blind spot and do the fluorescein dye test.

  g. Although papilledema increases the size of the blind spot, papilledema per se does not generally impair visual acuity until weeks to months after papilledema starts.

PAPIL-LEDEMA	PSEUDO-PAPIL-LEDEMA	TABLE 3-2 Differentiation of true and pseudopapilledema (reference only)	Papil-ledema	Pseudo-papil-ledema
		Disc characteristics		
+	0	Hyperemic, pink color (vascular distension)	___	___
+	0	Physiologic cup present (early)	___	___
+	0	Sparing of temporal margin (early)	___	___
0	+	High point of elevation central (see Fig. 4-19)	___	___
0	+	Drusen (hyaline bodies) submerged in children, exposed in adults, gray-yellow translucent color of disc; applies only to blond Caucasians	___	___
		Vessel characteristics		
+	0	Dilated veins	___	___
0	+/0	Venous pulsation present	___	___
+	0	Disc obscures origin of vessels	___	___
0	+	Arteries appear tortuous, show preretinal branching, and the disc does not obscure the origin of the vessels	___	___
0	+	Prominent choroidal vessels (from lack of retinal pigment)	___	___
+	0	Hemorrhages	___	___
0	+	*Hyperopia*	___	___
+	0	*Enlarged blind spot*	___	___
+	0	*Fluorescein dye test:* shows leaky vessels on and around disc	___	___

3. To summarize the differential diagnosis of papilledema and pseudopapilledema, complete Table 3-2.

E. *Summary of procedures to diagnose papilledema*

1. Make careful clinical notes, or better, make drawings or photographs. Describe the following:

   a. The color of the disc.

   b. Degree of blurring of disc margins and location of blurring. Record any measurable elevation of the disc as the diopter difference between the elevation of the disc margin and the adjacent retina.

   c. Condition of the physiologic cup.

   d. Venous congestion and pulsation.

   e. Peripapillary wrinkles and folds.

   f. Hemorrhages or exudates.

2. Measure the Pt's visual acuity.

3. Chart the blind spot in the visual field.

4. Consider the common anomalies confused with papilledema, as outlined in Table 3-1.

5. Consult an ophthalmologist about the fluorescein dye test.

6. Make careful serial examinations.

F. *Optic atrophy, primary and secondary*

1. *Definition.* Optic atrophy means any condition in which the nerve fibers that originate in the retina and penetrate the optic disc have degenerated or disappeared.

2. *Pathogenesis of optic atrophy* (anterograde or retrograde axonal degeneration)

   a. If a lesion destroys retinal neurons or their optic nerve fibers as they course to the optic papilla, the fibers undergo *wallerian (anterograde)* degeneration and disappear. If a lesion interrupts optic fibers in the optic nerve, chiasm, or tract, the fibers undergo *retrograde* degeneration and disappear back to their retinal neurons of origin. Thus with either retinal or optic nerve lesions, the optic papilla becomes denuded of nerve fibers, which brings us to a profound secret: the optic nerve fibers and retinal neurons are transparent and colorless. Why then doesn't the normal optic disc appear white, being backed by the white lamina cribrosa of the sclera? The answer is that the color of the disc is the color of the capillaries which accompany the nerve fibers and nourish them. Why does the physiologic cup appear white? _____

Ans: No nerve fibers and, therefore, no capillaries cover the physiologic cup. The white lamina cribrosa stands out.

   b. Such loss of capillarity follows a general rule: whenever the parenchymatous elements of an organ degenerate, so does its blood supply. Compare the capillarity of the pre- and postmenopausal ovary. With optic atrophy or retinal destruction, the arteries and veins also become smaller.

3. *Primary optic atrophy.* Disappearance of the nerve fibers and capillaries exposes the full extent of the chalk-white lamina cribrosa which then appears as a flat white disc with a cooky-cutter sharp border against the retina, a condition called *primary* optic atrophy. From Fig. 3-15, select the disc which shows primary optic atrophy: ☐ A/ ☐ B/ ☐ C/ ☐ D/ ☐ E/ ☐ F.

☑ D

4. *Secondary optic atrophy* follows long-standing disc lesions such as chronic papilledema or papillitis. The optic nerve fibers disappear, but connective tissue proliferation incited by the lesion causes the disc to become gray with

TABLE 3-3 Differential diagnosis of primary from secondary optic atrophy	
Primary optic atrophy	Secondary optic atrophy
Follows acute or chronic lesions of optic nerve or retina	Follows chronic lesion of optic papilla, usually papilledema or papillitis
Disc is chalk-white with cookie-cutter sharp borders	Disc is gray with shaggy borders from connective tissue proliferation
Lamina cribrosa exposed	Lamina cribrosa obscured
Arteries and veins reduced in size if optic atrophy is severe and prolonged	Arteries thin; veins may be dilated
May affect only one sector of the disc	Usually affects entire disc

☑ *Secondary*

shaggy, ragged borders due to glial scarring. In both primary and secondary optic atrophy, the nerve fibers crossing the disc disappear, but connective tissue proliferates on the disc only in ☐ primary/ ☐ secondary optic atrophy.

5. Table 3-3 summarizes the differential features of primary and secondary optic atrophy.

☑ *E*

6. From Fig. 3-15, select the disc which shows secondary optic atrophy: ☐ A/ ☐ B/ ☐ C/ ☐ D/ ☐ E/ ☐ F.

G. *Differential diagnosis of papilledema, papillitis, and acute retrobulbar neuritis.* Inflammatory or toxic processes may attack the optic papilla, so-called *papillitis.* Inflammatory, toxic, or demyelinating processes may affect the optic nerve behind the optic bulb, so-called *acute retrobulbar neuritis* (Fig. 3-18).

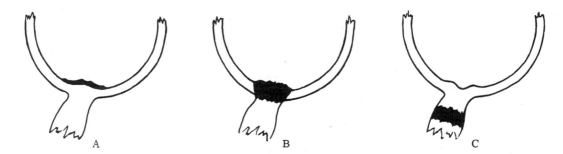

FIG. 3-18. Sites of lesions affecting the optic papilla and nerve. (*A*) Papilledema. (*B*) Papillitis. (*C*) Retrobulbar neuritis.

1. With the ophthalmoscope alone the Ex may not be able to distinguish papillitis from papilledema, but with papillitis the Pt loses vision, whereas with *papilledema* the Pt retains vision.

2. With acute retrobulbar neuritis, the disc and vessels look normal early in the course of the disease, but if the process destroys nerve fibers in the optic nerve, what happens to the nerve fibers and capillaries on the disc? _____.

Ans: The nerve fibers and capillaries degenerate and disappear.

The optic disc then has the ophthalmoscopic appearance called _____ _____ atrophy.

Primary optic

3. *Notice this critical fact:* The degeneration of optic nerve fibers and capillaries takes many days to several weeks to occur. Thus, the Ex will not see any atrophy in acute retrobulbar neuritis. Even though the Pt has no vision, the optic disc may look normal: the Pt sees nothing and neither does the Ex.

4. Summary of the differential effects of papilledema, papillitis, and acute retrobulbar neuritis on ophthalmoscopic appearances and visual acuity:
   a. If the physician sees a swollen disc, and the Pt sees as usual: papilledema.
   b. If the physician sees a swollen disc, and the Pt doesn't see well: papillitis.
   c. If the physician sees nothing abnormal, but the Pt's vision is blurred: acute retrobulbar neuritis.
   d. Thus, to put these statements in their tersest form:

       (1) If both the patient and physician see something, the diagnosis is
           _____.

       (2) If the physician sees something, and the patient doesn't, the diagnosis is _____.

       (3) If neither physician nor Pt sees anything, the diagnosis is
           _____.

Papilledema

Papillitis

*Acute retrobulbar
  neuritis*

FURTHER READING FOR OPHTHALMOSCOPY

Atlee W Jr: Talc and cornstarch emboli in eyes of drug abusers. *JAMA,* 1972; 51:49–51.

Bajandas FJ, Cline LB: *Neuro-ophthalmology Review Manual* (3d ed). Slack, New Jersey, 1988.

Bender MB, Rudolph SH, Stacy CB: *The Neurology of the Visual and Oculomotor Systems,* in Joynt RJ (ed): *Clinical Neurology.* Philadelphia, Lippincott, 1991.

Brown G, Tasman WS: *Congenital Anomalies of the Optic Disc.* New York, Grune and Stratton, 1983.

Chester E: *The Ocular Fundus in Systemic Disease.* Chicago, Year Book Medical Publishers, 1973.

Hayreh SS: *Anterior Ischemic Optic Neuropathy.* New York, Springer-Verlag, 1975.

Levin BE: The clinical significance of spontaneous pulsations of the retinal vein. *Arch Neurol,* 1978; 35:37–40.

Miller NR: *Walsh and Hoyt's Clinical Neuro-ophthalmology* (4th ed). Baltimore, Williams & Wilkins, 1982.

Nover A (translated by Blodi FC): *The Ocular Fundus: Methods of Examination and Typical Findings.* Philadelphia, Lea & Febiger, 1980.

Rosen E, Savir H: *Basic Ophthalmoscopy: Ophthalmoscopic Diagnosis in Systemic Disorders.* New York, Appleton-Century-Crofts, 1971.

Roy FH: *Ocular Differential Diagnosis* (4th ed). Philadelphia, Lea & Febiger, 1989.

Learning Objectives for Chapter Three

I. Introduction to the optic system

1. Make a drawing of a cross section of the eyeball at the level of the optic disc and fovea centralis (Fig. 3-1).
2. State which nerves provide afferent fibers for vision and somatic sensation from the eye.
3. Describe the visual pathway from receptor to receptive cortex.
4. Distinguish between the retinal image and the visual image (Fig. 3-2).
5. Describe what is meant by the statement that the mind projects the visual image to the usual site of origin of the light rays that strike the retina.

II. The visual fields

1. Explain the concept of the retina as a dual receptor. Describe the difference in the location of the rods and cones and relate them to their functions and to the central and peripheral fields of vision.
2. Describe a simple method for self-demonstration of the limited field of central vision for acuity and color vision.
3. Describe how to locate the perimeter of your own peripheral visual field.
4. State which part of the peripheral field permits the widest angle of vision and which permits the least, and

state which anatomic structure limits the height of the visual field.

5. Describe the nomenclature for the quadrants of the normal visual field of one eye (Fig. 3-3).

6. Diagram the pathway for the visual fields and describe with proper nomenclature the visual field defects resulting from lesions at various levels along the pathway (Figs. 3-4 and 3-5).

7. State how a tumor expanding upward against the center of the chiasm from the pituitary fossa would affect the visual fields (Fig. 3-5B).

8. Describe in principle the course of the geniculocalcarine tract.

9. State the effect of a temporal lobe lesion on the visual fields.

10. State the lobes of the brain that the geniculocalcarine tract traverses or borders on (Fig. 3-6).

III. Clinical testing of central vision

1. Describe how to test central vision at the bedside in a cooperative normal older child or adult and in young children or mentally retarded Pts.

2. State the indication for a tangent screen examination and describe in principle how it is done (Fig. 3-7).

3. Describe the difference between a scotoma and a patterned visual field defect.

4. Describe how to demonstrate your own blind spot in the visual field (Fig.3-8).

5. State what retinal structure causes the blind spot (Fig. 3-9).

6. Describe some lesions which may enlarge the blind spot or cause scotomas.

IV. Technique for confrontation testing of the peripheral visual fields

1. Demonstrate how to test the peripheral visual fields by confrontation (Fig. 3-10).

2. Explain why the Ex tests the extent of the peripheral fields by placing the finger at the midpoint of the quadrants, rather than exactly on the vertical or horizontal axes.

V. Suppression of vision

1. Describe how to demonstrate physiologic suppression of vision in the overlapping nasal fields of the two eyes (Fig. 3-12).

2. Explain the cause and prevention of suppression amblyopia (amblyopia ex anopsia).

3. Distinguish between visual inattention (suppression) on simultaneous bilateral stimulation and a hemianopic visual field defect. State the site of the lesion usually responsible for visual inattention.

4. Describe the neuro-ophthalmologic findings in cortical blindness, the site of the lesion, and the radiographic procedure of choice to identify the lesion.

VI. Ophthalmoscopy

1. Make and label a drawing of the normal optic fundus as seen through an ophthalmoscope (Fig. 3-15A).

2. Explain why the Ex, when facing the Pt, looks through the ophthalmoscope with the right eye into the Pt's right eye, but uses the left eye in testing the extent of the visual field of the Pt's right eye.

3. Describe how to use a "proprioceptive link" to steady the Pt and the Ex for ophthalmoscopy (Fig. 3-13).

4. State what type of lens is used to see the surface of the cornea and the superficial media of the eye.

5. Make drawings to show the extreme variations in the size of the physiologic cup in normal individuals (Fig. 3-14).

6. Explain why the central part of the normal optic disc (the physiologic cup) appears white, whereas the periphery appears orange-pink.

7. Describe how to distinguish retinal arteries from veins.

8. State the normal ratio of arterial diameter to venous diameter (A-V ratio) in the retina.

9. State the ratio of the width of the stripe of light reflected from the artery to the width of the artery.

10. State which border of the optic disc usually shows the most pigment.

11. State which border of the optic disc normally appears sharper than other borders.

12. State which part, the medial or lateral, of the optic papilla normally appears paler than the other.

13. Describe how to locate the macula and fovea centralis and describe their normal appearance.

14. Describe the texture of the normal retina as seen through the ophthalmoscope.

15. Describe the ophthalmoscopic features of papilledema, pseudopapilledema, primary optic atrophy, and secondary optic atrophy and pick them out from a series of illustrations (Fig. 3-15).

16. Describe the pathogenesis of papilledema.

17. Name several conditions of the optic papilla that need to be differentiated from papilledema (Table 3-1).

18. Describe procedures other than unaided ophthalmoscopy to detect true papilledema.

19. Describe how to distinguish pseudopapilledema from true papilledema (Table 3-2).

20. Describe the appearance of the optic disc in primary and secondary optic atrophy and distinguish between the pathogenesis of these conditions.

21. Describe the ophthalmoscopic findings in papilledema, optic neuritis, and acute retrobulbar neuritis, and state the effect each lesion has on vision.

22. State when optic atrophy may become evident by ophthalmoscopy after a retrobulbar lesion or compression of the optic nerve or chiasm.

23. Discuss the effect of partial or incomplete optic nerve lesions on visual acuity, color vision, visual fields, and the appearance of the optic disc.

Chapter Four

Examination of the Peripheral Optomotor System

In examining and treating motor anomalies (of the eye), one never loses an uneasy feeling of incompetence until he has become thoroughly familiar with the physiologic fundamentals from which the signs and symptoms of those anomalies are to be derived. Therefore, a discussion of motor anomalies of the eyes should begin with a synopsis of the physiology of the sensorial and motor apparatus of the eyes.

Alfred Bielschowsky (1871–1940)

I. Ocular alignment and diplopia

A. The goals of the optomotor system

The optomotor system *finds, fixates, focuses, aligns* on, and *follows* visual targets. Whether the eyes are fixed or moving, or the target is fixed or moving, each eye must continually *foveate*. To foveate means to align each eye so that the central ray falls on the fovea. The entire retinal image of the two eyes falls on corresponding retinal points, which promotes visual acuity and a single (fused) mental image. The optomotor mechanisms must foveate when the eyes hold still and during all movements, including head tilts, and vergences (convergence-divergence). Ultimately these optomotor mechanisms secure the advantages of binocular stereoscopic vision for survival.

B. Ocular alignment, the visual axes, and diplopia

1. To examine the alignment of the two eyes, start with the Pt looking straight ahead, the so-called *primary position* of the eyes. The point of fixation in the primary position is theoretically at infinity (Fig. 4-1).
2. A line drawn from the fovea centralis of one eye to the center of the visual field of that eye defines the *visual axis*. Such a line normally passes through the center of the refractive media of the eye to strike the fovea centralis. It is the "line of sight" of that eye. In Fig. 4-1, the line F-∞ defines the _____.

Visual axis

☑ *Essentially parallel (Fig. 4-1).*

3. When the eyes are in the primary position, fixating on infinity, the visual axes are ☐ convergent/ ☐ essentially parallel/ ☐ divergent.

*The light vertical rule on the left side of the text sets off an answer column. Cover the answers with a card until you have responded to the text. Then after each response, slide the card down to check your answer.

The heavy vertical rule denotes optional material.

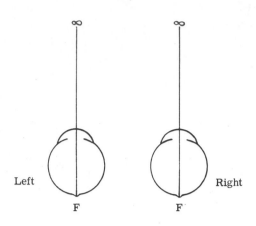

FIG. 4-1. Visual axes when the eyes are in the primary position, fixating on infinite distance. *F* is the fovea.

4. In Fig. 4-2, draw the visual axes when the eyes fixate on a point nearer than infinity. Use a colored pencil.

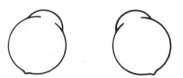

FIG. 4-2. Blank for drawing the visual axes when the eyes fixate on a near point.

5. When looking at a near point, the eyes converge. Because each eye adducts, the central light ray from the fixation point falls on the fovea and macula, the region of maximum visual acuity.

C. *Try this experiment to demonstrate the visual axis of the dominant eye*
   1. Fixate on the doorknob and place your index fingertip 20 cm away, so that the knob appears to ride on top of the finger.
   2. Alternately wink the right and left eyes as you fix on the doorknob. What happens to the appearance of the finger?_____

Ans: *It shifts to one side on closing one eye, if you strictly maintain your original fixation.*

   3. Balance the doorknob on your fingertip again, but this time fixate on your fingertip. Alternately wink the right and left eyes. What happens to the appearance of the doorknob?_____
   _____

Ans: *It shifts to one side on closing the eye.*

   4. *Explanation:* The shift occurs because you *primarily* fixate along the visual axis of the *dominant* eye; the other eye focuses *secondarily*.

D. *Self-production of diplopia*
   1. Try this experiment to produce diplopia
      a. Fixate on some definite, distant point across the room, such as a doorknob.

    b. Hold up the tip of your index finger about 20 cm directly in front of your eyes. Hold the finger so that the doorknob appears to balance on the fingertip.

    c. Fixate *first* on the doorknob, *then* on the very tip of your finger several times. Stop with your gaze firmly on the fingertip and *attend* to the image of the doorknob. Record what happens to the image of the doorknob.

Becomes doubled _____

    d. Now fixate *first* on the fingertip and *then* the door knob, while attending to the image of the finger. What happens to the appearance of the finger?

Becomes doubled _____

2. The previous experiment disclosed diplopia, *physiologic* diplopia. Fig. 4-3 shows why.

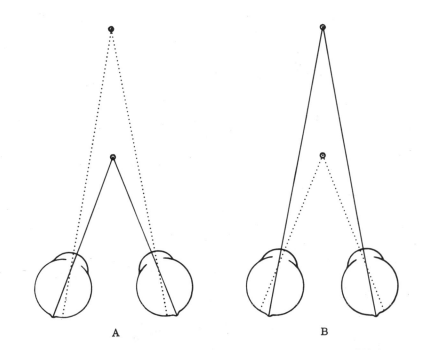

FIG. 4-3. Changes in the angulation of the visual axes (solid line) when the eyes shift from a near fixation point (*A*) to a distant one (*B*).

    a. *Explanation of physiologic diplopia.* In Fig. 4-3, rays from only one distance, the fixation point, strike the fovea. All other rays deviate from the fovea in proportion to their distance from the fixation point. Only the rays coming in along the visual axes strike correspondingly on the fovea centralis of each eye.

    b. Why don't we have diplopia all the time? Recall that you had to consciously *attend* to the point of *non*fixation to get diplopia. Ordinarily, we have learned to suppress physiologic diplopia. It only appears when we make a determined effort to break through its physiologic suppression. To state it another way, we can say that we only *attend* to the non-diplopic images.

3. *The canthal compression experiment to experience pathologic diplopia*

    a. Place the tip of your right index finger upon your right lateral canthus, as shown in Fig. 4-4.

    b. Fixate on your left index finger held upright at arm's length.

    c. Gently press on your canthus with your right index finger. By varying the pressure, you will be able to experience diplopia. If you do not pro-

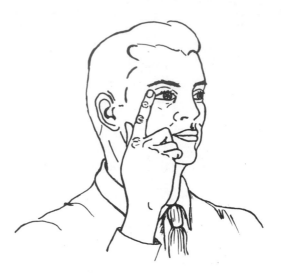

FIG. 4-4. Position of finger for lateral canthus compression to produce diplopia when the eyes gaze at the opposite finger.

    duce diplopia when looking at your finger, look across the room at a distant object.

    d. Try the experiment again, holding the outstretched finger horizontally this time. With the finger vertical or horizontal, you should obtain diplopia. It may be greater with the finger in one position than another, and it may vary each time you try the experiment, depending on the way the eyeball is displaced. Also hold the outstretched finger horizontally and try to get diplopia by pressing lightly on your eyeball through the upper lid with your other finger.

4. While your right finger compresses your lateral canthus, decide whether you get more diplopia with the finger vertical or horizontal and then move the finger from center to side, or up and down, in whichever direction gives the most diplopia.

    a. What happens to the distance between the diplopic images as you move your target finger away from its starting position? _____

Ans: The distance between the diplopic images varies.

    b. While experiencing diplopia by pressing your lateral canthus, try to identify which image is faulty. It can be identified by:

        (1) Alternating the pressure on the eye, causing the faulty image to move while the other image remains on target.

        (2) Winking the displaced eye.

        (3) Noticing which image is the sharpest.

        (4) Can you explain why the image from the displaced eye is not as sharp as from the nondisplaced eye? _____

_____.

Ans: The eye that is not displaced receives the central rays from the visual target directly on the macular cones, the site of sharpest vision. The retinal image in the displaced eye falls off of the macula, onto the rods (Fig. 4-6).

5. Work through Fig. 4-5 to understand how binocular fixation brings the retinal images onto corresponding parts of the retinas of the two eyes. Begin by drawing in the visual axes. To prove you understand the drawing, try to reproduce it.

6. *Explanation of diplopia from eyeball displacement by canthal compression*

    a. For description, the visual image of the normally aligned eye is called

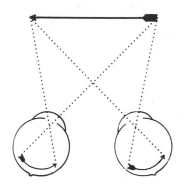

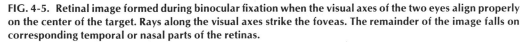

FIG. 4-5. Retinal image formed during binocular fixation when the visual axes of the two eyes align properly on the center of the target. Rays along the visual axes strike the foveas. The remainder of the image falls on corresponding temporal or nasal parts of the retinas.

the *true* image; of the abnormal eye, the *false* image. Of course, one image is no more "true" or "false" than the other, because both are visual images imposed on the afferent data by the mind.

    b. Consider now the diplopia produced with the target finger vertical. (Even if you failed to get diplopia this way, you can still follow the explanation.) With the finger vertical in the midline, you got one, or with

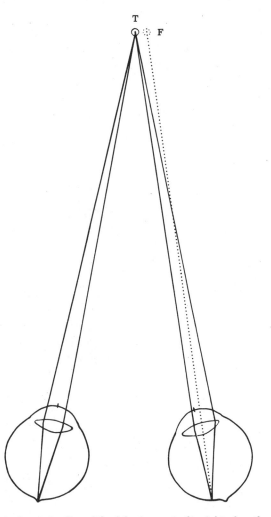

FIG. 4-6. Diagram to explain the projection of the false image to the right when the right eye is turned in (or fails to abduct). T = true image; F = false image. With a colored pencil, draw the visual axis of each eye, from fovea centralis through the center of the cornea.

practice, two results: one image was projected to the *right* or the *left* of the true position of the finger. Whichever direction the false image was projected depends on how the eyeball happened to be displaced. Study Fig. 4-6.

7. Explain why the false image appears to the right of the true image in Fig. 4-6._____

_____

_____

Ans: Since the right eye failed to ab̲duct to align with the left as it ad̲ducts, the retinal image of the right eye falls on the nas̲al half of the retina and, by learning, the mind projects the visual image to the right (temporal) side.

8. The eyeball displacement experiment shows that unless the eyes align properly to bring the retinal images onto corresponding retinal areas, the penalty is diplopia and decreased visual acuity.

II. The actions of the individual extraocular muscles (EOM)

NOTE: Every general physician must know how to detect ocular malalignment and must remember that the lateral rectus muscle has only one action, abduction of the eye, and the medial rectus only one action, adduction. All other EOMs have multiple actions, depending on the position of the eye. If the time for the neurologic examination (NE) course is short, photocopy Fig. 4-18, which summarizes these actions, paste it in your handbook for reference, and skip to section II.J. If you wish to understand the actions of the the EOM, work through the text, which calls for you to make two simple models. The second model uses paper strips to simulate the ocular muscles, enabling you to reason out their actions and recall them when needed. I find that many students automatically reject model-making as a waste of time. Let me say this: you will never really understand the ocular rotations unless you experience the actions by seeing them happen and feeling them with your own fingers. It might interest the skeptics among you to know that Leonardo da Vinci (1452–1519), who dissected many human bodies to learn about the actions of muscles, devised the method of tugging on tapes attached to the insertion of muscles to teach himself how the muscles worked. To *experience* the actions of the muscles, get these things to make the models: 1. An olive, or small ball of clay, or even a wad of gum. 2. Toothpicks or applicator sticks. 3. Several straight pins. 4. Scissors. 5. A table tennis ball or similar ball that you can stick pins into.

A. Axial rotation of the eyeball
The eye must be able to aim its visual axis to any point within the perimeter of movement. To achieve infinitely variable movement within that perimeter, the eyeball rotates *axially,* around three axes: a vertical axis (V); a lateral axis (L); and an anteroposterior axis (A-P) (Fig. 4-7).

B. Two teaching models
1. To visualize the axial rotation of the eyes, get a stuffed olive, a piece of clay, or a wad of gum, and insert three toothpicks at right angles as in Fig. 4-7. Rotate each of the three toothpicks. Then and only then, as your fingers feel it, will you understand that ocular rotation is *axial* rotation, not eccentric rotation. In Fig. 4-8 check the eye which shows the correct, axial rotation.

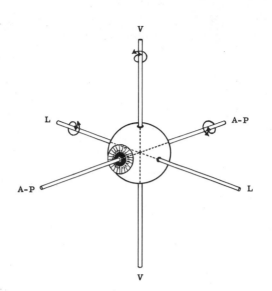

FIG. 4-7. The three rotational axes of the eye. V = vertical; L = lateral; A-P = anteroposterior.

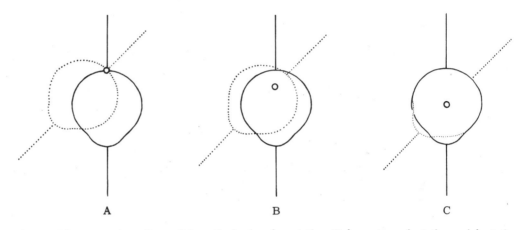

| A | B | C |

FIG. 4-8. Diagram to show the possible methods of ocular rotation. Only one type of rotation, *axial* rotation, is correct. It is shown by ☐ *(A)*/ ☐ *(B)*/ ☐ *(C)*.

☑ *C*

2. On a table tennis ball or small rubber ball, draw a cornea and pupil and the points of emergence of the three axes (Fig. 4-9). Label the three axes. Then place the ball on the mouth of a bottle (Fig. 4-9).

C. The four rectus muscles: the medial, lateral, superior, and inferior recti
The simplest way to move the eyes around two axes is by four muscles (Fig. 4-10). Label the axes, learn the names of the four rectus muscles, and note their insertion in relation to the axes.

D. Action of medial and lateral rectus muscles
1. Cut two strips of paper. Mark them MR and LR for medial and lateral recti. Draw an arrow along the strips to represent the vector or line of pull of the contracting muscle (see the arrow in Figs. 4-9 and 4-11). Stick a pin through the anterior end of each strip, and into the ball. *Stick the pin slightly anterior to but exactly in line with the lateral axis.* Now put the ball on the mouth of a bottle. Align the strips to pull exactly straight back, as in Fig. 4-9. Pull and relax the medial and lateral recti strips and observe the exact

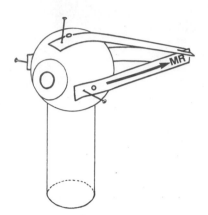

FIG. 4-9. Table tennis ball mounted to rotate on a bottle mouth, with paper strips pinned in place to simulate ocular muscles.

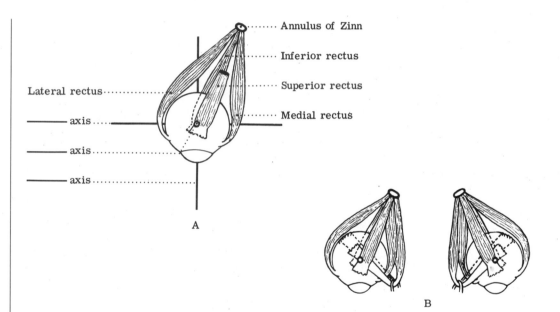

Lateral

Vertical

A-P

FIG. 4-10. Origin and insertion of the ocular muscles. (*A*) Right eye as seen from above, showing the rectus muscles. (*B*) Both eyes seen from above, showing all the ocular rotatory muscles and their sites of origin and insertion when the eyes are in the primary position.

Vertical

A-P

Lateral

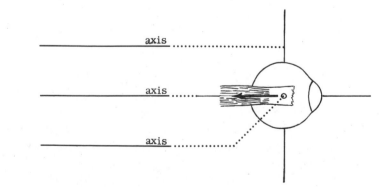

FIG. 4-11. Lateral view of the right eye to show the direct pull of the lateral rectus muscle over the lateral axis.

axial rotation of the ball around the vertical axis. Study Fig. 4-11 and label the axes.

2. From your model, and only from your model (have you made the model?), will you fully appreciate this fact: you have to pull exactly straight back, along the vector arrow in Fig. 4-11, or the eye will wobble around some other axis rather than showing precise axial rotation around the vertical axis.

3. Since the medial and lateral recti pull exactly straight back, they have one and only one action: to adduct or abduct the eye. The actions of the medial and lateral recti rotate the eye around the _____ axis. The other ocular rotatory muscles have an off-center relation to the ocular axes and thus display more than one effective action.

Vertical

E. Action of the superior rectus muscle

1. In Fig. 4-10 note that contraction of the superior rectus would rotate the eye *upward* around the _____ axis. This is the primary action of the muscle.

Lateral

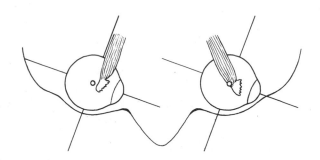

FIG. 4-12. Right eye and superior rectus muscle as seen from above. Notice how the position of the eye changes the relation of the muscle insertion to the vertical axis and, therefore, changes the effective action of the muscle.

2. The angulation of the superior and inferior recti causes a difference in the strength of the primary action, and permits secondary and tertiary actions, depending on the position of the eye. To understand how the actions of some of the ocular muscles change as the eyes rotate, you must know the origin and insertion of the muscles in relation to the axes of the eyeball.

3. The recti all originate from the *annulus of Zinn,* which is attached to the optic foramen. In Fig. 4-10 note that from their origin, the recti angle ☐ laterally; ☐ medially.

4. Notice in Fig. 4-10*B* that the superior rectus runs somewhat ☐ medial to/ ☐ lateral to the vertical axis.

   a. We have already seen that the superior rectus has the primary action of rotating the eye ☐ upward/ ☐ downward around the lateral axis.

   b. To analyze the other actions of the superior rectus, pin another strip of paper to the ball, inserting the pin *anteromedial* to the vertical axis, exactly as in Fig. 4-9. Angle the strip along the normal line of pull of the muscle as shown in Fig. 4-13*B* and notice the effect on the ball when the strip is pulled.

   c. Because its line of pull is slightly medial to the vertical axis, the superior rectus has a secondary action of rotating the eye *medially* around the vertical axis. The muscle whose sole action is medial rotation of the eye is the _____ rectus. This action is also termed __duction.

✓ *Laterally*

✓ *Medial to*

✓ *Upward*

Medial; adduction

5. To better visualize the secondary action and tertiary actions of the superior rectus, imagine the right eye in a position of extreme adduction, as in Fig. 4-13. Pull on the superior rectus strip after the right eyeball has adducted, as in Fig. 4-13*A*.

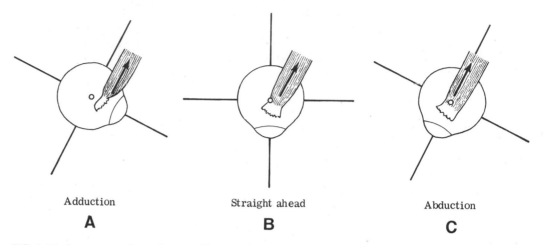

Adduction	Straight ahead	Abduction
A	**B**	**C**

FIG. 4-13. Eyes as seen from above to illustrate the relation of the pull of the superior rectus muscle to the ocular axes when the right eye adducts and abducts.

6. Now it is observable that the superior rectus can elevate the eye and adduct it, and in addition can tilt the vertical axis inward. Intilting of the vertical axis is called *intorsion,* as shown in Fig. 4-14.

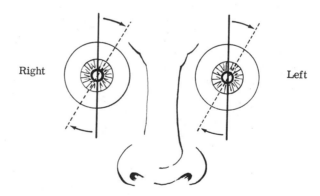

Right   Left

FIG. 4-14. Torsion of the eyes. The right eye is undergoing *in*torsion; the left, extorsion. The torsions are named *in-* or *ex-*, depending on whether the top of the vertical axis tilts in (medially) or out (laterally).

☑ *Intorsion*

Extorsion
A-P

7. In Fig. 4-14, the right eye has rotated around the A-P axis, tilting the top of the vertical axis *in*. Therefore, it is called ☐ intorsion/ ☐ extorsion.
8. In the left eye, the top of the vertical axis tilts *out*. Therefore, it is called _____ torsion.
9. The torsions involve rotation of the eye around the _____ axis. Use your toothpick model to visualize this action (Fig. 4-7).
10. When the eye is *abducted,* the point of insertion of the tendon of the superior rectus shifts laterally, as shown in Fig. 4-14*C*.
11. Would the superior rectus act to adduct or intort when the eye is abducted? ☐ Yes/ ☐ No.

Ans: Find out from your model.

12. With the eye abducted, the superior rectus pulls directly over the vertical axis. It dissipates none of its strength in adduction or intorsion. Therefore,

the superior rectus elevates the eye most strongly when the eye is ☐ adducted/ ☐ straight ahead/ ☐ abducted.

13. In what position of the eye would the superior rectus have the weakest action of elevation? _____

14. In summary, the primary action of the superior rectus is _____ of the eye. This action is strongest when the eye is _____.
    a. The secondary and tertiary actions are _____ and _____ of the eye.
    b. In what direction would you ask the Pt to look to test the strongest elevating action of the right superior rectus? _____

☑ *Abducted*

Adduction
Elevation
Abducted
Adduction
Intorsion

Up and to the right

F. *Action of the inferior rectus muscle*

1. The *inferior rectus* muscle has the same direction of origin and insertion as the superior rectus (Fig. 4-10). The primary action of the inferior rectus is to ☐ depress/ ☐ elevate the eye.

2. Its secondary action would be to _____ the eye.

3. You will have to analyze its tertiary action carefully. Pin a strip to the eye to represent the inferior rectus and consider its action with the eye *adducted*. Then when the inferior rectus contracts, the top of the vertical axis would be tilted ☐ internally/ ☐ externally

4. Internal tilting of the vertical axis is called _____. External tilting is called _____.

5. What is the only eye movement in which the superior and inferior recti could rotate the eye in the same direction? _____

6. The superior and inferior recti are ineffective adductors until the medial rectus muscle, the most critical muscle for adduction, has already begun to act.

7. To test the strongest action of the right inferior rectus as a depressor, in what direction would you ask the patient to look? _____

8. In summary, list the primary and supplementary two actions of the inferior rectus muscle. _____ _____

☑ *Depress*
Adduct

☑ *Externally*
Intorsion
Extorsion

Adduction

Ans: Down and to the right

Depress, extort and adduct

G. *Action of the superior oblique muscle*

1. The superior oblique originates from the lesser wing of the sphenoid bone, just above the annulus of Zinn. It threads its tendon through a trochlea (pulley) attached to the rim of the bony orbit (Fig. 4-15*A*). When the tendon runs to the eye, it inserts *posteriorly* to allow the superior oblique to have an effective pull when contracting. In so attaching, the tendon runs somewhat *medial* to the vertical axis, like the superior and inferior recti. Cut another paper strip and attach it to correspond to the line of pull of the tendon.

2. The vector diagram of Fig. 4-15*B* resolves the arrow **R-B** into effective components.
    a. Vector **R-A** ☐ depresses/ ☐ elevates the eye around the _____ axis.
    b. Vector **R-C** ☐ abducts/ ☐ adducts the eye around the _____ axis, and ☐ intorts/ ☐ extorts the eye around the _____ axis.
    c. Therefore, vector **R-B** acts to _____, _____, and _____ the eye.

☑ *Depresses; L*

☑ *Abducts; V;*
☑ *Intorts; A-P*

Depress, abduct, intort

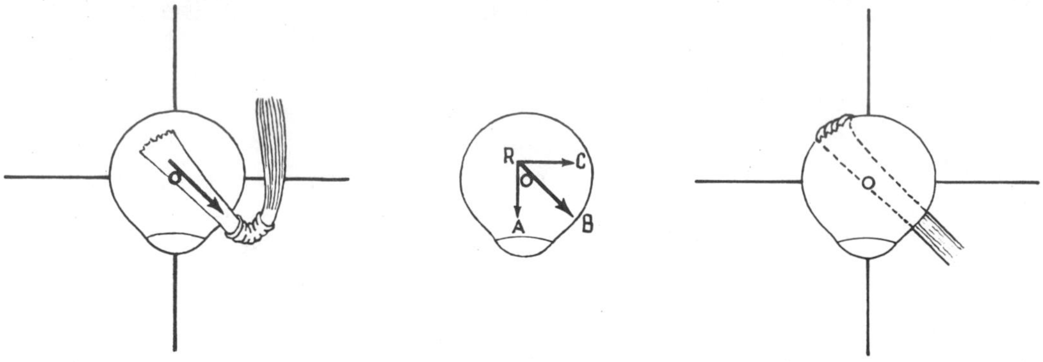

A. Superior Oblique B. Vector diagram C. Inferior Oblique

FIG. 4-15. Right eye, as seen from above, to illustrate the actions of the superior and inferior oblique muscles. The arrow in A represents the line of pull of both muscles, which is somewhat medial to the vertical axis. Notice that vector R-B originates *posterolateral* to the vertical axis.

☑ *Depress*
☑ *Abduct*
☑ *Intort*

3. To recapitulate. Contraction of the superior oblique, when the eye starts in the primary position, causes:
   a. A *primary* action to ☐ depress/ ☐ elevate the eye.
   b. A *secondary* action to ☐ adduct/ ☐ abduct/ ☐ elevate the eye.
   c. A *tertiary* action to ☐ intort/ ☐ extort the eye.
4. When the eye is in the primary position, the line of pull of the superior oblique tendon runs *medial* to the vertical axis (arrow in Fig. 4-15*A*). Complete Fig. 4-16 to show the relation of the vertical axis of the eye to the line of pull of the superior oblique tendon when the eye is *adducted.*

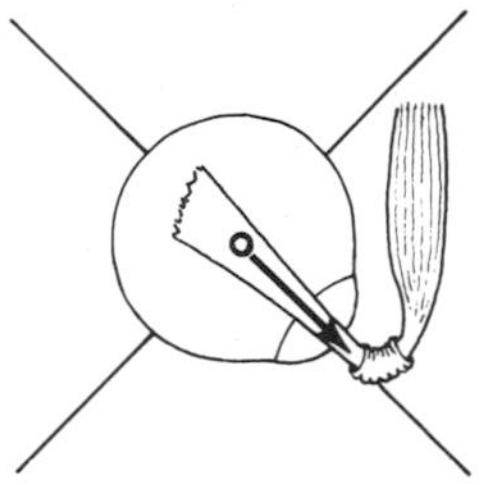

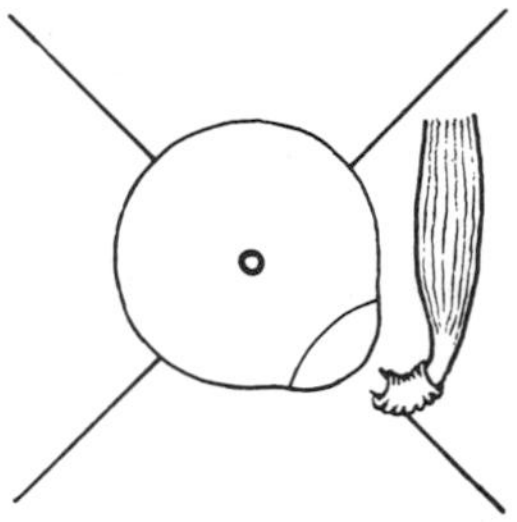

FIG. 4-16. Blank to be completed to show the relation of the vertical axis to the line of pull of the superior oblique tendon when the eye is adducted.

Abduct
Intort

Adduction

In and down

5. When the eye is *adducted,* the line of pull of the tendon of the superior oblique is directly over the vertical axis. Therefore, none of the action of the muscle is dissipated in the other actions which are to ________________ and to ________________ the eye.
6. In what position of the eye does the superior oblique have the strongest *primary* action of downward rotation of the eye? ________________
7. Hence, the clinical test for the strongest action of the superior oblique is to ask the Pt to look ________________________________.

H. Action of the inferior oblique muscle

1. The inferior oblique muscle, in contrast to the other ocular muscles, originates from the medial inferior rim of the bony orbit. It is the only ocular muscle to originate anteriorly. It inserts on the posterior part of the eyeball.

In order to attain sufficient length, it wraps further around the eye than the other muscles.

2. The inferior oblique muscle passes posteriorly, somewhat *medial* to the vertical axis, and its obliquity and alignment with the vertical axis is like that of the superior oblique (Fig. 4-15*C*).

Elevates

Abduction

Extorsion

Abduction

   a. The *primary* action is exactly antagonistic to the superior oblique. The inferior oblique _____ the eye.
   b. The *secondary* action is _____, acting in harmony with the superior oblique.
   c. The *tertiary* action is _____, antagonistic to the superior oblique.
   d. What is the only action in which the superior and inferior oblique could pull with each other?_____

3. The obliques can only abduct strongly after the lateral rectus has already started to rotate the eye laterally. When the lateral rectus is paralyzed, the obliques cannot initiate abduction and the eye cannot be abducted. We run squarely into a problem. Intorsion, the so-called tertiary action of the superior oblique, is clinically one of its most important actions. Therefore, in classifying intorsion as a tertiary action, we do not dismiss it to a negligible action.

I. A vector diagram of ocular muscle action
   1. In the blanks of Fig. 4-17, place the initials of the muscles represented by the vector arrow numbers.

1. LR

2. IR

3. SR

4. MR

5. IO

6. SO

1._____

2._____

3._____

4._____

5._____

6._____

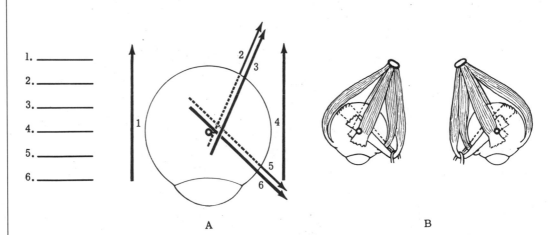

A   B

FIG. 4-17. Eyes, as seen from above. (*A*) Composite vector diagram to show the effective direction of pull of the muscles when the right eye is in the primary position. Fill in blanks 1 to 6 with initials corresponding to the muscle represented by the vectors. (*B*) Composite drawing of all of the ocular rotatory muscles. Match them with the vectors shown in *A*.

2. The vector diagram combined with a knowledge of origin and insertion provides a basis for you to remember forever the actions of the ocular muscles. We can state that when the eye is in the primary position, the pull or vector of all the ocular muscles is *medial* to the vertical axis except for the _____ _____ muscle.

Lateral rectus

3. Because four of the ocular muscles pull "off center," pull *medial* to the vertical axis, they display their particular secondary and tertiary actions. The four muscles that pull off center when the eye is in the primary position are the _____.

Ans: Superior and inferior oblique, and the superior and inferior recti.

TABLE 4-1 Summary of eye movements of individual muscles			
Muscle	Primary action	Secondary	Tertiary
Medial rectus	Adducts		
Lateral rectus	Abducts		
Superior rectus	Elevates	Adducts	Intorts
Inferior rectus	Depresses	Adducts	Extorts
Superior oblique	Depresses	Abducts	Intorts
Inferior oblique	Elevates	Abducts	Extorts

Medial and lateral recti

4. The two muscles that always pull "on center" and therefore have only primary actions are the _____.

5. Cover the answers in Table 4-1 and recite them. Use drawings or the ball model where necessary to deduce the answers.

J. Yoking of ocular muscles

NOTE: If the student did not do sections II.A to J use Table 4-1 and Fig. 4-18 for the following frames.

1. The ocular muscles of the two eyes collaborate with each other to keep the eyes aligned. If a Pt has diplopia on looking to the left, you would suspect weakness of the *ad*ductor of the right eye or the *ab*ductor of the left eye.

   Lateral rectus

   a. The strongest *ab*ductor of the left eye is the muscle whose only function is abduction, the _____ muscle.

   Medial rectus

   b. The strongest *ad*ductor of the right eye is the muscle whose only function is adduction, the _____ muscle.

   c. Those muscles of the two eyes that act in unison for conjugate gaze in any direction are said to be *yoked*.

2. Suppose a Pt complains of diplopia only when he looks *up* and to the *left*.

   Superior rectus

   a. When the left eye is *ab*ducted, the strongest elevator is the _____.

   Adduction
   Intorsion

   b. When the right eye is *ad*ducted the elevating power of its superior rectus is diverted to the secondary action of the muscle, _____, and to the tertiary action of the muscle, _____.

   Inferior oblique

   c. As the superior rectus loses its elevator strength during adduction, another muscle converts its action solely to elevation. That muscle is the _____ _____.

   ☑ *Decreases*
   ☑ *Increases*

   d. During adduction of an eye, the elevator action of the superior rectus ☐ decreases/ ☐ increases, while the elevator action of the inferior oblique simultaneously ☐ decreases/ ☐ increases.

   Superior rectus

   e. Thus for upward gaze to the left, the muscle which elevates the left eye, the _____ muscle, is "yoked" to a muscle of the right eye. The yoked muscle of the right eye which replaces the vanishing elevator action of the right superior rectus, as the eye adducts is the _____ muscle.

   Inferior oblique

   f. Which muscle has the strongest *depressant* action when the eye is adducted? _____

   Superior oblique

   g. Which muscle has the strongest *depressant action* when the eye is abducted? _____

   Inferior rectus

   h. A Pt, looking to the right, has diplopia when he looks down. Which yoked muscles would you suspect of weakness: either the _____ muscle of the right eye or the _____ muscle of the left eye.

   Inferior rectus
   Superior oblique

3. It will now be apparent that the muscles yoked for conjugate eye movements must have *equal* stimulation by the nervous system. Thus, if the right lateral rectus is innervated (stimulated) to rotate the right eye to the right, the left medial rectus is innervated (stimulated) equally. This principle is called *Hering's law* (Ewald Hering, 1834–1918). State Hering's law in your own words.

_____

_____

Ans: During conjugate eye movements, the yoke muscles receive equal innervation (stimulation).

4. *A summary of the yoke muscles.* If you did pages 114–123, complete Fig. 4-18 by reasoning out and writing in the initials of the muscles *most important* for the movement indicated by the arrows. If you did not do those pages, simply copy in the correct initials for reference.

1. SR	4. IO	7. SR
2. LR	5. MR	8. LR
3. IR	6. SO	9. IR

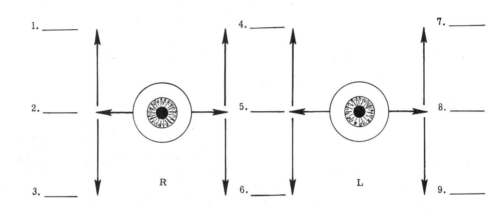

FIG. 4-18. Yoking of strongest actions of ocular muscles in moving the eyes in the cardinal directions of gaze. In blanks 1 to 9, place the initials of the muscle whose strongest action is indicated by the arrow. Then read across the diagram, e.g., 1 to 4 to 7, to see which muscles act in pairs for conjugate eye movements. Thus, in looking to the right and up, the superior rectus muscle (1) of the right eye is yoked with the inferior oblique muscle (4) of the left eye.

K. *Oppositional action of pairs of ocular muscles of one eye and the tonic innervation of the extraocular muscles*

1. The medial and lateral recti of one eye exemplify a general law of the EOMs: the muscles of one eye act in agonist-antagonist pairs. Each movement of the eye in any direction can be counteracted by one or more muscles which act in exactly the opposite direction.

2. An electromyographic needle inserted into the EOMs records a continuous play of muscle contractions, called *tonic innervation.* The contractions continue even with the eyes seemingly at rest, that is, in their *primary position,* looking straight ahead, or when deviated in any direction. All other skeletal muscles are electrically silent when the part they move is at rest.

3. Since each of the agonist-antagonist pairs of EOMs receives a tonic, equal play of nerve impulses, the pull of one muscle balances the pull of the other, like opposing rubber bands under slight tension. Thus, *the position of the eyes is always positively determined.*

4. After paralysis of one EOM, the eye deviates in the direction of pull of the intact, oppositional muscle, which continues to receive its tonic innervation. If the lateral rectus is paralyzed (VIth nerve palsy), the eye will then deviate ☐ medially/ ☐ laterally.

 ☑ *Medially*

L. Review of actions of the extraocular muscles. To insure your understanding of the actions of the EOMs, take a moment to review these points:

1. List the six ocular rotatory muscles and their origin and insertion in relation to the axes of ocular rotation.
2. The muscles (or the tendon in the case of superior oblique) all insert *distal* to the way they approach the globe (Fig. 4-17).
3. Only one muscle, the lateral rectus, has its vector pulling *lateral* to the vertical axis (Fig. 4-17).
4. Only one muscle, the inferior oblique, originates anteriorly.
5. Reason out the position of the eye when only one muscle is paralyzed. The eye turns away from the pull of the paralytic muscle because the intact muscles act unopposed.
6. Reason out the position of the eye when only one muscle is intact.
7. Distinguish between the *possible* movements of the muscle according to the mechanics of origin and insertion, and the *strongest* movements of the muscle when the eye is rotated into the optimum position for the muscle to exert the strongest pull.

III. Clinical tests for ocular malalignment and the range of eye movement

A. Initial inspection of limbus to eyelid relationships

Initially inspect the relation of the limbus to the lid margins as the Pt fixes straight ahead. Gross malalignments of the eyes are readily apparent, but first impressions may be misleading if the lids are asymmetrical, or if the Pt has some degree of canthus dystopia, as do many young children. Proceed with the corneal reflection test, which is the best single bedside method for detecting ocular malalignment.

B. Technique for the corneal light reflection or Hirschberg test

(Use a partner if available, but the instructions assume that you have no partner and will use a hand mirror.)

1. Darken the room and locate a single distant light source such as a light bulb or your otoscope light.
2. Face the light source and gaze straight ahead into the mirror, holding it as far away as possible to avoid convergence. Observe that a single, bright diamond of light reflects off of each cornea. By slight mirror movements try to center these diamonds simultaneously on the two corneas. What is the exact location of the corneal light reflections with respect to the true geometric center of each cornea? _____

Ans: *Generally, after being centered as carefully as possible, the points of corneal light reflection fall slightly medial to the true corneal centers. The reason is that the visual axes do not quite coincide with the geometric anteroposterior axes, which diverge slightly (Fig. 4-19).*

3. While watching your corneal light reflections, move the mirror slightly to one side (or have your partner move his eyes). The points of light reflection from each cornea then displace the same distance from the corneal centers, to end on corresponding corneal points, if ocular alignment is normal in all fields of gaze. Move your mirror around full range, chasing the points of reflection over the surfaces of the corneas and noting the correspondence of the points of each eye.

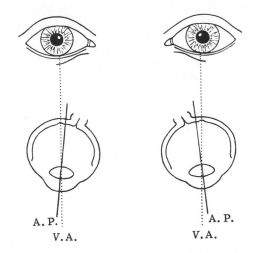

FIG. 4-19. Diagram to show why the corneal light reflections are slightly medial to the true geometric centers of the corneas. The Pt is looking straight ahead at infinite distance. The fixation reflexes have automatically aligned the visual axes parallel to each other, to bring the parallel light rays from infinity onto the foveas. The true, geometric anteroposterior axis of the eyes now diverge slightly. A.P. = anteroposterior axis; V.A. = visual axis.

4. Thus, the examiner (Ex) checks for ocular malalignment in two ways:
   a. Abnormal relation of the corneal limbus to the margins of the eyelids.
   b. Noncorrespondence of the points of corneal light reflection.
5. Why do you look for *non*correspondence of the corneal light reflections and *ab*normality of the limbus relation rather than for correspondence and normality? _____

Ans: As a first principle of physical diagnosis, expect every finding to be abnormal until proved otherwise. If you missed this answer, reread page 32.

C. *Technique for evaluating the range of movement of the eyes*
   1. During the history the Ex judges the range of volitional eye movements.
   2. Commence the examination proper with the Pt sitting. Gently press on top of the Pt's head with one hand, fixing the head in position by a "proprioceptive link" between Ex and Pt, permitting only the eyes to move. Mentally retarded or demented Pts have difficulty separating eye and head movements.
   3. Ask the Pt to fixate on your finger, which you hold up in the midline, about 50 cm away, at station 1 in Fig. 4-20. Request the Pt to follow your finger horizontally with the eyes to station 2, the extreme end of lateral gaze. In

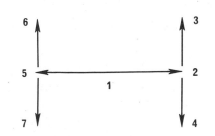

FIG. 4-20. The H is described by the Ex's finger in testing the Pt's ocular motility. The numbers indicate the end stations where the Pt fixes the gaze for the Ex to inspect for malalignment and for nystagmus. The Ex commences inspection with the Pt's eyes at station 1, the primary position.

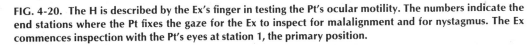

testing *horizontal* eye movements hold the finger *vertically* and in testing *vertical* movements hold the finger *horizontally.* Then the Pt can better appreciate any minimal separation of diplopic images that might occur.

4. Hold the finger at station 2 and inspect the corneal light reflections and the relation of the limbus to lid margins, canthi, and caruncles. Look for nystagmus (discussed in Chap. 5).

5. Next, move to stations 3 and 4 at the extremes of lateral upward and downward gaze. Repeat the observations of step 3.

6. Move your finger back to the horizontal plane and across to station 5, and repeat all observations and maneuvers at 6 and 7.

7. Finally, move your finger back to station 1, basically completing an H-shaped figure (Fig. 4-20). Instruct the Pt, "Look right at my finger," as you move it in to touch the bridge of the Pt's nose, observing for convergence and the accompanying pupilloconstriction. Usually, one eye breaks off of convergence when the finger is several centimeters away from the nose.

8. Fig. 4-21 shows the normal range of eye movements. Notice that upward gaze has the least range. Diffuse brain disease of any type impairs the relatively restricted upward movements before other movements.

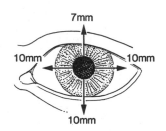

FIG. 4-21. The range of ocular movements as expressed in mm. Upward movement is the most restricted.

9. Since the Pt may have experienced diplopia while observing your finger, ask the Pt about it. Select the best-phrased question:
   a. ☐ You are seeing two fingers in place of one, aren't you?
   b. ☐ Do you have diplopia?
   c. ☐ Did you see one or two fingers?

☑ *c*

10. Students frequently make type 9*a* and 9*b* errors. The first question may force an erroneous answer, since the Pt expects the doctor to know what will happen. The second question uses a technical term unfamiliar to the Pt. What generalization can you make about the phrasing of questions?

_____

_____

_____

Ans: Avoid questions that imply the answer or use technical terms. Ask questions which allow the Pt to report freely, and as exactly as possible, whatever is experienced.

11. If the Pt does complain of diplopia, the Ex darkens the room and watches the corneal light reflections as the Pt pursues a tiny light, such as an otoscope lamp, through the "H" configuration (Fig. 4-20).

D. *The cover-uncover test for ocular malalignment*

1. After inspecting the eyes in the primary position and through the whole range of movement, do the cover-uncover test (Fig. 4-22).

2. Place your thumb between the Pt's eyes, as shown in Fig. 4-22.

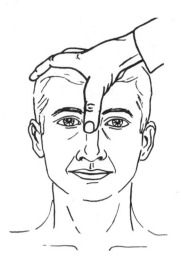

FIG. 4-22. **Resting position of the Ex's thumb for the cover-uncover test.**

3. Instruct the Pt to stare at a distant point. Strongly encourage the Pt to maintain fixation, which is essential.
4. Move the thumb first in front of one eye, then *back to the bridge of the nose* and then over the other eye. You do not have to occlude all vision with your thumb, only *central* vision. You must watch for deviation of *one* or *both* eyes and for noncorrespondence of the corneal light reflections.
5. *Interpretation of the cover-uncover test.* Normally, when both eyes are locked together in fixation, neither eye moves; *the Pt has no ocular malalignment.* If an eye moves when central vision is occluded, the alignment lock of the two eyes is deficient.

E. *The heterotropias: manifest ocular deviations and what to call them*
1. General terms for ocular malalignment are *heterotropia, strabismus,* and *squint.* The ophthalmologist speaks of "heterotropia," the neurologist speaks of "strabismus." The layman speaks of "squints"—or "cross-eye" for convergent strabismus, and "wall-eye" for divergent strabismus. Well, you have to know everyone's lingo.
2. *Definition:* heterotropia (manifest strabismus) is any ocular deviation detected by observing noncorrespondence of the corneal light reflections when the eyes are in any position. This is an ☐ operational/ ☐ interpretational definition.

Ans: ☑ *Operational. Heterotropia is defined in terms of the maneuver or operation by which one can identify it. An operational definition states what operations you do, the actual steps and actions required, to verify something through your own senses.*

a. Suppose we stated that "Heterotropia is any deviation of the visual axis of an eye from the fixation point." This would be an ☐ operational/ ☐ interpretational definition.

Ans: ☑ *Interpretational. This definition, based on an imaginary "visual axis," is an interpretational definition. It does not state the operations by which any observer may personally discover heterotropia.*

b. The physician must clearly distinguish operational from interpretational definitions. Most dictionary definitions uncritically mix operation and interpretation. Suppose you wish to find the length of a meter. Some dictionaries will advise you that a meter is one ten-millionth of the distance between the equator and the poles, measured on a meridian of the Earth.

Well, don't try to pace that off! That obviously *interprets* the length of a meter. Try this definition: a meter is the distance between two transverse lines on a platinum-iridium bar kept at the National Bureau of Standards, when the bar is at 0°C. The operation required to discover the length of a meter is implicit in the definition. What you do is to observe the distance between the two lines and mark it off on your own bar. Now that simple operation enables you to derive or verify and actually experience the length of a meter. In other words, if you do *this,* you will find out *that.*

    c. As operationally defined by the best test for it, heterotropia means any manifest ocular deviation detected by _____

_____

Ans: Inspecting the eyes for noncorrespondence of the corneal light reflections.

3. The heterotropias are named according to the direction of deviation of the errant eye:

    Exotropia: eye deviates outward (laterally)
    Esotropia: eye deviates inward (medially)
    Hypertropia: eye deviates upward
    Hypotropia: eye deviates downward

☑ *Out*
Exotropia
Right esotropia

4. To give the full name, designate the right or left eye. Thus, left exotropia means that the left eye deviates ☐ in/ ☐ out/ ☐ up/ ☐ down.
5. If both eyes deviate outward, the Pt would have bilateral _____.
6. If the right eye deviates inward, the Pt would have _____.
7. The Pts in Fig. 4-23*A* to *D* were asked to fixate straight ahead in each case. In designating whether the right or left eye is affected, remember that you are facing the Pt. In all of the ocular illustrations, the eyes will face you or be faced downward on the page to simulate the actual circumstance of looking at a Pt.

  F. Analysis of the cover-uncover test in monocular heterotropia

    1. Commence with Fig. 4-24*A,* step 1. Notice that step 1 is at the *bottom* of the figure. The Pt was instructed to look straight ahead. Being allowed free

A. R esotropia

B. L esotropia

C. L exotropia

D. R hypertropia

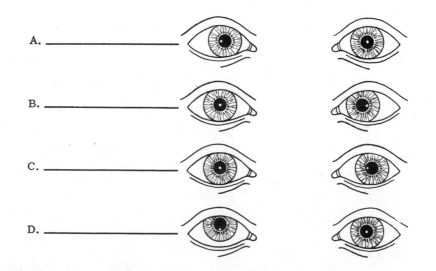

A. _____

B. _____

C. _____

D. _____

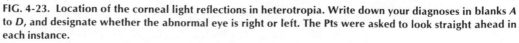

FIG. 4-23. Location of the corneal light reflections in heterotropia. Write down your diagnoses in blanks *A* to *D*, and designate whether the abnormal eye is right or left. The Pts were asked to look straight ahead in each instance.

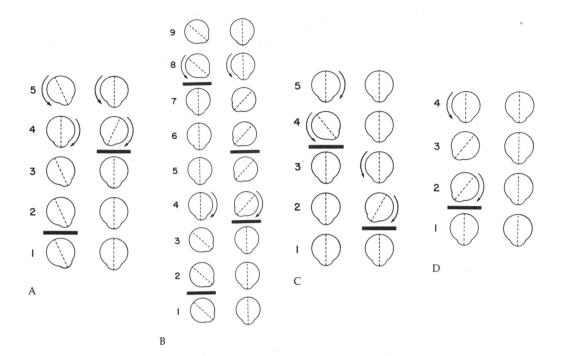

FIG. 4-24A–D. Results of the cover-uncover test for ocular malalignment. See text for explanation. *(After Jampolsky, 1964.)*

☑ *Right esotropia*

vision, the Pt fixates with his left eye, his dominant eye. This Pt appears to have the ocular malalignment called ☐ right/ ☐ left _____.

2. In step 2, the Ex's thumb occludes central vision of the right eye. The ocular alignment of neither eye changes.
3. In step 3, the Ex replaces the thumb on the bridge of the Pt's nose. The eyes maintain the same angulation of the visual axes.
4. In step 4, the Ex reinstructed the Pt to maintain fixation on the original distant point, and covered the Pt's left eye. The Pt's right eye then shifts to bring the central light ray onto the fovea, and the left eye rotates inward. (This inward movement will be explained later.)
5. In step 5, the Ex replaces the thumb on the bridge of the Pt's nose. The eyes shift to return fixation to the dominant left eye.
6. A Pt with right exotropia instead of esotropia would show a similar sequence of events. If you would like, draw the events of right exotropia alongside Fig. 4-24*A*, steps 1 to 5. In any event, go back through Fig. 4-24*A* without using the instructions in the text.
7. Suppose the Pt in Fig. 4-24*A*, step 1, had diplopia when looking straight ahead.

☑ *Nasal*

   a. The parallel rays from a distant object would strike the ☐ nasal/ ☐ temporal side of the retina of the right eye.

☑ *Right*

   b. Then the visual image would be projected by the mind into the field which would normally stimulate the nasal side of the retina. Thus, the false image would be projected to the ☐ right/ ☐ left of the true image.

G. *Analysis of the cover-uncover test in alternating heterotropia*

☑ *Right esotropia*

1. Work through Fig. 4-24*B*. In step 2 the Pt ostensibly has the ocular malalignment called ☐ right/ ☐ left _____.
2. Subsequent steps in Fig. 4-24*B* show that the Pt alternates fixation. In step 1 the Pt fixates with the left eye, and in step 5 the Pt fixates with the right

Esotropia

Alternating exotropia

eye. Since the right and left eyes alternately deviate inward, the heterotropia is called *alternating* _____.

3. Work through Fig. 4-24*B*, imagining that the Pt's eyes deviated out rather than in. This heterotropia would be called _____ _____.

H. *The cover-uncover test for heterophorias, the latent rather than the manifest ocular deviations.*

1. When a normal person looks at infinity, the visual axes are parallel. The two retinal images "fuse" into one mental image. Binocular vision requires fusion of central vision and is developed with maturation of the infant. Fusion-fixation reflexes operate to keep both eyes "on target" whenever the normal person's eyes are open. In some Pts, the eyes appear straight during preliminary testing, and show normal motility, but when central vision is covered in one eye, the eye deviates. When the cover is removed, reestablishing central vision, the fusion-fixation reflexes immediately realign the eye. Ocular deviations appearing *only* when central vision is blocked and disappearing when central vision is reestablished are called *heterophorias*.

Heterotropia
Heterophoria
Block (cover)

2. An ocular deviation apparent when the Pt is permitted free central vision is called <u>hetero</u>_____, while a deviation apparent *only* when central vision is occluded is called <u>hetero</u>_____.

3. The critical operation of the cover-uncover test is to _____ central vision.

4. What maneuver must always restore ocular alignment to distinguish heterophoria from heterotropia? _____

Ans: *Uncovering the occluded eye.*

☑ *Esophoria*

Esotropia

Exophoria

Hyperphoria

5. *Inward* deviation or *adduction* of the eye only during occlusion of central vision is called ☐ exophoria/ ☐ hyperphoria/ ☐ esophoria.

6. Manifest inturning of an eye when the Pt has free central vision is called _____.

7. *Abduction* of an eye *only* during occlusion of central vision is called _____.

8. Upward deviation of an eye *only* during occlusion of central vision is called _____.

9. Mnemonic: if you have trouble keeping your *t*ropias and *ph*orias straight, try to remember *t* for *t*ropia for manifes*t*ly *t*urned eye.

10. Fig. 4-24*C* depicts the cover-uncover test in heterophoria. Work through it. The latent deviation in Fig. 4-24*C* is called alternating _____.

Ans: *Esophoria. (Since esophoria virtually always involves both eyes, the adjective <u>alternating</u> is usually eliminated.)*

☑ *Right esotropia*

☑ *Intermittent*

a. Suppose in step 5 of Fig. 4-24*C* that the right eye had not returned to proper alignment on removal of the cover. Such a manifest inward deviation, not corrected all of the time by central vision, would be called ☐ right/ ☐ left _____.

b. If one of the Pt's eyes aligns sometimes when the cover is removed, but does not align at other times, the condition is called ☐ intermittent/ ☐ alternating heterotropia.

11. Complete the definitions in *a* and *b* by stating the clinical maneuvers that disclose heterophoria and heterotropia.

☑ *Manifest*

    a. Heterotropia is a ☐ manifest/ ☐ latent ocular deviation detected by inspection for _____

_____

_____ .

Ans: Noncorresponding corneal light reflections and abnormal relation of the corneal limbus to the eyelid margins.

☑ *Latent*

    b. Heterophoria is a ☐ manifest/ ☐ latent ocular deviation detected by _____

_____ .

Ans: Seeing the eye shift when its central vision is blocked during the cover-uncover test.

12. Now try to name the abnormality in Fig. 4-24*D*. Pay particular attention to step 3. Since the Pt starts and finishes with apparently straight eyes, the deviation of one eye is only intermittent. Therefore, the abnormality in Fig. 4-24*D* is called _____

_____ .

Ans: Intermittent right exotropia.

13. The abnormality in Fig. 4-24*D* is a *tropia* rather than a *phoria* because

_____

_____ .

Ans: The right eye remained manifestly deviated even after restoration of central vision.

  I. Clinical classification of heterotropia

    1. *Introduction.* To determine the cause of heterotropia, try to classify it into one of two types:

      a. The *paralytic* type, caused by a neuromuscular lesion.

      b. The *nonparalytic* type, usually caused by lesions which impair central vision in one eye and therefore impair fixation: refractive errors, opacification of the cornea or lens (refracting media), or macular lesions.

    2. *Effect of paralytic heterotropia caused by nerve or muscle lesions on yoke muscles*

☑ *Away from*

      a. When an ocular muscle is paretic or paralytic, the intact muscles act unopposed. Hence, the eye deviates ☐ away from/ ☐ toward the direction of pull of the afflicted muscle.

☑ *Increase*

      b. When the Pt looks in the direction of pull of the afflicted muscle, the normal eye moves more than the afflicted eye. Hence, the degrees of heterotropia and diplopia ☐ increase/ ☐ decrease when the Pt looks in the direction of action of the afflicted muscle.

☑ *Left*

      c. When turning in the direction of pull of the afflicted muscle, the *weak* eye rotates too little, while the *normal* eye may rotate too far. With a lateral rectus paralysis on the *right,* the Pt's ☐ right/ ☐ left eye would adduct too far when the Pt looks to the right. Explain this result by Hering's law._____

_____

See <u>d</u>

      d. According to Hering's law, the nervous system stimulates the yoke muscles equally. If a muscle is weak, the Pt automatically overstimulates in an attempt to rotate the afflicted eye. The normal yoke muscle receives the same excessive stimulus and contracts too strongly.

      e. *Use of the cover-uncover test in the analysis of neuromuscular heterotropia.* Study Scobee's lucid description to understand *primary* and *secondary* deviation of the eyes when the paretic and sound eye are alternately covered or uncovered.

Primary deviation *is the deviation of the eye with the paretic muscle when the sound eye is fixing. Secondary deviation is the deviation of the sound eye when the eye with the paretic muscle is fixing. In paresis, secondary deviation is greater than primary deviation.*

As an example of primary deviation, suppose the left lateral rectus is paretic, right eye dominant, and the patient fixes upon some object straight ahead with the right eye. The right medial rectus and the right lateral rectus are normal muscles and require but a normal innervation to maintain fixation with the right eye. According to Hering's law, similar normal innervations go to the yoke muscles of the right lateral rectus and the right medial rectus—to the left medial rectus and the left lateral rectus. The left lateral rectus is paretic and responds in subnormal fashion to normal stimuli; the left medial rectus is normal and thus not properly opposed by the subnormal tonus of its paretic antagonist. The left medial rectus will, therefore, seem to overact since it will pull the left eye inward toward the nose in adduction. The deviation produced is small but definite and is a left esotropia. This is deviation of the paretic eye with the sound eye fixing—primary deviation.

As an example of secondary deviation, suppose the left lateral rectus is paretic, left eye dominant, and the patient fixes upon some object straight ahead with the dominant left eye. The left lateral rectus, in order to perform its usual functions, must be excessively innervated because it is paretic; its yoke muscle, the right medial rectus, receives the same excessive innervation according to Hering's law. The right medial rectus is a normal muscle receiving an excessive innervation and it makes an excessive response, pulling the right eye well inward in adduction. This is a deviation of the sound eye with the paretic eye's fixing—secondary deviation. In paresis, secondary deviation is greater than primary deviation and the reason should now be obvious.

Richard Scobee

3. *Effect of neuromuscular heterotropia on head position*
   a. The Pt with heterotropia tends to compensate for an afflicted muscle by turning or tilting his head. The head posture compensates for or keeps the eyes in such a position as to avoid the action of the affected muscle. Thus, with a right superior oblique palsy, the Pt has weakness of ☐ intorsion/ ☐ extorsion of the right eye, an action for which the superior oblique is mainly responsible.

☑ *Intorsion*

   b. The unopposed action of the extortors would cause the eye to be in a position of extorsion. In compensation, therefore, the Pt with a right superior oblique palsy tilts his head to the ☐ right/ ☐ left to prevent diplopia.
   (If the answer is unclear, review Fig. 4-14.)

☑ *Left*

   c. A persistent head tilt is called *torticollis.* Oblique muscle palsy is only one of its many causes.
4. *Effect of heterotropia on vision in infants*—suppression amblyopia (amblyopia exanopsia)
   a. Infants with heterotropia learn to suppress the image from the errant eye. If suppression continues for the first years of life, the Pt ultimately becomes completely blind in the deviating eye, even though the retina and visual pathways are structurally intact. So strong are the suppressive forces that rid the visual image of confusing elements that the child can rarely regain vision, after suppression blindness has set in.
   b. This *suppression amblyopia* (amblyopia ex anopsia) is a preventable

cause of monocular blindness, treated by the simple expedient of placing a patch intermittently over the sound eye to require the Pt to use the errant eye. Suppression amblyopia occurs not only with heterotropia but also with many monocular disorders of retinal image formation—refractive errors, opacification of the refracting media, or retinal lesions. Never neglect ocular deviations or other impediments to vision because of a naive expectation that the infant will simply grow "out" of it. The infant may grow more and more "into" it. Do a complete ocular and funduscopic examination on every infant, and refer the Pt for ophthalmologic or neurologic consultation.

J. *Nonparalytic or concomitant heterotropias*

1. With muscular paresis or paralysis, the eyes do not move concomitantly— one eye moves *more* or *less* than the other. Hence, we can classify paralytic heterotropia as *nonconcomitant*. In *concomitant heterotropia* or nonparalytic heterotropia, the eyes are malaligned at rest, but upon movement, they retain the same malalignment, the same degree of deviant angulation.

☑ *Concomitant*

2. If the eyes maintain the same degree of deviation in all directions of gaze, the heterotropia is ☐ concomitant/ ☐ nonconcomitant.
3. Concomitant heterotropia may be intermittent, but when present, the deviation is the same in all directions of gaze. What happens to the angulation of the eyes in heterotropia due to neuromuscular lesions, when the eyes move? _____
_____
_____

Ans: The angle of deviation of the two eyes increases when the eyes move in the direction of action of the afflicted muscle.

4. The cause of concomitant heterotropia is usually a disturbance in image formation in one macula—cloudiness of the cornea, a severe refractive error, a cataract, or a macular lesion. In some cases, it is as if a new macula is established, off center from the true macula, and then the visual axis is aligned on the new macula. The Pt alternates in fixating with the normal eye and the abnormal one, but the angle of deviation remains fixed. The Pt learns to suppress vision from whichever eye is not in use at the moment for fixation, much as you can learn to use a monocular microscope or an opthalmoscope with both eyes open. Thus, the Pt alternately fixes with one eye and suppresses vision from the other eye. When fixation alternates between the two eyes, suppression amblyopia does not occur.

5. *The clinical characteristics of concomitant heterotropia*

☑ *Same*

   a. The deviation of the ocular axes is ☐ the same/ ☐ different for the primary position and in all directions of gaze.
   b. In contrast to nonconcomitant heterotropia, the primary and secondary deviations disclosed by the cover-uncover test are ☐ equal/ ☐ unequal in concomitant heterotropia.

Ans: ☑ Equal. (If they weren't equal at all times the Pt would have nonconcomitant heterotropia.)

   c. When either eye fixates alone, it shows a full range of motility. None of the individual muscles is paralyzed.

☑ *Nonconcomitant*

6. The term *paralytic heterotropia* is essentially synonymous with ☐ concomitant/ ☐ nonconcomitant heterotropia.

Concomitant

7. The term *nonparalytic* heterotropia is essentially synonymous with _____ heterotropia.

P	N-P
√	
	√
√	
	√
	√
√	
√	

TABLE 4-2 Differential diagnosis of paralytic and nonparalytic heterotropia*		
1	2	3
Paralytic (nonconcomitant)	Nonparalytic (concomitant)	Clinical characteristic
		Ocular deviation changes with eye movement
		Full movement when each eye is tested after covering the other
		Secondary deviation greater than primary
		Secondary and primary deviations equal
		Frequently has opacity or severe refractive error in one eye
		Has diplopia if heterotropia comes on after early age
		Often has compensatory head turning or tilting

*The rules given here cover the majority of the cases. When heterotropia is of long standing, fibrosis and contracture of the affected muscles may change the deviation patterns given here. Other confounding factors are eccentric fixation and fusional problems at the cortical level.

8. Complete Table 4-2 by making a check in the left-hand columns (1 and 2) if the characteristic in column 3 applies.

K. *The laws of diplopia and the clinical analysis of diplopia*
1. Repeat the canthal compression experiment and obtain diplopia with the finger vertical. Move the finger to the right and left, studying the distance between the true and false images. You should find a null point straight ahead where the images are virtually superimposed. Identify the false image by its haziness. This is one law of diplopia: *the aberrant or "false" image is always hazier than the "true" image.*
   a. If the false image projects to the *right* of the finger, the distance between the images increases as you move the finger to the ☐ right/ ☐ left side.
   b. If the false image projects to the *left,* the distance between the images increases as you move to the _____ side.
   c. If you follow the images too far laterally, one disappears. Can you discover an explanation (look for the simplest one). _____

☑ *Right (Fig. 4-6)*

Left

Ans: The nose blocks the light rays from entering one eye.

2. As you move your finger away from the midpoint, the distance between the true and false images ☐ increases/ ☐ decreases/ ☐ stays the same. Go to the next frame for the explanation, unless you would like to try to work it out yourself.

☑ *Increases*

3. *Explanation for the increasing distance between the diplopic images*
   a. In Fig. 4-25A, the left eye, aligned on target, receives the real image on its fovea. The mind projects the visual image back to the true target position (T1). The deviated right eye receives the real image on the nasal side of the fovea. The mind projects the visual image to the right of the true target position (F1).
   b. In Fig. 4-25B, the mobile left eye follows the target to the right (T2). The paralytic right eye remains imprisoned in its original position, and

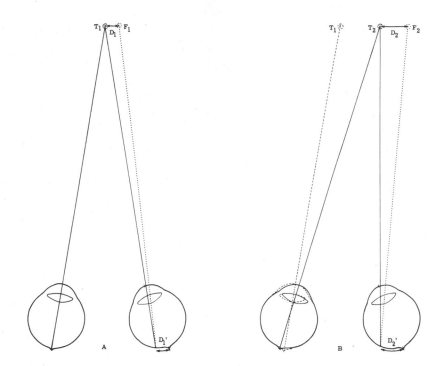

FIG. 4-25. Illustration of a law of diplopia—the distance between the true and false images increases when the Pt looks in the direction of projection of the false image. T1 = true image; F1 = false image; D1 = distance 1; D2 = distance 2.

as the target moves rightward, the real image moves leftward (nasally) on the retina. The mind projects the visual image more and more rightward. Thus D2 > D1.

4. No matter which way the false image deviates, it moves away from the true image. The true image remains centered on target. This is another law of diplopia: *the false image is projected peripheral to the true image.*

5. If the false image is to the right of the true image, as in Fig. 4-25*A*, the eye is deviated to the left (or has not rotated sufficiently to the right). The false image projects in the ☐ same/ ☐ opposite direction as eye deviation.

   a. If the false image projects *above* the true image, the afflicted eye is deviated ☐ upward/ ☐ downward.

   b. If the false image is to the *left,* the afflicted eye is deviated to the ☐ right/ ☐ left.

6. This is another law of diplopia: *the false image projects in the* ☐ same/ ☐ opposite *direction as the direction of eye deviation.*

7. In Fig. 4-25, with projection of the false image to the right, the right eye has failed to abduct to center its visual axis on target. Thus, the diagram simulates paralysis of the _____ _____ muscle.

8. This is another law of diplopia: *the false image projects* ☐ toward/ ☐ away from *the of action of the paretic muscle.* Thus when the Pt looks in the direction of action of the paretic muscle, the distance between the diplopic images ☐ increases/ ☐ decreases.

9. State the four laws of diplopia in respect to image projection.

   a. The law stating whether the true or false image is the sharpest. _____

   _____

   b. The law of peripheral projection. _____

   _____

   c. The law of projection opposite to the eye deviation. _____

   _____

☑ *Opposite*

☑ *Downward*

☑ *Right*

☑ *Opposite*

Lateral rectus

☑ *Toward*

☑ *Increases*

Frame K.1

Frame K.4

Frame K.6

Frame K.8

    d. The law relating the false image to the pull of the paretic muscle. ____
_____

10. It should now be clear that the use of the corneal light reflection test and the laws of diplopia, permit you to diagnose the faulty muscle. You need not memorize these laws, since you can recover them whenever needed by pressing on your lateral canthus, the Aladdin's lamp for diplopia.

L. *A summary of the procedures for testing a Pt who has diplopia*
    1. *Observe the corneal light reflections.* Observe them when the eyes are straight ahead and when they are held in the various directions of gaze.
    2. *Identify the position of maximum diplopia.* As you move your finger or examining light through all fields of gaze, have the Pt report when the two images are maximally separated. A colored glass placed over one eye helps to keep track of the two images during motility testing. The point of maximum separation identifies the action of the weak muscle.
    3. *Identify the eye which produces the false image.* The eye which produces the false image has the faulty muscle. The false image is the peripheral image. It is identified by occluding vision alternately in the two eyes. When the normal eye is occluded, the sharp, central image disappears. When the abnormal eye is occluded, the hazy, peripheral image disappears.
    4. *Reason out the muscle responsible for the deficient ocular action.*

M. *Analyze these Pts*
    1. This Pt complains of double vision on looking to the left. Testing discloses that image separation is greatest on left lateral gaze.

Medial rectus
Lateral rectus

      a. The muscles pairs responsible for left lateral gaze are the _____ _____ muscle of the right eye, and the _____ _____ muscle of the left eye.

☑ *Left*
☑ *Left lateral rectus*

      b. On occlusion of the right eye, the central image ("true" image) disappears. On occlusion of the left eye the peripheral image ("false" image) disappears. Therefore, the afflicted eye is the ☐ left/ ☐ right eye and the afflicted muscle is the ☐ right/ ☐ left _____ _____ muscle.

    2. This Pt complains of double vision when looking up. The images separate the most when the Pt looks up and to the left.

Superior rectus
Inferior oblique

      a. This direction of gaze is achieved by the _____ _____ muscle of the left eye and the _____ muscle of the right eye.

☑ *Left*
☑ *Left superior rectus*

      b. On occlusion of the right eye, the central image disappears. On occlusion of the left eye, the peripheral image disappears. Therefore, the afflicted eye is the ☐ right/ ☐ left and the afflicted muscle left is the ☐ right/ ☐ left _____ _____.

      c. Common causes of diplopia on vertical gaze are orbital trauma, hyperthyroidism, myasthenia gravis, neoplastic infiltration or inflammation of the orbit, and IIId or IVth nerve lesions.

IV. Refraction and accommodation

A. *Refraction by negative and positive lenses*
    1. To understand lenses, start with a prism. The law of the prism is that *it bends light rays toward its base* (Fig. 4-26*A*).

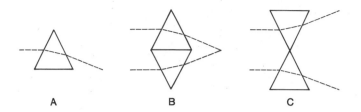

FIG. 4-26. The law of the prism states that a prism deflects light rays towards its base. Two prisms with bases *in* make a converging (positive) lens, or bases *out,* a diverging (negative) lens.

> *a.* Two prisms, placed base *in,* form a *positive* or *converging* lens (Fig. 4-26*B*).
>
> *b.* Two prisms, placed base *out,* form a *negative* or *diverging* lens (Fig. 4-26*C*).
>
> *c.* Rounding of the sides of the prism into the familiar lens shape reduces chromatic and spherical aberration.
>
> 2. In bending light rays, a prism or lens bends violet light more than red, thus causing *chromatic* aberration because the rays do not fall on one focal point, but are spread out. Any defect in the curvature of the lens causes *spherical* aberration (astigmatism).
>
> 3. A pinhole aperture screens out the more peripheral light rays, which must undergo more refraction than the central rays, thus reducing chromatic and spherical aberration (Fig. 4-27*D*).

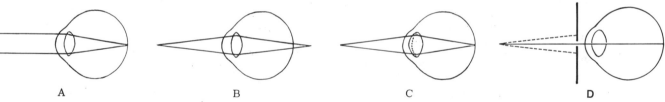
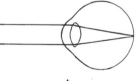

FIG. 4-27. Schematic cross sections of the eye to show the focal point of light rays in various conditions of refraction. (*A*) Emmetropic eye. Parallel rays from a distant object focus on the retina. (*B*) Emmetropic eye in which no adjustment has been made to accommodate for near vision. The light rays from the near point diverge as they travel to the eye, and they focus behind the retina. (*C*) Emmetropic eye accommodated for near vision. The lens has thickened, increasing its power of refraction. The divergent rays now focus upon, rather than behind, the retina. (*D*) A pinhole allows only the central light ray to enter the eye. The peripheral rays, which require refraction, are blocked.

> *B. Light refraction by the normal eye.* The refracting media of the eye includes the cornea and lens. Study refraction by the emmetropic (normal) eye in Fig. 4-27*A–C.*
>
> *C. The accommodation reflex*
>
> 1. Accommodation for near vision requires three actions and three muscles.
>
> > *a.* The eyes converge to aim the visual axes onto the near fixation point, an action accomplished by the medial rectus muscles (Fig. 4-3).
> >
> > *b.* As the eyes converge, the sphincter action of the *pupilloconstrictor* muscle of the iris causes cormiosis (pinhole effect, Fig. 4-27*D*), reducing spherical and chromatic aberration.
> >
> > *c.* The third action is thickening of the lens, increasing its ability to refract the more divergent rays from the near fixation point. Contraction of the *ciliary muscle,* a sphincter, relaxes the suspensory ligament of the lens, allowing it to thicken by its natural elasticity.

TABLE 4-3 The accommodation reflex and the muscles that accomplish it	
List the three events of the accommodation reflex	List the responsible muscles
	(skeletal)
	(smooth)
	(smooth)

Convergence; medial recti

Cormiosis; pupilloconstrictor muscle

Lens thickening; ciliary muscle

2. Thus, during accommodation for near vision, three distinct events occur: the visual axes _____ onto the fixation point, the pupils _____, and the lenses _____.

Ans: Converge, constrict, thicken

3. Although volition initiates the act of looking at a near object, neural mechanisms lock the three events of accommodation into a single *accommodation reflex.* Thus, whenever a person voluntarily converges the eyes, neural circuits automatically cause pupilloconstriction and lens thickening. Complete Table 4-3.

D. *Myopia and hyperopia*
1. Learn Fig. 4-28.
2. A person with sharp vision for far away *and* close objects is ☑ emmetropic/ ☐ myopic/ ☐ hyperopic.
3. For far vision, the emmetropic person's muscles of accommodation are ☐ active/ ☐ relaxed.
4. A person with sharp vision for far objects, but blurred vision for close

☑ *Emmetropic*

☑ *Relaxed*

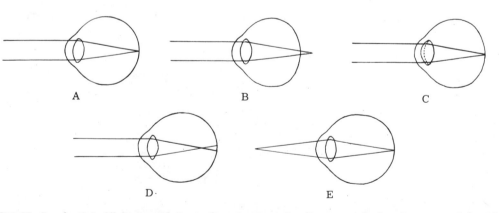

FIG. 4-28. Focal point of light rays relative to the anteroposterior diameter and refractive power of the eye. (*A*) *Emmetropia.* The diameter of the normal eye is proper relative to its refracting power. Parallel rays from a distant source focus on the retina without accommodation. Divergent rays from a near source require lens thickening in order to be focused on the retina. (*B*) *Hyperopia.* The diameter of the eye is too short relative to its refracting power. Parallel rays focus behind the retina. (*C*) *Hyperopia with accommodation.* The lens of the hyperopic eye must thicken, increasing its focusing power, to bring parallel rays to focus on the retina. When looking at a near object, the hyperopic person has no accommodation reserve. (*D*) *Myopia.* The diameter of the eye is too long relative to its refracting power. Parallel rays focus in front of the retina. (*E*) *Myopic eye focusing on near object.* Divergent rays from the near object focus properly on the retina with little or no accommodation.

☑ *Hyperopia*
☑ *Behind* (*Fig. 4-28B*)

☑ *When looking at close and far objects*

☑ *Myopia*

☑ *In front of*

objects, is said to be "farsighted." The technical term for farsightedness is ☐ emmetropia/ ☐ myopia/ ☐ hyperopia.

5. The hyperopic eye focuses parallel rays ☐ behind/ ☐ in front of/ ☐ upon the retina.
   a. The hyperopic Pt requires some activity of the accommodation reflex to thicken the lens ☐ only when viewing far objects/ ☐ only when viewing close objects/ ☐ when looking at close and far objects.
   b. Normally, however, the accommodation reflex should be active only during near vision. The hyperopic Pt requires some degree of accommodation at all times, to bring the focal point forward onto the retina.
6. A person with blurred vision for distant objects, but sharp vision for near objects is "nearsighted." The technical term for nearsightedness is ☐ emmetropia/ ☐ myopia/ ☐ hyperopia.
   a. The myopic eye focuses parallel rays from far objects ☐ in front of/ ☐ upon/ ☐ behind the retina.
   b. Which of the three events of the accommodation reflex actually work against the myopic Pt who is attempting to look at a near object?

   _____

   Explain: _____

Ans: Lens thickening works against the myope. The near object's rays diverge more before striking the lens and therefore move the focal point backwards, nearer the desired focal point on the retina. Lens thickening, however, moves the focal point <u>forward</u>.

7. On scrap paper, draw three eyeballs and show the focal point of parallel rays in emmetropia, hyperopia, and myopia. Compare with Fig. 4-28*A*, *B*, and *D*.

E. *Relation of refractive errors to heterotropia and heterophoria.*
(To be done only if optional section H, page 130, was completed.)
1. During the first several months of life, infants must develop binocular fixation and fuse the images from the two eyes. Adding to the relatively poor vision of the infant is the fact that the A-P diameter of the eyeball is too short relative to its refracting power. With maturation, the eyeball expands.

☑ *Hyperopic*

Myopic

2. Since the infant's eyeballs tend to be too short in relation to the focal point of the lens, the infant is ☐ myopic/ ☐ emmetropic/ ☐ hyperopic.
3. As the eyeball increases in diameter with maturation, the hyperopia tends to change to emmetropia. If the child is emmetropic at birth instead of hyperopic, he would become _____ as the diameter of the eye increases with growth.
4. Because of the small diameter of the eyeball relative to the focusing power of the lens, infants tend to keep their lenses thickened. In other words, they tend to accommodate all of the time. As the maturing infant or young child turns its attention to the close, detailed inspection of near objects, extra demands are placed on accommodation. The need for accommodation may overcome the hyperopic child's capacity for it.

☑ *Esophoria*

Esotropia

   a. Since one of the accommodation mechanisms is convergence of the eyes, the hyperopic child at first will show only a latent tendency to crossing of the eyes, which would be called ☐ esotropia/ ☐ esophoria.
   b. If the hyperopia is severe, the esophoria may convert to a manifest internal deviation of an eye, which would be called _____.
   c. Thus, refractive errors or neuromuscular lesions may cause crossed eyes. Two eyelid anomalies in children may give a spurious appearance of crossed eyes because the medial margin of the limbus appears to be too

close to the medial eyelid margins. These anomalies are _____ and _____.

Ans: Dystopic canthi and epicanthal folds (Fig. 1-6).

✓ *More*

✓ *Drift apart*

Exophoria; exotropia

✓ *Hyperopia*

✓ *Myopia*

✓ *Myope*

5. Consider the infant who is going to be myopic at maturity. As his eyeball enlarges with age, he becomes ☐ more/ ☐ less myopic. Therefore the nervous system adjusts by reducing accommodation.
    a. With an underactive accommodation mechanism, the child's eyes would tend to ☐ drift apart/ ☐ converge too much.
    b. At first the child might show only a latent tendency to drift apart, which would be called _____ or later, if manifest, _____.
6. Tropias and phorias commonly accompany refractive errors.
    a. Esophoria or esotropia in a child would raise the question of the refractive error called ☐ myopia/ ☐ emmetropia/ ☐ hyperopia.
    b. Exophoria or exotropia in a child would raise the question of ☐ myopia/ ☐ emotropia,/ ☐ hyperopia.
7. Which child would complain of increasing inability to read the chalkboard at school, requiring differentiation of neurologic and ophthalmologic causes for blurred vision, the ☐ myope or ☐ hyperope?

F. *Presbyopia, blurred vision, myopia, and hyperopia*
    1. At around 42 years of age, normal adults experience blurred vision when they try to read newsprint or look at near objects. The differential diagnosis then involves a neurologic versus an ophthalmologic disorder.
    2. The usual cause is *presbyopia,* the loss of elasticity of the lens due to aging. The lens will no longer thicken to increase its refractive power during accommodation. When this happens, the Pt will lose the ability to see close objects, particularly newsprint.
        a. Who would suffer blurred near vision from presbyopia first and more severely, the *hyperope* or the *myope.* Explain: _____

Ans: The presbyopic hyperope suffers first and more severely from blurred near vision, because the hyperope is already straining the accommodation mechanism. Any loss of elasticity will reduce refraction and thus reduce the ability to see close objects. The myope doesn't need much accommodation and therefore doesn't suffer much when it fails.

        b. Would placing a pinhole in front of the eye of the presbyopic hyperope improve near vision and would it help in differentiating loss of visual acuity due to presbyopia from loss due to a lesion of the macula or optic nerve? Explain: _____

Ans: A pinhole will block off the more peripheral rays from the near object, thus allowing only the central rays to reach the retina. The pinhole thus becomes a tiny pupil, tinier than that obtainable by normal pupilloconstriction. The pinhole eliminates the need to increase refraction by lens thickening. Hence restoration of visual acuity by the pinhole proves that the disorder is one of refraction, not a retinal or optic nerve lesion.

    3. *The parallax test for positive or negative corrective lenses*
        a. The *parallax test* provides a quick way to test whether the Pt's glasses correct for hyperopia or myopia. For the parallax test, hold the glasses over any visual target, such as a vertical line, and move the glasses to the right and left alternately.
        b. If the lens is *divergent (negative),* the line will appear to move *in the direction* that you move the glasses. Myopia requires a *divergent* or *neg-*

☑ *Backward*

ative lens to move the focal point ☐ backward/ ☐ forward onto the retina.

    c. If the lens is *convergent (positive)*, the line will appear to move in the *opposite* direction to the movement of the glasses. Hyperopia requires a *convergent* or *positive* lens to bring the focal point ☐ backward/ ☐ forward onto the retina.

☑ *Forward*

4. Now to prove that you understand all of the foregoing, answer this question: why does a presbyopic myope remove his glasses to read newsprint, while a presbyopic hyperope (who previously had fairly adequate accommodation) puts his glasses on to read but removes them for far vision. The question, put in another form, is which, the presbyopic myope or the presbyopic hyperope, benefits from half-frame positive or bifocal lens?

Ans: At some point, the teacher and the text must fade away. The text contains the answer. Search it out.

SUGGESTED READING FOR OCULAR MOTILITY AND STRABISMUS

Bajandas FJ, Cline LB: *Neuro-ophthalmology Review Manual* (2d ed). Slack, New Jersey, 1987.

Burger L, Kalvin N, Smith J: Acquired lesions of the fourth cranial nerve. *Brain,* 1970; 93:567–574.

Davson H: *The Eye,* vol 3, *Muscular Mechanisms* (2d ed). New York, Academic, 1969.

Glaser JS: *Neuro-ophthalmology* (2d ed). Philadelphia, Lippincott, 1990.

Helveston EM: A two-step test for diagnosing paresis of a single vertically acting extraocular muscle. *Am J Ophthal,* 1967; 64:914–915.

Helveston EM, Ellis FD: *Pediatric Ophthalmology Practice,* (2d ed). St. Louis, CV Mosby, 1984.

Jampolsky A: Strabismus, in Holt, L. (ed): *Pediatric Ophthalmology.* Philadelphia, Lea & Febiger, 1964.

Miller NR: *Walsh and Hoyt's Clinical Neuro-ophthalmology* (4th ed). Baltimore, Williams & Wilkins, 1982.

Reinecke R, Miller D: *Strabismus. A Programmed Text* (3d ed). New York, Appleton-Century-Crofts, 1987.

Roy FH: *Ocular Differential Diagnosis* (4th ed). Philadelphia, Lea & Febiger, 1989.

Sanders E, deKeizer RJW, Zee DS (eds): *Eye Movement Disorders.* Dordrecht, Martinus Nijhoff-DR W. Junk Publishers, 1987.

Scobee R: *Disturbances of Ocular Motility.* Section in Instruction, Home Study Courses, American Academy of Ophthalmology and Otolaryngology. Omaha, Douglas Printing Co, 1951.

V. Innervation of the ocular muscles

A. Classification of ocular muscles into intraocular and extraocular

1. Each eye has 11 ocular muscles: three *intra*ocular smooth muscles and 8 *extra*ocular muscles, 1 smooth and 7 skeletal. Since the EOMs derive from somites, they are innervated only by somite nerves (III, IV, and VI). Learn Fig. 4-29.

2. One ocular-related muscle, the orbicularis oculi, a sphincter which closes the eyelids, is classed with the facial muscles, because it is derived from a branchial arch and innervated by cranial nerve VII.

B. Peripheral innervation of the extraocular muscles. Six nerves innervate the eye, four of which are motor (Table 4-4).

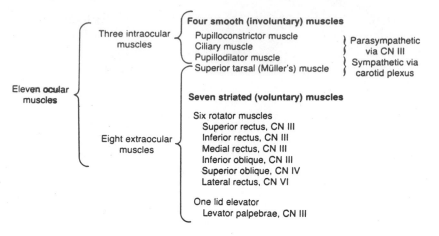

FIG. 4-29. The 11 ocular muscles and their innervation.

1. Of the four essentially motor nerves, three convey sensory efferent (SE) fibers, III, IV, and VI. Two of the three somatomotor nerves serve one extraocular muscle each: VI innervates the lateral rectus, and IV innervates the superior oblique, while the IIId nerve serves the remaining EOMs and two of the three intraocular muscles. Only III also conveys parasympathetic fibers (VE), which innervate the intraocular, smooth pupilloconstrictor, and ciliary muscles.

2. The fourth motor nerve, the *carotid sympathetic nerve,* innervates only one intraocular muscle, the pupillodilator muscle and one extraocular, the superior tarsal.

3. Learn cranial nerves III, IV, and VI in Table 4-4, and then test yourself with frames 4 to 12.

4. *The IVth cranial nerve*

   Trochlear

   a. Nerve IV is called the _____ nerve.

TABLE 4-4 Innervation of the eye by its six nerves

Number and name of nerve	Innervation	Clinical effects of interruption of nerve
Efferent		
CN III (oculomotor nerve)	Striated muscle: superior, medial, and inferior recti; inferior oblique	Diplopia, eye abducted and turned down
	Levator palpebrae	Ptosis (paralysis of volitional lid elevation)
	Smooth muscle: pupilloconstrictor; ciliary muscle	Pupil dilated and fixed to light; loss of lens thickening
CN IV (trochlear nerve)	Striated muscle: superior oblique	Diplopia, most severe on looking down and in; eye extorted; head tilted to side opposite paralyzed eye
CN VI (abducens nerve)	Striated muscle: lateral rectus	Diplopia, most severe on looking to side of paralysis; eye turned in (adducted)
Carotid sympathetic nerve	Smooth muscle: superior tarsal and pupillodilator	Horner's syndrome (ptosis, miosis, hemifacial anhidrosis, vasodilation)
Afferent		
CN II (optic nerve)	Visual afferents	Blindness
CN V (trigeminal nerve)	Proprioceptive afferents	No known clinical effect
	Corneal/conjunctival afferents	Anesthesia of cornea with loss of corneal reflex

Superior oblique
Depression
Abduction; intorsion

Abducens
Lateral rectus
Abduct

Oculomotor

b. Nerve IV innervates the only EOM to have a trochlea, the _____
_____ muscle.

c. The superior oblique muscle has three actions: _____
_____, and _____.

5. *The VIth cranial nerve*
   a. Nerve VI is called the _____ nerve. It innervates the
   _____ _____ muscle.
   b. The only action of lateral rectus is to _____ the eye.

6. *The IIId cranial nerve*
   a. Nerve III is called the _____ nerve.
   b. The EOMs innervated by III are _____
   _____.

Ans: Medial, superior and inferior recti, inferior oblique, and levator palpebrae.

Lateral rectus,
*   superior oblique,*
*   superior tarsal*
Levator palpebrae

c. Nerve III innervates two intraocular muscles and all EOMs, except for
_____.

d. In addition, III innervates a muscle that elevates the eyelid, the
_____ _____ muscle.

VI. Examination of the pupils

A. *Technique of pupillary examination*
   1. Commence in a room with normal illumination, not brightly lit or in direct sunlight. Ask the Pt to gaze at a distant point, to avoid pupilloconstriction from the accommodation reflex.
   2. Compare the size of the two pupils, and record the pupillary size in millimeters. Check for anisocoria. Benign congenital anisocoria in which the pupils react normally is relatively common. The pupils of neonates are small. The pupils enlarge in size through childhood and the early teen years and again are relatively small in the elderly. Look for faint rapid oscillations of the pupillary margins, called hippus, which may be benign or reflect a metabolic encephalopathy. Inspect the limbus for a Kayser-Fleischer ring or an arcus senilis.
   3. Darken the room, leaving only a faint background illumination. Observe whether the pupils dilate promptly.
   4. Check the *direct* and *consensual pupillary light reflexes.*
      a. Request that the Pt continue to look at a distant point, not directly at the light, and beam a flashlight slowly in from the sides to illuminate each eye separately. Observe whether *both* pupils constrict promptly and equally to unilateral illumination. After the prompt initial constriction, the pupils normally dilate slightly.
         (1) Direct constriction of the pupil in the eye stimulated by light is called the *direct light reflex.*
         (2) The *consensual* constriction of the opposite pupil when light stimulates only one eye is the *consensual light reflex.* Normally, the direct and consensual responses are equal.
      b. Do not shine the flashlight abruptly into the Pt's eyes from directly in front, for two reasons:
         (1) The Pt will automatically look at the light and accommodate for near vision.
         (2) The bright light will cause discomfort, particularly if the Pt has photophobia.

5. For the *swinging flashlight test,* alternately swing the light from one eye to the other at 3- to 5-second intervals, and watch for equal reactions of both pupils. If the Pt has an afferent defect in one optic nerve, the pupils will dilate as the light swings from the normal to the affected eye (Marcus Gunn pupil), rather than maintaining the same degree of constriction (Thompson and Corbett, 1989).
6. While the room is dimly lit, do the ophthalmoscopic examination.
7. Whenever a question exists about the duration of an ocular finding, such as anisocoria or ptosis, ask the Pt to bring in an old facial photograph.

B. *Pathway for the pupillary light reflexes*
1. Figure 4-30 shows the pathway for the *direct* and *consensual light reflexes.*

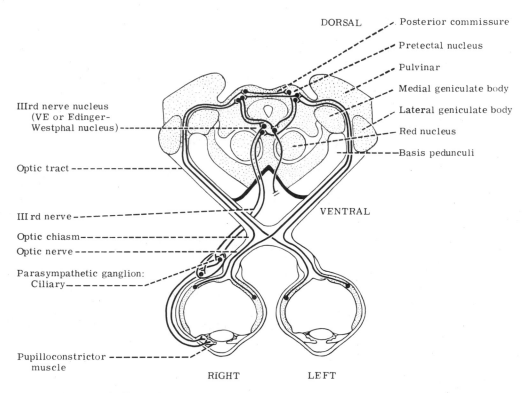

FIG. 4-30. Diagram of afferent (optic nerve) and efferent (IIId nerve) pathway for pupilloconstriction. R stands for the receptor which, in this case, is the retina. The mesencephalon has been transected through its rostral part, encroaching on the geniculate bodies and pulvinar nuclei of the diencephalon. Learn this pathway *(Adapted from E. Crosby, T. Humprey, and E. Lauer: Correlative Anatomy of the Nervous System, New York, Macmillan, 1962.)*

2. Learn this pathway as if your life depended on it: someone else's may sometime. Evaluation of the pupillary reflexes is essential in coma, cerebrovascular disease, brain tumors, and head injuries. Study Fig. 4-30 this way:
   a. Learn the names down the left side. Those on the right are for general orientation.
   b. As is typical of reflex arcs, the pupillary reflex arc has a *receptor, afferent limb, central nuclear synapse(s),* an *efferent limb,* and an *effector.* Start at R, the receptor for light. Always start at the receptor to analyze any reflex. Trace the path of impulses through the brainstem and back to the effector muscles.
   c. Notice the alternate ipsilateral-contralateral course of axons through the optic chiasm.

    d. Notice that after the nerve impulses reach the mesencephalon, they are distributed *bilaterally* to the VE nucleus of III, called the Edinger-Westphal nucleus. Hence light stimulation in one eye will cause both pupils to constrict equally. The consensual pupillary constriction equals the direct.

    e. Efferent axons travel to the eyes via both IIId nerves. Notice that according to the general plan of the parasympathetic system, the ganglion of synapse of the VE axon is near the end organ, the ciliary and pupilloconstrictor muscles. The same efferent pathway serves in pupilloconstriction to light and in accommodation.

3. On scrap paper draw the axonal pathways for the pupillary light reflex.

4. If a Pt has no direct light reflex in the left eye, but has a consensual light reflex on the left when the right eye is illuminated, the lesion is in the ☐ right optic tract/ ☐ left IIId nerve/ ☐ left optic nerve.

Ans: ☑ *Left optic nerve*

5. Describe the result of the swinging flashlight test in the foregoing Pt _____

Ans: See frame A.5, above.

    C. Physiology and pharmacology of the pupils

1. The eyeball contains three intraocular muscles, all smooth muscles: the *pupillodilator,* the *pupilloconstrictor,* and the *ciliary.*

    a. The *pupilloconstrictor* and *pupillodilator* muscles of the iris adjust the diameter of the pupil.

       (1) The *pupillodilator* muscle fibers run radially out from the pupillary margin, like spokes in a wheel.

       (2) The *pupilloconstrictor* muscle fibers form a sphincter around the pupillary margin.

    b. The *ciliary* muscle, is likewise a sphincter. It adjusts the diameter of the lens by relaxing its suspensory ligament, to allow the lens to thicken by its own elasticity; however, the ciliary muscle does not control the pupil.

2. *Role of smooth muscle.* If we consider the role of smooth muscle generally—in the bowel, bronchi, blood vessels, ureters, bladder, etc.—we can recognize that smooth muscle functions to adjust the diameters of the apertures or passageways of the viscera. Curiously, however, the one viscus whose *sole* function is to change its diameter, the heart, is striated, not smooth muscle. Striated muscle is specialized for quick, powerful *phasic* contractions, smooth muscle for slow, *tonic* contractions.

3. *Tonic oppositional action of the pupilloconstrictor and pupillodilator muscles*

    a. Like the EOMs which act in tonically innervated, oppositional pairs, the pupilloconstrictor and pupillodilator muscles actively oppose each other.

    b. The pupilloconstrictor muscle is *parasympathetic* and *cholinergic;* the pupillodilator is *sympathetic* and *adrenergic.* Normally the outflow of tonic innervation by sympathetic and parasympathetic impulses balances out. After the pupil adopts any new size, the vector acting to *increase* pupillary diameter equals the vector acting to *decrease* it. Thus a tug-of-war between the constrictor and dilator muscles always positively determines pupillary size.

    c. If a lesion or drug interrupts one system, either sympathetic or parasympathetic, the other acts unopposed, and the pupil assumes the size dictated by the tonic innervation that reaches the intact muscle.

☑ *Pupillodilation*

☑ *Pupilloconstriction*
   (cormiosis)

☑ *Sympathetic*

☑ *Parasympathetic*

☐ *Parasympathetic*
   blocking agent

(1) Parasympathetic denervation results in ☐ pupillodilation/ ☐ pupilloconstriction.

(2) Sympathetic denervation results in ☐ pupilloconstriction/ ☐ pupillodilation.

4. *Pupillodilation (mydriasis)*

   a. The ophthalmologist never presumes to be able to do a complete funduscopic examination without dilating the pupil. Pharmacologically, pupillodilation can result from mimicking the ☐ sympathetic/ ☐ parasympathetic nervous system, or by blocking the ☐ sympathetic/ ☐ parasympathetic nervous system.

   b. After sympathomimetic or parasympathetic blocking drugs have dilated the pupil, exposure to light will make the Pt uncomfortable, a symptom called *photophobia.* Which drug would also interfere with lens thickening by paralyzing the ciliary muscle (cycloplegia)—a ☐ sympathomimetic/ or a ☐ parasympathetic blocking agent?

   c. Although pupillodilator drugs (mydriatics) cause temporary blurring of vision, they are necessary to see the periphery of the fundus. The pupils of infants and Pts with deeply pigmented irises respond slowly to mydriatics:

      (1) For infants: cyclopentolate (Cyclogyl) 1% ophthalmic solution, two drops in each eye every 15 min for three doses.

      (2) Older Pts: one or two drops in each eye. Repeat in 15 to 20 minutes.

   d. Since pupillodilation increases intraocular pressure, check the intraocular pressure of adults over 40 by tonometry, before instilling mydriatics. Two percent of all adults over 40 years of age have glaucoma.

5. *Overall determinants of pupillary size*

   Although the amount of light normally is the major determinant of pupillary size, many other factors are also active:

   a. Age. Small pupils in infants, large in adolescents, and small again in the elderly.

   b. Anatomic integrity of pupillary innervation.

   c. Local disease of the eye and iris.

   d. Local ocular or systemic drugs which affect the autonomic nervous system.

   e. Emotionality. When the sympathetic nervous system predominates, pupillodilation and tachycardia occur.

   f. Sleep and drowsiness. When the parasympathetic nervous system predominates, pupilloconstriction and bradycardia occur.

D. *Analyze these Pts*

   1. A 51-year-old woman was admitted to the hospital because of hypertension. She has had no visual complaints, and the intern recorded normal eyes. Your examination a few hours after the initial examination by the intern discloses a dilated right pupil, but no ptosis, heterotropia, fundus lesions, loss of vision, or other ocular signs. She has no direct or consensual pupillary light reflex on the right, and no pupilloconstriction in accommodation. The direct and consensual response of the left pupil to light is normal, and it constricts during accommodation. The best inference is:

      a. ☐ The Pt is blind in the right eye and has a right IIId nerve lesion.

      b. ☐ The Pt has an intact right optic nerve, but has complete interruption of the right IIId nerve.

      c. ☐ The Pt has had eyedrops placed in the right eye to dilate the pupil.

Ans: ☑ *c. Alternative a is excluded because the Pt is not blind and has a consensual reflex on the* left, *proving that the afferent pathway, the optic nerve, from the right retina is intact; b is excluded because of no ptosis or ocular malalignment; c is all that is left. The reason for this frame is that the commonest cause of dilated, nonreactive pupils in medical student practice in teaching hospitals is that the intern or resident has used—properly— eyedrops to dilate the pupil for an adequate funduscopic examination. The intern erred, however, in dilating only one pupil. The more general implication of the frame is that in ''thinking through'' a reflex arc, you must include* both *the neuromyal junction and the effector as possible sites of mischief. And the final lesson—always record on the chart that the pupils have been dilated.*

2. This 24-year-old male is somnolent because of a head injury, but he is arousable. His left eye is turned down and out and does not turn on command although the other eye moves on command. When the Pt attempts to look to the right and down, the left eye intorts strongly, but remains turned down and out. His left pupil is dilated and fixed (nonreactive) to light or in accommodation. No eye drops were used. The right pupil shows a direct and a consensual response to light and reacts normally in accommodation. This Pt most likely has a lesion of his ☐ left optic nerve/ ☐ right optic nerve/ ☐ left IVth nerve only/ ☐ left IIId nerve./ ☐ The ocular findings cannot be explained by a single nerve lesion.

Ans: ☑ *Left IIId nerve*

a. Because of the importance of pupillary signs, avoid mydriatic eyedrops in Pts with impaired consciousness.
b. Name two contraindications to pupillodilator drugs. _____
_____.

Ans: Glaucoma and impaired consciousness.

E. The syndrome of parasympathetic paralysis of the eye (internal ophthalmoplegia)
  1. The muscles innervated by the VE, parasympathetic axons of III are:
    a. ☐ intraocular/ ☐ extraocular.
    b. ☐ smooth/ ☐ skeletal.

☑ *Intraocular*
☑ *Smooth*

  2. The VE axons of III are the only efferent pathway for active pupilloconstriction. Since the VE and SE axons of III originate from the same nucleus and travel in the same peripheral nerve, lesions affecting III generally involve both sets of axons, but important exceptions occur. State the symptoms and signs that would be caused by a pure parasympathetic paralysis of the eye._____
_____

Ans: Blurring of near vision (ciliary muscle paralysis) and dilated pupil, not reactive to light or in accommodation (pupilloconstrictor muscle paralysis).

F. The syndrome of sympathetic paralysis of the eye and face (Bernard-Horner or Horner's syndrome)
  1. As is typical of all sympathetic pathways, the *central* sympathetic pathway to the eye begins in the hypothalamus. It descends through the brainstem tegmentum to the VE column of the spinal cord (Fig. 4-31).
  2. As also typifies the sympathetic system, the *peripheral* pathway begins in the VE cell column of the spinal cord. The VE column extends from T-1 to L-2 to L-3. Mnemonic: T-1 to L-2 to L-3. Axons to the eye derive from T-1 and T-2.

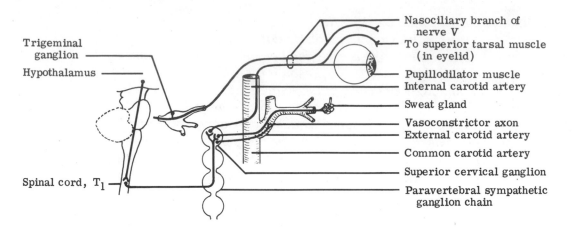

Trigeminal ganglion

Hypothalamus

Spinal cord, T_1

Nasociliary branch of nerve V

To superior tarsal muscle (in eyelid)

Pupillodilator muscle
Internal carotid artery

Sweat gland

Vasoconstrictor axon
External carotid artery

Common carotid artery

Superior cervical ganglion

Paravertebral sympathetic ganglion chain

FIG. 4-31. Diagram of sympathetic pathway from the hypothalamus (part of the diencephalon) to the pupillodilator and superior tarsal muscles, sweat glands of the face, and the smooth muscle of the carotid arteries.

3. As is also typical, the primary VE sympathetic axons exit with a spinal nerve to synapse in a paravertebral ganglion. The secondary axons, from the paravertebral ganglion, then hitchhike as a plexus along blood vessels or nerves to their effectors. The carotid sympathetic plexus innervates the sweat glands of the face and the smooth muscles of the blood vessels of the carotid system. Learn Fig. 4-31, starting at the hypothalamus.

4. The sympathetic and parasympathetic systems differ in the location of the ganglion containing the secondary axon.
   a. The ganglia of the sympathetic nervous system are located in the paravertebral chain.
   b. By contrast, the ganglia of the parasympathetic nervous system are located in or near the organ innervated.

Superior tarsal; pupillodilator

5. The two ocular muscles innervated by sympathetic axons are _____ (extraocular) and _____ (intraocular).

6. *Pt analysis.* A 21-year-old man has suffered a stab wound in the neck interrupting the sympathetic innervation to one side of his face. Run down the right-hand labels of Fig. 4-31 to compile a list of signs that would occur.

_____

_____

Ans: Ipsilateral pupilloconstriction (cormiosis), ptosis, anhidrosis, and flushing (vasodilation).

7. These four features of sympathetic facial denervation constitute the *Bernard-Horner* or *Horner's syndrome.* Although enophthalmos is also described as part of this syndrome in man, this sign is inconstant and more apparent, because of ptosis, than real.

8. Explain why miosis occurs after sympathetic denervation of the eye.

_____

_____

Ans: The pupillodilator and pupilloconstrictor muscles are in tonic opposition. After pupillodilator muscle paralysis, the pupilloconstrictor muscle acts unopposed.

9. After sympathetic paralysis, the miotic pupil will constrict further in response to light or accommodation, because then the muscle receives an additive constrictor stimulus, rather than simply a "tonic" stimulus.

10. *Separation of the components of Horner's syndrome.* The number of signs of sympathetic facial denervation vary depending on the location of the lesion along the sympathetic pathway.

Ptosis; cormiosis

a. If the lesion interrupts the sympathetic pathway *distal* to the origin of the external carotid artery, the only sympathetic denervation signs the Pt will show are _____ and _____.

b. If the lesion interrupts the sympathetic pathway *proximal* to the external carotid artery (between the hypothalamus and the carotid artery), the Pt will show, in addition to ptosis and cormiosis, the other two features of Horner's syndrome: _____ and _____.

Ans: Hemifacial (ipsilateral) anhidrosis; vasodilation

11. *Clinical testing of the ocular sympathetic pathway:* the spinociliary reflex
    a. To test the sympathetic pathway to the eye, pinch the skin over the face (cranial nerve V afferent) or neck (C-2 or C-3 afferent) firmly for 5 seconds. Both pupils should dilate briskly—the *faciociliary* or *spinociliary (ciliospinal)* reflex.
    b. Should you do the test in a dark or light room, and with the Pt looking at a near or distant target? Explain: _____
    _____
    _____

Ans: Do the test in subdued light and with the Pt looking in the distance, to avoid the strong pupilloconstriction due to light and accommodation that could mask a mild sympathetic pupillary paralysis.

12. *Causes of Horner's syndrome.* Apart from direct trauma, important causes include neoplastic or inflammatory masses in the neck, base of the skull, or orbit; and vascular diseases of the carotid artery, such as aneurysms. A newly acquired Horner's syndrome requires a search for such lesions. Congenital or neonatal Horner's syndrome, such as due to birth

TABLE 4-5 Differential diagnosis of Argyll Robertson and Adie's pupils

Characteristic	Argyll Robertson pupil	Adie's myotonic pupil
Laterality	Usually bilateral	Usually unilateral (aniscocoria)
Size	Cormiosis	Mild corectasia
Pupillary outline	Irregular	Regular (normal circle)
Response to light	None (neither direct nor consensual)	Very slow direct and consensual response; remains myotonically contracted after light is removed
Response to dark	No pupillodilation	Slow pupillodilation, with delay in constriction on reexposure to light
Response to accommodation	Constricts	Constricts very slowly and remains myotonically constricted after accommodation is relaxed
Response to mydriatics	Poor or none	Responds normally
Systemic features	Virtually pathognomonic of syphilis. If the patient has tabes dorsalis, his muscle stretch reflexes will be absent.	Benign disorder, often associated with absent muscle stretch reflexes—"Adie's syndrome"

injury of the brachial plexus with traction on nerve roots, will result in a defect in iris pigmentation and iris heterochromia.

G. *Abnormal pupillary reflexes with absent muscle stretch reflexes*
1. Two important syndromes of abnormal or dissociated pupillary response to light and accommodation, with absent muscle stretch reflexes are tabes dorsalis with an Argyll Robertson pupil (Sir Douglas Argyll Robertson, 1837–1909) and Adie's myotonic pupil (William Adie, 1886–1935) (Table 4-5). The A-R pupil may also occur in neurosyphilis without tabes dorsalis.
2. Diabetes mellitus may also cause abnormal pupillary reflexes and absence of muscle stretch reflexes, as may several other disorders. What you must know is how to test pupillary responses and stretch reflexes and then how to consult a reference for the implication of abnormalities. The basic issue is compulsive thoroughness in the examination. After reading through Table 4-5, you will see why you must routinely test pupillary constriction to light *and* in accommodation.

SUGGESTED READING FOR PUPILLARY REACTIONS

Adie W: Tonic pupils and absent tendon reflexes: A benign disorder sui generis; its complete and incomplete forms. *Brain,* 1932; 55:98–113.

Hollenhorst R: The pupil in neurologic diagnosis. *Med Clin N Am,* 1968; 52:871–884.

Reeves A, Posner J: The ciliospinal response in man. *Neurology,* 1969; 19:1145–1152.

Slamovits TL, Glaser JS: The pupils and accommodation, in JS Glaser (ed): *Neuro-ophthalmology.* Philadelphia, Lippincott, 1990.

Spector RH, Bachman DL: Bilateral Adie's tonic pupil with anhidrosis and hyperthermia. *Arch Neurol* 1984; 41:342–343.

Thompson HS, Corbett JJ: Swinging flashlight test. *Neurology,* 1989; 38:154–156.

Zinn K: *The Pupil.* Springfield, CC Thomas, 1972.

VII. Clinical evaluation of ptosis

A. *Elevation of the eyelid*
1. *Two muscles elevate the eyelid,* thus adjusting the vertical diameter of the palpebral fissure: the superior tarsal and the levator palpebrae muscles.
   a. The superior tarsal muscle, a smooth muscle, acts *tonically* to elevate the eyelid. It is innervated by _____.
   b. The levator palpebrae muscle, a skeletal muscle, acts *tonically* and *phasically* to elevate the eyelid. It is innervated by _____.
2. *Try this experiment to understand eyelid elevation*
   a. Look straight ahead into your mirror. The combined tonic action of the superior tarsal muscle and the levator palpebrae muscle sets the height of your palpebral fissure. Elevate and lower the mirror while observing the rise and fall of your upper lids, but do not allow your head to move.
   b. Now try to elevate and lower your eyelids without moving your eyes, and try to elevate and lower your eyes without allowing your upper lid to move. Can you separate the eyeball and eyelid movements? ☐ Yes/ ☐ No

The carotid sympathetic nerve

Cranial nerve III

Ans: By now you know not to look here for answers that you should derive yourself!

    c. Activation of the levator palpebrae causes the quick or phasic rise and fall of the eyelid during vertical eye movements. Although eyelid elevation is linked automatically as an associated movement to the ocular muscles which elevate the eyeball, the levator palpebrae is a skeletal muscle. Inhibition of its action in the CNS allows the lid to drop with gravity when the eye looks down.

3. *Levator palpebrae paralysis causes:*
    a. Severe ptosis, greater than with superior tarsal ptosis.
    b. Paralysis of lid elevation during upward gaze.
4. Will the lid elevate when the Pt with sympathetic ptosis looks up? ☐ Yes/ ☐ No. Explain. _____

       _____

Ans: ☑ *Yes. The levator palpebrae is intact and will elevate the lid by its phasic contraction.*

5. *Differentiation of sympathetic and IIId nerve ptosis:* complete Table 4-6 by placing a ✓ sign in column 2 *or* 3.

B. *The causes of ptosis*
1. Sometimes ptosis is neither the result of a IIId nerve lesion nor the result of a sympathetic denervation. In myasthenia gravis, levator palpebrae weakness results from defective cholinergic transmission at the neuromyal junction. Ptosis from nerve or neurohumoral transmission lesions is called *neuropathic* ptosis. Ptosis may occur in primary muscle diseases such as dystrophy, *myopathic* ptosis. Sometimes ptosis is congenital and may or may not be associated with other anomalies. After injury or inflammation, lid edema may cause ptosis. The point is this: in analyzing ptosis, or any other neurologic sign, you must "think through" the possible lesion sites, down to and including the effector, and integrate the sign with other physical signs and the history. The lesion may be:
    a. *Central:* at the hypothalamus, brainstem, or spinal cord.
    b. *Peripheral:* along the course of the IIId or sympathetic nerves.
    c. *Neuromyal:* at the nerve-muscle junction.

III	*Symp.*
	✓
✓	
	✓
✓	
	✓
✓	

TABLE 4-6 Differential diagnosis of IIId nerve and sympathetic ptosis

1	2	3
Feature	Present with IIId nerve lesion	Present with sympathetic lesion
Cormiosis		
Corectasia		
Reaction to light and accommodation		
Usually have heterotropia		
Elevation of eyelid on upward gaze		
Normal sweating		

   d. Local, within the muscle itself, myopathic, congenital, inflammatory, or
      traumatic.
   e. Dehiscence of the levator muscle aponeurosis.
2. Thus ptosis is not simply one thing or another: it is a puzzle to be solved.
   Every sign generates a range of differential diagnostic possibilities, which
   the Ex must sort through in an orderly fashion. The most important point
   of distinction is that ptosis due to levator paralysis is almost always accompanied by other signs of IIId nerve interruption, and ptosis due to superior
   tarsal paralysis is almost always accompanied by other signs of sympathetic
   denervation.

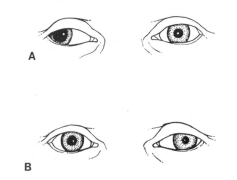

FIG. 4-32. Two Pts with ocular abnormalities. Describe and diagnose them.

C. Analyze these Pts
   1. The 34-year-old woman in Fig. 4-32*A* suddenly noticed double vision. She
      was unable to adduct, elevate, or depress her right eye, but it did intort when
      she attempted to look down and to the left. The right eyelid did not elevate
      on volitional upward gaze. The right pupil neither reacted directly nor con-
      sensually to light. The left pupil did react directly and consensually. All
      other neurologic functions were intact. These findings indicate a lesion
      affecting _____
      _____.

*Ans: Right IIId nerve. Cerebral angiograms showed an aneurysm of the right
posterior communicating artery, which had compressed the IIId nerve just
after its exit from the midbrain.*

   2. The 21-year-old woman in Fig. 4-32*B* complained of deep pain behind her
      left eye for several months. She also noticed diplopia on looking to the left.
      For some weeks her left eyelid had drooped. Examination showed ptosis that
      was corrected on upward gaze, miosis, and mild weakness of abduction of
      the left eye. All other neurologic findings remained intact. At her doctor's
      request, the Pt brought in old facial photographs which proved that the pto-
      sis was new. Can the findings be explained by involvement of only one nerve?
      If not, what nerves are implicated?_____
      _____.

*Ans: The Pt had sympathetic ptosis. The pain and ocular palsy required
involvement of other nerves. Because this Pt had only ptosis and miosis
without hemifacial anhidrosis, the lesion must have affected her
sympathetic pathway <u>distal</u> to the origin of her external carotid artery.*

   a. Normal eye movements and the absence of exophthalmos tend to
      exclude a lesion within the orbit itself.
   b. The pain location and the neurologic findings implicated a lesion at the

base of the skull, affecting pain fibers of V. Abductor weakness implicated a lateral rectus palsy. Hence some lesion was progressively attacking successive cranial nerves. The conjunction site of the sympathetic pathway and the VIth nerve is at the cavernous sinus region. This region receives its sensory innervation from V. Inspection of the nasopharynx disclosed a soft tissue mass. Radiographs of the skull base showed bony erosion. A biopsy disclosed a nasopharyngeal carcinoma. It had infiltrated the base of the skull and cavernous sinus and encircled the internal carotid artery, where it had interrupted the carotid sympathetic and VIth nerves. Painful ophthalmoplegia due to cavernous sinus lesion is called the Tolosa-Hunt syndrome.

SUGGESTED READING FOR PTOSIS

Callahan MA. *Beard's Ptosis* (4th ed). Birmingham, Aesculapius, 1990.

Campbell J, Okazaki H: Painful ophthalmoplegia (Tolosa-Hunt variant): Autopsy findings in a patient with necrotizing intracavernous carotid vasculitis and inflammatory disease of the orbit. *Mayo Clin Proc,* 1987; 62:520–526.

VIII. Summary of ocular examination for vision and the peripheral optomotor system: now as shall be our habit, return to the Summarized Neurologic Examination and rehearse part V.A.

Learning Objectives for Chapter Four

I. Ocular alignment and diplopia

1. Explain the concept and function of foveation.
2. Describe the *primary position* of the eyes.
3. Make a diagram to show the visual axis of a normal eye (Fig. 4-1).
4. Diagram the difference in the visual axes of the eyes during near and distant vision (Fig. 4-3).
5. Describe how to demonstrate the dominant eye.
6. Describe self-experiments to demonstrate physiologic and pathologic diplopia.
7. Explain the concept of true and false images in diplopia.
8. Explain why the diplopic (false) image produced by displacing your eyeball by compression of your lateral canthus was less sharp than the (true) image from the nondisplaced eye.

II. The actions of the individual extraocular muscles (EOMs)

1. Describe the axes of rotation of the eyeball and distinguish axial from eccentric rotation (Figs. 4-7 and 4-8).
*2. List the EOMs, their origins and insertions, and by means of a table tennis ball model illustrate their actions (Fig. 4-9).

*3. Make a diagram to show the difference in the actions of the superior rectus and the superior oblique muscle when the eye is adducted, straight ahead, and abducted (Figs. 4-12 and 4-13).
*4. Make a composite vector diagram which summarizes the line of pull of the EOMs of one eye and shows that all muscles pull medial to the vertical axis, except the lateral rectus (Fig. 4-17).
5. Make a tabular summary of the ocular rotatory muscles and list their primary, secondary, and tertiary actions (Table 4-1).
6. Explain the concept of yoking of ocular muscles, state Hering's law, and draw a figure which summarizes the yoke muscles (Fig. 4-18).
7. Name the muscles which turn the eye up and in, and contrast them with the muscles which turn the eye up and out.
8. Explain why an eye deviates in a predictable direction after paralysis of one of its EOMs.

III. Clinical tests for ocular malalignment and the range of eye movement

1. Describe and demonstrate how to check the corneal light reflections.

2. Explain why the corneal light reflections fall a little to the medial side of the true geometric center of the corneas with the eyes in the primary position (Fig. 4-19).
3. Describe why inspecting the corneal light reflections is a more reliable test for ocular malalignment than inspecting the limbus-lid relations.
4. Demonstrate how to test the range of eye movements (Fig. 4-20).
5. State which direction of eye movement has the weakest range normally and suffers most in aging or diffuse brain disease (Fig. 4-21).
6. Demonstrate how to do the cover-uncover test for ocular malalignment (Fig. 4-22).
7. Explain and give examples of the difference between an operational and an interpretational definition.
8. Give an operational definition of heterotropia and outline the terms used to describe the various directions of eye deviation.
9. From a series of illustrations, diagnose the state of ocular alignment from the corneal light reflections (Fig. 4-23).
10. From a series of diagrams of the results (Fig. 4-24*A*–*D*), describe and interpret the cover-uncover test.
*11. Distinguish between heterotropia and heterophoria and describe the results of the cover-uncover test in heterophoria.
*12. Explain why the Pt shows a greater ocular deviation when fixating with the paretic eye than when fixating with the sound eye (e.g., explain why the secondary deviation is greater than the primary deviation).
13. Describe the effects of heterotropia on vision in infants and on head position.
14. Define suppression amblyopia (amblyopia ex anopsia). Describe how it may arise and be prevented.
15. Describe the direction of the head tilt to compensate for the weakness of intorsion and to minimize the diplopia from a right superior oblique muscle palsy.
*16. Describe the clinical differentiation between paralytic (nonconcomitant) and nonparalytic (concomitant) heterotropia (Table 4-2).
17. Explain these laws of diplopia:
    a. The false image is fuzzier than the true image.
    b. The false image projects peripheral to (or away from) the true image.
    c. The false image projects *opposite* to the direction of deviation of the paralytic eye.
    d. The false image projects *toward* the direction of action of the paralytic muscle.
    e. The distance between the true and false images increases as the eyes move in the direction of action of the paralytic muscle (Fig. 4-25).

IV. Refraction and accommodation

1. Make a diagram to show the action of negative and positive lenses, illustrating the law of the prism (Fig. 4-26).
2. Describe the triad of actions that constitute the accommodation (near) reflex. Name the muscles which produce each of these actions (Table 4-3).
3. Make a diagram showing the point of focus of parallel light rays in a myopic, emmotropic, and hyperopic eye (Fig. 4-27).
4. Describe the relation between myopia and hyperopia and eso- and exophorias and eso- and exotropias.
5. Describe the age of onset of presbyopia and its differential affect on vision in myopes and hyperopes.
6. Describe the effect of a pinhole aperture on myopia, hyperopia, and presbyopia.
7. State whether a pinhole aperture corrects blurred vision due to a macular or optic nerve lesion.
8. Describe how to use the parallax test to determine whether the Pt's glasses correct for hyperopia or myopia.
9. Explain why a presbyopic myope removes eyeglasses to read newsprint, whereas a presbyopic emmetrope and particularly a presbyopic hyperope must use eyeglasses for near vision.

V. Innervation of the ocular muscles

1. Name and classify the 11 intra- and extraocular muscles. (Fig. 4-29).
2. Give the name and number of the cranial nerves which innervate the ocular muscles. Reason out and describe the clinical deficits due to interruption of each of these nerves (Table 4-4).
3. Name the nucleus of origin for each of the cranial nerves which innervates eye muscles and state which division of the brainstem contains it.

VI. Examination of the pupils

1. Demonstrate how to examine the pupils.
2. Explain why a Pt should look at a distant point when you test the pupillary light reflexes.
3. Describe the age-dependent changes in the baseline size of the pupils.
4. Explain the difference between the corneal light reflection test and the pupillary light reflex.
5. Define the direct and consensual pupillary light reflexes.
6. State whether in a normal person the direct and consensual pupilloconstrictions are equal or unequal and explain neuroanatomically.
7. Explain why the Ex should not abruptly shine the flashlight into the Pt's eyes from directly in front.
8. Diagram the pathways of the pupillary light reflex (Fig. 4-30).
9. Describe the effect of interruption of one optic nerve or one IIId nerve on the direct and consensual pupillary light reflexes.
10. Describe the result of the swinging flashlight test in a Pt with interruption of one optic nerve.
11. Name the pharmacological class of the neurotransmitter for each intraocular and extraocular muscle.

12. Describe what happens to pupillary size after interruption or blocking of either the parasympathetic or sympathetic nervous system and explain why this change in size occurs.
13. State whether a sympathomimetic or parasympathetic blocking drug will affect accommodation and explain why.
14. Explain why a mydriatic is used in the examination of the eye and describe the effect on the Pt's vision.
15. State the effect of a pupillodilator drug on intraocular tension. State the age range of Pts most likely to suffer from this effect.
16. Describe several factors that determine pupillary size at any given moment.
17. Diagram the parasympathetic pathway from the brain to the intraocular muscles. State the clinical deficits resulting from the internal ophthalmoplegia due to interruption of this pathway (Fig. 4-30).
18. Diagram the sympathetic pathway to the eye and contrast the location of the parasympathetic and sympathetic ganglia (Figs. 4-30 and 4-31).
19. Describe Horner's syndrome and the differences in signs dependent on interruption of the sympathetic pathway at various sites between the CNS and orbit.
20. Describe the faciociliary and spinociliary (ciliospinal) reflex.
21. What are some important causes of acquired Horner's syndrome? State how to distinguish congenital from recently acquired Horner's syndrome by inspecting the irises.
22. Name three disorders characterized by abnormal pupils and absent muscle stretch reflexes.
23. Contrast the Argyll Robertson and Adie's myotonic pupils (Table 4-5).
24. Explain why you should test for pupilloconstriction, to light and in accommodation, in the routine examination.

VII. Clinical evaluation of ptosis

1. Name the two muscles which elevate the eyelid, and name their nerve supply.
2. Describe the clinical features which differentiate IIId nerve ptosis from sympathetic ptosis (Table 4-6).
3. Describe how to "think through" the efferent pathway in analyzing ptosis.

Chapter Five

Examination of the Central Optomotor Systems

I. Central systems for the control of eye movements

A. Five major eye movement systems. Five systems of pathways direct volitional and reflex eye movements. Selection of a visual target is volitional. After that, fixation, fusion, following, vergences, and the control of refraction proceed more or less automatically (Table 5-1).

1. *Fixation (position maintenance) system.* Proper fixation of both eyes on the visual target permits fusion of both retinal images into one visual image. Retino-occipito-tegmental and retino-occipito-fronto-tegmental pathways mediate fixation and fusion.

2. *Saccadic system.* Saccade means to jerk or reign in. It describes eye movements by means of rapid, incremental jerks, like a rachet.

    a. *Self-demonstration of saccadic volitional movement.* Look straight ahead, and while keeping your head completely still, move your eyes all of the way to the right. Now very slowly and deliberately try to move your eyes as continuously and smoothly as possible all of the way to the left. You will find that they move by jerks, that is, saccades. You cannot move your eyes smoothly by volition.

    b. Saccadic eye movements include all volitional horizontal and vertical eye movements, the kickback phase of induced nystagmus (caloric or optokinetic), and rapid eye movements (REM) in sleep. Fronto-tegmental pathways mediate such saccades.

3. *Smooth pursuit system*

    a. *Self-demonstration of smooth pursuit.* Again keeping your head still throughout, move your eyes all of the way to the right, but this time hold up your finger, fixate on it, and move it slowly all of the way across from right to left, allowing your eyes to pursue it. This time you will experience smooth rather than saccadic movement.

    b. Retino-occipito-tegmental pathways reflexly mediate smooth pursuit. *This system keeps the eyes on the visual target when the target moves. The eye counterrolling system keeps the eyes on the visual target when the head moves.* Drug intoxication, major psychoses, and diffuse cortical

---

*The light vertical rule on the left side of the text sets off an answer column. Cover the answers with a card until you have responded to the text. Then after each response, slide the card down to check your answer.

The heavy vertical rule denotes optional material.

TABLE 5-1 Five major eye movement systems	
System	Function or characteristic
1. Fixation (position maintenance system)	Fixates eyes on target, maintains them on target, and locks the eyes in unison to fuse the two retinal images into one visual image (occipital lobe)
2. Saccadic system	Produces all volitional movements and the fast phase of reflex eye movements (frontal lobe)
3. Smooth pursuit system	Keeps eyes on moving target (occipital lobe)
4. Vergence system	Converges or diverges eyes for near or distant targets (occipital lobe)
5. Counterrolling system	Vestibular and neck proprioceptive system. This system counterrolls the eyes to keep them fixed on the visual target in compensation for head movement. It produces postural information to align the eyes, head, neck, and trunk.

diseases (as in mental retardation and dementia) impair smooth pursuit of a moving object (Yee, Baloh, Marder et al, 1987).

4. *Vergence system.* This system *converges* or *diverges* the eyes to insure fusion of the two retinal images and appropriate refraction when the person looks at near or distant objects.

5. *Eye counterrolling system*

   a. *Self-demonstration of counterrolling of the eyes.* Hold your finger up at arm's length, directly in front of you. Then move your head while volitionally fixating on the finger. You eyes will reflexly counterroll *against* the direction of head movement to maintain fixation on the chosen visual target.

   b. In the alert Pt, two systems collaborate to counterroll the eyes when the head moves:

      (1) The ocular fixation system.

      (2) Proprioceptive motion receptors in the vestibular system and neck. The proprioceptors mediate counterrolling via pathways through the brainstem to the optomotor nuclei (III, IV, and VI).

   c. In the comatose Pt, who cannot fixate, the Ex can move the Pt's head (doll's eye maneuver) to test the integrity of the vestibuloproprioceptive counterrolling reflex. (See Chap. 12 on the unconscious Pt).

6. *Mnemonic note:* Now, I haven't just loaded on you five more things to memorize. *To remember these five eye movement systems, simply hold up your finger and choose to look at it; then move it and follow it.* Your eyes will *saccade* onto it, and your brain automatically *converges, fixates,* and *focuses* the eyes on the visual target, and *fuses* the visual images. If you move your finger, your eyes *follow (pursue)* it, and if you move your head, your *fixation* and *counterrolling* systems keep your eyes on target. Most acts of vision normally enlist all five systems.

B. *The corticopontine pathway for horizontal eye movements*

   1. A pathway for contralateral conjugate horizontal eye movements begins in the posterior part of the frontal lobe and parietal lobe and runs to the pontine tegmentum (Bender, 1980) (Fig. 2-31).

   2. The pathway terminates in the *paramedian pontine reticular formation,* which integrates the equal innervation of the medial and lateral recti as required by Hering's law. The connecting link is the medial longitudinal fasciculus (MLF) (Bronstein, Morris, du Boulay et al, 1990).

3. *Effects of interruption of the horizontal conjugate gaze pathway*

Interruption of the cortical pathway for horizontal movements *rostral* to its decussation results in deviation of the eyes *ipsilateral* to the lesion, because the opposite pathways are intact and continue to convey tonic innervation. The Pt is unable to initiate saccades to move the eyes past the midline contralaterally (Bender, 1980). Interruption *caudal* to the decussation, results in deviation to the side *contralateral* to the lesion.

4. *Effects of interruption of the MLF*

a. When the Pt attempts to look to the left after unilateral interruption of the right MLF (tip of the arrow in Fig. 2-31), the right eye will not adduct (Ross, DeMyer, 1966), and the Pt experiences diplopia.

b. In addition to adductor paralysis during left lateral gaze, the Pt would also show an oscillation of the left eye, a feature which cannot be deduced from the diagram. Such ocular oscillations are called *nystagmus*. Because of the nystagmus, the Pt will experience oscillopsia (apparent oscillation of the object viewed). Hence, a second sign of the MLF syndrome is monocular nystagmus of the *abducting* eye. At rest the eye has no nystagmus. It occurs only during abduction.

c. These two signs, paralysis of the *adducting* eye and nystagmus of the *abducting* eye, appear *only* on gaze to the *opposite* side of the MLF lesion. The eyes adduct normally to convergence or on vertical gaze. The corticobulbar pathways for convergence and vertical eye movements thus run directly into the mesencephalon, to the LMNs of the IIId and IVth nuclei, rather than looping down into the pons and returning in the MLF.

☑ *Looking right*

d. After a *left*-sided MLF lesion the only direction of gaze in which the Pt would have diplopia, oscillopsia, and heterotropia would be ☐ looking right/ ☐ looking left. (To reason out the answer from Fig. 2-31, draw in the pathway from the left cerebral hemisphere with colored pencil.)

e. *Summary of the MLF syndrome*

(1) The signs of a unilateral MLF lesion occur only when the Pt attempts to look away from the side of the lesion. All other eye movements, including convergence, conjugate vertical gaze, and pupillary responses are normal.

Diplopia; oscillopsia
Adduct

(2) The *symptoms* of interruption of one MLF consist of _____ and _____.

(3) During horizontal gaze, the Pt is unable to _____ the eye ipsilateral to the lesion.

Nystagmus;
☑ *abducting*

(4) The Pt shows monocular _____ of the ☐ abducting/ ☐ adducting eye, contralateral to the lesion.

f. List the signs of a bilateral MLF lesion at the level indicated by the arrow in Fig. 2-31. _____

Ans: Monocular nystagmus of the leading (abducting) eye on attempted gaze to either side; paralysis of adduction of the following eye on attempted gaze to either side. All other eye movements and pupillary responses are preserved.

g. Would a Pt with a bilateral MLF lesion be able to converge the eyes during accommodation? ☐ Yes/ ☐ No. Explain: _____

Ans: ☑ Yes. The convergence pathways run directly into the midbrain without looping down into the MLF.

C. *Bilateral destruction of the corticotegmental pathway for horizontal gaze*
1. After bilateral destruction of the cortical horizontal gaze pathway the Pt loses all saccades and cannot move the eyes voluntarily to either side. After vestibular stimulation the eyes will move to the sides, and when the Pt fixates straight ahead and the head is turned, the eyes counterroll to remain on target.
2. In addition to the paralysis of volitional horizontal movements, the fixation reflexes tend to become overly tenacious. The Pt cannot voluntarily break fixation by moving the eyes, only by blinking or moving the head to interrupt the afferent arc that maintains the fixation reflex.

D. *Pathways for vertical eye movements*
1. Pathways for vertical eye movements arise diffusely from frontal and occipital cortex. Like the convergence pathways, they project directly to the pretectal and tectal region and to oculomotor nuclei, without looping down into the pons and reflecting back along the MLF (Bender, 1980).
2. The cortical pathway for conjugate *upward* eye movements runs into the tegmentum *dorsal* to the pathway for *downward* movements.
   a. *Parinaud's syndrome.* Dorsal compression of the midbrain tectum, as from a pineal tumor, will selectively impair *upward* vertical movements (Parinaud's syndrome) before affecting downward gaze. Convergence palsy and pupillodilation are commonly present.
   b. *Bell's phenomenon* consists of the eyeballs automatically rotating upward and somewhat outward as an associated movement when the Pt closes the eyelids by orbicularis oculi contraction, as during volitional movements or sleep. After interruption of the UMN pathways for volitional upward movement, the presence of Bell's phenomenon on attempted eyelid closure proves that the LMNs for the upward movement are intact. Bell's phenomenon occurs in 85 percent of normal individuals, but the Ex will see Bell's phenomenon best after paralysis of the orbicularis oculi muscles due to interruption of the VIIth cranial nerve, which is called *Bell's palsy* (Sir Charles Bell, 1774–1842).
3. The pathway for conjugate *downward* eye movements runs into the midbrain tegmentum, dorsomedial to the red nucleus, where a lesion may selectively affect it, sparing vertical and horizontal eye movements (Jacobs, Heffner, Newman, 1985; Ross, 1986).

E. *Comparison of UMN and LMN lesions of the ocular system*
1. Interruption of optomotor nuclei or cranial nerves III, IV, or VI paralyzes individual EOMs. No reflex or volitional act can make the paralyzed muscle contract. The Pt suffers diplopia and strabismus.
2. Interruption of *internuclear* pathways, such as the MLF, paralyzes only that pathway's movements. Other reflexes or volitional pathways can still activate the ocular muscles. The Pt has diplopia only when that pathway should participate, as in the MLF syndrome.
3. Interruption of *supranuclear* pathways, the UMNs of the optomotor system, impairs conjugate eye movements, not the actions of the individual EOMs. The Pt does not have diplopia. Even after paralysis of volitional conjugate eye movements, reflexes, such as from vestibular stimulation, can activate the eyes.
4. Cortical or corticobulbar pathway lesions, as we have seen, paralyze volitional conjugate eye movements. Reflexes can still activate the muscles. We can conclude that ocular movements illustrate the previously announced

☑ *Movements*
☑ *Muscles*

epigram that UMN lesions paralyze ☐ movements/ ☐ muscles while LMN lesions paralyze ☐ movements/ ☐ muscles.

5. In fact, the MLF syndrome helps to emphasize that when an individual muscle is paralytic for only one movement and participates in others, the responsible lesion cannot be in the LMN.

F. *The concept of a head and eye centering center*
   1. We have discovered that many competing vectors determine the position of the eyes at any given instant. These include:
      a. The will or intent of the bearer of the eyes, the emotional state, the survival requirements and advantage-seeking possibilities of the circumstances, and the attractiveness of the visual display.
      b. The position of the head in relation to space, movement, gravity, and the activity of the vestibular system.
      c. The illumination and conditions of vision.
      d. The distance of the visual target and the refractive capability of the eyes.
      e. The demands of binocular fixation and image fusion.
   2. Vectors competing for the control of eye movements originate at every level of the neuraxis: cerebral cortex, basal motor nuclei, diencephalon, reticular formation, cerebellum, and even the rostral part of the spinal cord. Hence lesions at all of these levels can influence the movement and position of the eyes. The result is that for every eye position some forces act to keep the eyes there, and others act to move them. All of these forces, in the aggregate, result in the tonic innervation of the intra- and extraocular muscles, keeping them forever in a state of positive oppositional tension that positively determines eye position. To avoid chaos, some mechanism must integrate and balance these vectors. While no specific head and eye centering exists as such in one specific site, the concept of an eye and head centering "thermostat" that balances the right and left vectors, and the up and down vectors, explains a number of clinical phenomena.
   3. *Self-demonstration of the tendency to center the eyes and head.* The tendency for centering of the eyes and head is considerable. You can stare straight ahead, more or less vacantly or vapidly for some period, with no discomfort. Such staring spells are common, even in infants. But if you stare fully to one side, or up or down with your eyes, discomfort soon requires them to return to the primary position. To experience the centering tendency do this:
      a. Seat yourself comfortably. Then without turning your head, turn your eyes as far as possible to the left and keep them there as long as possible, gazing at one point. Blink as necessary but do not break fixation, and as you keep the eyes deviated attend to your own sensation. Time how long you can maintain the eyes in the deviated position. As an alternative try looking *up* as long as possible.
      b. After some brief period of increasing discomfort, you will find it necessary to return your eyes to the primary position, sometimes after as little as 30 seconds. You may feel the discomfort as anxiety, vertigo, blurred vision, or even headache. In any event, notice that you felt a considerable relief when your eyes returned to the primary position. Something about the organism wants its eyes and head straight ahead. In fact many mentally retarded and demented Pts cannot sustain deviation for even 30 seconds, a sign which can be included in the category of *motor impersistence.*
   4. Deviation of the eyes for any reason, volitional or reflex, triggers a reflex

saccade that kicks the eyes back to the primary position, unless kept deviated by volition, as in the foregoing experiment. Overcoming the saccadic kickback reflex is what requires the volitional effort of the eye deviation experiment.

5. Normally the right cerebral hemisphere tends to drive the head and eyes to the left, balanced by the left hemisphere trying to drive them to the right (Fig. 5-1*A*). The vector from one hemisphere actively opposes and counterbalances the vector from the other. An *up* vector also counterbalances a *down* vector. The net result is to keep the eyes positively centered in the primary position (Fig. 5-1*A*).

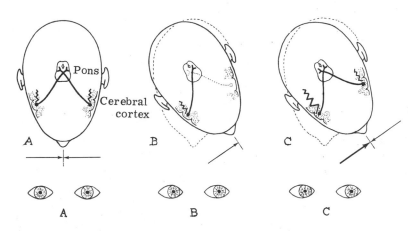

FIG. 5-1. The head and eye turning center (conjugate gaze center) in the posterior part of the frontal lobe. The arrows beneath the figures represent the strength of the vector originating on one side, acting to turn the head and eyes to the opposite side. Below each head is shown the position of the eyes. Notice the corticobulbar pathway to the pons and that it decussates. Relate this pathway to the MLF in Fig. 2-31. (*A*) Normal resting condition. The vectors are equal and the head and eyes are straight ahead. (*B*) A lesion has destroyed the conjugate gaze center on the left. The right center acts unopposed. The head and eyes deviate to the left. (*C*) An epileptogenic lesion has caused an excessive discharge of impulses from the right conjugate gaze center. The vector from the right hemisphere overpowers the one from the left. The head and eyes deviate to the left.

6. *The net effects of the centering vectors are tonic innervation and the reflex saccades that kick the eyes back to the primary position whenever they deviate from it for any reason.* Conversely, any Pt with persistent deviation of both eyes in any direction from the primary position has a neurologic lesion affecting the central pathways. If only one eye deviates when the eyes should be in the primary position, the lesion is in the LMN or neuromuscular apparatus.

G. *Effect of destructive cerebral lesions on the position of the eyes and head*
   1. A sudden massive infarct of one cerebral hemisphere, say the *left,* will interrupt the corticobulbar and corticospinal tracts, causing a complete *right* hemiplegia. The lesion nullifies the vector arising in the *left* hemisphere that should continually strive to turn the eyes and head to the *right* (Fig. 5-1*B*).
   2. What would you expect the position of the head and eyes to be in the foregoing Pt? ☐ midline/ ☐ turned to the left/ ☐ turned to the right. Explain:

_____

_____

_____

Ans: ☑ *Turned to the left. The lesion has eliminated the vector from the left hemisphere that tries to turn the head and eyes to the right. The vector from*

*the right hemisphere would be acting unopposed. Therefore, the head and
eyes would turn to the left, opposite to the hemiplegic side.*

3. The head and eye deviation are most prominent in the acute phase of the lesion (De Renzi et al., 1982; Fijssen et al. 1991). The head and eye centering mechanisms reset themselves quickly, but the hemiplegia endures.

H. *Effect of irritative lesions on the position of the head and eyes*

1. Some cerebral lesions irritate cortical neurons, causing them to discharge excessively. Such an irritative lesion is called an *epileptogenic focus* because it initiates epileptic seizures. Stimulation of cortical tissue by an electrode has the same effect. Suppose you have observed a Pt with a focal epileptic seizure which began by turning of the head and eyes to the *left*. You would anticipate that the Pt had an epileptogenic focus in the ☐ right/ ☐ left frontal lobe (Fig. 5-1*C*).

☑ *right*

2. *During* the epileptic discharge, the excess of impulses overcomes the normal vector from the opposite side. *After* the epileptic cataclysm has subsided, the cortical neurons which have been discharging excessively are metabolically exhausted and temporarily nonfunctional. Immediately *after* an epileptic seizure caused by a right-sided cerebral lesion, to which side would the head and eyes be turned? ☐ right/ ☐ left Explain: _____

_____

*Ans: ☑ Right. Since the right center for turning the eyes and head is
exhausted, the left acts unopposed. The head and eyes turn to the right,
opposite to the direction that they turned during the seizure.*

I. *The sylvian aqueduct syndrome*

Concentrated in the tissue around the sylvian aqueduct, in the midbrain tectum and pretectal area that merges with the diencephalon, are a number of nuclei and pathways that control the actions of the eyes: upward and downward gaze, vertical ocular alignment and verticality of the head and eyes, pupillary size, palpebral fissue height, vergences, and the ocular muscles innervated by III and IV.

TABLE 5-2 Sylvian aqueduct syndrome and related findings

Sylvian aqueduct syndrome per se
   Pupillary changes: anisocoria, corectopia, absence of light reaction
   Impairment of upward gaze
   Convergence nystagmus
   Paralysis of divergence or convergence
   Retractory nystagmus, usually inconstant
   Vertical nystagmus on gaze upward or downward
   Palsy of extraocular muscles of III or IV
   Lid retraction, "reptilian stare"
   Obliquity of head

Midbrain signs in addition to aqueduct syndrome
   Minimal to severe impairment of consciousness
   Unilateral or bilateral IIId nerve palsy
   Quadriparesis and upper motor neuron signs of hyperreflexia and extensor plantar
      responses
   Decerebrate rigidity
   Central neurogenic hyperventilation

Combinations of these ocular signs localize the lesion (Table 5-2) (Baloh et al, 1985; Keane, 1990; Oliva and Rosenberg, 1990).

References for Central Control of Eye Movements

Baloh RW, Furman JM, Yee RD: Dorsal midbrain syndrome: Clinical and oculographic findings. *Neurology,* 1985; 35:54–60.

Bender MB: Brain control of conjugate horizontal and vertical eye movements. A survey of the structural and functional correlates. *Brain,* 1980; 103:23–69.

Bronstein AM, Morris J, du Boulay G, Gresty MA, Rudge P: Abnormalities of horizontal gaze. Clinical, oculographic and magnetic resonance imaging findings. I. Abducens palsy. *J Neurol Neurosurg Psychiat,* 1990; 53:194–199.

Bronstein AM, Rudge P, Gresty MA, du Boulay G, Morris J: Abnormalities of horizontal gaze. Clinical, oculographic and magnetic resonance imaging findings. II. Gaze palsy and internuclear ophthalmoplegia. *J Neurol Neurosurg Psychiat,* 1990; 53:200–207.

De Renzi E, Colombo A, Faglioni P, Gibertoni M: Conjugate gaze in stroke patients with unilateral damage. *Arch Neurol,* 1982; 39:482–486.

Jacobs L, Heffner RR, Jr, Newman RP: Selective paralysis of downward gaze caused by bilateral lesions of the mesencephalic periaqueductal gray matter. *Neurology,* 1985; 35:516–521.

Keane JF: The pretectal syndrome. *Neurology,* 1990; 40:684–690.

Oliva A, Rosenberg ML: Convergence-evoked nystagmus. *Neurology,* 1990; 40:161–162.

Ross RT: Paralysis of downward gaze. *Neurology,* 1986; 36:1540–1541.

Ross AT, DeMyer W: Isolated syndrome of the medial longitudinal fasciculus in man. *Arch Neurol,* 1966; 15:203–205.

Tijssen CC, van Gisbergen JAM, Schulte BPM: Conjugate eye deviation: Side, site, and size of the hemispheric lesion. *Neurology,* 1991; 41:846–850.

Yee RD, Baloh RW, Marder SR, et al: Eye movements in schizophrenia. *Invest Ophthalmol Vis Sci,* 1987; 28:366–374.

Further Reading

Bach-y-Rita P, Collins C (eds): *The Control of Eye Movements.* New York, Academic, 1971.

Gay A, Newman N: Eye movements and their disorders: An analytical evaluation, in Critchley M (ed): *Scientific Foundations of Neurology.* Philadelphia, F.A. Davis, 1972.

Glaser JF (ed): *Neuro-ophthalmology* (2d ed). Lippincott, Philadelphia, 1990.

J. *The asymmetric tonic neck reflex (ATNR):* the integration of the contralateral visual field, proprioception, and volitional movement, or how the infant discovers its own hand.
  1. *Technique to elicit the asymmetric tonic neck reflex*
     a. With the infant *supine* and *quiet,* gently and slowly turn the infant's head to one side, holding it there for at least 30 seconds. Then turn the infant's head back fully to the opposite side (Fig. 5-2).
     b. Normally the infant *extends* the arm and leg on the side to which the head is turned, and *flexes* the contralateral extremities. Remember the expected result of the head-turning maneuver by the rule that *as the head looks to one side the hand extends into that visual field.*
     c. Careful observation discloses that normal infants spend much time in the ATNR posture, but they can readily elude it. It is most prominent between the ages of 2 and 4 months, at a time when the infant is learning to fixate and reach for objects.
  2. *Physiologic basis of the ATNR.* Slow head-turning elicits the ATNR by stimulating position sense receptors in the neck (fast head-turning elicits a

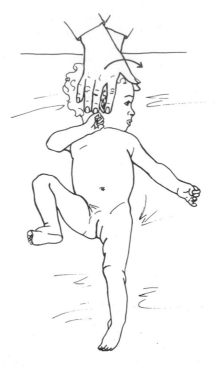

FIG. 5-2. Posture of the extremities during a tonic neck reflex. The Ex has forcefully turned the infant's head to the left.

vestibular reflex). The afferent pathway of the reflex runs *rostrally* into the brainstem reticular formation and then *caudally* into the spinal cord by reticulospinal pathways.

3. *Interpretation of the ATNR*

   a. Since the head and eyes look to the side of the extended hand, we can interpret the ATNR as the forerunner of eye-hand coordination. The reflex causes the infant to discover its own extending hand as indicated by sight and proprioception. If the hand encounters an object, the grasp reflex closes the fingers on the object. The eyes then learn to direct via the pyramidal tract the hand as it explores space and learns to grasp visual targets. Here again is demonstrated the unity of a visual field, proprioception, and the control of movement in one hemisphere, as related to the opposite side of space. It marvellously substantiates the law of contralateral sensorimotor innervation (Chap. 2).

   b. The reflex is interpreted as a primitive behavior. It disappears as cerebral pathways establish dominance over the primitive reflexes during maturation. Any undue persistence of the ATNR posture, either when spontaneously assumed by the infant or when induced by an Ex predicts poor motor development. The more obligatory the response and the longer it persists in infancy, the more abnormal the infant. When strong and persistent it interferes with sitting and volitional movement. It indicates that UMN dominance over the primitive reflexes is not proceeding according to the normal developmental timetable.

4. The ATNR may reappear in older children or adults who suffer high brainstem lesions interrupting corticobulbar and other descending motor pathways; in these Pts cerebral dominance over the brainstem is lost.

5. *Summary of the ATNR*

   a. When the head of an infant is turned to one side, the ipsilateral extrem-

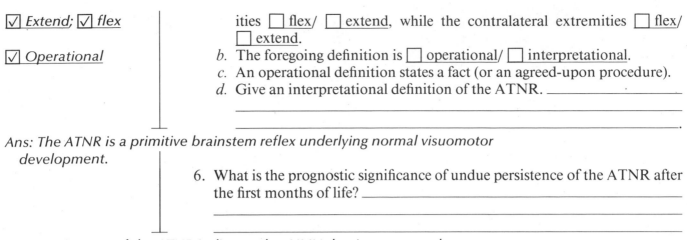

✓ *Extend;* ✓ *flex*

✓ *Operational*

ities ☐ flex/ ☐ extend, while the contralateral extremities ☐ flex/ ☐ extend.

b. The foregoing definition is ☐ operational/ ☐ interpretational.

c. An operational definition states a fact (or an agreed-upon procedure).

d. Give an interpretational definition of the ATNR. _____

_____

_____

Ans: The ATNR is a primitive brainstem reflex underlying normal visuomotor development.

6. What is the prognostic significance of undue persistence of the ATNR after the first months of life? _____

_____

Ans: Persistence of the ATNR indicates that UMN dominance over the brainstem reflexes is not proceeding according to the normal developmental timetable. The infant is likely to show permanent deficits in UMN control of movement.

FURTHER READING FOR THE ASYMMETRIC TONIC NECK REFLEX

Capute AJ, Shapiro BK, Pasquale AJ, Accardo J, et al.: Motor functions: associated primitive reflex profiles. *Develop Med and Child Neurol,* 1982; 24:662–669.

Magnus R: Cameron Prize Lectures on some results of studies in the physiology of posture. *Lancet,* 1926, 2:531–536; 585–588.

II. Nystagmus

A. *Definition and causes.* Nystagmus consists of involuntary, rhythmic to-and-fro oscillations of the eyeballs. It reflects disruption of the intricate feedback circuits of the brainstem that control the various, competing optomotor systems. It is distinguished from *opsoclonus,* which is a rapid, chaotic, non-rhythmic jerking of the eyeballs. Nystagmus may result from

1. Ocular lesions which interfere with fixation.
2. Vestibular end organ lesions.
3. Central nervous system (CNS) lesions in the *nystagmogenic zone,* which consists of
   a. The rostral end of the spinal cord.
   b. The brainstem tegmentum up to the midbrain-diencephalic junction.

B. *Symptoms of nystagmus*

1. Symptoms may or may not accompany nystagmus. The presence of *symptoms* depends on the age of onset, acuteness of the lesion, and type of nystagmus. Recall that heterotropia of congenital or early origin usually causes no diplopia. Similarly, nystagmus of congenital or early origin may cause no symptoms.
2. The *symptoms* are nausea, vertigo, and oscillopsia.
   a. *Nausea* (with or without vomiting).
   b. *Vertigo:* a sensation of movement, generally a feeling of rotation or spinning of self or environment (Chap. 8).
   c. *Oscillopsia:* oscillating vision, apparent oscillation of objects viewed.

C. *Analysis of the signs of nystagmus.* Describe nystagmus as to its *form*, *type*, and *direction*.

   1. *Form.* Classify the nystagmus according to the form of the eye movement. Nystagmus form

     ☐ Horizontal

     ☐ Vertical

     ☐ Rotatory

     ☐ Mixed

     a. To remember the forms of nystagmus, ask yourself this: What are the *possible* forms of eye movement as related to the three axes of rotation?

       (1) *Horizontal* (lateral) eye movements are rotations around the _____ axis of the eyeball.

Vertical
Lateral

       (2) *Vertical* movements are rotations around the _____ axis.

A-P

       (3) *Rotatory* movements (torsions) are rotations around the _____ axis.

     b. Hence, the *forms* of nystagmus are:

     Nystagmus forms

Horizontal
Vertical
Rotatory (torsional)
Mixed

     ☐ _____

     ☐ _____

     ☐ _____

     ☐ _____

   2. *Type.* Observe whether the eye excursions are of a *jerk* or *pendular* type. Jerk nystagmus has a *fast* and *slow* component. Pendular nystagmus is like a pendulum: the excursions are of equal velocity. It is a tick-tock or metronomic movement.

Pendular
Jerk

     a. If to = fro, the Pt has _____ nystagmus.

     b. If to ≠ fro, the Pt has _____ nystagmus.

   3. *Direction.* If the Pt has jerk nystagmus, identify the *direction* of the nystagmus. The direction is usually named according to the direction of movement of the fast component.

Right

     a. If the nystagmus has the fast component to the right side, we say the direction is to the _____.

     b. If the direction of the fast component is always to one side, the nystagmus is said to be *unidirectional.* If the direction of the fast component changes with the direction of eye movement, the nystagmus is *bidirectional.*

     c. Nomenclature note: The convention in the past has been to name jerk nystagmus according to the direction of the fast movement. Physiologically, the important event is the deviation or slow phase, as in caloric or optokinetic nystagmus. Once deviation occurs, the saccadic kickback is automatic.

   4. *The effect of eye movement on nystagmus.* Determine whether the nystagmus changes in *rate, amplitude,* or *direction* as the eyes are moved through the various fields of gaze. Generally speaking, jerk nystagmus increases in amplitude when the Pt looks in the direction of the fast component.

D. *Differentiation of nystagmus of various origins*

   1. If you can describe the *form, type,* and *direction* of nystagmus you need not memorize the almost endless kinds and causes. Dendrograms and tables will provide the probable diagnosis (Figs. 5-3, 5-4, and 5-5). Familiarize yourself with the dendrograms and tables but do not memorize. Notice that *pendular*

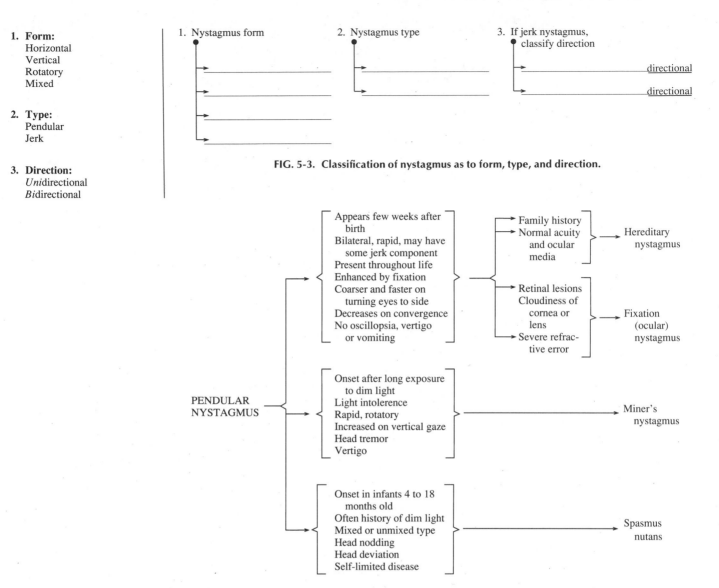

1. **Form:**
   Horizontal
   Vertical
   Rotatory
   Mixed

2. **Type:**
   Pendular
   Jerk

3. **Direction:**
   *Uni*directional
   *Bi*directional

FIG. 5-3. Classification of nystagmus as to form, type, and direction.

FIG. 5-4. Differential diagnostic dendrogram for pendular nystagmus (reference only).

nystagmus implies an ocular cause or lesion. *Jerk* nystagmus implies a *vestibular* or *neural* lesion.

2. *Differentiation of spontaneous vestibular nystagmus* (Table 5-3). Do not memorize.

3. *Differentiation of positional vestibular nystagmus* (Table 5-4). Do not memorize.

4. *Electronystagmography.* For more refined analysis, spontaneous nystagmus or that induced by caloric irrigation or positional change can be recorded by electronystagmography (Chap. 13).

FURTHER READING FOR NYSTAGMUS

Baloh RW, Sakala SM, Yee RD et al: Quantitative vestibular testing. *Otolaryngol Head Neck Surg* 1984; 92:145–150.

Hornrubia V, Brazier MAB (eds): Nystagmus and Vertigo: Clinical Approaches to the Patient with Dizziness. Vol 24, UCLA Forum in Medical Sciences, 1982.

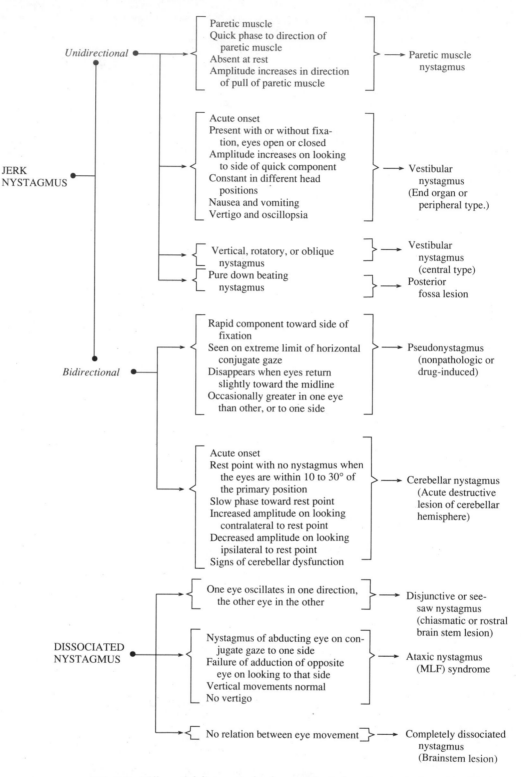

FIG. 5-5. Differential diagnostic dendrogram for jerk nystagmus (reference only).

III. Summary of the laws of ocular motility as applied to the clinical examination

A. *Laws governing the actions of the ocular muscles*

    1. *The law of on-center/off-center pull of the extraocular muscles.* The ocular muscles which pull "on-center" have only one primary rotatory action,

TABLE 5-3 Vestibular nystagmus

Symptoms or sign	Peripheral (end-organ)	Central (nuclear)
Direction of nystagmus	Unidirectional; fast phase opposite lesion	Bidirectional or unidirectional
Purely horizontal nystagmus without torsional component	Uncommon	Common
Vertical or purely torsional nystagmus	Never present	May be present
Visual fixation	Inhibits nystagmus and vertigo	No inhibition
Severity of vertigo	Marked	Mild
Direction of spin	Toward fast phase	Variable
Direction of pastpointing	Toward slow phase	Variable
Direction of Romberg fall	Toward slow phase	Variable
Effect of head-turning	Changes Romberg fall	No effect
Duration of symptoms	Finite (minutes, days, weeks) but recurrent	May be chronic
Tinnitus or deafness	Often present	Usually absent
Common causes	Infection (labyrinthitis), Meniere's disease, neuronitis, vascular disorders, trauma, toxicity	Vascular, demyelinating, and neoplastic disorders

SOURCE: From Glaser, 1990.

TABLE 5-4 Differences between peripheral and central positional nystagmus

	Peripheral (extra-axial)	Central (intra-axial)
Latency	2–20 seconds	None
Persistence	Disappears within 50 seconds	Lasts longer than one minute
Fatigability	Disappears on repetition	Repeatable
Positions	Present in one position	Present in multiple positions
Vertigo	Always present	Occasionally absent, with only nystagmus present
Direction of nystagmus	One direction	Changing directions in different positions
Incidence	Common (85% of all cases)	Uncommon (10–15% of all cases)

whereas those that pull "off-center" cause primary, secondary, and tertiary rotations. The line of pull or vector of all EOMs runs *medial* to the vertical axis, except for the lateral rectus muscle (Fig. 4-17). *Corollary:* the muscles which pull off-center change their actions depending on the position of the eye (Figs. 4-12, 4-13, 4-15, and 4-16).

2. *The law of positive tonic oppositional innervation of the intra- and extraocular muscles.* All intraocular and extraocular muscles of one eye act in oppositional pairs. (The ciliary muscle would seem to be an exception, but its opposition is the elasticity of the lens.) When the eye is still in any position, all of its extraocular muscles receive continuous tonic innervation that positively determines the position. *Corollary:* paralysis of one ocular muscle causes that eye to assume the position, or the pupil to assume the size, dictated by the pull of the intact, tonically innervated, oppositional, muscle. A nuclear, nerve, or neuromuscular lesion paralyzes individual ocular muscles, causing strabismus and diplopia. Persistent monocular deviation is always peripheral, whereas persistent conjugate (binocular) deviation is central in origin.

B. *Laws governing the central control of eye movements*

1. *The law of conjugate ocular fixation and movement.* The eyes fixate and move conjugately. *Corollary:* failure of conjugate fixation and conjugate movement is always abnormal and requires investigation.

2. *Hering's law of equal innervation of the corresponding EOMs.* When the two eyes move, the collaborating muscles in the two eyes must receive equal innervation to keep the eyes yoked conjugately, so that the maculae align on the target and the retinal images fall on corresponding points.

3. *The law of different pathways for horizontal and vertical conjugate eye movements.* The supranuclear pathway for conjugate horizontal movements arises in the posterior frontal and the parietal cortex and loops down into the pontine tegmentum and back up to the midbrain through the MLF (Fig. 2-31). In direct contrast, the pathways for vertical movements arise more diffusely from the cortex and run directly into the pretectum and midbrain without looping down into the pons. The pathway for conjugate upward eye movements runs into the midbrain dorsal to the pathway for conjugate downward movements. *Corollary:* focal lesions may differentially affect the horizontal and vertical gaze pathways and may differentially affect either the upward or downward gaze pathways.

4. *The law of control of saccades by the fronto-parieto-tegmental pathway.* The fronto-parietal optomotor pathways (Fig. 2-31) mediate all saccadic eye movements: the saccades that move the eyes volitionally and those that restore them to the primary position after deviation by vestibular or optokinetic reflexes and REM sleep. *Corollary:* since fast and slow movements (slow pursuit and vestibular deviation) arise in different pathways, focal lesions may affect one set of pathways and not the other.

5. *The law of a positive eye and head centering mechanism.* The head and eyes remain in or tend to return to the primary position because of active centering mechanisms (Fig. 5-1). If the eyes deviate from the primary position for any reason, saccadic kickback tends to restore the eyes to the primary position. *Corollary:* any *persistent* deviation of the eyes horizontally or vertically indicates an unbalanced centering mechanism, caused by a destructive lesion or by excessive drive in one of the centering systems.
   a. Unbalanced *destruction* of one supranuclear pathway for eye movements results in persistent conjugate deviation of the eyes in the direction *opposite* to the one mediated by the affected pathway (Fig. 5-1).
   b. Unbalanced irritation of one supranuclear pathway for eye movements will cause persistent conjugate deviation in the same direction mediated by that pathway (Fig. 5-1).

6. *The law of occipital control of visually mediated reflexes.* The occipital lobe controls the visually mediated reflex eye movements: fixation, fusion, following, vergences, and optokinetic nystagmus. All require an intact afferent arc through the retina and intact occipito-tegmental or occipito-fronto-tegmental pathways.

7. *The law of competition between reflex control and volitional demand.* Fixation, fusion, following (pursuit), and vergences operate reflexly but can be overcome by or subjugated to volitional demand. *Corollary:* interruption of the volitional pathways may allow reflex mechanisms to become overactive, particularly fixation reflexes, and then the Pt cannot move the eyes from a visual target without blinking or moving the head.

8. *The counterrolling law.* When the head moves, proprioceptive reflexes, arising in the vestibular system and neck, and fixation reflexes counterroll the eyes against the direction of movement, thus tending to keep the eyes

locked on the visual target. *Corollary:* failure of the eyes to counterroll indicates failure of one or more of these systems. When unconsciousness negates volitional movements and fixation, failure of the eyes to counterroll in response to vestibular stimulation by head turning (doll's eye test) or caloric irrigation, means interruption of the vestibular connections through the brainstem tegmentum.

C. *Summary of clinical tests for central eye movement disorders* (Table 5-5)

IV. Summary of the eye examination

A. Now we have to unite the individual fragments of the eye examination into a coherent routine. I would have no trouble convincing you to practice if you were a tennis player wanting to improve his strokes or an actor. A great actor, preparing to play the role of a physician, would practice hour after hour to capture the exact nuances of professional behavior. Ours, too, is a performing art. Do you always want to look like a beginner? If not, practice with another student until you can offer a professional performance to your patient. Then you can say with Blaise Cendrars:

> *I have deciphered all the confused texts of the wheels and I have assembled*
> *the scattered elements of a most violent beauty.*

TABLE 5-5 Outline of clinical tests for central eye movement disorders	
Type of eye movement	Method of examination
1. Spontaneous movements during ordinary behavior and ordinary environmental stimuli	Inspection while taking the history. Look for malalignment, range, and persistence of eye movements, and for hyperkinesias such as nystagmus.
2. Volitional fixation and volitional movements	Examiner observes steadiness and range of eye movements after commanding patient to fixate on a distant object straight ahead and then to move the eyes to the *right, left, up,* and *down.*
3. Visual reflex ocular movements	
a. Smooth pursuit	The patient's eyes pursue the examiner's finger as it moves through the full range of ocular movements.
b. Vergences	The examiner directs the patient to look at near and distant objects and to follow the examiner's moving finger in toward the patient's nose.
c. Reflex fixation	The patient fixates straight ahead and the examiner turns the patient's head slowly to the right, left, up, and down.
d. Alignment lock	As the patient fixates straight ahead the examiner alternately covers and uncovers first one, then the other eye, and looks for deviation in alignment after monocular occlusion of vision (cover-uncover test).
*e. Optokinetic nystagmus (OKN)	Patient fixates on rotating drum or a moving striped strip.
4. Nonvisual reflex ocular movements	
†a. Caloric nystagmus	Irrigation of ears with hot or cold water
†b. Positional nystagmus	Placing the patient's head in various postures
†c. Contraversive eye-turning test (Doll's eye test, oculocephalic test)	Quick turning of the patient's head by the examiner's hands; used in comatose patients
†5. Associated eye movement (Bell's phenomenon)	The examiner holds the patient's eyelids open and observes the involuntary upward movement of the eyes that occurs when the patient attempts to close the lids.

*Not discussed in this text
†Discussed later in text

B. Part V, A,1-5 of the Summarized Neurologic Examination organizes the scattered elements of the eye examination. Practice, *practice,* until they unite into one beautiful, flowing sequence for testing cranial nerves II, III, IV, and VI and their central pathways.

C. The five steps that you have just rehearsed constitute a minimum routine examination. Pts with ocular complaints or in whom you suspect a brain disorder may need a more thorough analysis of ocular motility mechanisms. Use Table 5-5 as a reference as needed to supplement Part V, A of the summarized examination. Notice that steps 1 to 3 apply to the conscious, cooperative Pt, while steps 4 to 5 depend on reflex or associated movements not under conscious control.

Learning Objectives for Chapter Five

I. Central systems for the control of eye movements

1. Define a saccade and list the eye movements that are saccadic.
2. State the five major eye movement systems and the pathways involved. (Mnemonic: hold up your finger, look at it, and move it.)
3. Diagram the pathway for volitional conjugate horizontal eye movements, from cortex to ocular muscles (Fig. 2-31).
4. Describe the signs and symptoms after interruption of one medial longitudinal fasciculus (MLF).
5. Explain why an eye that fails to adduct because of an MLF lesion will adduct during convergence.
6. Describe the effect on eye movements of bilateral interruption of the corticobulbar pathway for volitional horizontal conjugate gaze.
7. Contrast the pathways for volitional vertical eye movements and convergence with the horizontal movement pathway.
8. Describe the difference in the location of pathways for upward gaze and downward gaze at the pretectal-midbrain level.
9. Describe Parinaud's syndrome and associated findings.
10. Describe how to use Bell's phenomenon to eliminate a LMN lesion in a Pt with paralysis of volitional upward gaze.
11. Explain how the aphorism that "UMN (supranuclear) lesions paralyze movements whereas LMN lesions paralyze muscles" applies to the optomotor system.
12. By means of a vector analysis, explain the concept of an eye and head centering center.
13. Explain the effect of an acute destructive lesion of a cerebral hemisphere on the position of the head and eyes, as contrasted to an irritative, epileptogenic lesion of the same hemisphere (Fig. 5-1).
14. Describe several neuro-ophthalmologic findings that would localize a lesion in the pretectal-tectal-tegmental region surrounding the sylvian aqueduct (sylvian aqueduct syndrome).
15. Describe how to elicit the asymmetric tonic neck reflex, the response expected, and the clinical interpretation of the results.
16. Explain how the asymmetric tonic neck reflex fits in with the law of contralateral cerebral sensorimotor innervation.

II. Nystagmus

1. Define nystagmus.
2. State the difference in the symptoms of congenital nystagmus and acutely acquired nystagmus following a vestibular or central lesion.
3. Classify nystagmus as to form, type, and direction.
4. State which type of nystagmus implies an ocular lesion and which type a vestibular or neurologic lesion.
5. Describe several maneuvers to induce eye movements after paralysis of UMNs to prove that the LMNs are intact. (Hint: Table 5-5 contains them, although not formally listed as such.)

III. Summary of the Laws of Ocular Motility as applied to the Clinical Examination

Explain the clinical applications of each of the laws of ocular motility listed in Section III, A and B.

IV. Summary of the Eye Examination

Demonstrate the standard NE of vision and ocular motility (Section V of the Summarized NE and Table 5-5).

Chapter Six

Motor Examination of Cranial Nerves V, VII, IX, X, XI, and XII

To those I address, it is unnecessary to go farther, than to indicate that the nerves treated of in these papers are the instruments of expression, from the smile upon the infant's cheek to the last agony of life. . . .

Sir Charles Bell (1774–1842)

I. Vth cranial nerve motor function: Chewing

A. Functional anatomy of chewing
1. The Vth nerve chews. It innervates *all* and, for clinical purposes, *only* the chewing muscles: the *masseter, temporal,* and *lateral* and *medial pterygoids.* Nerve V innervates no salivary glands or smooth muscle.
2. *Jaw closure.* Place your fingertips about 2 cm above and in front of the angle of the mandible. Bite hard and relax several times. The muscle felt, the *masseter,* is the only chewing muscle that the Ex can adequately palpate. The pull of the chewing muscles in closing the jaw is relatively direct and uncomplicated.
3. *Lateral jaw movement.* Move your jaw from side to side. Chewing requires not only jaw closure but also a *lateral,* grinding action caused by contraction of the *lateral* pterygoid muscles (Ramfjord and Ash, 1966).
   a. In Fig. 6-1 notice the *origin* of the lateral pterygoid muscles from the skull base and their *insertion* near the mandibular condyle. The origin of the muscle from the base of the skull is immobile. When the muscle contracts, only the mandible can move. The vector diagram shows that the mandible moves straight forward when both muscles contract equally (Fig. 6-1).
   b. If only the *right* lateral pterygoid muscle contracts, the mandibular tip moves to the ☐ right/ ☐ left.
   c. If the Pt can move the jaw to the right but not to the left, the lateral pterygoid muscle on the ☐ right/ ☐ left is paralyzed.
   d. As a second action, the lateral pterygoid muscles aid in opening the jaw because of their insertion on the neck of the mandible (Fig. 6-2).

☑ *Left*

☑ *Right*

*The light vertical rule on the left side of the text sets off an answer column. Cover the answers with a card until you have responded to the text. Then after each response, slide the card down to check your answer.

The heavy vertical rule denotes optional material.

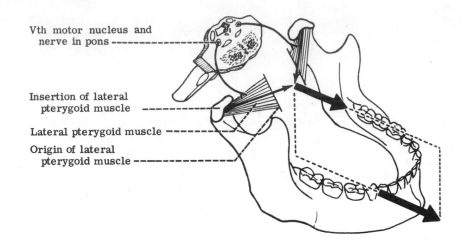

Vth motor nucleus and nerve in pons

Insertion of lateral pterygoid muscle

Lateral pterygoid muscle

Origin of lateral pterygoid muscle

FIG. 6-1. Innervation and action of the lateral pterygoid muscles. If both muscles contract equally, the tip of the mandible moves forward in the midline. If only one muscle contracts, the tip moves forward and to the opposite side. Study the vector diagram (arrows between the muscles).

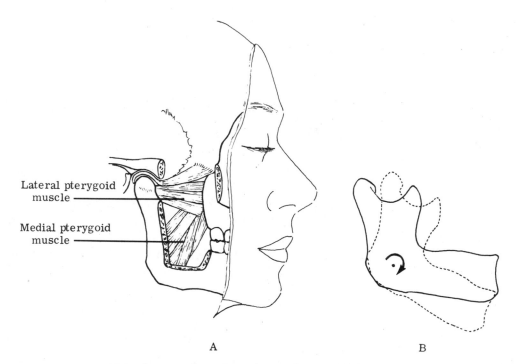

Lateral pterygoid muscle

Medial pterygoid muscle

A   B

FIG. 6-2. (*A*) Action of lateral pterygoid muscles to depress the tip of the mandible when the patient forcefully opens the jaw. The forward pull of the lateral pterygoid muscles acts to open the jaw because the jaw is suspended so as to rotate around a lateral axis, as shown by the curved arrow in *B*.

Lateral pterygoid

☑ *Right;* ☑ *down*

☑ *Left*

e. If the Pt's mandible moves forward and down in the *midline* on jaw opening, both _____ _____ muscles have contracted equally.

f. If the *left* lateral pterygoid muscle contracts, the tip of the mandible moves not only to the ☐ right/ ☐ left but also ☐ up/ ☐ down.

g. If the Pt's jaw deviates to the *left* on forceful opening, the weak muscle is the ☐ right/ ☐ left lateral pterygoid muscle.

4. Name the two major actions of the lateral pterygoid muscles. _____

_____

Ans: Lateral movement and opening of the jaw.

5. The remaining mandibular muscles innervated by the Vth nerve all act to close the jaw. The names of these muscles are: _____

_____ .

Ans: Masseter, temporal, and medial pterygoid.

B. *Lower motor neuron (LMN) lesions of V*
1. Unilateral destruction of the perikarya or axons of the Vth nerve causes complete paralysis of all of the ipsilateral chewing muscles.
2. The denervated muscle undergoes atrophy. *Atrophy* and *paralysis* are the two outstanding signs of LMN lesions. Which chewing muscle can you can most readily palpate to check for atrophy? _____

Masseter

C. *Upper motor neuron (UMN) innervation of V*
1. Pursuant to general principles of UMN innervation, one cerebral hemisphere sends UMN axons to the contralateral Vth nerve nucleus. However, the principle of contralateral motor innervation requires some qualification, because not all muscles customarily act unilaterally. The proximal (axial) muscles for many movements, such as trunk extension, vertical head movements, chewing, and swallowing, act with bilateral symmetry much or all of the time. Compare your ability to contract half of your diaphragm, half of your anal sphincter, and half of your abdomen to your ability to flex a finger. Although some axial muscles can act unilaterally, such as the abdominal, they customarily act bilaterally. The law of contralateral innervation holds most strictly for movements, such as those of the hand, which has as their outstanding characteristic free, independent unilateral movement. Hence, we find that:
   a. The proximal (axial) muscles which ordinarily act symmetrically have ☐ mostly ipsilateral/ ☐ bilateral/ ☐ mostly contralateral UMN innervation.

☑ *Bilateral*

   b. The distal (appendicular) muscles which ordinarily act unilaterally have mainly ☐ ipsilateral/ ☐ bilateral/ ☐ contralateral UMN innervation.

☑ *Contralateral*

2. Because of bilateral UMN innervation, unilateral UMN lesions do not cause a severe or enduring unilateral paralysis of the chewing muscles (Willoughby and Anderson, 1984). UMN lesions do not selectively paralyze individual muscles or sets of muscles innervated by one peripheral nerve.

D. *Clinical tests of the Vth nerve motor function*
NOTE: Do these tests on yourself as they are described.
1. Inspect the temples and cheeks for atrophy of the temporalis and masseter muscles. The temporal muscle fills out the temple. Even when the Pt bites, the muscle is difficult to palpate, but after temporalis muscle atrophy, the temple sinks in (Fig. 1-9I).
2. Palpate both masseters for atrophy. Ask the Pt to clench the teeth together strongly and then palpate both muscles for simultaneous comparison as they mound up.
3. Test for the strength of jaw closure by having the Pt clench the teeth strongly. Place the heel of one palm on the tip of the Pt's mandible and the other on the Pt's forehead. Press hard on the tip of the mandible. You must help support the Pt's head with your opposite hand because jaw closure is a very strong movement, and you do not want to test the strength of head extension and jaw closure at the same time. *The principle is to test only the strength of one muscle or set of muscles at a time.*

4. Test the lateral pterygoids by having the Pt forcefully open the jaw. Note whether its tip aligns with the notch between the upper medial incisor teeth. Then ask the Pt to move the jaw from side to side. Finally ask the Pt to hold the jaw forcefully to the side as you try to push it back to the center with the heel of your palm. What do you do with your opposite hand to stabilize the Pt's head and neck? _____

Ans: Press against the opposite cheekbone. If you are doing these tests on yourself or a partner, as I have requested, all of these answers will be self-evident.

Censored

5. To insure that you know what to do, test Vth nerve motor function on yourself and on a partner. Don't just sit there: get up off of your _____ and do it! The text cannot substitute for the proprioceptive experience provided by use of your own hands. A word of caution: do not be jerky or too forceful in testing jaw muscles, particularly in elderly or edentulous Pts. The temporomandibular joint may dislocate.

E. Analyze this Pt

☑ *LMN;* ☑ *left*

Examination of a 46-year-old man with difficulty in chewing disclosed atrophy and paralysis of the left temporal and masseter muscles. When he opened his jaw, it deviated to the left. He could not move it forcefully to the right. No other muscles were weak. The evidence points to ☐ LMN/ ☐ UMN lesion on the ☐ right/ ☐ left/ ☐ both side(s).
Explain: _____

Ans: The paralysis affects only the muscles of a single nerve, V. The paralysis is complete, and the muscles are atrophic. Since the atrophic and paralyzed muscles are on the left, the lesion interrupts the left Vth nerve.

REFERENCES FOR Vth NERVE MOTOR FUNCTION

Ramfjord S, Ash M, Jr: *Occlusion.* Philadelphia, Saunders, 1966.
Willoughby EW, Anderson NE: Lower cranial nerve motor function in unilateral vascular lesions of the cerebral hemisphere. *Br Med J,* 1984; 289:791–794.

II. VIIth cranial nerve motor functions: Facial movements

A. Functional anatomy of facial movements

V

1. The VIIth nerve moves the face. In generalizing that VII innervates *all* facial muscles, we mean all of the facial muscles proper (Fig. 6-3). Cranial nerve V innervates mandibular muscles.
2. Look into a mirror and make every possible facial movement, including wiggling your nose and ears. Work through Table 6-1, remembering that *every* facial movement tests the integrity of VII.
3. *Two functions of the facial muscles.* The facial muscles perform two roles—expressing emotions and guarding the facial apertures.
    a. Expression of emotions such as frowning, smiling, and mimicking.
    b. Controlling and guarding *every* facial aperture: the palpebral fissures, oral fissure, nares, and external auditory canals.

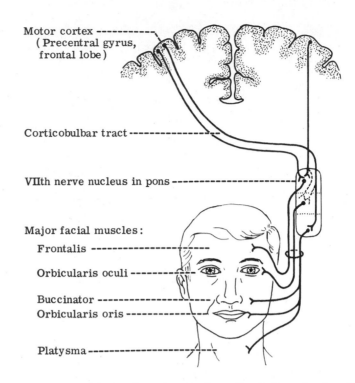

FIG. 6-3. UMN and LMN innervation of the facial muscles. The dotted lines indicate that the orbicularis oculi muscles receive a variable number of crossed and uncrossed axons. Therefore, the degree of weakness of the muscle varies after UMN lesions.

4. *Innervation of the stapedius muscle.* Having accepted that VII and its muscles guard the facial apertures, we can extend the guardianship notion to the middle ear, where VII innervates the *stapedius* muscle. It acts to dampen excessive movement of the ossicles during loud sounds. After paralysis of the stapedius muscle, the Pt may experience ordinary sounds as uncomfortably loud.

TABLE 6-1 Clinically important movements and muscles innervated by the VIIth cranial nerve

Movements	Muscles
1. *Wrinkle up* your forehead, as in looking up as far as possible	Frontalis
2. *Close* your eyes as tightly as possible	Orbicularis oculi, the sphincter of the palpebral fissure
3. *Close* your lips tightly as possible	Orbicularis oris, the sphincter of the oral fissure
4. *Pull back* the corners of your mouth strongly, as in smiling. At the same time palpate your cheeks	Buccinator
5. *Pull down* the corners of your mouth strongly, as in pouting. At the same time palpate the anterolateral aspect of your neck and observe it in the mirror	Platysma

B. *Intra- and extraaxial anatomy of cranial nerve VII*

1. Learn Fig. 6-4, and compare it to the generalized brainstem section in Fig. 2-14.

2. Notice the peculiar internal loop of VII around the VIth nerve nucleus. Using a colored pencil, draw in the course of the VIth and VIIth nerves on the opposite side of Fig. 6-4.

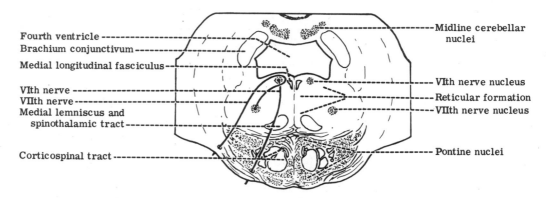

FIG. 6-4. **Transverse section of the pons at a caudal level to include the VIth and VIIth cranial nerve nuclei. The VIth and VIIth nerves, along with the VIIIth, exit at the pontomedullary sulcus.**

Tectum; cerebellum
(Fig. 2-14)

3. In accordance with general principles of brainstem nomenclature, the longitudinal plate that forms the roof of the pons is called the _____. It contains the deep nuclei that belong to the _____.

4. The second longitudinal division of the pons, the _____, contains the cranial nerve nuclei. The three motor nuclei of the pons are for cranial neves _____, _____, and _____.

Tegmentum; V; VI; VII
Basis; corticospinal

5. The most ventral longitudinal zone of the pons is the _____. Through it run the _____ tracts to the LMNs of the spinal cord.

6. Before exiting from the pons, the VIIth nerve fibers loop around the _____th nerve nucleus.

VI

7. Three cranial nerves exit at the pontomedullary sulcus. In ventrodorsal order, these nerves are _____, _____, and _____.

Ans: VI, VII, VIII. (Review Fig. 2-22 if you erred.)

8. As typifies peripheral nerves, the VIIth nerves do not cross the midline. Study only the LMNs of VII in Fig. 6-3. We will return to the UMN innervation later.

9. If a lesion destroys the VIIth nerve nucleus, the intraaxial course of the axons, or the peripheral nerve trunk, the result is paralysis of *all* ☐ ipsilateral/ ☐ contralateral facial muscles.

☑ *Ipsilateral*

10. The only clinically testable sensory function of VII is taste (Chap. 8). See Fig. 9-6 for the full peripheral distribution of VII.

C. *Upper motor neuron innervation of VII*

1. A demonstration of the degree of unilaterality of facial movements will help to unravel the pattern of UMN paralysis and will fix it in your memory *forever*. As you watch in your mirror make the movements in Table 6-2.

TABLE 6-2 Tests for unilaterality of facial movements	
Movement	Result
Retract one corner of your mouth at a time	*Every* normal person can do it: the movement is *unilateral*
Wink one eye at a time. Watch in your mirror for simultaneous contraction of the opposite orbicularis oculi muscle	*Most* can do it, but some will be unable to wink one eye without the other. When one eye winks, the opposite orbicularis oculi contracts to some degree
Elevate one eyebrow at a time	*Few* will be able to do it, but everyone can elevate them together. The movement is essentially *bilateral*

☑ *Lip retraction*

☑ *Forehead elevation*

    a. The freest unilateral facial movement usually is ☐ forehead elevation/ ☐ eyelid closure/ ☐ lip retraction.

    b. The least free unilateral facial movement usually is ☐ forehead elevation/ ☐ eyelid closure/ ☐ lip retraction.

    c. The utility of the various facial movements plausibly explains the gradient of unilaterality. Notice when eating that you make unilateral lip movements to manipulate food and clear it from your cheeks. Indeed, one of the chief discomforts of a facial palsy is that food lodges in the cheek. Unilateral forehead movements offer no such utility. Although usually the eyes blink together, sometimes you do need to close only one. Thus, the utility of unilateral eyelid action falls between that of mouth retraction and forehead wrinkling.

☑ *Mainly from the controlateral hemisphere*

2. Body parts such as the hand and lip which have the freest, most independent unilateral movements derive their UMN innervation ☐ equally from each hemisphere/ ☐ mainly from the contralateral hemisphere/ ☐ mainly from the same hemisphere.

3. Proximal, customarily symmetrical movements such as chewing and swallowing receive about the same number of UMN axons from each hemisphere, in a ratio, let us say, of 50/50. Free, independent unilateral movements are innervated by crossed and uncrossed UMN axons in a ratio of, let us say, 90/10. For movements with an intermediate degree of unilateral independence, the ratio might be 60/40, and so on.

4. Now predict the pattern of facial muscle weakness after unilateral destruction of one corticobulbar pathway. The Pt would show *most* paralysis of ☐ forehead wrinkling/ ☐ eyelid closure/ ☐ lip retraction, and *least* paralysis of ☐ forehead wrinkling/ ☐ eyelid closure/ ☐ lip retraction.

☑ *Lip retraction*
☑ *Forehead wrinkling*

5. *Facial weakness after acute, severe interruption of UMNs*

    a. After a large, acute UMN lesion, such as a massive cerebral infarct, eyelid closure is usually paretic (incomplete paralysis), and there is paralysis of lip retraction. Rarely, even the frontalis muscle is somewhat paretic. Because such a Pt has weakness of eyelid closure, the Ex who does not understand the gradient of unilaterality of facial movement erroneously diagnoses a lesion of the *ipsi*lateral facial nerve rather than the *contra*lateral corticobulbar tract.

    b. In the *acute* phase, shortly after a severe UMN lesion, lip retraction contralateral to the lesion will be paralytic both during volitional movement *and* during emotional expression, such as smiling. In the *chronic* phase of the UMN lesion, especially if the Pt has bilateral UMN lesions, lip retraction may remain weak during volitional action, but may be prominent or even exaggerated during emotional expression (Monrad-Krohn phenomenon). See *pseudobulbar palsy* in section III.F.

D. *Clinical testing of VIIth cranial nerve motor function*
  1. Facial inspection begins as you first meet the Pt and continues while taking the history.
     a. Notice the overall play of facial muscles during ordinary speech and during emotional expression. Facial movements may be too much or too little. Many disorders, such as muscular dystrophy (Fig. 1-9XX), parkinsonism, and depression, reduce all facial movements, a condition called "masked facies," in which the face is immobile—as though the Pt wore a mask.
     b. Excessive or involuntary movements seen on inspection of the face include *blepharospasm,* which may close the eyelids so tightly that the Pt cannot see; *hemifacial spasm,* in which all of the muscles innervated by one of the VIIth nerves twitch paroxysmally; and *tics, chorea,* and *athetosis,* as described in Chap. 7.
     c. Next, search for asymmetry of facial movements, asymmetry of blinking, and asymmetry of the movement and depth of the nasolabial folds. The most reliable way to detect mild unilateral weakness of lip retraction after partial UMN lesions is to watch for asymmetry of the depth and movement of the nasolabial folds, the prominent skin creases beginning just lateral to the lips and bowing upward to the nose. Using your mirror, observe these two creases when your lips are at rest, and when you speak and smile. Slight congenital asymmetries are common.
  2. Work through Table 6-3 with a partner. Often the Ex finds it quicker to illustrate the desired movements as well as to give the commands. In working through Table 6-3, pay particular attention to the strength of eyelid closure.
  3. Can you open your partner's eyelids against a maximum effort at closure?

Ans: Don't go to Aristotle for the answer: get it from your own experience on your partner or yourself!

E. *Analysis of Pts with facial weakness*
  1. Each Pt in Fig. 6-5 was asked to pull back the corners of her mouth, as in smiling, and simultaneously to close her eyes tightly. Make sure that you understand that the side which shows some action, which "draws to one

TABLE 6-3 Summary of methods for testing the motor function of cranial nerve VII		
Command	Test	Muscle tested
(1) "Wrinkle up your forehead," or "Look up at the ceiling."	Inspect for asymmetry	Frontalis
(2) "Close your eyes tight and don't let me open them."	Inspect for asymmetry of wrinkles; try to pull eyelids apart	Orbicularis oculi
(3) "Pull back the corners of your mouth."	Inspect for asymmetry of nasolabial fold	Buccinator
(4) "Wrinkle up the skin on your neck," or "Pull down hard on the corners of your mouth."	Inspect for asymmetry	Platysma

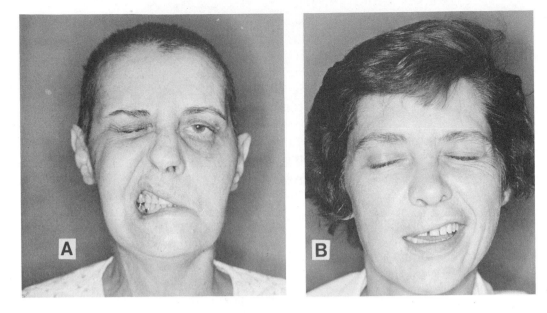

FIG. 6-5. Two patients with facial palsies. Each had been asked to close her eyes tightly and to pull back the corners of her mouth, as in smiling.

side," is the normal one. The side which does nothing is the abnormal one. The Pt with a facial palsy may state in the history that the face "drew to one side," as if that were the abnormal not the normal action. Systematically inspect all facial movements of the Pt, but especially compare both sides of each face for asymmetry of facial movement and for differences in the bulk of the chewing muscles.

See next frame

2. Describe the abnormalities in the Pt in Fig. 6-5*A*. _____

_____

☑ *Left VIIth nerve*

a. Pt A cannot close the left eyelid, as shown by lack of contraction of the orbicularis oculi muscle and absence of any "crow's feet" wrinkles around the eye. The mouth retractors on the left are paralyzed. When this Pt looked up, the left half of her forehead failed to wrinkle. This pattern of total paralysis of all facial muscles on one side implicates a lesion of the ☐ right/ ☐ left VIIth nerve/ or the ☐ right/ ☐ left corticobulbar tract.

V

b. The cognoscente of physical diagnosis will also have detected the hollowing of Pt A's left temporal foss and the concavity over the left masseter muscle, indicating atrophy of the chewing muscles and thus a lesion of the _____th cranial nerve. If you missed this finding, remember that you must compare both halves of the body, specifically looking for just such asymmetries. Pt A had been operated on to remove an acoustic nerve tumor, a neurinoma. The tumor, expanding in the cerebellopontine angle, had already destroyed the Vth and VIIth cranial nerves, but full abduction of her left eye indicated sparing of cranial nerve _____.

VI

c. Did you also notice Pt A's very short hair? It was just growing back after having been shaved off for the operation on her acoustic neurinoma.

d. This Pt was one of a minority (15 percent) who fail to show Bell's phenomenon on attempting to close the eyelids.

3. Describe the abnormalities of Pt B's face in Fig. 6-5*B*. _____
_____

   a. The right side of Pt B's mouth failed to retract, and eyelid closure on the right was weak, as shown by the wider exposure of the upper eyelid and lack of wrinkling around the right eye. This "crow's feet" wrinkling on the normal side results from the purse-string, sphincter action of the orbicularis oculi muscle. When Pt B looked up, her forehead acted equally on both sides. Thus, on the right side of the Pt's face, forehead movements were active, eyelid closure was weak, and mouth retraction was paralyzed. This gradient of weakness of the facial movement on the right side of the Pt's face indicates a lesion of the _____
_____.

Ans: Corticobulbar tract originating from the left cerebral hemisphere. This is a UMN facial palsy.

   b. Patient B has an UMN facial palsy because of infarction of her left cerebral hemisphere due to occlusion of *her* left middle cerebral artery.

FURTHER READING FOR VIIth NERVE MOTOR FUNCTION

Auger RG, Piepgras DG, Laws EL, Jr: Hemifacial spasm: Results of microvascular decompression of the facial nerve in 54 patients. *Mayo Clin Proc,* 1986; 61:640–644.

Graham MD, House WF (eds): *Disorders of the Facial Nerve. Anatomy, Diagnosis and Management.* New York, Raven, 1982.

May M (ed): *The Facial Nerve.* New York, Thieme Medical Publishers, 1986.

III. IXth and Xth cranial nerve motor functions

A. Peripheral distribution of IX and X (Learn Figs. 6-6 and 6-7.)

B. Lower motor neuron innervation of the pharynx and larynx

   1. The skeletal muscles supplied by IX and X originally were derived from branchial arches. The branchial efferent nucleus for IX and X, called the *nucleus ambiguus,* is located in the ☐ mesencephalon/ ☐ pons/ ☐ medulla.

☑ *Medulla*

   2. Nerve IX supplies only one muscle exclusively (stylopharyngeus). Since this muscle participates with X in swallowing, its isolated function cannot be tested clinically. The remaining motor fibers of IX supply the pharyngeal constrictors. Since the pharyngeal constrictors of IX act as a unit with X in swallowing, the isolated function of the individual constrictors cannot be tested at the bedside.

   3. Nerve X innervates the *palatal* muscles, with assistance from V; the *pharyngeal* constrictors, with assistance from IX; and the *laryngeal muscles,* without any assistance *(palate, pharynx, larynx).*

   4. Since even complete interruption of V has little clinical effect on palatal function, V can be disregarded. Hence, the motor functions of the palate, pharynx, and larynx are innervated by cranial nerves _____ and _____.

IX; X

   5. Sensation from the palate and pharynx is mediated by IX and X and from the larynx by X alone. Hence, IX and X are both the *motor* and *sensory*

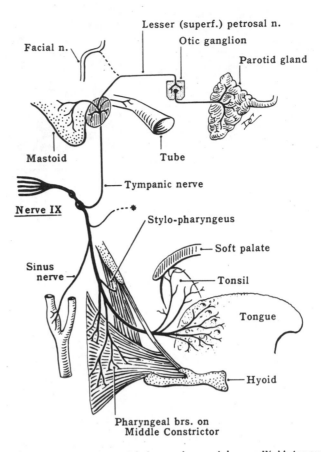

FIG. 6-6. Innervation of the palate, tongue, and pharynx by cranial nerve IX. Motor axons innervate the stylopharyngeus and middle pharyngeal constrictor muscles. Sensory axons mediate taste from the tongue, the afferent arc of the swallowing reflex, and the vasomotor, cardioinhibitory, and respiratory reflexes of the carotid body and sinus. *(From J. C. B. Grant: An Atlas of Anatomy, 5th ed. Baltimore, Williams & Wilkins, 1962.)*

X

sentinels of the palatal orifice, but _____ alone is the sensorimotor sentinel of the larynx.

C. *Swallowing*

1. Swallowing, a very complex act, requires coordination of cranial nerves and respiratory muscles. The tongue initiates the act of swallowing by throwing a bolus of food back into the palatal archway which then reflexly stimulates the pharyngeal constrictors. Tongue movements are innervated exclusively by the _____ th cranial nerve (if you don't know, sort through the nerves I and XII until you come to the right one).

XII

2. Hold your jaw open and try to swallow while your lips are open. You may succeed after a struggle, but normal swallowing requires closure of the lips and jaw. Cranial nerve _____ innervates jaw closure, and cranial nerve _____ innervates lip closure.

V
VII

3. Thus, swallowing requires the collaboration of cranial nerves _____
_____ .

V, VII, IX, X, XII

D. *Clinical physiology of the soft palate*

1. By the action of the levator veli palatini muscle innervated by X, the soft palate swings upward and backward to contact the posterior wall of the pharynx, sealing off the *naso*pharynx from the *oro*pharynx. See Fig. 6-8.

2. Unless the soft palate elevates properly, *liquid* will escape into your nose when you drink, and *air* will escape into your nose when you speak. The

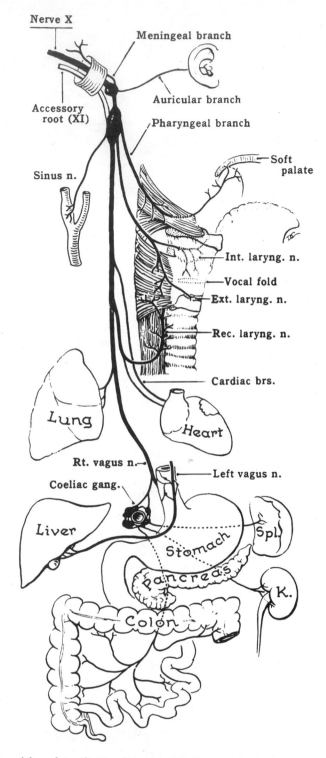

Nerve X

Meningeal branch

Accessory root (XI)

Auricular branch

Pharyngeal branch

Sinus n.

Soft palate

Int. laryng. n.

Vocal fold

Ext. laryng. n.

Rec. laryng. n.

Cardiac brs.

Lung

Heart

Rt. vagus n.

Left vagus n.

Coeliac gang.

Liver

Spl.

Stomach

Pancreas

K.

Colon

FIG. 6-7. Innervation of the palate, pharynx, larynx, and thoracicoabdominal viscera by cranial nerve X. The palatal branch innervates the levator veli palatini muscle which lifts the palate. The pharyngeal and laryngeal branches mediate sensory and motor functions of these structures. *(From J. C. B. Grant: An Atlas of Anatomy, 5th ed. Baltimore, Williams & Wilkins, 1962.)*

result is "nasal" swallowing and "nasal" speech. Since physicists define both liquids and gases as fluids, we can agree that the function of the soft palate is to rightly divide the flow of fluids between the oropharynx and nasopharynx. Looking further, we can say that the branchial musculature of the throat also controls the fluid traffic at the oropharyngeal and naso-pharyngeal openings.

IX, X

V
VII

> a. Thus, the fluid dynamics of the *oro*pharyngeal, *naso*pharyngeal, laryngeal, and esophageal orifices are mainly controlled by cranial nerves _____ (with some assistance from V, VII, and XII).
> b. Cranial nerves IX and X innervate, guard, and control the internal apertures of the head much as cranial nerves _____ (sensory) and _____ (motor) innervate the external apertures (eyes, mouth, ears, and nares).

3. The nasopharyngeal airway remains open until the palate elevates. The palate elevates whenever it would be advantageous to block anything that is in your oropharynx from getting into your nasopharynx. Thus the palate elevates when you

> a. Swallow.
> b. Whistle or trumpet.
> c. Speak.

E. *Upper motor neuron innervation of IX and X*

Equal (50/50)

1. The palate, pharynx, and vocal cords act with bilateral synchrony. Knowing this fact, you can predict that the numbers of crossed and uncrossed UMN fibers from each cerebral hemisphere would be about _____.
2. Because of the bilateral UMN innervation, unilateral UMN lesions that cause hemiplegia only rarely cause unilateral weakness of the palate; however, Pts with acute hemiplegia frequently show mild dysarthria (about 60 percent) and mild dysphagia.

F. *Bulbar and pseudobulbar palsy: the nomenclature of muscular paralysis from LMN and UMN lesions of the cranial nerves*

1. Clinical jargon includes many different terms for UMN and LMN paralysis, terms which bear the imprint of medical history. The earlier anatomists visualized the medulla as a bulb-like expansion of the spinal cord. Thus, the medulla was called the "bulb." LMN paralysis from a lesion of the bulb or its nerves was called "bulbar paralysis." Paralysis of bulbar speech and swallowing mechanisms after UMN lesions was called "pseudobulbar," or "false" bulbar paralysis, because the lesion was not truly in the bulb or its nerves. The UMNs to the bulb were called "corticobulbar fibers." By usage, the term *corticobulbar fibers* has expanded to include *all* cortical efferent fibers to all cranial nerve motor nuclei, III to XII. But we only use *bulbar paralysis* to apply to LMN paralysis of the bulbar cranial nerves, e.g., IX, X and XII. Well, "A foolish consistency is the hobgoblin of little minds" (Ralph Waldo Emerson [1803–1882]).

✓ LMN
✓ IX to XII

2. Thus, "bulbar paralysis" means only an ☐ LMN/ ☐ UMN lesion of cranial nerves ☐ IX to XII/ ☐ III to XII.
3. *The syndrome of pseudobulbar palsy*

> a. After acute, bilateral interruption of the corticobulbar fibers, as with bilateral cerebral infarction, the Pt becomes mute, and loses the ability to speak or swallow at all. In the recovery phase or with gradual lesions of the corticobulbar tracts, the Pt shows a characteristic, virtually pathognomonic syndrome termed *pseudobulbar palsy*. The Pt initiates speaking or swallowing very slowly, and the words are slurred. The voice has a peculiar strained pitch and quality. The Pt may swallow or chew reflexly but cannot initiate these acts volitionally and may yawn automatically but cannot open the mouth volitionally. The Pt exhibits extreme emotional lability, crying one moment, laughing the next, like turning on and off a faucet. The face appears immobile most of the time, as though it were a wooden mask; but when the Pt cries or laughs, the

facial movements expressing the emotion become exaggerated; and, strangely, when queried, the Pt may not feel the emotion that the muscles express. Thus, the pathways that activate the muscles for emotional expression differ from those for volitional movement, but we do not know their exact course.

☑ *Both volitional and emotional movements*

b. LMN lesions of cranial nerves would cause loss of ☐ emotional movements only/ ☐ volitional movements only/ ☐ both volitional and emotional movements.

c. Acute bilateral UMN lesions would cause loss of both volitional and emotional facial movements initially, but in the chronic stage emotional expression may be _____.

Exaggerated

4. Summarize the clinical features of pseudobulbar palsy and state the pathways affected. _____

_____

_____

_____

Ans: Check against frame 3. Did you miss anything?

5. Table 6-4 lists the many different terms for UMN and LMN paralysis. Clearly, the terms UMN and LMN convey the concept concisely and informatively.

FURTHER READING FOR PSEUDOBULBAR PALSY

Asfora WT, Desalles AF, Abe M, Kjellberg RN: Is the syndrome of pathological laughing and crying a manifestation of pseudobulbar palsy? *J Neurol Neurosurg Psychiat*, 1989; 52:523–525.

Grattan-Smith PJ, Hopkins IJ, Shield LK, Boldt DW: Acute pseudobulbar palsy due to bilateral focal cortical damage: The opercular syndrome of Foix-Chavany-Marie. *J Child Neurol*, 1989; 4:131–136.

Langworthy O, Hesser F: Syndrome of pseudobulbar palsy. Anatomic and physiologic analysis. *Arch Intern Med*, 1940; 65:106–121.

Lieberman A, Bensen D: Control of emotional expression in pseudobulbar palsy. *Arch Neurol*, 1977; 34:717–719.

Mao C-C, Coull BM, Golper LAC, Rau MT: Anterior operculum syndrome. *Neurology*, 1989; 39:1169–1172.

IV. Speech production

A. The five basic mechanisms of speech

1. Speech requires a *bellows,* provided by the lungs and respiratory muscles, to express a stream of air through the larynx and upper airway.
2. Speech requires *phonation* by the vocal cords.

TABLE 6-4 Synonyms or near synonyms for muscular paralysis from UMN and LMN lesions	
UMN paresis or paralysis	LMN paresis or paralysis
Central	Peripheral
Pseudobulbar	Bulbar
Suprasegmental	Segmental/nuclear
Supranuclear	Infranuclear

3. Speech requires *articulation* by palate, tongue, lips, and to some extent the mandible.
4. Speech requires *resonance,* provided by the pharyngeal, oral, and nasal passages.
5. Speech requires *neural direction* of the foregoing mechanisms via UMNs and LMNs. Chapter 11 discusses cerebral disorders of speech.

B. *Phonation: role of cranial nerve X.* Galen (130–200 A.D.) of Pergamum was troubled by the squealing of piglets during surgical experiments. But he was troubled even more by his own ignorance, which drove him to continue his work. Since he had no anesthetic, he eliminated the squealing and dispelled a share of his own ignorance with one stroke. After verifying that the voice came from the larynx, he found that he could silence it by cutting the recurrent laryngeal nerves—and that is how we learned what these nerves do.

C. *Articulation of speech*
1. *Phonation versus articulation.* After the larynx phonates, speech sounds require *articulation.* Hence, to make vocal sounds is to *phonate,* while to shape sounds into speech is to *articulate.* To distinguish clearly between phonation and articulation, whisper a sentence. When whispering, you do not phonate at all, but you can articulate every word with perfect clarity. Normal speech may be regarded as a mixture of voiced and nonvoiced sounds.
2. *Labial sounds.* While watching your lips in a mirror, recite loudly each letter of the alphabet, and after each one, try to make the sound without any lip movement. In Table 6-5, check the sounds which require strong labial action.
3. *Lingual sounds.* Complete Table 6-6 by reciting the alphabet loudly and checking the sounds which require strong lingual actions.

TABLE 6-5 Letter sounds requiring strong lip action (labials)			
	Strong labial		Strong labial
A		N	
B		O	
C		P	
D		Q	
E		R	
F		S	
G		T	
H		U	
I		V	
J		W	
K		X	
L		Y	
M		Z	

TABLE 6-6 Letter sounds requiring strong tongue-tip elevation (linguals)			
	Strong lingual		Strong lingual
A		N	
B		O	
C		P	
D		Q	
E		R	
F		S	
G		T	
H		U	
I		V	
J		W	
K		X	
L		Y	
M		Z	

4. *Vowel sounds*

   a. Compare the tongue action of *D*, *G*, and *J* sounds, strong linguals, with the position of the tongue during vowel sounds: A, E, I, O, and U. To understand tongue action during vowel sounds, do this: press down on your tongue with a tongue blade as you recite the vowels.

   b. Vowels require palatal elevation. The palate does not completely seal off the nasopharynx during most speech sounds. Instead, it merely reduces the nasopharyngeal aperture, detouring most of the air through the mouth, the path of least resistance. Only a few sounds require complete palatal closure.

      (1) Plosives: *K* or hard *G*, as in good.

      (2) Vowels: sustained "EEEEE . . ." or "Ah . . ."

   c. Clinicians traditionally test for palatal elevation by asking the Pt to say, "Ahh. . . ." The vowel *E* requires tighter palatal closure, but the Pt can say "Ah" easier with the mouth open to permit palatal inspection. A good test sentence for palatal function is one combining consonant and vowel sounds: "We see three geese."

5. *Plosive sounds*

   a. Plosives require momentary impounding of air and sudden release. Try this experiment: cup your palm and hold it about 3 cm in front of your mouth. Loudly say, "Puh, Puh, Puh . . ." "Guh, Guh, Guh . . ." "Em, Em, Em . . ." and "Kuh, Kuh, Kuh. . ."

   b. In all but one of these sounds, you felt a *strong* puff of air in your palm. The sound not requiring forceful air expulsion and therefore not a plosive was _____.

em (M)

   c. In order to divert all of the air through your mouth, for plosives, the palate must effectively seal the nasopharynx off from the oropharynx. Therefore, if the patient articulates vowels and plosives well, the velopharyngeal (palatal) valve closes well.

6. *Sibilants and fricatives*

   a. *Sibilants* are hissing or whistling sounds. Cup your palm over your mouth and sustain a forceful "SSS . . ." of a prolonged "Hisssss. . . ." Do you feel a stream of air against your palm? ☐ Yes/ ☐ No.

☑ *Yes*

   b. *Fricatives* are high frequency frictional or rustling sounds. Cup your hand to your mouth and forcefully pronounce "V, V, V . . ." "Z, Z, Z . . ." and "F, F, F FF, FF, FF. . . ."

   c. Try the sibilants and fricatives again, without using tongue or lips at all. Can you say them? ☐ Yes/ ☐ No.

☑ *No*

   d. To produce sibilants and fricatives, you must force a strong stream of air through a small aperture formed by lips, tongue, and teeth. In order to divert air from the nose into the mouth, the velopharyngeal valve must close more or less completely.

7. *Voiceless consonants.* Many speech sounds, such as sibilants and plosives, require no phonation. Examples of such *voiceless consonants* are *Shhhh*, *P*, *T*, and *K*. Hence, all speech sounds require ☐ articulation/ ☐ phonation, but not all speech sounds require ☐ articulation/ ☐ phonation.

☑ *Articulation*
☑ *Phonation*

D. *Nomenclature for disorders of speech and swallowing*

   1. *Aphonia* is the inability to phonate. Abnormal phonation, such as hoarseness, is *dysphonia*. *Mutism* is the inability to speak. Neuromuscular disorders may cause mutism, but commonly it implicates a block at the level of the cerebrum or mind, as in dementia or *hysterical* mutism, or an afferent block, as in *deaf* mutism. In *elective* mutism a child, for example, may refuse to speak at all in public or at school but talks readily at home.

2. *Dysarthria* is faulty articulation of speech sounds. It may result from central lesions of the brain or cerebellum, intoxication (such as alcohol), or neuromuscular disorders. The key to the definition of dysarthria is a defect in the articulation of speech sounds, not in the content of speech, words, syntax, rhythm, or vocabulary. Chapter 11 discusses the further speech disorders called *dysprosody* and *dysphasia.*

3. *Dysphagia* (phagein = to eat, e.g., macrophage) is difficulty in swallowing. It may be caused by central or neuromuscular lesions, mechanical disorders such as an esophageal fistula, or emotional illnesses, such as globus hystericus when the Pt cannot swallow because of a delusion of a lump or mass in the throat.

E. *Hyponasal and hypernasal speech*
1. *Hyponasal* speech is too little escape of air through the nose.
   a. Pinch your nostrils together and say "Good morning."
   b. Lack of nasal escape of air transforms "Good morning" into "Good bordig." It is what you say when your nasal mucous membranes are swollen by a cold. This would be ☐ hypernasal/ ☐ hyponasal speech.

2. *Hypernasal* speech is too much escape of air through the nose. It indicates that the palate has not sealed off the oropharynx, either because of palatal weakness or mechanical defects, such as from a cleft palate (velopharyngeal incompetency; velum = curtain = soft palate). The Pt produces palatal sounds poorly.

3. A patient with *hyper*nasal speech would have ☐ incompetent velopharyngeal closure/ ☐ nasal obstruction, while a patient with *hypo*nasal speech would have ☐ incompetent palatal closure/ ☐ nasal obstruction.

4. *An unfortunate, common, but preventable error:*
   a. Failure to distinguish between hyper- and hyponasal speech leads to serious errors in treatment. When the palate elevates, it contacts the dorsal pharyngeal wall (Fig. 6-8). In children, the adenoid tissue, which occu-

☑ *Hyponasal*

☑ *Incompetent velopharyngeal closure;* ☑ *nasal obstruction*

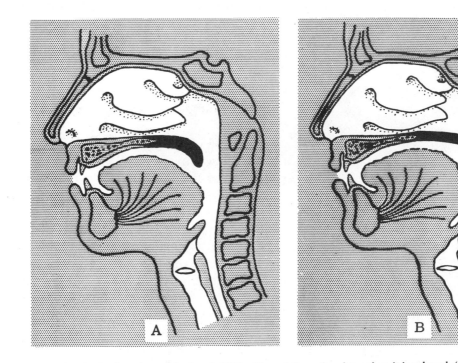

FIG. 6-8. Sagittal section of the head. (A) Position of the soft palate when it is relaxed. (B) Position of soft palate when it is elevated, occluding the nasopharynx from the oropharynx.

☑ *Hyponasal*

pies the posterior pharyngeal wall, may hypertrophy and then bulge forward into the pharyngeal lumen. Hypertrophy of the adenoid would tend to cause ☐ hyponasal/ ☐ hypernasal speech.

b. Some Pts with neurogenic palatal weakness or submucous palatal clefts will have hypernasality. The Ex may erroneously conclude that enlarged adenoids are at fault. Actually, the adenoid *reduces* the need for velopharyngeal closure. Removal of the adenoids of a Pt with hypernasal speech will make it ☐ better/ ☐ worse. Explain: _____

_____.

Ans: Worse! Removal of the adenoid tissue increases the distance the palate has to elevate to shut off the nasopharynx. The weak palate is now even less capable of preventing nasal escape of air.

c. This example shows what happens if a knife is in the wrong person's hand: he'll remove adenoids for hypernasal speech, snip a lingual frenulum for "tongue-tie" when the problem is not lingual articulations at all, or extract a uterus for backache.

F. *Stuttering*
   1. All of us suffer from pauses and repetitions when we speak, the toddler more than the adult. When the pauses and repetitions impede communicative speech, the Pt is a stutterer. The Pt usually falters and repeats the first syllable of words, sometimes the middle or last syllables.
   2. Although emotional stress makes the stuttering worse, the cause of stuttering is still unknown. It apparently results from defective central processing of speech. The standard bedside NE discloses no evidence of neurologic dysfunction per se in stutterers.

G. *Clinical testing of the motor function of cranial nerves IX and X*
   1. *Speech*
      a. During the history, the Ex appraises the Pt's speech almost automatically. If it is perfectly normal in all respects, no further speech testing is required. Otherwise, test the articulation mechanisms individually.

Soft palate (velopharyngeal valve)
Tongue (linguals)
Lips (labials)

      b. Test competency of articulation by the soft tissues, the soft palate, tongue, and lips, with the *KLM* test.
         (1) *Kuh, Kuh,* tests the function of the _____.
         (2) *La, La,* tests the function of the _____.
         (3) *Mi, Mi,* tests the function of the _____.
      c. Any infant or young child who does not speak requires thorough audiologic examination.
   2. *Swallowing.* If the Pt has dysarthria or dysphagia, provide a glass of water to swallow (Nathadwarawala et al. 1992.)
   3. *Neurologic examination of the palate and larynx*
      a. While the Pt says "Ahh," inspect the tonsillar pillars for asymmetry as they arch upwards and medially to form the palate. Look at the arch, the arch above, not the uvula. Students commonly mistake an asymmetrically hung uvula for palatal palsy. Let the uvula hang as it will. See Fig. 6-9, and then study your own palatal action in the mirror.

☑ *Right (the right side is the one that fails to elevate)*
IX
X

      b. Fig. 6-9*A* depicts a normal person saying "Ah . . ." Fig. 6-9*B* depicts a person with palatal palsy. Which side is paralyzed in *B*? ☐ right/ ☐ left.
      c. An additional test for anatomic elevation of the palate is the *gag reflex.* Touch one tonsillar pillar then the other with a tongue blade. The afferent arc of the gag reflex is primarily cranial nerve _____.
      The efferent arc is cranial nerve _____.

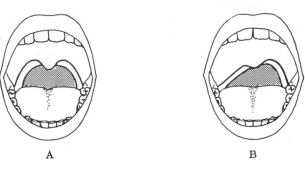

FIG. 6-9. Palatal arch. (*A*) Appearance of palatal arch when a normal subject says, "Ah. . . ." (*B*) Appearance of palatal arch when a patient with unilateral palatal weakness says, "Ah . . . ," indicating a weak levator veli palatini muscle on the right side.

☑ *UMNs*

    d. If the palate fails to elevate when the Pt says "Ah," but does elevate during the gag reflex, the Pt would have to have a lesion of the ☐ UMNs/ ☐ LMNs or muscles.

    e. If the history or examination disclose no evidence of dysarthria or dysphagia, omit the gag reflex. It is uncomfortable and unnecessary.

    f. Incompetent palatal elevation may result from UMN or LMN lesions; congenital malformations, such as cleft palate, myopathies, or local lesions in the soft tissue; and palatopharyngeal discrepancy in size. Palatal incompetence is not simply one thing *or* another. Like every sign, it is a puzzle to be solved.

  4. *Hoarseness and unilateral vagal lesions*

    a. A number of mechanical or neurogenic disorders of the larynx may cause hoarseness, but vocal cord paralysis may cause little hoarseness in some Pts. Therefore, merely listening to the voice or examining only the palate constitutes an incomplete examination. If the Ex suspects Xth nerve dysfunction, direct inspection of the cords by laryngoscopy is required (Blitzer et al., 1992).

    b. Unilateral vocal cord paralysis usually causes a breathy or raspy voice and a flutter of the voice because of vibration of the flaccid cord; it may also cause stridor and anoxia. Additionally, paralysis of the cricothyroid muscles, the pitch adjustor muscles (innervated by the superior laryngeal nerve), results in a monotone sound, without changes in pitch. Interruption of the entire vagus nerve results in dysphagia as well as dysphonia, because of paralysis of the pharyngeal constrictors.

  5. The Ex will learn to recognize many speech disorders, particularly disorders in rhythm, force, and timber of the voice, only by listening to Pts, not from a text. The speech affliction is often characteristic and even pathognomonic of some diseases or disorders. In *cerebral palsy,* the cry or the speech has a characteristic slow, rachety onset and a harsh, tight, and irritating dysphonic quality, diagnosable without even seeing the Pt. In the *cat's cry syndrome* (cri du chat), the infant sounds like a cat in heat. The Pt's karyotype confirms the diagnosis: the fifth chromosome lacks a short arm. In *hypothyroidism,* the voice is deep and raspy. In *paralysis agitans* (parkinsonism), the muscular rigidity dampens the normal inflections and modulations of the Pt's voice: the sound is all on one plane, "plateau speech." *Cerebellar disease* causes the opposite: the Pt overaccentuates some sounds, and underaccentuates others; the voice scans from one peak of volume to another, so-called "scanning speech." And finally the commonest dysarthria of all, the slurred, scanning speech due to intoxication with alcohol or other drugs.

H. *A summary of ancillary diagnostic procedures for mutism, aphonia/ dysphonia, dysarthria, and dysphagia.* Whenever the Pt, particularly an infant or child, presents with disorders in speaking or swallowing, consider:
1. Audiologic investigation. The Pt who does not hear correctly does not speak correctly.
2. Direct laryngoscopy.
3. Plain radiographs of the oropharyngeal airway.
4. Radiographic cinematography, often with a "barium swallow," to visualize the palate and throat in action.

FURTHER READING FOR DISORDERS OF SPEECH PRODUCTION

Aronson AE: *Clinical Voice Disorders* (3d ed). New York, Thieme Medical Publishers, 1990.

Blitzer A, Brin MF, Sasaki CT, et al: *Neurologic Disorders of the Larynx.* New York, Thieme Medical, 1992.

Nathadwarawala KM, Nicklin J, Wiles CM: A timed test of swallowing capacity for neurological patients. *J Neurol Neurosurg Psychiatr,* 1992; 55:822–825.

Pollack MA, Shprintzen RF, Zimmerman-Manchester KL: Velopharyngeal insufficiency. The neurological perspective. A report of 32 cases. *Dev Med and Child Neurol,* 1979: 21:194–201.

V. XIth cranial nerve motor functions

A. *Functional anatomy*

Spinal accessory

1. Nerve XI has two parts, a *spinal* and an *accessory.* Hence, it is called the _____ _____ nerve.
2. The *spinal* part supplies the *sternocleidomastoid* and rostral portions of the *trapezius* muscles. The *accessory* part is accessory to the vagus, supplying fibers which arise in the nucleus ambiguus of the medulla and merely hitch-hike along the proximal part of XI before joining X for distribution to the pharynx and larynx. In testing the function of XI clinically, we test the spinal part. Study Fig. 6-10.

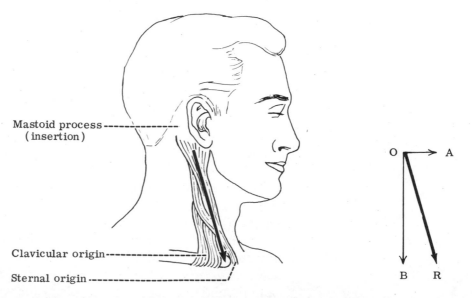

FIG. 6-10. Origin and insertion of the sternocleidomastoid muscle. On the right is a vector diagram of its action. The oblique arrow (*O-R*) is the actual line of pull. It can be resolved into a *horizontal* vector (*O-A*) acting to thrust the head forward and turn it to the opposite side, and into a *vertical* vector (*O-B*) acting to tilt the head to the same side as the muscle.

Sternum
Clavicle; mastoid

☑ *Right*

☑ *Left*

☑ *Yes*

☑ *Forward*
☑ *Opposite*
☑ *Same*

☑ *Away from*

B. *The sternocleidomastoid (SCM) muscle*
1. The SCM muscle originates from the _____ and the _____ and inserts into the _____ process.
2. Palpate both SCMs as you forcefully turn (turn, not tilt) your head to the *left*. Which SCM contracts most? ☐ right/ ☐ left/ ☐ neither.
3. With your chin up, forcefully tilt (tilt, not turn) your head to the left. Which SCM contracts most? ☐ right/ ☐ left/ ☐ both equally.
4. Press back on your forehead with one hand while you thrust your head forward. Palpate both SCM muscles with your other hand. Do they both contract equally? ☐ Yes/ ☐ No.
5. To avoid memorization, simply palpate yourself to recall SCM's three actions: to *thrust* the head forward, to *turn* it, and to *tilt* it.
   a. The SCM muscle *thrusts* the head ☐ forward/ ☐ backward.
   b. The SCM muscle *turns* the head to the ☐ same/ ☐ opposite side.
   c. The SCM muscle *tilts* the head to the ☐ same/ ☐ opposite side.
   d. The action of one SCM muscle in turning the head, like the action of one lateral pterygoid muscle in turning the mandible, results in turning ☐ toward/ ☐ away from the side of the muscle.

C. *The trapezius muscle*
1. The trapezius muscle *originates* in the midline from the occiput and the spinous processes of all cervical and thoracic vertebrae. It *inserts* into the clavicle and scapula.
2. Nerve XI innervates only the rostral part of the trapezius muscle, the part that lifts the shoulders.

D. *Upper motor neuron innervation of cranial nerve XI*
1. After acute interruption of the UMNs of the pyramidal tract rostral to the medulla, the head tends to turn to the side of the lesion (Fig. 5-1) because of weakness of the SCM muscle *ipsilateral* to the lesion. On the hemiplegic side, the SCM and perhaps other cervical muscles that turn the head to the opposite side are the only ones that retain their strength (Willoughby and Anderson, 1984). In contrast, the trapezius muscle and of course the extremity muscles on the hemiplegic side are paralyzed. Thus these paralyzed muscles receive the classical *contralateral* UMN innervation.
2. The course of the UMN innervation to the SCM muscle is still unclear. The clinical evidence suggests that the UMN fibers to one SCM muscle derive mainly from the ipsilateral hemisphere and that they run directly without decussating to the LMNs for the SCM or that the pathway undergoes a double decussation to end up ipsilateral to the hemisphere that activates them (Gandevia and Applegate, 1988; Marcus, 1989).

E. *Clinical testing of the muscles innervated by cranial nerve XI.*
1. Inspect the SCM and trapezius muscles for size and asymmetry.
2. Next palpate the muscles at rest and as they exert their actions.
3. To test the strength of SCM and trapezius muscles, try the maneuvers listed in Table 6-7 on yourself and another person.
4. In step 1, why should you press on the Pt's cheek, rather than the mandible?

_____

_____

_____

Ans: You do not want to test lateral pterygoid and SCM. Test only one muscle at a time whenever possible. Moreover strong lateral pressure on the jaw

☑ *Right SCM*

Press forward over vertebra prominens (C-7)
☑ *SCM*

TABLE 6-7 Clinical tests of the motor function of cranial nerve XI	
Commands to patient	Examiner's maneuver
1. "Turn your head to the left; hold it there, and don't let me push it back."	Place your right hand on the left cheek of the patient, your left hand on his right shoulder to brace him and try to force his head to the midline. Repeat with the patient's head turned to the right. With the patient's head turned to the left, you test the ☐ right SCM/ ☐ left SCM/ ☐ trapezius muscle when you try to return the head to the midline.
2. "Push your head forward as hard as possible."	Place one hand on the patient's forehead and push backwards. What do you do with your other hand to brace the patient? _____ _____ In this maneuver you test the action of both ☐ SCM/ ☐ trapezius muscles, which thrust the head forwards.
3. "Try to touch your ears with the tips of your shoulders. Hold them there and don't let me push them down."	Place your hands on both of the patient's shoulders and press down. Observe from in front and in back, and watch for scapular winging which may occur with trapezius or serratus anterior weakness.

may dislocate the temporomandibular joint, particularly in an edentulous or elderly Pt.

FURTHER READING FOR XIth NERVE MOTOR FUNCTION

Gandevia SC, Applegate C: Activation of neck muscles from the human motor cortex. *Brain,* 1988; 111:801–813.

Marcus JC: The spinal accessory nerve in childhood hemiplegia. *Arch Neurol,* 1989; 46:60–61.

Willoughby EW, Anderson NE: Lower cranial nerve motor function in unilatral vascular lesions of the cerebral hemisphere. *Br Med J,* 1984; 289:791–794.

VI. XIIth cranial nerve motor functions

A. *Functional anatomy of the tongue*

Hypoglossal

    1. Nerve XII controls *all* and *only* tongue movements. Because it runs under the tongue, XII is called the _____ nerve.

    2. *Action of the genioglossus muscle*

        a. To understand how XIIth nerve lesions affect tongue movements, learn the actions of the genioglossus muscles. Notice in Fig. 6-11 that each genioglossus muscle is triangular. Its *apex* originates from the apex of the mandible, which is hard, unyielding, and immobile. Its *base* fans out to insert into the base of the tongue, which is soft, fleshy, and mobile. Genioglossus contraction, therefore, must pull the base of the tongue ☐ forward/ ☐ backward.

☑ *Forward (Fig. 6-11)*

Genioglossus

☑ *Right*

☑ *Opposite*

3. If the tongue protrudes in the midline, both right and left _____ muscles contract equally.
4. If the Pt attempts to protrude the tongue in the midline, and it deviates to the right, the weakness affects the ☐ right/ ☐ left genioglossus muscle.
5. Compare the action of the genioglossus in Fig. 6-11 with that of the lateral pterygoid muscle in Fig. 6-1. Clearly the mechanics of tongue and jaw protrusion are identical. Midline protrusion is the result of balanced muscular action. Compare the action of these two muscles with the SCM. All three muscles, when contracting unilaterally, turn the part they operate to the ☐ same/ ☐ opposite/ side.

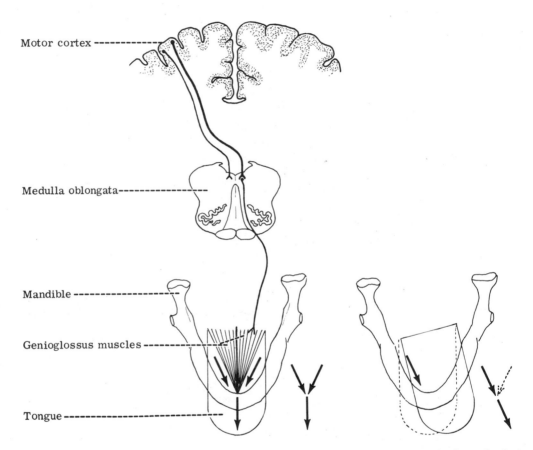

Motor cortex

Medulla oblongata

Mandible

Genioglossus muscles

Tongue

FIG. 6-11. Action and innervation of the genioglossus muscle. The diagram to the the right shows the deviation of the tongue when only the right genioglossus muscle contracts, pulling the *base* of the tongue forward on the right and protruding and deviating the *tip* of the tongue to the left.

☑ *Left; genioglossus*

☑ *Right; lateral pterygoid*
☑ *Left; SCM*

6. The muscle which turns the tongue to the *right* is the ☐ right/ ☐ left _____ muscle.
7. The muscle which turns the mandible to the *left* is the ☐ right/ ☐ left _____ muscle.
8. One muscle which turns the head to the *right* is the ☐ right/ ☐ left _____ muscle.

B. Lower motor neuron lesions of XII

Notice in Fig. 6-11 that each XIIth nerve innervates one half of the tongue. although we have mentioned only the genioglossus, the bulk of the tongue is muscle. After interruption of the XIIth nerve, the muscle fibers on the *ipsilateral* half of the tongue undergo atrophy. Therefore the signs of unilateral XIIth nerve interruption are *ipsilateral atrophy* and *ipsilateral deviation* of the tongue on attempted midline protrusion. Infarcts of the basis of the medulla may interrupt the XIIth nerve and the adjacent pyramidal tract (Currier, 1976).

C. *Upper motor neuron innervation of XII*

1. Notice in Fig. 6-11 that the hypoglossal nucleus receives crossed and uncrossed UMN fibers. Using a colored pencil, draw in the UMN and LMN innervation from the *left* motor cortex. Notice the somewhat thicker line representing crossed fibers, indicating a slightly greater percentage of decussated corticobulbar fibers. In this respect, the UMN innervation of the tongue most closely resembles the innervation of ☐ forehead elevation/ ☐ eyelid closure/ ☐ lip retraction.

2. In 10 to 15 percent of Pts the tongue deviates after a unilateral corticobulbar lesion. Thus if the tongue deviates after say a *right* hemisphere lesion, the tongue would deviate to the ☐ right/☐ left when protruded. Use Fig. 6-11 to reason out the answer.

3. In hysterical hemiplegia, if the tongue deviates, it typically deviates to the side *opposite* to the putatively paralyzed extremities (Keane, 1986).

4. Because the corticobulbar fibers for branchial nuclei and the corticospinal fibers run more or less together through the brainstem, isolated interruption of just the corticobulbar fibers to the tongue is unlikely. Thus if the UMN lesion affects tongue movements, the Pt usually shows an UMN type of facial palsy, with dysphagia, dysarthria, and usually frank hemiplegia.

D. *Clinical testing of XII*

1. *Inspection of the tongue at rest*

   a. Inspect the tongue for the most reliable sign of a XIIth nerve lesion, hemiatrophy. However, diseases that affect LMNs bilaterally, such as amyotrophic lateral sclerosis, result in bilateral atrophy of the tongue.

   b. Palpation may help resolve questionable hemiatrophy. Wearing a rubber glove, palpate each half of the tongue between your thumb and index finger.

2. *Testing tongue motility and deviation*

   a. Say to the Pt, "Stick your tongue straight out as far as possible and hold it there." Check for alignment of the median raphe of the tongue with the notch between the medial incisor teeth. Check the alignment of your own tongue in a mirror.

   b. Then, if the history or findings suggest a bulbar problem, ask the Pt to move the tongue alternately to the right and left, and to try to touch the tip of the tongue to the tip of the nose and the tip of the chin. On protrusion the tongue tip should extend well beyond the teeth. Many disorders may impair tongue motility:

      (1) Weakness due to UMN or LMN interruption.
      (2) Myopathy.
      (3) Rigidity, as in parkinsonism.
      (4) Apraxia (Chap. 11), mental retardation, dementia, or a major mental illness such as depression or schizophrenia.

3. *Tongue strength.* Tongue strength per se is difficult to evaluate. Have the Pt press tongue-against-cheek while you press your finger against the cheek. Keep your tongue in cheek while you evaluate this rather unreliable test.

4. *Involuntary movements of the tongue*

   a. Rippling of a normal tongue frequently indicates incomplete relaxation. Ask the Pt to make some tongue movements and then inspect it again after he relaxes it. Rippling of one half of the tongue, if that half is weak

---

☑ *Eyelid closure*

☑ *Left*

and atrophic, suggests fasciculations (see Chap. 7); this supports the diagnosis of an LMN lesion, but pathologic fasciculations and normal rippling are difficult to distinguish by clinical inspection.

    b. Pts with involuntary movements such as chorea or athetosis (Chap. 7) cannot maintain a still tongue when it is protruded. Ask the Pt to hold the tongue protruded and still for 30 seconds.

    c. Infants with mental retardation or cerebral palsy often display an action called *tongue thrusting.* Whenever food is put into the infant's mouth, the tongue thrusts it back out, impairing nutritional input.

    E. Distinguishing unilateral upper motor neuron and lower motor neuron weakness of the tongue

      1. If the tip of the tongue deviates, the Pt has either a *UMN* or an *LMN lesion.* Suppose the tongue deviates to the *left.* If the lesion is UMN it involves the ☐ right/ ☐ left hemisphere. The weakness is usually ☐ severe/ ☐ moderate.

☑ *Right/*
☑ *Moderate*

      2. The clinical distinction between unilateral UMN and LMN weakness of the tongue rests on supporting evidence of UMN signs in other movements or upon positive evidence of LMN involvement. The best evidence of a unilateral XIIth nerve lesion would be _____

Ans: Ipsilateral atrophy and considerable ipsilateral deviation on protrusion.

    F. Pt analysis

      1. The Pt in Fig. 6-12 was asked to stick out his tongue. Describe any abnormalities. _____

Ans: The tongue shows right-sided atrophy, and deviation of the tip to the right.

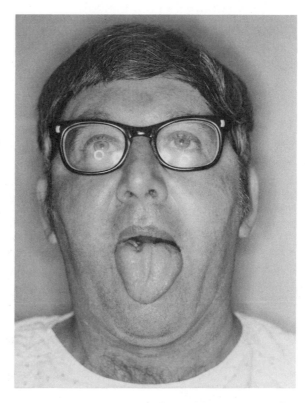

FIG. 6-12. This patient was asked to stick his tongue straight out.

☑ *Right*
☑ *XIIth nerve*

2. These clinical findings indicate interruption of the ☐ right/ ☐ left ☐ XIIth nerve/ ☐ corticobulbar tract.

3. The Pt in Fig. 6-12 had a glioma of the medulla oblongata that destroyed the fibers of the XII nerve in their intraaxial course.

REFERENCES FOR THE MOTOR FUNCTION OF THE XIIth NERVE

Currier RD, The medial medullary syndrome. *Neurology,* 1976; 42:96–104.
Keane JR: Wrong-way deviation of the tongue with hysterical hemiparesis. *Neurology,* 1986; 36:1406–1409.

VII. Multiple cranial nerve palsies, pathologic fatigability, and myasthenia gravis

A. *Signs and symptoms of multiple cranial nerve palsies.* If a Pt complains of diplopia, dysphagia, dysphonia, or dysarthria, particularly if these complaints are intermittent, or if the Ex finds an unexplained ocular, facial, or bulbar palsy, such as ptosis, strabismus, or mild hypernasal speech, suspect myasthenia gravis. Myasthenics may have little or no deficit when rested, as when first arising in the morning, but as the day wears on, or as they use their cranial nerve muscles to look, talk, swallow, or chew, the weakness becomes increasingly severe. This *pathologic fatigability* of muscles, particularly of cranial nerve muscles, is virtually pathognomonic of myasthenia gravis. Myasthenic Pts have a deficit in cholinergic transmission at the motor endplates of skeletal muscle. The diagnosis depends on clinical demonstration of the pathologic fatigability, repetitive nerve stimulation that shows a decremental response, proving that a cholinergic drug will restore strength, and the demonstration of antibodies that block acetyl choline receptors at motor endplates of the skeletal muscles.

B. *Bedside tests for pathologic fatigability of cranial nerve muscles*
1. The clinical tests chosen depend on the particular muscles implicated by the Pt's history, and whether the muscles display some evident weakness at the time of examination. If the Pt complains of double vision or ptosis, select the eye muscles, or if the complaint involves dysphagia, dysarthria, or dyspnea, select the oropharyngeal and breathing muscles. To bring out latent weakness of such muscles or of a muscle not overtly weak, require the Pt to make repetitive or prolonged contractions. *Make sure that you enlist the Pt's full cooperation and effort.*
2. To test for ptosis or diplopia, carefully measure the height of the palpebral fissure and record the range of eye movements. Pay particular attention to the range of upward eye movement, the ocular movement that has the least range and is frequently weak in myasthenics. Ask the Pt to follow your finger up and down through a full range of movement 100 times. Then measure the height of the palpebral fissure and again record the range of eye movements. Test lateral eye movements by noting the distance between limbus and lateral or medial canthi before and after repetitive exercise, or have the Pt hold the eyes in a deviated position for a timed period. Test oropharyngeal function by actually timing how long the Pt can read or count aloud without weakness of the voice, and then have the Pt try to swallow a glass of water. Test fatigability of the tongue by having the Pt waggle it from side to side 100 times. For masseter weakness, request the Pt to chew

gum or paraffin a given number of times, such as 100. Test palatal function by timing how long the Pt can sustain an "EEEE. . . ." Test breathing by measuring vital capacity before and after a timed period of hyperventilation. As a quick, quantitative, test for breathing insufficiency, requiring no apparatus and useful in myasthenia or other neurologic disorders in lieu of spirometry, ask the Pt to take a full, deep breath and to count aloud from one upward. Control the rate of counting by tapping your finger at the rate of one per second. The average adult Pt should reach at least 30. Try this test yourself. The point of all such tests is to select some quantifiable or measurable endpoint to prove that repetitive use of the muscle causes pathologic fatigability.

C. *Procedure for the edrophonium test on an adult for cholinergic responsivity*
  1. Determine some measurable endpoint, as just discussed in section A.
  2. Have cardiopulmonary resuscitation equipment available, as when giving any intravenous medication, and provisions for relief of bladder or bowels.
  3. Draw up a mL of 10 mg/mL edrophonium in a tuberculin syringe. Draw up 0.4 mg of atropine in another syringe to counteract any excessive reaction to the edrophonium.
  4. Draw up 1 mL of sterile saline solution in another tuberculin syringe to serve as a placebo control.
  5. Anchor an intravenous needle with flexible tubing to connect to the syringes.
  6. Describe the test procedure to the Pt, but do not state whether the injection will make the Pt stronger or weaker. Forewarn the Pt that some subjective responses may occur, consisting of symptoms and signs of cholinergic stimulation. The cholinergic effect on skeletal muscles consists of a feeling of tightness in previously weak muscles, such as the ocular muscles, and fasciculations. The sympathetic effect consists of sweating. The parasympathetic effects consist of blurred vision (pupilloconstrictor and ciliary muscles), salivation (salivary gland stimulation), bradycardia, abdominal cramping and diarrhea, and urinary urgency and urination (pelvic parasympathomimetic). By reviewing all of the cholinergic endings in the peripheral motor system—skeletal, sympathetic, and parasympathetic— you will have an organizing principle to remember all of these effects, rather than memorizing them as a list. Then invoke the rostrocaudal principle to "think through" the parasympathetic end organs of the oral, ocular, thoracic, and abdominopelvic cavities.
  7. Have an assistant inject 0.1 mL of sterile saline every 30 seconds for five injections, while you measure whatever you have chosen to measure. Placebo-reacting patients may show very dramatic effects, including fainting, but the injection will produce no measurable improvement in motor function in Pts with organic disease.
  8. Next inject edrophonium at the rate of 0.1 mL (1 mg) every 30 seconds either until you obtain some measurable improvement or until the Pt becomes uncomfortable. If no response occurs at the end of the first 10 injections, add another syringe. Thus you must proceed to one or the other of these two endpoints of discomfort or improvement, or you may not have given sufficient edrophonium to adequately test the Pt. Some myasthenics have an extreme tolerance for the medication. *A very common error in tests such as these is to give a set, predetermined amount of medication, rather than titrating the dose against endpoints.* The same holds when giving anticonvulsant drugs to arrest status epilepticus.

D. *Electrical tests for pathologic fatigability in myasthenia gravis.* Electrical testing for myasthenia requires repetitive stimulation of a peripheral nerve while recording the amplitude of the action potentials generated in the muscle fibers. Myasthenics show a decrement in the amplitude of muscular contraction after repetitive electrical stimulation of the nerve. The repetitive nerve stimulation test (Jolly test) provides entirely objective data. It eliminates the need for the Pt's active, willful participation, required by the repetitive exercise tests.

E. *Summary of common causes for multiple cranial nerve palsies or weakness of multiple ocular and faciobulbar muscles*
   1. Myasthenia gravis.
   2. Landry-Guillain-Barre-Strohl polyradiculopathy syndrome (including C. Miller Fisher variant).
   3. Chronic basilar meningitis.
   4. Diabetes mellitus.
   5. Neoplasms along the base of the skull and nasopharynx.
   6. Botulism.
   7. Myotonic dystrophy (diffuse weakness of all cranial nerve muscles with predilection for temporal and sternocleidomastoid muscles and relative sparing of EOMs) (Fig. 1-*I*).

VIII. The neurology of breathing

A. *Functions of the breathing apparatus*
   1. *Gas exchange for respiration*
      a. Homeostatic control of blood gases and pH.
      b. Clearing the airway by coughing and sneezing.
   2. *Speech.*
   3. *Emotional expression* (sighs, laughter, and crying).
   4. *Sucking/blowing.*

B. *The neuroanatomy of breathing*
   1. *Origin of the drive to breathe.* We may regard the drive to breathe as arising in two sources in the brain: the *forebrain* and the *brainstem reticular formation.* The isolated spinal cord by itself cannot produce any drive to breathe. That must descend from the brain. Thus separation of the spinal cord from the brain by transection at the medullocervical junction causes complete and irreversible apnea.
   2. *The forebrain and the control of volitional and emotional breathing*
      a. The forebrain mediates the *volitional* control of breathing via the pyramidal tracts, particularly for speech.
      b. The forebrain also mediates the *emotional* control of breathing, in particular for laughing and crying, through descending pyramidal and nonpyramidal pathways. Other common examples of emotional expression through control of breathing are hyperventilation attacks in anxiety, breath-holding spells in infants, and sighing.
   3. *The reticular formation and the control of automatic breathing*
      a. Reticulospinal tracts, arising in the medullary reticular formation, control *automatic,* essentially homeostatic breathing, for the control of blood gases and pH.
      b. The *caudal* half of the reticular formation, from midpons to the medullocervical junction, generates the rhythmic drive to breath; controls the related reflexes served by the caudal cranial nerves—swallowing,

chewing, rooting, sucking, coughing, and hiccoughing; and mediates the control of blood pressure and pulse. Bilateral lesions of the caudal reticular formation permanently impair or abolish automatic breathing and the related reflexes.

c. The medullary reticular formation sends the single most important pathway for survival, the *reticulospinal pathway*. It activates the LMNs of the muscles of respiration, essentially the diaphragm and intercostal muscles. The reticulospinal tracts decussate at the medullocervical junction, just ventral to the obex, and descend in the ventrolateral quadrants of the spinal cord to activate the phrenic and intercostal motoneurons (Fig. 6-13).

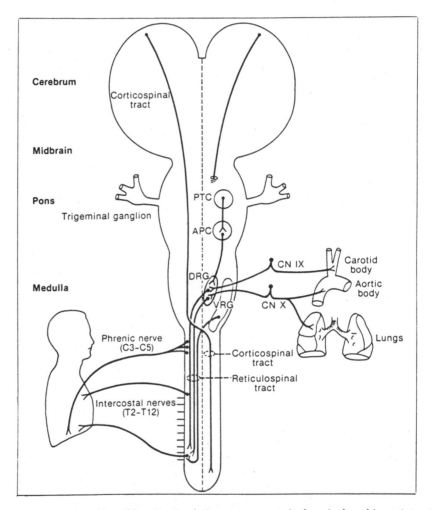

FIG. 6-13. Neuroanatomy of breathing. By stimulating motoneurons in the spinal cord from C-3 to T-12, the corticospinal tracts control volitional breathing and the reticulospinal tracts control automatic breathing. **PTC** = pneumotaxic center; **APC** = apneustic center; **DRG** = dorsal respiratory group of neurons, mainly inspiratory, associated with the dorsal motor nucleus of the vagus nerve; **VRG** = ventral respiratory group of mixed inspiratory-expiratory neurons associated with the nuclei ambiguus and retroambigualis. *(From W. DeMyer: Neuroanatomy. Media, PA, Harwal, 1988.)*

d. The *phrenic* nerves are the single most important nerves in the body. If they are intact and the drive to breathe descends through the reticulospinal tracts, the Pt can maintain breathing by diaphragmatic action alone, even after spinal cord transection paralyzes all of the intercostal muscles. Study Fig. 6-14, an infant who suffered spinal cord transection during a breech delivery. The infant shows dorsiflexed wrists secondary

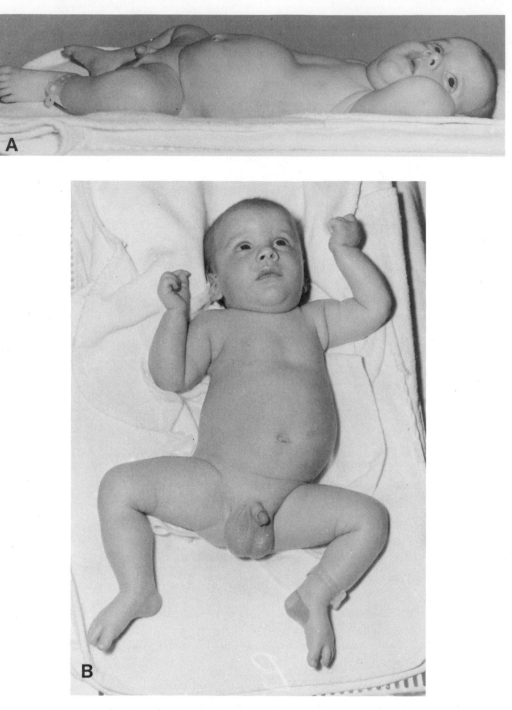

FIG. 6-14. Eight-week old infant showing the characteristic posture and breathing action after spinal cord transection at C-7 level, due in this instance to breech delivery. See text for description. *(Reproduced by permission from W. DeMyer: Anatomy and clinical neurology of the spinal cord, in R. J. Joynt: Clinical Neurology, rev. ed, Chap. 43. Philadelphia, Lippincott, 1990.*

to intact extensor muscles and paralyzed flexors. The extensor muscle motoneurons are slightly rostral to the level of the flexors and are spared. The phrenic nerve that arises from C-2 or C-3 to C-5 is also spared, but the lesion has interrupted all ascending and descending spinal pathways at the C-7 level, thus depriving the intercostal muscles of pyramidal and reticulospinal activation. Because of the descent of the diaphragm without intercostal action, the chest sucks in and the abdomen protrudes when the infant inspires, as the picture shows, so-called "abdominal breathing." The legs show the characteristic flexed leg posture that follows chronic spinal cord transection (paraplegia in flexion) (Fig. 6-14).

C. *Ondine's curse and the dichotomy between volitional and automatic breathing*
   1. *Ondine's curse*
      a. Consider a Pt with intact pyramidal tracts but interruption of the reticulospinal pathways. Such a condition may arise from:
         (1) Bilateral destruction of the medullary reticular formation.
         (2) Interruption of the reticulospinal tracts at the obex (Fig. 6-13).
         (3) Interruption of the reticulospinal tracts as they descend in the ventrolateral quadrants of the spinal cord white matter (Fig. 2-4).
      b. The Pt without a reticulospinal pathway has no automatic respiration but continues to breathe while awake because of the respiratory drive generated in the waking forebrain, transmitted through the pyramidal tracts. Sleep removes the respiratory drive arising in the forebrain. Thus with no automatic breathing to take over, apnea ensues when the Pt goes to sleep and the Pt may die. This condition, *Ondine's curse,* condemns the Pt to death if he goes to sleep. To breathe and thus to live, the Pt must remain perpetually awake, never to enjoy Keats' "sleep full of sweet dreams and quiet breathing."
      c. By contrast, interruption of the pyramidal tracts, with the reticulospinal tracts intact, abolishes volitional control of breathing; however, automatic breathing, via the reticulospinal tracts, keeps the Pt alive, whether awake or asleep. Such Pts with bilateral pyramidal tract destruction also show the pseudobulbar palsy syndrome described in section III.
   2. *Other types of sleep apnea.* Both adults and children commonly suffer sleep apnea, which may have various causes—some obstructive and others neurogenic. In the sudden infant death syndrome (SIDS or crib death) the infant fails to breathe when it is asleep and is found dead by a parent. This may represent a failure of the automatic drive to breathe, but the exact mechanism is still uncertain (Kinney, Brody, and Finkelstein, 1991).
   3. Describe the two major pathways that transmit the drive to breathe and state how interruption of each affects volitional and automatic breathing.

Ans: See Fig. 6-13.

D. *Hypoventilation in hemiplegia.* Since some Pts have a greater number of decussating axons in the pyramidal tract than others, hemiplegia may cause significant paralysis of the contralateral intercostal muscles and diaphragm, even though these muscles customarily act symmetrically (Przedborski, Brunko, Hubert et al, 1988). The Ex must consider UMN paresis of the muscles of respiration in Pts with acute hemiplegia.

REFERENCES FOR THE NEUROANATOMY OF BREATHING

Kinney HC, Brody BA, Finkelstein DM et al: Delayed central nervous system myelination in the sudden infant death syndrome. *J Neuropath Exp Neurol,* 1991; 50:29–48.
Przedborski S, Brunko E, Hubert M et al: The effect of acute hemiplegia on intercostal muscle activity. *Neurology,* 1988; 38:1882–1884.

FURTHER READING FOR THE NEUROANATOMY OF BREATHING

Harper RM, Hoffman HJ: *Sudden Infant Death Syndrome: Risk Factors and Basic Mechanisms.* New York, Demos Publications, 1988.

Weiner WJ (ed): *Respiratory Dysfunction in Neurologic Disease.* New York, Futura Publishing, 1980.

IX. A localizing diagnosticon for brainstem symptoms and signs

Fig. 6-15 summarizes the clinical effects of brainstem lesions. One important, classical localizing combination is paralysis of a cranial nerve in midbrain, pons, or medulla *ipsilateral* to the lesion, and motor or sensory signs *contralateral,* due to interruption of a decussating tract, i.e., right VIth nerve palsy and left-sided pyramidal signs caused by a lesion of the basis pontis.

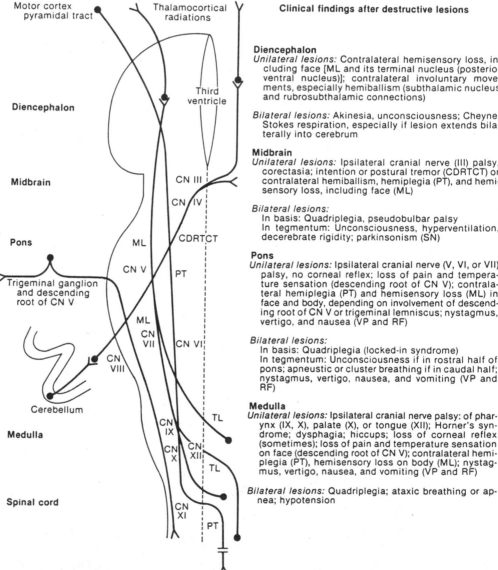

FIG. 6-15. Localizing diagnosticon for brainstem lesions (exclusive of central ocular pathways). CDRTCT = cerebello-dentato-rubro-thalamo-cortical tract; ML = medial lemniscus; PT = pyramidal tract; TL = trigeminal lemniscus; Roman numerals = cranial nerve nuclei; SN = substantia nigra; VP = vestibular pathways; RF = reticular formation. *(From W. DeMyer: Neuroanatomy. Media, PA, Harwal, 1988.)*

X. Sequential screening examination of the motor functions of all of the cranial nerves

A. Preliminary observations

And now the crucial test: can you sit down with a Pt and actually and systematically examine cranial nerve motor function? If you did your job when taking the history, you have already observed the Pt's eye movements and blinking, noted the degree and symmetry of other facial movements, and inspected the relation of the lids to palpebral fissures. You have looked for en- or exophthalmos, listened to phonation, and the articulation of labials, linguals, and palatals, and noted the spontaneous swallowing of saliva. If these are all normal, the Pt can't have too much wrong with cranial nerve motor function, but you must do a formal examination anyhow.

B. Motor examination of all of the cranial nerves in 45 seconds

The formal examination of cranial nerve motor function begins with the eyes. We test

TABLE 6-8 Method for rapid sequential screening of the motor function of the cranial nerves

Nerves	Commands to patient by examiner	Observations and tests by examiner
III, IV, VI	"Follow my finger."	Move finger through the pattern described in Chap. 4 and pictured in Fig. 4-20 and watch for asymmetrical corneal light reflections, lid-limbus relations, nystagmus, and pupilloconstriction during convergence. Inquire about diplopia.
	"Look up at the ceiling."	Watch for asymmetry or absence of forehead wrinkling and eyebrow elevation.
VII	"Close your eyes tight and don't let me open them."	Look for asymmetry of wrinkles radiating from lateral canthi and try to force lids open with your fingers.
	"Draw back the corners of your mouth" or "Smile."	Look for asymmetry of the nasolabial folds. Have patient make labial sounds if speech sounded abnormal.
	"Draw down the corners of your mouth hard."	Look for asymmetry of movement and for wrinkling of skin on neck from platysma action.
V	"Bite your jaws together hard."	Palpate the masseter muscles.
	"Open your jaw as wide as possible."	Look for deviation of the tip by sighting on the notch between the medial two incisors.
	"Hold your jaw to one side."	Try to push it back. Repeat test to the opposite side.
XII	"Stick out your tongue as far as possible."	Look for deviation, atrophy, and fasciculations. Test for lingual articulations if speech sounded abnormal.
	"Move your tongue from side to side."	Look for weakness or slowness of movement.
X	"Say, Ah."	Look for asymmetrical palatal elevation. Test for palatal articulations and do gag reflex if speech or swallowing were abnormal.
XI	"Turn your head to one side and don't let me push it back."	Try to push head back to midline. Inspect and palpate SCM muscles. Repeat maneuver to opposite side.
	"Touch your ear with your shoulders."	Try to press the patient's shoulders back down.

motility last in the ocular sequence for a reason. We can then flow smoothly through the entire cranial nerve motor examination, yes, III to XII, in just 45 seconds, in a normal cooperative Pt. No, the 45 seconds is not a misprint. Get a partner and rehearse the commands and observations in Table 6-8 today, tomorrow, and every day until you meet the 45-second criterion.

FURTHER READINGS FOR THE MOTOR FUNCTION OF THE CRANIAL NERVES

DeMyer W: *Neuroanatomy.* Media, PA, Harwal Publishing, 1988.
Samii M, Janetta PJ (eds): *The Cranial Nerves.* New York, Springer-Verlag, 1981.
Wilson-Pauwels L, Akesson EJ, Stewart PA: *Cranial Nerves: Anatomy and Clinical Comments.* Philadelphia, B.C. Decker, 1988.

Learning Objectives for Chapter Six

I. Vth cranial nerve motor functions: Chewing
1. State in one word the motor function of the Vth nerve.
2. Name the chewing muscles innervated by the Vth nerve.
3. Describe the actions of the lateral pterygoid muscles and describe the effect of paralysis of one lateral pterygoid muscle on jaw movement (Figs. 6-1 and 6-2).
4. Describe the UMN (corticobulbar) innervation of the Vth nerve nucleus.
5. Demonstrate the steps in the clinical examination of the chewing muscles.
6. Demonstrate how to place your hands to test the strength of the lateral pterygoid muscle.
6. Describe the clinical findings on inspection, palpation, and strength testing of a Pt after complete unilateral interruption of the motor division of the Vth cranial nerve.

II. VIIth cranial nerve motor function: Facial movements
1. List the major movements of your own face (exclusive of the mandible) and name the muscles responsible (Table 6-1 and Fig. 6-3).
2. On a cross-sectional drawing of the pons, show the origin and intraaxial course of the VIth and VIIth cranial nerves (Fig. 6-4).
3. Describe the pattern of facial muscle paralysis after a VIIth nerve (LMN) lesion as contrasted with a corticobulbar tract (UMN) lesion. Relate the side of the paralysis to the side of the LMN or UMN lesion.
4. State which facial movements a normal person can most easily make unilaterally and which least easily (Table 6-2). Relate this observation to the degree of unilaterality or bilaterality of the UMN innervation of the movements.
5. Explain why an acute UMN lesion will sometimes

cause paresis of the orbicularis oculi muscle, as well as paralysis of the lower part of the face.
6. Describe the clinical observations you make to detect mild UMN palsy of the face.
7. Recite the commands to test movements of the facial muscles (Table 6-4).
8. Describe whether it is easy or difficult to open a normal person's forcefully closed eyelids.
9. Describe what happens to the strength of the orbicularis oculi muscle in LMN and acute UMN lesions.
9. Describe the discrepancy between volitional and emotional facial movements, such as smiling, often seen in the chronic stage after UMN lesions affecting the face.
11. Describe "masked facies" and mention some disorders that cause it.
12. List several types of involuntary movements which can be seen by inspecting the Pt's face.

III. IXth and Xth cranial nerve motor functions
1. State which cranial nerves provide clinically significant motor and sensory nerve fibers for the palate, pharynx, and larynx.
2. Describe the act of normal swallowing. State what cranial nerves participate and the actions of the muscles they innervate.
3. Describe the action of the soft palate in swallowing (Fig. 6-8), and state which cranial nerve is mainly responsible for its action.
4. Produce two sounds which require complete palatal closure.
5. State whether severe and enduring unilateral palatal palsy would implicate an UMN or LMN lesion and explain why.
6. Describe pseudobulbar palsy and distinguish between bulbar and pseudobulbar palsy.

IV. Speech production

1. Distinguish between *phonation* and *articulation.*
2. Demonstrate how to use yourself to recall the sounds which require strong labial or lingual action.
3. Define ·fricative, sibilant, voiceless consonant, and plosive.
4. Define aphonia/dysphonia, anarthria/dysarthria, aphagia/dysphagia.
5. Distinguish between *hyper*nasal and *hypo*nasal speech and relate them to the size of the nasopharyngeal opening.
6. Explain why removal of adenoid tissue may worsen the speech of a Pt who has hypernasal speech.
7. Recite three sounds that you ask the Pt to make that test palatal, lingual, and labial articulations, respectively.
8. State which cranial nerves innervate the muscles responsible for labial, lingual, and palatal sounds.
9. Make a drawing to show the appearance of the palate of a Pt with a unilateral palate palsy. State what sound the Pt should make when you inspect the palatal arch for weakness (Fig. 6-9).
10. Describe how to elicit the gag reflex. State which cranial nerves mediate the afferent and efferent arc of the reflex.
11. Describe the effects of unilateral vocal cord paralysis on the Pt's voice.
12. State several neurologic, neuromuscular, or anatomic causes for deficient velopharyngeal closure.
13. State the only way to conclusively identify paralysis of a vocal cord.
14. State which sensory cranial nerve you must always test in an infant or young child with delayed speech or significant dysarthria.

V. XIth cranial nerve motor functions

1. Explain why the XIth nerve is called the *spinal accessory* nerve.
2. Name the two clinically testable muscles innervated by the XIth nerve.
3. Describe the three actions of the sternocleidomastoid muscle and demonstrate how to use yourself to remember these actions.
4. Demonstrate the clinical examination of the sterno-cleidomastoid and trapezius muscles (Table 6-7 and preceding paragraph).
5. Explain whether to press on the Pt's cheek or mandible to test the strength of head rotation by the sternocleidomastoid muscle.

VI. XIIth cranial nerve motor functions

1. By means of a vector diagram, explain the action of the genioglossus muscle (Fig. 6-11).
2. Explain this statement: "The lateral pterygoid, sterno-cleidomastoid, and the genioglossus muscles all turn the part they operate to the opposite side."

3. State the typical signs of LMN XIIth nerve palsy and the findings that distinguish LMN from UMN weakness of the tongue.
4. Demonstrate the steps in the clinical examination of the motor functions of the tongue.

VII. Multiple cranial nerve palsies, pathologic fatigability, and myasthenia gravis

1. Describe the most frequent presenting symptoms of Pts with pathologic fatigability of multiple cranial nerve muscles.
2. Name the neuromuscular disease you should suspect when the Pt has these complaints.
3. Describe the neurochemical defect in myasthenia gravis.
4. Describe how to decide which muscles to test for pathologic fatigability in a Pt suspected of myasthenia gravis.
5. Describe in principle the clinical, electrical, and pharmacologic tests for pathologic fatigability of muscles.
6. Describe several quantitative bedside tests for pathologic fatigability.
7. Describe a simple, quantitative, apparatus-less bedside test for respiratory insufficiency.
8. State the pharmacologic action of edrophonium.
*9. Describe the procedure for the edrophonium test and state what precautions you take to insure the Pt's safety and comfort during the edrophonium test.
*10. Describe the symptoms and signs that may occur during an edrophonium test. Describe the organizing principles for remembering these effects.
*11. Describe the endpoints you use to decide how much edrophonium to give and when to terminate the test. Explain why you titrate the dose of edrophonium to one of these endpoints rather than giving a preset dose.

VIII. The neurology of breathing

1. State the functions of the breathing apparatus.
2. Describe the origins of the drive to breathe.
3. Give examples of emotional expressions that employ the breathing apparatus.
4. Describe the role of the pontomedullary reticular formation in breathing and list the breathing-related reflexes mediated through it and the medullary cranial nerves.
5. Describe the origin, course, and LMNs of termination of the reticulospinal pathways for breathing (Fig. 6-13).
6. Name the single most important peripheral nerve for the maintenance of breathing, and the spinal cord segments from which it arises.
7. Describe the pathways that mediate automatic and volitional breathing.
8. Describe which pathway is responsible for automatic breathing during sleep and describe the nature of Ondine's curse.

9. Describe the posture of a Pt with a C-7 level cord transection and the characteristic action of the chest and abdomen when such a Pt breathes (Fig. 6-14).

IX. A localizing diagnosticon for brainstem symptoms and signs
   1. List in rostrocaudal order the three parts of the brainstem, and the cranial nerve motor nuclei contained in each (Fig. 6-15).
   2. Commencing with the midbrain and working caudally, describe the typical unilateral-contralateral signs seen after unilateral lesions of the midbrain, pons, and medulla (Fig. 6-15).

X. Sequential screening examination of the motor functions of all of the cranial nerves
   Starting with the ocular movements, recite the commands and demonstrate the maneuvers used to screen the motor functions of *all* of the cranial nerves (III to XII) in serial order in less than one minute (Table 6-9).

Chapter Seven

Examination of the Somatic Motor System (Excluding Cranial Nerves)

But the expression of a well-made man appears not only in his face,
It is in his limbs and joints also, it is curiously in the joints of his hips and wrists.
It is in his walk, the carriage of his neck, the flex of his waist, and knees . . .
To see him pass conveys as much as the best poem, perhaps more.

Walt Whitman (1819–1892)

I. Inspection of the body contours, postures, and gait

A. _Initial inspection_

1. The motor examination begins as soon as you meet the Pt. Study every activity: how the Pt sits, stands, walks and gestures; the postures; and the general level of activity. Unobtrusive observation of the Pt's spontaneous activity often discloses more than formal tests, particularly in infants or mentally ill Pts.

2. To start the formal examination, have the Pt undress and stand under an overhead light. Undergarments may remain in place, in deference to modesty, but at some time during the examination you must look under them. If you leave one-third of the body covered, you can do only two-thirds of an examination. Before the cock crows, one of you will violate this commandment that thou shalt undress every Pt. Your own anxieties about viewing a nude Pt may exceed those of the Pt about being viewed nude. After all, the Pt came to you expecting an examination.

3. Next, ponder, yes _ponder,_ the Pt's somatotype or body build, comparing the Pt's body contours and proportions, with the standard normal figure of a person of like age and sex. From abnormalities in the Pt's _gestalt,_ sometimes from just a glance at the silhouette, the examiner (Ex) can diagnose an immense number of syndromes, such as arachnodactyly, achondroplastic dwarfism, and Down's syndrome.

---

*The light vertical rule on the left side of the text sets off an answer column. Cover the answers with a card until you have responded to the text. Then after each response, slide the card down to check your answer.

The heavy vertical rule or asterisk denotes optional material.

4. Next, scrutinize the size and contours of the Pt's muscles, looking for atrophy or hypertrophy. Then, look for body asymmetry, joint malalignments, fasciculations, tremors, and involuntary movements. Proceed in an orderly, rostrocaudal, neck-shoulder-arm-forearm-hand-chest-abdomen-thigh-leg-foot-toe sequence, and continually compare right and left sides.

B. *Station and gait testing*
1. Next, observe the Pt's *station,* the steadiness and verticality of the standing posture. Then test the *gait* by asking the Pt to walk freely across the room. Look for unsteadiness, a broad-based gait, and lack of arm swinging. Ask the Pt to walk on the toes, heels, and in tandem (heel-to-toe along a straight line). Request a deep knee-bend. Ask a child to hop on each foot and to run. *Watching the Pt walk is the single most important part of the entire neurologic examination (NE).* An essay at the end of Chap. 8 details gait analysis, after the student has a better concept of what to look for.
2. Now, rehearse the five steps of section VI.A of the Summarized Neurologic Examination. Yes, I'll ask you to demonstrate them by and by.

II. Principles of strength testing

NOTE: To learn strength testing, get another student, and do the strength tests on each other. How else can you learn to match your strength against another's? And something else: remove your outer garments in order to see the muscles and tendons in action.

A. *The matching principle:* select those movements that just about match the Ex's arm and hand strength. Even if an iron bar loses much of its strength, it may remain too strong for your hands to bend. Contrariwise, wet tissue paper offers too little resistance. To gauge strength accurately, select movements that are neither too strong for you to possibly overcome, nor too weak for you to judge their resistance. Those movements in which the Pt's resistance just about matches your own arm and hand strength are ideal.

B. *The length-strength principle:* muscles are strongest when they act from their shortest position and have little or no strength when they act from their longest position.
1. To understand the length-strength law, work through Fig. 7-1*A* to *D* to test biceps and triceps strength. The Ex pulls or pushes on the Pt's wrist with one hand while stabilizing the Pt's elbow or shoulder with the other hand. In all strength tests, the participants should exert maximum power, but they should pull to a peak in a slow crescendo without jerking.
2. Relate the strength of the biceps and triceps muscles to their length: these muscles are strongest when acting from their ☐ shortest/ ☐ intermediate/ ☐ longest position.

☑ *Shortest*

3. Now test the flexor and extensor strength of your partner's neck. In testing these movements, place one hand on the Pt's forehead or occiput and the other on the front or back of the Pt's chest to provide bracing and counterpressure.
4. Test the strength of the neck flexors when your partner starts with the head strongly extended. Then you resist the neck flexion with your hands. Compare the neck flexor strength when your partner starts with the head tightly flexed, chin on chest. Then you try to extend it. The neck flexors are strong-

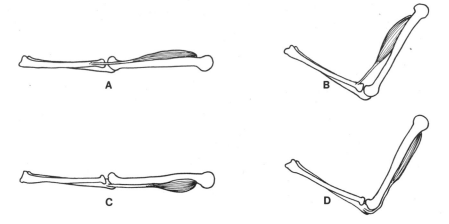

FIG. 7-1. Relation of length to strength of muscles.

✓ *Flexed*
✓ *Shortest*

est with the neck ☐ flexed/ ☐ extended, in which position the flexor muscles are ☐ shortest/ ☐ longest.

5. Next compare the maximum strength of the neck extensors with that of the neck flexors. One action, extension or flexion is, by far, stronger than the other. Determine which.

6. To see whether we have discovered a general length-strength law, test the quadriceps femoris and hamstring muscles with the knee flexed and extended. With the knee extended, the quadriceps femoris muscle is ☐ Strongest; ☐ weakest and ☐ shortest/ ☐ longest.

Ans: ✓ *Strongest;* ✓ *shortest (thus confirming the length-strength law)*

NOTE: The kinesiologist's length-strength law that the muscles are strongest when shortest differs from Starling's law of the heart that the strength of cardiac contraction increases as the resting length of the cardiac muscle fibers increases.

7. In general, to test muscles of weak or modest strength more accurately, start with the Pt's part in a position of strength, e.g., neck flexed. But to test very strong muscles, place them at a disadvantage to bring them within your range of strength. Thus to reduce the strength of the normally powerful triceps muscle to bring it within the testing range, test the Pt with the elbow ☐ bent/ ☐ extended. Explain: _____

Ans: ✓ *Bent. With the elbow bent the triceps is longest and therefore weakest.*

C. *The antigravity muscle principle: how to remember the strongest of opposing sets of muscles*

1. Muscles work in opposing, *agonist-antagonist* pairs. One of the opposing pairs is immensely stronger than the other, e.g., neck extension is far stronger than flexion. Without a general law to recall the strongest of opposing sets of muscles, we face the oppressive task of memorizing each set individually. If we look at a quadruped, or, better, at a man in quadrupedal position, the solution leaps out at us (Fig. 7-2). The immensely powerful muscles all belong to the postural antigravity system of a quadruped.

2. Stand up and assume the posture of Fig. 7-2*A* and *B*. Of particular importance, assume posture *B*. Notice then how the triceps muscle locks the upper extremities against collapse from the pull of gravity and how the quadriceps femoris locks the lower extremities. The neck extensors erect the head. Buttocks and back extensors erect the trunk, holding it from col-

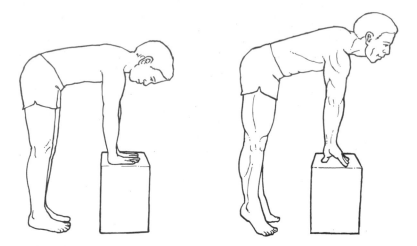

FIG. 7-2. Man in quadrupedal posture. (*A*) Relaxed. (*B*) Rising on fingers and toes.

lapse by gravity when the individual stands, or equally important, when leaping or locomoting. When a person is leaping or locomoting, the hands and feet flex *downwards.* The muscles which support or lock the standing posture against collapse by the pull of gravity and which leap and locomote against gravity constitute the *antigravity muscle system.* Invariably, the strength of these antigravity locking, locomoting, and leaping muscles greatly exceeds their antagonists.

3. Using the principle of the superior strength of the antigrativy locking, locomoting, and leaping muscles, predict the strongest of these opposing movements:

   ☐ wrist extension/ ☐ flexion
   ☐ trunk extension/ ☐ flexion
   ☐ foot dorsiflexion/ ☐ plantar flexion
   ☐ toe extension/ ☐ flexion.

☑ *Flexion*
☑ *Trunk extension*
☑ *Plantar flexion*
☑ *Flexion*

4. Confusion may arise in applying the antigravity theory to some actions like arm abduction. When abducting, the arm acts against the pull of gravity, but the abductor muscles do not support the standing skeleton against collapse by gravity when the animal stands, leaps, or locomotes; hence, the arm elevator and abductors are not postural antigravity muscles and, quite to the contrary, their opponents are. Consider as examples of postural antigravity muscles the pectoral and latissimus dorsi muscles. The pectoral muscles prevent the forelimbs from straddling out when the animal stands. (Imagine the leverage acting to spread a giraffe's legs.) The latissimus dorsi muscles pull the forelimbs backwards, thrusting the shoulders forward and upward, i.e., against gravity, when the quadruped leaps or locomotes. Consequently, the strength of these adductor and flexor muscles acting at the shoulder far exceeds their opponents, the abductor-extensor muscles. Applying this consideration to the hip, which would be stronger? ☐ hip abductors/ ☐ hip adductors. Explain: _____

Ans: ☑ *Hip adductors. Read the last paragraph again if you can't explain the answer. As a further example consider the action of dorsiflexing and plantar flexing the foot when walking. The dorsiflexors lift the foot against the pull of gravity, but merely act to clear the toes and set the foot in place again so that the powerful plantar flexors can again act to support the posture, leap, or locomote.*

5. The antigravity theory predicts not only the strongest muscles, but also how much stronger they are. Your arm and hand strength cannot even begin to overcome the antigravity muscles when set in their strongest positions, with the head and trunk extended; jaw closed; arms and knees extended; wrists, fingers, feet, and toes flexed (Fig. 12-10). But your arm and hand strength just about equals or barely overcomes the non-antigravity muscles when set in their strongest position, with the head flexed, jaw open, arms abducted, hips flexed, and wrist and feet dorsiflexed.

6. As a final bonus, the antigravity theory explains the very important posture called *decerebrate rigidity,* seen in comatose Pts, when the Pt assumes the position dictated by contraction of the whole system of antigravity muscles (Fig. 12-13).

III. The sequence and technique to test for muscular weakness

A. *The rostrocaudal sequence*

1. Test muscles in the natural rostrocaudal order since it requires no memorization. After testing cranial nerve muscles, simply continue in the neck-shoulder-arm-forearm-hand-chest-abdomen-thigh-leg-foot-toe sequence, and continually compare right and left sides.

2. Throughout all strength testing and the whole NE, the Ex should engage the Pt's competitive spirit in order to get maximum effort. Challenge the Pt: "I am trying to test how strong you are. Do your best on each test. Don't let me win."

3. Preceding strength testing, the Ex has an opportunity to test for *range of motion* of the joints, if the history suggests a need to do so. To test range of motion, the Ex asks the Pt to move the joint through its full range of motion, and then the Ex may attempt to passively manipulate the joint.

B. *Testing the strength of neck flexors and extensors*

1. Extensors are ordinarily too strong for the Ex's arm and hand strength.

2. In what position does the Ex ask the Pt to place the head to bring the strength of the relatively weak neck flexors up into the best range to test? ☐ flexed/ ☐ extended

☑ *Flexed*

C. *Testing the strength of shoulder girdle muscles*

1. *Trapezius* has been tested with the cranial nerves.

2. Test free shoulder and arm movements by having the Pt extend the arms forward, to the sides, and then over the head. Inspect from front and back. Look for scapular movement, particularly winging of the dorsal border away from the rib cage.

3. After testing *free movement* of arm abduction and elevation, test the *strength* of these movements. Have your Pt (or partner) hold the arms straight out to the sides (abducted). Push down on them as the Pt resists. Where do you push? That depends on you. If you are a strong man and the Pt a woman, push down *proximally* at the elbows to reduce your leverage. If you are a woman and the Pt a man, push down *distally,* on the forearms or wrists, to increase your leverage. Select a point where your strength in pushing down about equals that of the standard person of the height, weight, age, and sex of your Pt. Here you must build your own catalog of experience. Work through Table 7-1.

TABLE 7-1 Method of testing shoulder girdle strength	
Action	Commands and maneuvers
Arm elevation	Command patient to hold the arms straight out to the sides. Press down on both arms at a point where you expect your strength to approximate the patient's.
Arm adduction downward	With the arms extended to the sides, the patient resists your efforts to elevate them.
Arm adduction across the chest	With the arms extended straight in front, the patient crosses the wrists. You try to pull them apart.
Scapular adduction	With the hands on the hips, the patient forces the elbows backwards as hard as possible. Standing behind the patient, the Ex tries to push them forward.
Scapular winging	Have the patient try a push-up or lean forward against a wall, supporting the body with outstretched arms.

4. Arm abduction is complex, requiring *supraspinatus* action to initiate the act, *deltoid* action to carry the arm to shoulder height, and *scapular* rotation to continue the elevation to the vertical position. The serratus anterior and trapezius muscles hold the scapula in place against the chest wall. Serratus anterior paralysis (long thoracic nerve) results in winging of the scapula away from the chest wall.

D. *Testing the strength of upper arm muscles:* flexion and extension of the elbow.
   1. *Elbow flexors.* The Pt tightly flexes the forearm. Brace one hand against the Pt's shoulder. With the other hand grasp the Pt's wrist and attempt to straighten the Pt's forearm. This matches your biceps against the Pt's. When average person contests average person of the same age and sex, the battle is a deadlock, therefore, just about ideal for testing.
   2. *Elbow extensors.* If you give the matter no thought, you might try to test the triceps with the elbow locked in extension. But the triceps, an antigravity muscle, is tremendously strong, and average person against average person, the locked-out elbow wins easily. If, however, the Pt's locked-out arm yields, the Pt's triceps is significantly weak. For a subtler test, start with the Pt's elbow flexed, as in testing the elbow flexors, but this time grasp the wrist and oppose extension of the forearm by the Pt. This maneuver puts the triceps at a disadvantage, and average person against average person, the Ex will win, but barely. Since this test pits nearly equal strengths, it discloses slight loss of triceps power better than the arm extended position.

E. *Testing the strength of forearm muscles:* flexion and extension
   1. *Wrist flexors.* The Pt makes a fist and holds the wrist flexed against your efforts to extend it. By hooking your fingers around the Pt's fist and flexing your own wrist you can pit your own wrist flexion against the Pt's. Brace the Pt's wrist with your other hand. Other forms of manual opposition will not overcome the wrist flexors, because they are very strong antigravity muscles. (Visualize a quadruped leaping.)
   2. *Wrist extensors.* Rest the Pt's forearm on his thigh or a table top for support. The Pt then holds the wrist cocked-up (dorsiflexed) as you try to press it down with the butt of your palm on the Pt's knuckles. With the Pt's wrist

in extension, the relatively weak wrist extensors just about match your arm and hand strength.

F. *Testing the strength of finger muscles*

   1. Carefully inspect and palpate the thenar and hypothenar eminences for size and asymmetry. Look for atrophy of interosseous muscles. Most old people show obvious interosseous atrophy.
   2. *Abduction-adduction of the fingers.* Test by carefully figuring out how to match your strength against the Pt's.
      a. Start with the first dorsal interosseous muscle. Palpate it in your own hand as the mass of tissue alongside the second metacarpal bone, in the web between your thumb and index finger. The first dorsal interosseous muscle moves the index finger *away* from the middle finger and towards the thumb. Palpate your own muscle during that action.
      b. To test a Pt's dorsal interosseous muscle press the terminal phalanx of your *right* index finger alongside the resisting terminal phalanx of the Pt's *right* index finger, matching muscle to muscle (Fig. 7-3).
      c. Work through the fingers, learning how to match your finger abductors and adductors against the Pt's.

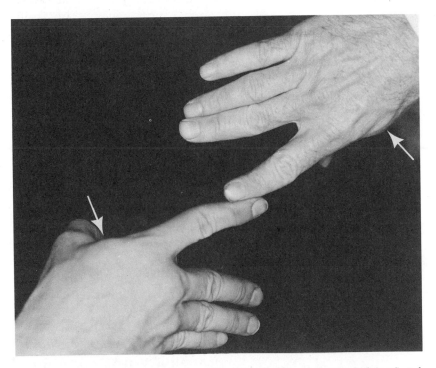

FIG. 7-3. Method of matching the Ex's finger strength against the Pt's. Notice the bulging first dorsal interosseous muscles (arrows) of both Ex and Pt.

   3. *Finger extension.* The Pt holds out the hand with palm down, fingers hyperextended. Simply turn your hand over so that the dorsum of your fingernail presses against the dorsum of the Pt's. Then you can carefully match the extensor strength of each of your own fingers against the Pt's.
   4. *Finger flexion:* strength of the grip as a whole
      a. Ask the Pt to squeeze your fingers. Grasp the Pt's wrist with one hand to steady the arm and offer two fingers of your other hand for the Pt to grasp. To add an element of fun and competition to the test, particularly with a child, and to keep the Pt working at top strength, say, "Don't let

my fingers get away," as you try to extract your fingers from the Pt's grasp.

> b. Try this experiment. Grip a pencil as tightly as possible in your fist. Notice that your wrist automatically *dorsiflexes* slightly. Have your partner try to pull the pencil out of your grip when your hand is in the normal position it automatically assumes when you tighten your grip. Then, hold your wrist *flexed* as strongly as possible and *dorsiflexed* as strongly as possible, and ask the partner to pull the pencil out of your grip in each instance. Finger flexion is strongest when the wrist is ☐ strongly flexed/ ☐ partially dorsiflexed/ ☐ completely dorsiflexed.

☑ *Partially dorsiflexed*

> c. This experiment shows that partial dorsiflexion of the wrist allows the strongest grip. Partial dorsiflexion is the *functional position of the hand,* the position chosen when putting a cast on the forearm or wrist to treat a fracture or when splinting the wrist to maintain optimum hand position while the Pt recovers from paralysis. This so-called *functional position of the hand* is the position of complete shortening of the finger flexor muscles, and therefore the position that allows them to exert the strongest grip. Further flexion of the wrist merely slackens the flexor tendons of the fingers, without further shortening of the finger flexor muscles. Hence this action of the hand does not contradict the law that the muscles are strongest when acting from their shortest position. Now if you understand all of this, state into which position you would try to force an assailant's wrist to cause him to drop a knife? _____. Explain: _____

_____

Ans: Force the assailant's wrist into flexion. First, your hands have a chance to overpower the assailant's wrist extensors, and second, the assailant's flexed wrist can no longer grip the knife strongly, and it may fall free of his hand.

> G. *Testing abdominal muscle strength*
>
> 1. *Position.* With the Pt supine (face up), ask for a sit-up, or for the Pt to elevate the legs or the head. At the same time watch the umbilicus as the abdominal muscles contract.
>
> 2. *Try this experiment.* Lying supine, stick your index finger in your own umbilicus to palpate it during the foregoing actions. If the muscles of all four quadrants have equal strength, the umbilicus will remain centered. When the Pt attempts to raise the head or legs, what would happen to the position of the umbilicus if the *lower* abdominal muscles are weak, and the *upper* are intact? The umbilicus would migrate ☐ upward/ ☐ downward.

Ans: ☑ *Upward. (The intact muscles pull the umbilicus in their direction.)*

☑ *Toward*

> a. In general, if some abdominal muscles are weak, the umbilicus will migrate ☐ toward/ ☐ away from the pull of the intact muscles during strong abdominal contraction.
>
> b. The umbilical migration test aids greatly in localizing the level of spinal cord lesions. The umbilicus corresponds to the 10th thoracic segment of the spinal cord (Fig. 2-10). Spinal cord transection at the T-10 level paralyzes all muscles *caudal* to that level. Because of paralysis of the lower abdominal muscles, when a Pt with a T-10 level cord lesion contracts the abdominal muscles, the umbilicus migrates ☐ upward/ ☐ downward (Beevor's sign).

☑ *Upward*

> H. *Testing the large back muscles.* The average Pt's back is far too strong for the Ex to test by manual opposition. Two tests can be done.

1. With the Pt prone ask the Pt to arch the back and rock on the stomach. Inspect and palpate the paraspinal muscles.
2. Have the Pt bend forward at the waist and straighten up. If you try to oppose the Pt's straightening up from a bent waist, you may cause a back sprain or herniation of an intervertebral disc.

I. *Testing the strength of the hip girdle*
   1. *Hip flexion.* With the Pt sitting, ask the Pt to lift a knee off of the table surface and to hold the thigh in a flexed position. With the butt of your palm, try to push the knee back down. The flexors are relatively weak, non-antigravity muscles and must be given an advantage by the flexed position.
   2. *Thigh abduction and adduction*
      a. With the Pt sitting, have the Pt hold the legs *abducted* as you try to press them together with your hands on the lateral sides of the knees.
      b. Then have the Pt try to hold the legs *adducted* (squeezed together) as you place your hands on the medial sides of the knees to try to pull the knees apart. It is inconvenient for the Ex to try to test adductor strength when starting with the Pt's legs apart.
   3. *Hip extension.* With the Pt prone, have the Pt lift the knee from the table surface and hold it up. Place your hand on the popliteal space and try to press the knee back down.

J. *Testing the strength of the thigh muscles*
   1. *Knee extensors*
      a. The deep knee-bend has already tested the quadriceps, an immensely powerful antigravity muscle that ordinarily is too strong to test by manual opposition if it acts from its strongest position. To test the quadriceps, place it at a mechanical disadvantage, starting with the knee ☐ flexed/ ☐ intermediate/ ☐ straight.
      b. With the Pt prone, have the Pt try to touch the heel to the buttock to induce extreme flexion of the knee. Grasp the Pt's ankle and oppose extension. Compare the extensor strength of the two legs.
   2. *Knee flexors (hamstrings).* The Pt holds the knee at a 90-degree or more acute angle, while you try to straighten it by grasping the Pt's ankle.

☑ *Flexed*

K. *Testing the strength of the ankle and toe movements*
   1. Have the Pt *dorsiflex, invert,* and *evert* the feet. Inspect, palpate the leg, and check for the strength of these movements by manual opposition.
   2. *Plantar flexion* of the foot is ordinarily too strong to test by manual opposition. Since the Pt walked on the balls of the feet during the gait examination, you already know that the plantar flexors can lift the entire body weight of the Pt.
   3. The Pt holds the toes flexed or extended, as the Ex attempts to press them back to the neutral position. Which action of the big toe is strongest, ☐ extension/ ☐ flexion. Explain: _____
   _____.

Ans: ☑ *Flexion. Of course, flexion! Which action leaps or locomotes and which action merely lifts the foot into place for another leaping or locomoting action (Fig. 7-2)?*

L. *The screening tests for muscle strength during the routine physical examination versus a complete examination*
   1. Testing the strength of every muscle in every Pt would squander time. For

the screening NE, sample a few selected movements, as outlined in section VI, step C of the Summarized Neurologic Examination. Rehearse it.

2. Pts with neurologic symptoms and signs require a much more extensive examination. From the history and initial appraisal, the Ex selects the critical muscles for testing and the conditions under which to do the tests. For example, if the Pt complains of weakness after exertion, have the Pt climb stairs before testing. If the Pt's muscles "freeze up" when cold, put the arm in ice water and ask the Pt to make repetitive contractions. If the muscles cramp when the Pt writes, have the Pt write. So often, physicians fail to examine the Pt under the conditions which reproduce the symptoms.

3. The diagnosis of specific nerve injuries and entrapment neuropathies requires detailed testing of individual muscles and comparison with charts of segmental versus peripheral nerve innervation patterns (Table 2-1 and Figs. 2-10 and 2-11). Of the guides to muscle testing, the economical little pamphlet entitled *Aids to the Examination of the Peripheral Nervous System* (see References) fits easily in your bag. (For detailed references see D'Ambrosia, 1986; Hollingshead, 1969; Sunderland, 1978. For entrapment neuropathies see Dawson et al, 1990; Kopell and Thompson, 1987.)

M. Recording the strength examination

1. Table 2-1 lists the clinically testable muscles or movements. State in the medical record the movements actually tested. If on a later visit the Pt then displays weakness, the record will prove that you actually tested the muscles and did not overlook something.

2. Record muscle strength on a numerical scale from 0 to 5. Or, use a word scale, such as *paralysis, severe weakness, moderate weakness, minimal weakness,* and *normal.* A hand-held myometer or dynamometer can be used to further quantify strength (Wiles et al, 1990; van der Ploeg et al., 1991).

N. Review. Rehearse section VI.A, B, and C of the Summarized Neurologic Examination. Do you remember the steps? No? That's the reason to rehearse them now.

REFERENCES FOR THE STRENGTH EXAMINATION

Aids to the Examination of the Peripheral Nervous System. Medical Research Council (Great Britain) Memorandum no 45 (1st ed). London, Her Majesty's Stationery Office, 1976

D'Ambrosia RD (ed): *Musculoskeletal Disorders, Regional Examination and Differential Diagnosis* (2d ed). Philadelphia, Lippincott, 1986

Dawson DM, Hallett M, Millender LH: *Entrapment Neuropathies* (2d ed). Boston, Little, Brown, 1990

Hollingshead W: *Functional Anatomy of the Limbs and Back* (3d ed). Philadelphia, Saunders, 1969

Kopell H, Thompson W: *Peripheral Entrapment Neuropathies* (2d ed). Baltimore, Williams & Wilkins, 1987

Sunderland S: *Nerves and Nerve Injuries* (2d ed). New York, Churchill Livingstone, 1978

van der Ploeg RJO, Fidler V, Oosterhuis HJGH: Hand-held myometry: Reference values. *J Neurol Neurosurg Psychiatr,* 1991; 54:244–247.

Wiles CM, Karni Y, Nicklin J: Laboratory testing of muscle function in the management of neuromuscular disease. *J Neurol Neurosurg Psychiatry* 1990; 53:384–387.

IV. Results of direct percussion of muscle

It will not surprise the cognoscente in physical diagnosis that percussing follows inspecting, palpating, and strength-testing of muscle.

A. *Self-demonstration of percussion irritability of muscle*
   1. Bare your biceps muscle and strike its belly a sharp blow with the *point* of your (tomahawk type) reflex hammer. You will see a faint dimple or ripple at the percussion site. Strike a crisp blow and jerk the hammer out of the way because the ripple is very transient.
   2. The contraction of muscle fibers in response to a direct blow demonstrates the intrinsic irritability of the muscle fibers themselves. It is not a reflex and not dependent on innervation (Brody and Rozear, 1970). In fact percussion irritability remains, and may even increase, for a period of time after denervation of the muscle (Patel and Swami, 1969), because the denervated muscle fibers become hyperirritable (denervation hypersensitivity).

B. *Percussion myoedema.* Sometimes muscle percussion causes a persistent tiny hump, myoedema, at the percussion site. The sarcoplasmic reticulum is slow in the reuptake of calcium (Layzer, 1985). Myoedema occurs in some normal people and often in debilitation or dysmetabolic states like uremia and myxedema.

C. *Percussion myotonia.* Place your hand on the table, palm up. Crisply percuss your thenar eminence with the point of your percussion hammer. Normally the thumb bounces up a little due to percussion irritability, but if your thumb slowly rises up from your palm and holds up, you have got problems. You have *percussion myotonia.*

D. *Muscle contraction myotonia.* To demonstrate myotonia in another way, ask the Pt to make a tight fist, hold it for 10 seconds, and flip the fingers open as quickly as possible on command. The myotonic Pt cannot flip the fingers open rapidly, and the wrist involuntarily flexes because of sustained "after contraction" or delayed relaxation of the flexors. Myotonia also affects the ocular muscles (Dyken, 1966). Myotonia occurs in myopathies, mainly myotonia dystrophica (Harper, 1989) and myotonia congenita, and also in paramyotonia congenita and some types of periodic muscular paralysis associated with a disturbance in potassium metabolism (Brooke, 1986; Engel and Banker, 1986; Walton, 1988).

E. *Summary of muscle responses to percussion*
   1. List the three muscular responses to direct percussion: percussion _____, percussion _____, and percussion _____.

Ans: *Percussion irritability, percussion myoedema, and percussion myotonia.*

Irritability

   2. *Most* normal persons show percussion _____ of their muscles.

Myoedema

   3. *Some* normal persons show percussion _____.

Myotonia

   4. *No* normal persons show percussion _____. It indicates a primary disease of the muscle, hence a myopathy.
   5. Apart from the myotonic myopathies, percussion of most myopathic muscles, as in Duchenne's muscular dystrophy, after disease has impaired the contractile properties of muscle, demonstrates little or no contraction. Percussion irritability of muscle is *reduced* or *absent* in those myopathies which do not have myotonia but is *increased* after denervation.

REFERENCES FOR MUSCLE DISEASES (MYOPATHIES)

Brody IA, Rozear MP: Contraction response to muscle percussion: physiology and clinical significance. *Arch Neurol* 1970; 23:259–265.

Brooke MH: *A Clinician's View of Neuromuscular Diseases* (2d ed). Baltimore, Williams & Wilkins, 1986.

Dyken P: Extraocular myotonia in families with dystrophia myotonica. *Neurology* 1966; 16:738–740.

Engel AG, Banker BQ: *Myology.* New York, McGraw-Hill, 1986.

Harper PS: *Myotonic dystrophy* (vol. 21: *Major Problems in Neurology*). London, Saunders, 1989.

Layzer RB: *Neuromuscular Manifestations of Systemic Disease* (vol. 25: *Contemporary Neurology Series*). Philadelphia, F.A. Davis, 1985.

Patel A, Swami R: Muscle percussion and neostigmine test in the clinical evaluation of neuromuscular disorders, *N Engl J Med* 1969; 281:523–526.

Walton JN (ed): *Disorders of Voluntary Muscle* (5th ed). London, Churchill Livingstone, 1988.

V. Examination of muscle stretch reflexes

A. *Physiology of the muscle stretch reflexes (MSRs)*

1. Evolution has perfected muscle fibers for precisely one function: they are contractile engines. Whatever the stimulus—a nerve impulse, chemical agent, electricity, or mechanical deformation, such as by percussion—the fiber responds by contracting.

2. Stretch of the entire muscle demonstrates *reflex irritability* of muscle. The stretch-sensitive receptors for the MSRs are the *muscle spindles,* which consist of small bags of small muscle fibers (Lance and McLeod, 1981; Swash and Kennard, 1985). Think of the muscle spindles as "muscles within a muscle" (Fig. 7-4).

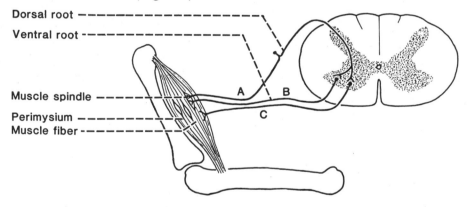

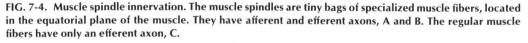

FIG. 7-4. Muscle spindle innervation. The muscle spindles are tiny bags of specialized muscle fibers, located in the equatorial plane of the muscle. They have afferent and efferent axons, A and B. The regular muscle fibers have only an efferent axon, C.

3. *Effects of stretch on the muscle spindles*

a. The muscle fibers of the spindle originate and insert into the perimysial connective tissue which ultimately is continuous with the tendons. If the joint in Fig. 7-4 *extends,* the tendon pulls on the perimysium and stretches the muscle spindles. Flexion of the joint causes relaxation of the muscle spindles.

b. In order for the muscle spindles to remain sensitive to stretch throughout the entire range of muscle length, they must readjust their length whenever the muscle length changes.

c. During *flexion* of the part, relaxing the tension, the muscle fibers of the spindles adjust to maintain their original tension by *contracting* slightly.

☑ *Relaxing*

     d. During *extension* of the part, the spindles adjust to maintain their original tension by ☐ relaxing/ ☐ contracting slightly.

  4. *Innervation of the muscle spindles*

     a. Each muscle spindle has its own *afferent* and *efferent* nerve supply to maintain its constant tension, depicted by axon A, afferent, and axon B, efferent, in Fig. 7-4. The regular muscle fibers, outside of the spindle have only *efferent* axons, depicted by C.

     b. In response to stretch, the spindles send an afferent volley into the neuraxis by axon A. In response to *slow* stretch, the spindles signal intermittently and asynchronously. The spindles quickly adapt to the new length and resume a baseline level of activity.

     c. If the stretch is *rapid,* essentially instantaneous, all spindles of the muscle, numbering hundreds, signal synchronously, sending a strong afferent volley into the neuraxis. The strong afferent volley stimulates the lower motor neurons (LMNs) to the regular muscle fibers. The resultant discharge of motor units causes a clinically evident muscular contraction, the *muscle stretch reflex (MSR).* The efferent axon is axon C, of Fig. 7-4.

☑ *Muscle spindles*
☑ *Regular muscle fibers*

     d. The event which initiates the MSR is stretch of the ☐ muscle spindles/ ☐ regular muscle fibers.

     e. The resultant twitch of the whole muscle is the result of contraction of the ☐ muscle spindles/ ☐ regular muscle fibers.

☑ *Reduced*

  5. When the MSR acts, the muscular contraction pulls the ends of the tendons closer together. The tension on the muscle spindles is momentarily ☐ reduced/ ☐ increased. Hence the spindles cease firing abruptly, and the MSR ends abruptly.

  6. When the muscle comes to rest at a new length, what adjustment takes place in the tension of the muscle spindles? _____.

Ans: They reset their tension to the baseline level.

  7. Explain why only a quick stretch elicits a MSR. _____

Ans: All spindles must fire rapidly and synchronously to discharge the LMNs. If the stretch is too slow, the spindles fire slowly and asynchronously, and they adapt to the new resting length without sending a sufficiently strong volley to discharge the LMNs.

Percussion

  8. Muscle fibers can be made to contract in response to stretch of the muscle membrane by direct percussion of the fiber. This phenomenon is called _____ irritability of the muscle.

Muscle spindles

  9. In contrast to percussion irritability, reflex irritability of muscle depends on a strong volley of afferent impulses initiated by the stretch of the specialized stretch receptors called _____.

  10. After interruption of all efferent axons to a muscle which would be lost, percussion irritability or the MSRs? Explain: _____.

Ans: Denervation of a muscle abolishes the MSRs, which depend on the integrity of the reflex arc (Fig. 7-4). Percussion irritability depends on the intrinsic property of muscle fibers. It is retained or even enhanced after denervation (Cannon's law of hypersensitivity of denervated end organs).

  11. Because of percussion irritability, the Ex percusses tendons, not the muscles directly. Direct percussion of the muscle not only causes direct contraction of the muscle fibers but also stretches spindles. The muscle twitches in either case, but clinically, the Ex cannot distinguish the cause.

The tap on the tendon can only elicit contraction by stretching the muscle spindles.

REFERENCES FOR PHYSIOLOGY OF MUSCLE STRETCH REFLEXES

Lance JW, McLeod JG: *A Physiological Approach to Clinical Neurology* (3d ed). London, Butterworths, 1981.

Swash M, Kennard C: *Scientific Basis of Clinical Neurology*. Edinburgh, Churchill-Livingstone, 1985.

B. *Technique for eliciting MSRs*
   1. *Holding the percussion hammer and delivering the blow*
      a. A percussion hammer permits you to strike a rapid blow, producing the instantaneous stretch of the numerous muscle spindles necessary to elicit a MSR. To deliver a crisp stimulus, you must learn to become a hammer *swinger,* not a hammer *pecker.* The same technique applies whether you use the Taylor tomahawk hammer pictured in this text or the round-tipped Tromner hammer.
      b. *Hammer pecking:* the wrong way to elicit the MSRs. Consider first the *wrong* technique, *hammer pecking.* The novice grips the hammer tightly with all of the fingers, and pecks at the target, using no wrist action. Recall how a baby holds a rattle tightly in its fist and bangs or pecks, using all arm action and no wrist action. Grip the handle of your reflex hammer tightly and peck the table top in this incorrect manner. (Go ahead, do it. Learn what is wrong so that you will know what is right.)
      c. *Hammer swinging:* the right way to elicit the MSRs. Pick up the hammer handle loosely, dangling it between the thumb and forefinger. The other fingers are free, like a lady holding a teacup. With a loose, floppy wrist, dangle the hammer, allowing it to swing like a pendulum. Think of the hammer handle as a bird: hold it too tightly and you crush it to death; hold it too loosely and it flies away. Fig. 7-5 shows how a loose wrist and loose finger grip permits a double whiplash effect, imparting the maximal terminal velocity to the hammer head by literally throwing it without actually releasing it.
      d. Simultaneous extension of the elbow added to the wrist swing adds further velocity to the tip of the hammer, delivering the crisp blow that instantaneously and simultaneously stretches all spindles to successfully elicit the MSR.
      e. Practice by holding your wrist a foot above a hard table top. Starting with the handle of the hammer laying back across the web between your thumb and forefinger (Fig. 7-5), whiplash the hammer head against the table top. *If the velocity of the hammer head is great enough and the wrist and grip loose enough, the hammer head bounces all of the way back up and falls backward across the crevice between your thumb and forefinger, thus returning to the starting position in Fig. 7-5.* Practice, practice, practice until you can get this limp-wristed, whiplash feeling of literally throwing or swinging the hammer tip, but without actually releasing the handle. As a hammer swinger, you will proudly elicit MSRs when your tight-fisted colleagues, with their incorrect hammer-pecking style, fail.
   2. *Eliciting the MSRs in the neurologic examination*
      a. Generally the Pt is sitting or reclining. The Pt places the part to be tested

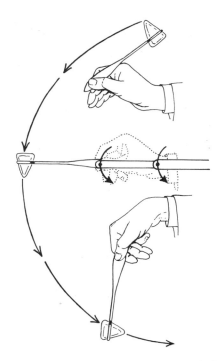

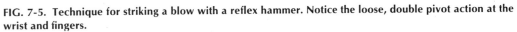

FIG. 7-5. Technique for striking a blow with a reflex hammer. Notice the loose, double pivot action at the wrist and fingers.

at rest, with the muscles relaxed. Usually the best position is intermediate between full extension and full flexion.

b. Work through Figs. 7-6 to 7-18, testing the reflexes on yourself where possible, and on a partner. Do the reflexes in pairs, directly comparing right and left sides. In testing the knee jerks (quadriceps reflex), the Pt should be sitting, with the legs dangling over the edge of a table. The Ex can then observe the degree of *pendulousness,* which usually amounts to 2 to 3 afterswings before the leg stops swinging.

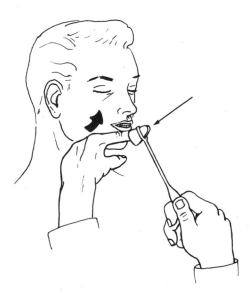

FIG. 7-6. *Jaw reflex.* With the Pt's jaw sagging loosely open, the Ex rests a finger across the jaw and strikes it a crisp blow. In Figs. 7-6 to 7-18, the *thin* arrow shows the direction of the percussion hammer *blow,* the thick arrow shows the response.

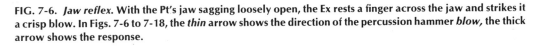

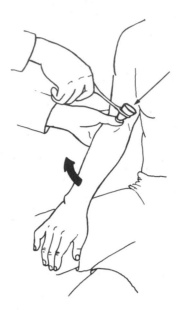

FIG. 7-7. *Biceps reflex.* The Ex's thumb places slight tension on the Pt's biceps tendon. The Ex strikes his thumbnail a sharp blow.

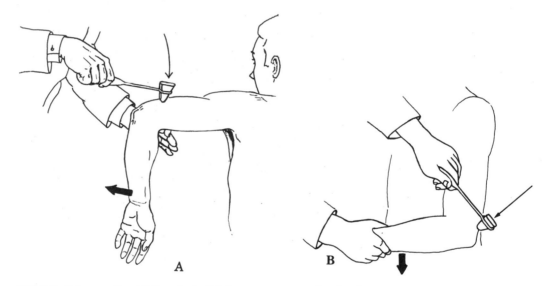

FIG. 7-8. *Triceps reflex.* (*A*) Dangle the Pt's forearm over your hand and strike the triceps tendon. (*B*) Cradle the Pt's forearm in your hand and strike the triceps tendon.

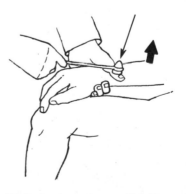

FIG. 7-9. *Brachioradialis reflex.* Cradle the Pt's forearm in one hand, placing the thumb on top of the radius. The hammer strikes the Ex's thumbnail rather than the Pt's radius. Don't whack away on the Pt's unprotected bone. Both forearms may be cradled simultaneously to compare more accurately the responses of the two arms.

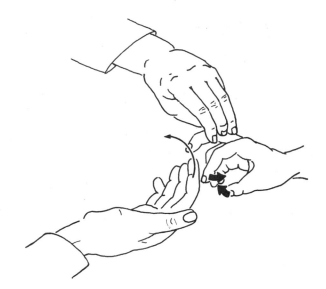

FIG. 7-10. *Finger flexion reflex* (Tromner's method). The Ex supports the Pt's completely relaxed hand and briskly flips the Pt's distal phalanx upward, as though trying to flip a handful of water high into the air. The Pt's fingers and thumb flex in response to the stretch of the finger flexor muscles.

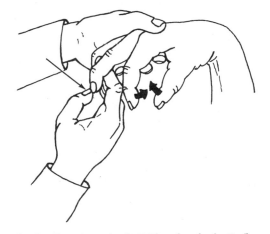

FIG. 7-11. *Finger flexion reflex* (Hoffman's method). With a thumb, the Ex flexes the distal phalanx of the Pt's finger, while pressing up with the index finger. Then the Ex releases the phalanx abruptly, allowing it to flip up sharply. The abrupt release and resultant extension of the phalanx stretches the flexor muscles, causing the fingers and thumb to flex. The Pt's MSRs must be very brisk for this method to work.

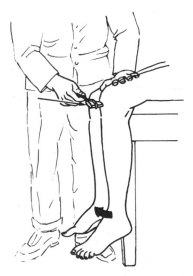

FIG. 7-12. *Quadriceps femoris reflex,* Pt sitting. The Ex strikes the patellar tendon a crisp blow. By placing a hand on the patients knee, the Ex feels, as well as sees, the magnitude of the response.

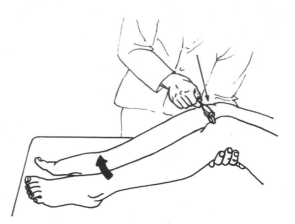

FIG. 7-13. *Quadriceps femoris reflex,* Pt supine. The Ex bends the Pt's legs to place slight tension on the patellar tendon. The blow then will deform the tendon and transmit a stretch to the muscle.

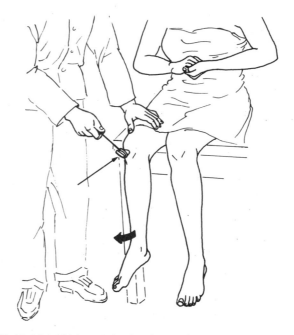

FIG. 7-14. *Pull method* (of Jendrassik) for reinforcing the quadriceps reflex. The Pt locks the hands and pulls apart hard while the Ex strikes the tendon.

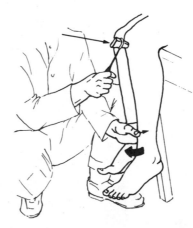

FIG. 7-15. *Counterpressure method* for reinforcing the quadriceps reflex. The Ex applies slight thumb pressure (small arrow) against the Pt's tibia. The Pt counteracts the thumb pressure by slight tension in the quadriceps femoris muscle. Then the Ex strikes the quadriceps tendon.

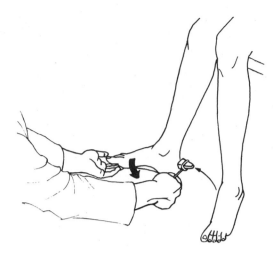

FIG. 7-16. *Triceps surae reflex,* Pt sitting. The Pt completely relaxes the leg. The Ex places slight tension on the Achilles tendon by dorsiflexing the foot. Try reinforcement if no reflex occurs.

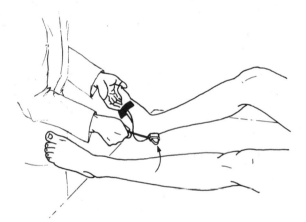

FIG. 7-17. *Triceps surae reflex,* Pt supine. With the Pt's knee bent and relaxed, the Ex dorsiflexes the Pt's foot to control the tension on the triceps surae muscle. Try reinforcement if no reflex occurs.

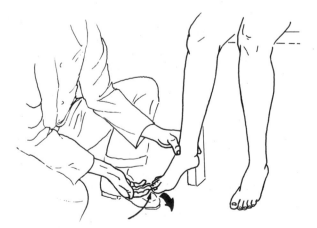

FIG. 7-18. *Toe flexion* reflex (Rossolimo's method). The maneuver is identical with the finger flexion method, Fig. 7-10.

    C. What to do if you get no response in your first attempts to elicit a MSR

      1. *Strike a crisper blow.* Make sure you have *swung* the hammer, not pecked with it. Pecking is the commonest error.

      2. *Change the mechanical tension on the muscle*

        a. Flex or extend the joint somewhat to alter the tension on the tendon.

        b. Compress the tendon slightly more, or slightly less, with your thumb (Fig. 7-7).

      3. *Try reinforcement*

        a. The Jendrassik maneuver for reinforcing a MSR. Slight innervation of the muscle under test increases the excitability of the LMNs for the MSR. For this purpose have the Pt make a strong voluntary contraction of a muscle you are *not* testing. Thus, failing to get a quadriceps femoris reflex after several trials, ask the Pt to lock the fingers together and pull hard as you tap the quadriceps tendon (Fig. 7-14). In this maneuver, the *Jendrassik maneuver,* the voluntary UMN innervation of the arm muscles "overflows" to increase the excitability of the LMN pool of the lower extremities (Gasser and Diamantopolous, 1964; Hagbarth et al, 1975; Lance and McLeod, 1981; Stam et al, 1989).

        b. The counterpressure method of reinforcement. If the Jendrassik maneuver fails, ask the Pt to tense very slightly the muscle being tested. Ask the Pt to just counterbalance the slight pressure you apply against the action of the muscle, as shown in Fig. 7-15. Too much tension in the muscle prevents the stretch stimulus from being effective.

      4. *Absence of the muscle stretch reflexes.* If all maneuvers fail, conclude that the MSRs are absent, which usually indicates a pathologic condition, with some exceptions, such as the finger and toe flexion reflexes. In infants or girls, whose tendons are not prominent, it may be difficult to elicit some MSRs, such as the biceps. Lack of patellar development in infants makes it mechanically difficult to stretch the tendon of the quadriceps femoris muscle by tapping its tendon. Position the infant's leg nearly straight, with the infant recumbent, and then tap the tendon.

    D. Analyze this clinical problem in eliciting MSRs.

      1. You wish to elicit the biceps reflex of a 38-year-old conscious woman. She is seated. Her arm should be positioned ＿＿＿＿＿＿＿＿＿＿＿＿＿＿＿＿＿＿＿＿＿＿＿.

Ans: Partially bent across her thigh (Fig. 7-7).

      2. Although you have struck a crisp blow, you got no MSR. List the maneuvers you must try before concluding that the patient has no biceps MSR.

＿＿＿＿＿＿＿＿＿＿＿＿＿＿＿＿＿＿＿＿＿＿＿＿＿＿＿＿＿＿＿＿＿＿＿.

Ans: Place more or less thumb pressure on the tendon. Reposition the elbow at a slightly different angle. Ask her to "tense" her leg muscles (extend her legs) for reinforcement. (The counterpressure method of reinforcement is inconvenient for arm reflexes.)

      3. In the same Pt, you are unable to elicit the quadriceps and triceps surae MSRs when the Pt is sitting. What maneuvers do you try before concluding she has no quadriceps MSR? ＿＿＿＿＿＿＿＿＿＿＿＿＿＿＿＿＿

＿＿＿＿＿＿＿＿＿＿＿＿＿＿＿＿＿＿＿＿＿＿＿＿＿＿＿＿＿＿＿＿＿＿＿.

Ans: Above all, strike the tendon a crisp blow. Next, request the Pt to lock her hands and pull as you strike the quadriceps tendon; then, ask the Pt to counterbalance the slight pressure you apply against the tibia. These are examples of the pull (Jendrassik maneuver) and counterpressure methods of reinforcement.

4. For the triceps surae MSR use the Jendrassik maneuver and then the counterpressure maneuver by having the Pt slightly plantar flex the foot as you press up on the sole with your finger, while tapping the Achilles tendon with the other hand. If these maneuvers fail to elicit quadriceps or triceps surae MSRs, place her supine and try different positions of flexion of her legs.

E. *Nomenclature of the MSRs*
1. Name the MSRs according to the muscles which respond or to the part which moves, e.g., the quadriceps MSR or the knee jerk (Fig. 7-12), or the triceps surae MSR or ankle jerk.
2. The fact that the MSR was elicited by tendon percussion led to the archaic, misleading name of "deep tendon reflexes" for the MSRs. This name implies that the receptor for the reflex is in the tendons. In fact, the tendon receptors *inhibit* the MSR. Sir William Gowers (1845–1915) stated in 1885:

> It seems, therefore, most desirable to discard the term "tendon reflex" altogether. The phenomena are, according to the explanation above given, dependent on a "muscle reflex" irritability, which has nothing to do with the tendons. If we wish to describe them by a general term, it will be best to employ "tendon-muscular phenomena," but the intervention of tendons is not necessary for their production; the one condition which all have in common is that passive tension is essential for their occurrence, and they may more conveniently be termed myotatic contractions (myo = muscle; teinein = to stretch). The irritability, on which they depend, is due to and demonstrative of a muscle reflex action which depends on the spinal cord.

3. Gowers synthesized a complex body of knowledge into a single word, *myotatic.* But his plea for rational, informative terminology has fallen unheeded. Each class of medical students is taught the "deep tendon reflexes" and almost universally fails to understand the spindle mechanism and the adequate stimulus required to elicit the MSRs.

F. *Recording the MSRs by using a stick figure*
1. Grade the MSRs on a scale of 1 to 4+, with 0 for *areflexia,* 1 for *hyporeflexia,* 2 and 3 for normal, and 4 or 4+ for hyperreflexia (Table 7-2).
2. Because of the wide range in normal persons, the absolute value assigned to the MSR is less important than asymmetry, or a discrepancy between one part of the body and another. A stick figure displays the MSRs, and as shown later, other reflexes for interpretation at a glance. Notice in Fig. 7-19*A*, a normal subject, that the finger and toe flexion MSRs (Figs. 7-10, 7-11, and 7-18) may not be obtainable.

⊥
   a. Describe the reflex pattern in Fig. 7-19*B*: _____

Ans: Hyperreflexia on the left.

TABLE 7-2 Grading of MSRs	
0	Areflexia
±	Hyporeflexia
1 to 3	Average
3+ to 4+	Hyperreflexia

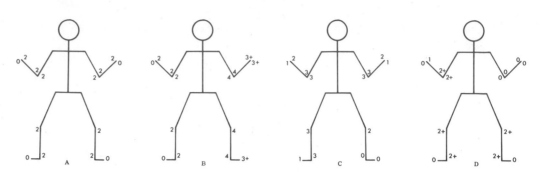

FIG. 7-19. Stick figure method of recording muscle stretch reflexes (MSRs).

⊥   *b.* Describe Fig. 7-19*C*: _____

Ans: Quadriceps hyporeflexia, triceps surae, and toe areflexia on the left.

⊥   *c.* Fig. 7-19*D*: _____

Ans: Areflexia left arm.

REFERENCES FOR CLINICAL EXAMINATION OF MUSCLE STRETCH REFLEXES

Gasser M, Diamantopoulos E: The Jendrassik maneuver. I. The pattern of reinforcement of monosynaptic reflexes in normal subjects and patients with spasticity or rigidity. *Neurology,* 1964; 14:555–560

Gowers W: *Diagnosis of Diseases of the Brain and of the Spinal Cord.* New York, William Wood, 1885

Hagbarth K-E, Wallin G, Burke D, Lofstedt L: Effects of the Jendrassik manoeuvre on muscle spindle activity in man. *J Neurol Neurosurg Psychiatry,* 1975; 38:1143–1153

Lance JW, McLeod JG: *A Physiological Approach to Clinical Neurology* (3d ed). London, Butterworths, 1981

Lanska DJ, Lanska MJ: John Madison Taylor (1855–1931) and the first reflex hammer. *J Child Neurol,* 1990; 5:38–39

Stam J, Speelman HD, van Crevel H: Tendon reflex asymmetry by voluntary mental effort in healthy subjects. *Arch Neurol,* 1989; 46:70–73

Wartenberg R: *The Examination of Reflexes.* Chicago, Year Book Medical Publishers, 1945

VI. Clinical and electromyographic signs accompanying areflexia and hyporeflexia after interruption of the reflex arc

A. *Areflexia and the reflex arc.* Areflexia is pathologic, excepting in toe and finger MSRs, and in some particular muscles in infants and females whose tendons are not strongly developed. Some persons with generalized hyporeflexia (or hyperreflexia) merely fall at one end of the normal range. *If that is the case, the muscles will be normal in size and strength and sensation will be normal.* In deciphering the cause of areflexia or hyporeflexia, you must *think through* the afferent and efferent limbs of the reflex arc (Fig. 7-20).

1. To think through a reflex arc, start with the stimulus and the receptor. The adequate stimulus is sudden stretch of the muscle. If you get no response, then ask this question: Was the stimulus adequate? Outline the clinical maneuvers to elicit a reflex when your first attempt fails. _____

_____

_____

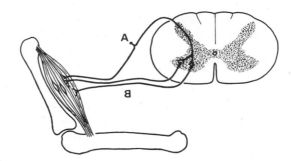

FIG. 7-20. Simplified diagram of the arc for the muscle stretch reflex. This reflex can be regarded as a closed ring, the muscle being both receptor and effector.

Ans: Deliver a crisper blow, alter tendon tension by finger pressure or repositioning the part, and try reinforcement.

☑ *Strongly*

☑ *Weakly*

2. The two methods of reinforcement are
   a. To have the Pt contract ☐ strongly/ ☐ weakly a set of muscle *not* being tested.
   b. To have the patient contract ☐ strongly/ ☐ weakly the muscle being tested.

3. Having applied the stimulus for the MSR properly, the next step in thinking through the reflex arc is to consider the integrity of the muscle spindles and afferent limb. We cannot directly check the integrity of the muscle spindle clinically, but we can test the afferent limb as a whole.
   a. Interruption of the nerve or dorsal root conveying spindle afferents would also interrupt other sensory afferents. Hence, areflexia from interruption of the afferent arc would also cause loss of sensation.
   b. Would interruption of the sensory afferents from the muscle cause paralysis? ☐ Yes/ ☐ No. Explain: _____

Ans: ☑ No. As long as upper motor neuron (UMN) and LMN pathways to the regular muscle fibers are intact, movement is possible. In tabes dorsalis, for example, the axons of the dorsal roots selectively degenerate. Since the afferent axons from the muscle spindles are lost, the Pt has areflexia and sensory ataxia but can move.

4. Knowing that the stimulus is proper and the *afferent* arc is intact, consider next the LMN and the *efferent* side of the arc. (We do not consider the synapses of the afferent axon on the LMNs because we do not know how to evaluate them clinically). The term *LMN* includes both the cell *body* of the neuron and its axon. Many diseases attack the bodies of LMNs. Poliomyelitis, one of the most specific, destroys LMNs, with less effect on the dorsal horns or afferent fibers. A poliomyelitis Pt loses MSRs because of destruction of the efferent arc, but the Pt retains sensation.

5. After the LMN cell body, the next level to consider is the ventral root and *efferent axon.* The efferent axon may be interrupted by mechanical lesions such as cuts or compression. Many toxic-metabolic disorders, such as lead poisoning, may predominantly affect efferent axons, causing a *motor neuropathy.* Other toxins, such as arsenic, regularly affect both afferent and efferent axons, causing a *sensorimotor neuropathy.* Irrespective of cause, irrespective of involvement of the afferent system, a lesion of the LMN cell body or axons has essentially the same effect on the muscle: weakness, atrophy, and loss of MSRs.

6. Consider next in the efferent arc the *neuromyal junction.*
   a. Two diseases of the neuromyal junction, causing defective impulse transmission, are *myasthenia gravis* and *botulinum infection.*
   b. Myasthenia is a disease of fluctuating intensity. Complete areflexia is unusual.
7. The final level of the reflex arc is the *effector,* the *muscle.* Many *myopathies,* including the muscular dystrophies and myositides, may cause areflexia. The afferent and efferent limbs of the reflex arc are preserved, but the diseased muscle cannot respond.
8. List the clinically significant stations in a reflex arc, beginning with the stimulus: _____
   _____
   _____

Ans: Receptor, afferent axons, LMN (including efferent axon), neuromyal junction, and effector.

B. *Effects of neuromuscular disease on muscle size*
   1. *Use hypertrophy and disuse atrophy of normal muscle*
      a. The size of normal muscle depends on *use.* If used, a muscle undergoes *use* hypertrophy: witness weightlifters. If not used, muscle undergoes *disuse atrophy.* For example, the muscles of a limb immobilized in a cast begin to undergo disuse atrophy within 24 hours. After removal of the cast, the muscles resume their work, undergo *use hypertrophy,* and regain their normal size.
      b. UMN lesions that result in paresis or paralysis reduce muscle use. Therefore the muscles undergo some degree of disuse atrophy, but the atrophy is slight in relation to the effect of LMN lesions or myopathies.
      c. If deprived of axons by LMN lesions, muscle fibers undergo *denervation* atrophy, a severe atrophy ending in death of the muscle fibers, unless reinnervation occurs.

Disuse
Denervation

      d. A normal muscle put at rest for prolonged periods of time undergoes _____ atrophy, whereas a muscle deprived of its nerve supply undergoes _____ atrophy.
   2. Myopathies, primary diseases of muscle, may also result in death of muscle fibers. This atrophy is called *myopathic* atrophy. List the three types of muscular atrophy:

Disuse
Denervation
Myopathic

      a. From prolonged inactivity, _____ atrophy.
      b. From LMN lesions, _____ atrophy.
      c. From primary diseases of muscle, _____ atrophy.
      d. In some myopathies, notably Duchenne's muscular dystrophy, some muscles go through a stage of *pseudo*hypertrophy, appearing larger for the first years and then later undergoing atrophy.
   3. *Differentation of aplasia, hypoplasia, and atrophy*
      a. *Aplasia* (amyoplasia) means that the muscle failed to develop at all. *Hypoplasia* means that the muscle has failed to develop to its normal size.
      b. *Atrophy* of whatever type (disuse, denervation, or myopathic) means that the muscle once had a normal size and then lost its bulk.
      c. These various terms enable the Ex to designate the mechanism of the reduction in muscle bulk.
   4. *Circumferential measurement of the extremities.* If the history or examination suggest a disorder that could affect muscle size, measure the greatest circumference of the part for documentation in the chart and to compare the right and left sides.

C. *Neuromuscular disease, motor units, and electromyography*

1. *Definition of a motor unit.* A *motor unit* is one LMN, its axon, and all of the muscle fibers it innervates.

   a. Each efferent axon from a motoneuron may innervate one or more muscle fibers. In some small muscles, such as the extraocular, each motor axon is thought to innervate only one muscle fiber. In large muscles, such as the gluteus maximus or quadriceps femoris, each motor axon may innervate hundreds of muscle fibers. Learn Fig. 7-21.

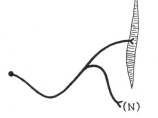

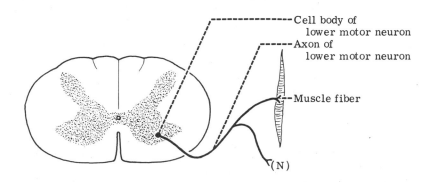

FIG. 7-21. **Cross section of spinal cord and motor unit. The motor unit consists of a motoneuron body, its axon, and all of the muscle fibers innervated by the axon. *N* varies from zero to hundreds of additional muscle fibers. The larger muscles have larger values of *N*. Encircle the portion of Fig. 7-21 which defines the motor unit and compare with the drawing in the answer colunn.**

✓ *All*

   b. If a normal LMN discharges a nerve impulse, ☐ some/ ☐ all/ ☐ none of the muscle fibers of the motor unit would be expected to contract.

2. *Motor units and fasciculations*

   a. The muscle fibers of the motor units are grouped together in a *fascicle* (fasciculus) of the muscle. If a single motor unit fires, the Ex can see the contraction of the fascicle of muscle fibers as a small ripple or twitch under the Pt's skin. Such a twitch is a *fasciculation.* You have all probably experienced twitching of an eyelid: that is a fasciculation. The Ex can see fasciculations, and the Pt can see and feel them.

   b. Define a motor unit. _____

Ans: A LMN, its axon, and all of the muscle fibers it innervates.

   c. If a single motor unit discharges what would the Ex see and what is the technical name for it? _____.

Ans: A small muscular twitch called a fasciculation.

3. *Electromyography (EMG)*

   a. Normally, motor units discharge only when stimulated by UMNs or other afferents. A needle inserted into a normal *resting* muscle and wired to an amplifier and oscilloscope records no electrical activity. When the motor units discharge, the oscilloscope screen displays numerous electrical potentials caused by depolarization of muscle fibers. The recording of the electrical activity from muscle is called *electromyography (EMG).* See Fig. 7-22.

   b. The surface membrane of a diseased LMN becomes unstable. The neuron then discharges spontaneous, random impulses, rather than discharging only in response to appropriate stimuli. All of the muscle fibers connected to the axon of the motoneuron contract, resulting in spontaneous fasciculations (Fig. 7-22*B*). Some normal individuals, who do not have neuronal disease, show *benign fasciculations,* particularly after exercise.

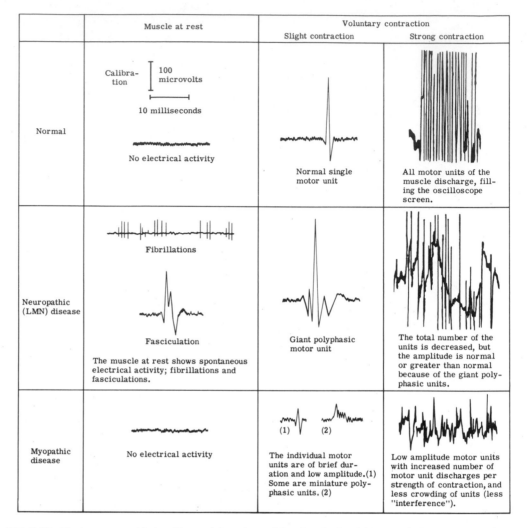

	Muscle at rest	Voluntary contraction	
		Slight contraction	Strong contraction
Normal	Calibration — 100 microvolts 10 milliseconds No electrical activity	Normal single motor unit	All motor units of the muscle discharge, filling the oscilloscope screen.
Neuropathic (LMN) disease	Fibrillations Fasciculation The muscle at rest shows spontaneous electrical activity; fibrillations and fasciculations.	Giant polyphasic motor unit	The total number of the units is decreased, but the amplitude is normal or greater than normal because of the giant polyphasic units.
Myopathic disease	No electrical activity	(1) (2) The individual motor units are of brief duration and low amplitude.(1) Some are miniature polyphasic units. (2)	Low amplitude motor units with increased number of motor unit discharges per strength of contraction, and less crowding of units (less "interference").

FIG. 7-22. **Electromyographic (oscilloscopic) tracings of the electrical activity recorded from muscle.** *(Courtesy of Dr. Mark Dyken.)*

4. *Wallerian degeneration and the electromyography of denervation*
   a. If the neuronal perikaryon dies its axon dies. The axon also dies if it is completely severed from its perikaryon. The process of dissolution of the dead axon and its myelin sheath is called *wallerian* degeneration (Augustus Waller, 1816–1870). See Fig. 7-23.
   b. After axonal severance and wallerian degeneration the denervated muscle fibers will not contract in response to volition, afferent stimuli, or

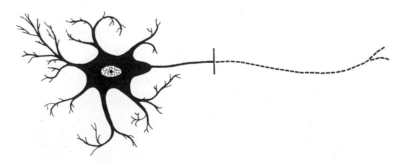

FIG. 7-23. **Neuron and axon to show wallerian (anterograde) degeneration of the distal, severed part of the axon that has lost contact with the metabolic machinery in the perikaryon.**

direct electrical stimulation of the peripheral nerve trunk. The Ex can still elicit a twitch of the denervated muscle fibers by direct percussion.

5. *Fibrillations*

   a. *Definition.* A *fibrillation* is a random, spontaneous contraction of an individual denervated muscle fiber. After denervation by wallerian degeneration of the motor axon, the muscle fiber undergoes a period of hyperexcitability (*Cannon's law of hypersensitity of denervated structures;* Walter Cannon, 1871–1945). It is as if the muscle fibers attempt to compensate for the lack of nerve impulses by making themselves easier to discharge. Thus, the membrane of the individual muscle fiber depolarizes spontaneously and the fiber contracts. The Ex cannot see fibrillations but an oscilloscope records them (Fig. 7-22).

   b. Spontaneous depolarization of the membranes of diseased LMNs causes visible muscular twitches called _____, whereas spontaneous depolarization of individual denervated muscle fibers causes _____.

Fasciculations

Fibrillations
Fasciculations

Fibrillations

   c. The Ex can see the motor unit twitches called _____, while the oscilloscope is required to "see" the individual muscle fiber contractions called _____.

6. After the death of LMNs, fasciculations cease. They occur only during the period when the neurons are abnormal, but the axons remain intact. Fibrillations begin about 3 weeks after denervation and continue for as long as the denervated muscle fibers remain alive, until the final stage of denervation atrophy, in which the muscle fibers die and disappear.

7. Define fasciculations and fibrillations. Include the operations by which they are detected and their pathophysiology. _____
_____
_____
_____
_____

Ans: Fasciculations are contractions of muscle fascicles, detected by clinical inspection or by characteristic EMG waves. They indicate a hyperexcitable state of the cell membrane of the LMNs, which depolarizes spontaneously, causing contraction of all muscle fibers of the motor unit. Fibrillations are spontaneous contractions of individual denervated muscle fibers, detected by characteristic EMG waves. They indicate a state of hyperexcitability of the muscle fibers following denervation.

8. *Giant polyphasic motor units* are another electromyographic sign of denervation (Fig. 7-22). These giant EMG waves are of greater amplitude and of more complex form than normal motor unit discharges. The denervated muscle fibers induce sprouting of new axonal terminals from a remaining intact axons. When that axon fires it activates not only its original number of muscle fibers but also the newly innervated adjacent muscle fibers. The larger number of muscle fibers firing causes the polyphasic potentials recorded by the EMG.

D. *Summary of the clinical and electromyographic syndrome of LMN lesions*

   1. The *clinical* syndrome of LMN lesions is *paresis* or *paralysis, atrophy,* and *areflexia* of the affected muscles.

   2. The *electromyographic* syndrome of LMN lesions is spontaneous individual motor unit discharges called _____, spontaneous contractions of individual muscle fibers called _____, and the appearance of giant _____.

Fasciculations
Fibrillations
Polyphasic motor units

E. *Differentiation of lesions at various sites in the reflex arc*

☑ *LMN lesions;*
  ☑ *myopathies*
☑ *LMN lesions*

1. Paresis or paralysis would accompany which one or more of the following? ☐ dorsal root lesions/ ☐ LMN lesions/ ☐ myopathies.
2. Denervation atrophy occurs with which one or more of the following? ☐ dorsal root lesions/ ☐ LMN lesions/ ☐ myopathies.

☑ *Dorsal root lesions*

3. Loss of sensation occurs with which one or more of the following? ☐ dorsal root lesions/ ☐ LMN lesions/ ☐ myopathies.

All three

4. Absence of MSRs occurs with which one or more of the following? ☐ dorsal root lesions/ ☐ LMN lesions/ ☐ myopathies.
5. Complete Table 7-3 to differentiate the various neuromuscular syndromes associated with lesions of the reflex arc. Notice that hypotonia (loose floppy limbs), occurs with lesions at any level of the reflex arc.

F. *Consider this Pt*

Three weeks before hospitalization a 52-year-old man became violently ill with nausea, vomiting, and bloody diarrhea. The gastrointestinal symptoms receded, but four days before admission, he began to have severe pain in his extremities and some leg weakness. Examination showed intact cranial nerves. He had slight paresis of his hand muscles and severe leg weakness, most pronounced distally. He was hyporeflexic in the arms, areflexic in the lower extremities. He had difficulty distinguishing pinprick and light touch over his hands, and his feet were almost anesthetic. He had no muscular atrophy on admission, but it became evident in 10 days. An EMG on admission disclosed no spontaneous activity indicative of fasciculations or fibrillations. A second EMG, done 3 weeks after hospitalization, disclosed fasciculations and numerous fibrillations in the muscles which were clinically weak and areflexic.

☑ *A combined*
  sensorimotor

1. This Pt had ☐ only a motor/ ☐ only a sensory/ ☐ a combined sensorimotor neuropathy.
2. From the history and examination the evidence for sensory neuropathy was: (Review the case protocol to sift out the answers.)

_____

_____

Ans: Symptoms of severe pain, distal sensory loss, and areflexia.

	Clinical signs	Probable diagnosis		
		Dorsal root lesion	LMN lesion	Myopathy
☑ *1*	Areflexia, hypotonia, loss of sensation. No atrophy, weakness, or EMG abnormalities.	☐ 1	☐ 2	☐ 3
☑ *2*	Weakness, areflexia, atrophy, hypotonia, fasciculations, and fibrillations. No sensory loss.	☐ 1	☐ 2	☐ 3
☑ *3*	Weakness, areflexia, atrophy, hypotonia. No sensory loss, fasciculations, or fibrillations.	☐ 1	☐ 2	☐ 3
☑ *3* *(myotonia dystrophica)*	Weakness, hyporeflexia, atrophy, hypotonia, percussion myotonia. No sensory loss, fasciculations, or fibrillations.	☐ 1	☐ 2	☐ 3
☑ *1* ☑ *2* *(sensorimotor neuropathy)*	Weakness, areflexia, atrophy, hypotonia, loss of sensation, fasciculations, and fibrillations.	☐ 1	☐ 2	☐ 3

TABLE 7-3 Clinical signs and probable diagnosis of lesions at the level of the reflex arc

TABLE 7-4 Time of onset of neurologic signs in acute motor neuropathies			
	Relatively early	Intermediate	Late
Paresis, paralysis, and areflexia	☐	☐	☐
Atrophy	☐	☐	☐
Fibrillations and fasciculations	☐	☐	☐

☑ *Early*

☑ *Intermediate*

☑ *Late*

3. The evidence for motor neuropathy was: _____
_____
_____ .

Ans: Initially, weakness and areflexia; later on, atrophy, fasciculations, and
   fibrillations.

4. The sensorimotor neuropathy preceded by a severe gastrointestinal disturbance suggested poisoning. There is often a lag between toxic exposure and
onset of a neuropathy. Chemical tests of the Pt's urine for lead, mercury,
and arsenic showed high arsenic levels. Questioning disclosed domestic
strife. The Pt's wife admitted giving him rat poison. The Pt was treated with
dimercaprol and made a satisfactory, but incomplete, recovery.
5. The onset of fasciculations and fibrillations about 3 weeks after the first
signs of LMN disease indicates the approximate time required for these
signs of denervation to appear. The full syndrome of LMN lesions takes
time to develop. Even after cutting a nerve with a knife, fibrillations usually
do not appear for 3 weeks or more. Some signs are early and persist for the
duration of the disease. Other signs appear later. Check the order that the
LMN signs appeared in this Pt to review the usual time sequence that they
occur in LMN disease in general (Table 7-4).
6. Would a Pt whose areflexia was caused by a lesion confined to the afferent
arc show muscular atrophy, fasciculations, and fibrillations? ☐ Yes/
☐ No. Explain: _____
_____
_____ .

Ans: ☑ No. Atrophy, fasciculations, and fibrillations indicate interruption of
   the efferent arc, a lesion of the LMN.

REFERENCES FOR ARSENIC POLYNEUROPATHY

Goebel HH, Schmidt PF, Bohl J et al: Polyneuropathy due to acute arsenic intoxication: biopsy studies. *J Neuropathol Exp Neurol,* 1990; 49:137–149.

VII. Clinical analysis of hyperactive muscle strength reflexes (MSRs) and clonus

A. *Causes of hyperreflexia*
   1. Hyperreflexia has many causes. Figure 7-24 illustrates yet again how each
   sign generates many diagnostic possibilities.
   2. To analyze any finding, always ask first, "Is it merely a normal variation?"
   Very brisk MSRs may still fall within the wide range of normal variation.

HYPERREFLEXIA

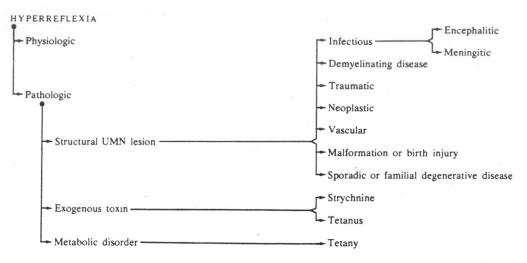

- Physiologic

- Pathologic

  - Structural UMN lesion ——————————————

    - Infectious ——————
      - Encephalitic
      - Meningitic
    - Demyelinating disease
    - Traumatic
    - Neoplastic
    - Vascular
    - Malformation or birth injury
    - Sporadic or familial degenerative disease

  - Exogenous toxin ——————————————
    - Strychnine
    - Tetanus

  - Metabolic disorder ——————————————— Tetany

FIG. 7-24. **Some common causes of hyperreflexia (reference only).**

The commonest cause of pathologic hyperreflexia is interruption of UMN pathways between cerebrum and LMNs. When UMN lesions cause increased MSRs on one side, the Ex should also find weakness on that side, thus a hemiparesis. The syndrome or pattern of signs, integrated with the history, produces the diagnosis.

B. *Clonus*

1. *Definition.* Clonus is a to-and-fro, rhythmic oscillation of a body part, elicited by a quick stretch. Clonus is yet another way to demonstrate hyperactive MSRs.

2. *Technique for eliciting clonus*

   a. Induce the Pt to relax completely. To elicit ankle clonus, flex the Pt's knee slightly to relax the triceps surae muscle.

   b. With your hand on the Pt's sole, briskly jerk the Pt's foot up and slightly outward. After the upward jerk, maintain finger pressure against the sole of the Pt's foot. The foot oscillates between flexion and extension for as long as the Ex maintains pressure (Fig. 7-25).

3. *The mechanism of clonus*

   a. The quick dorsiflexion of the Pt's foot stretches the triceps surae (Fig. 7-26*A*, thin arrow). The triceps surae responds with a single MSR, causing the foot to plantar flex (Fig. 7-26*B*, thick arrow).

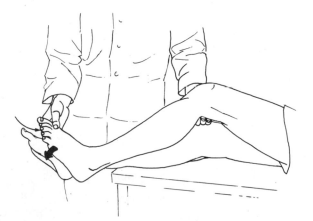

FIG. 7-25. **Method for eliciting ankle clonus. The Ex jerks upward and a little outward on the Pt's foot (thin arrow). The thick arrow is the downward response.**

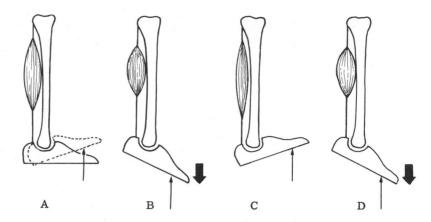

FIG. 7-26. Mechanism of ankle clonus. The thin arrow represents the light pressure applied by the examiner to the ball of the Pt's foot, the thick arrow the response.

    b. The Ex continues to apply light pressure against the ball of the Pt's foot, opposing plantar·flexion. When the foot plantar flexes from the first MSR and stops, the Ex's pressure immediately dorsiflexes the foot again (Fig. 7-26*C*, thin arrow). The restretching of the triceps surae causes plantar flexion again (Fig. 7-26*D*). As long as the Ex applies the proper pressure to elicit successive MSRs from the triceps surae, the foot continues to oscillate.

    c. When very active, clonus may persist without continued pressure by the Ex, suggesting that a central "pace-maker" may govern clonus (Dimitrivejic et al, 1980).

4. The same technique of applying a quick jerk elicits wrist, finger, or jaw clonus. Jerking downward on the patella with the leg completely straight and relaxed elicits quadriceps clonus. Try this test on your own leg.

5. Why must the Ex jerk the part briskly to elicit clonus? _____

_____

Ans: The muscle spindles have to be stretched rapidly enough to initiate a
   muscle stretch reflex.

6. *Clinical interpretation of clonus*

    a. Some normal individuals with physiologic hyperreflexia will have a few clonic jerks, called *abortive clonus.* In mature individuals, only *sustained clonus* is likely to be pathologic.

    b. Clonus is common in normal newborn infants. It may affect the jaw and extremities, and often is elicited by the infant's own movements (Shuper et al, 1991). Simply eliciting a MSR by tendon percussion may initiate a train of clonic after-jerks in such infants, or in any Pt with hyperreflexia, normal or pathologic.

7. Give an *operational* definition of clonus. (Include the maneuvers and what response occurs.) _____

_____

Ans: Clonus is a series of to-and-fro oscillations of a part initiated by a quick
   jerk and maintained by slight pressure. (Notice that this is purely descriptive
   and operational.)

8. Give a *pathophysiologic* and *clinical interpretation* of clonus? _____

_____

Ans: Clonus is a series of repetitive MSRs, indicating pathologic hyperreflexia, usually as a result of interruption of UMNs (the pyramidal tract), but it can occur in normal newborn infants.

REFERENCES FOR CLONUS

Dimitrivejic MR, Nathan PW, Sherwood AM: Clonus: the role of central mechanisms. *J Neurol Neurosurg Psychiatry,* 1980; 43:321–332.

Shuper A, Zalaberg J, Wertz R, Minouni M: Jitteriness beyond the neonatal period: a benign movement pattern in infancy. *J Child Neurol,* 1991; 6:243–245.

VIII. Disorders of muscle tone: hypertonia and hypotonia

NOTE: As developed to this point, the syndrome of UMN lesions consists of paresis or paralysis, hyperreflexia, and clonus. To understand *spasticity,* yet another component of the full UMN syndrome (Table 7-6), requires a general discussion of muscle tone.

A. Definition. Muscle tone is the *muscular* resistance (apart from gravity or joint disease) the Ex feels when manipulating a Pt's resting joint.

B. Self-demonstration of muscle tone
   1. Place your forearm flat on a table top, with your ulnar head resting directly on the table edge and with your wrist dangling freely over the table edge. Supinate your forearm so that your radius is on top. After relaxing this arm completely, grasp its hand with your other hand and flex and extend the wrist as fully as possible.
   2. As your active hand moves your relaxed hand, the active hand will feel slight resistance. This slight resistance to passive movement is *normal muscle tone.* (The ligaments set the ultimate range of joint movement.)
   3. Try now to relax your elbow and, with your other hand, flex and extend your forearm. Try these exercises with a partner.
   4. These exercises serve two purposes: to provide proprioceptive experience in judging muscle tone and to provide insight into the difficulty in relaxing a part completely. Do not lose patience when your Pts fail to relax. Keep working patiently to get the part completely relaxed before judging tone.

C. Origin of muscle tone. Normally the resistance of the muscle to passive movement has two components.
   1. The *elasticity* of the muscle, which ordinarily is slight unless the muscle is fibrotic.
   2. The *number and rate of motor discharges,* which is the critical variable. The number and rate of motor unit discharges depends on
      a. The stimulation of LMNs by muscle spindles and other receptors in skin, tendons, joints, and bone.
      b. The stimulation of LMNs by pyramidal and extrapyramidal pathways. Thus muscle tone depends on the activity of motor units as determined by the algebraic sum of diverse excitatory and inhibitory impulses from the peripheral nervous system (PNS) and central nervous system (CNS) on the LMNs.

    c. Since numerous pathways affect tone, and since the theories about it are complex and conflicting (Clemente, 1978; Glenn and Whyte, 1990), we will content ourselves with the operational findings and their clinical analysis. In this way, we will not err in giving explanation priority over the operational techniques to be learned.

  3. It is easy to surmise that the two possible alterations of tone are too much tone, *hypertonia,* and too little tone, *hypotonia.*

D. *Hypertonia.* The two most common hypertonic states are *spasticity* and *rigidity.* Less common is *paratonia (Gegenhalten).*

  1. *Spasticity,* as operationally defined, is an initial catch or resistance and then a yielding when the Ex quickly manipulates the Pt's resting extremity. It is a catch-and-yield sequence, like pulling an ordinary pocket-knife blade open. When first opened, the blade resists, but quickly yields as it straightens out. The similar phenomenon in muscle tone is called *clasp-knife spasticity* (Fig. 7-27).

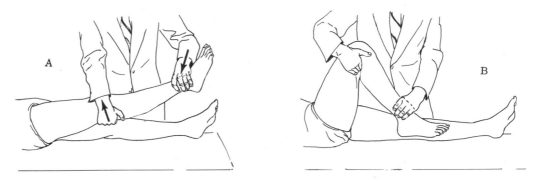

FIG. 7-27. Method for eliciting clasp-knife spasticity in the lower extremities. (A) The Ex lifts the Pt's leg with one hand, placing the other under the Pt's knee. As briskly as possible, in fact with a jerk, he simultaneously pushes *down* with the ankle hand and *up* with the other. (B) The spastic leg catches and then molds to the flexed position.

    a. The brisk movement required to elicit clasp-knife spasticity suggests that the stimulus has to engage the muscle spindles. According to this interpretation, the resistance felt is simply a muscle stretch reflex, which then fades out as the muscle spindles readjust. Oversensitivity of the MSR arc, centrally or peripherally, is the fundamental change, of which hyperreflexia, clonus, and spasticity are derivative. Although hyperreflexia, clonus, and clasp-knife spasticity usually parallel each other in intensity, occasionally one feature predominates out of proportion to the others. The pathophysiology of these variations is unknown. Clasp-knife spasticity is generally greater in the *flexors* of the upper extremities and *extensors* of the lower.

    b. The three phenomena presented to this point, which indicate a pyramidal tract or UMN lesion and act through an oversensitive MSR arc are

_____

_____.

Ans: Hyperreflexia, clonus, and clasp-knife spasticity.

  2. *Rigidity,* as operationally defined, is an increased muscular resistance felt throughout the entire range of movement when the Ex slowly manipulates a Pt's resting joint. It feels like bending solder, or a lead pipe. Hence, its name, *lead-pipe rigidity.* It involves the agonists and antagonists at the joints.

    a. The presence of lead-pipe rigidity indicates an extrapyramidal lesion, in the basal motor circuitry, more specifically in the dopaminergic projection from the substantia nigra to the striatum. The pathophysiology of lead-pipe rigidity is uncertain.

    b. The *cogwheel phenomenon* often occurs with the rigidity of parkinsonism. The Ex feels the rigidity as a series of rachet-like catches while slowly moving the elbow or wrist through their range of motion. It apparently reflects the superimposed beats of the parkinsonian tremor, even though the tremor may not be otherwise obvious.

3. *Paratonia* (Gegenhalten: gegen = against or towards; halten = to hold; therefore to hold against or resist)

    a. Definition. Paratonia is the resistance, equal in degree and range, that the Pt presents to each attempt of the Ex to move a part in any direction. It is a *pari passu* response.

    b. Self-demonstration of paratonia. Press your palms together and while maintaining the palms in contact with slight pressure, move both hands to the right and left, and up and down. Imagine one hand as the Pt's and the other as the Ex's. If one hand increases pressure, speeds up or detours, so does the other in equal degree. It is like leading and following in ballroom dancing. The balanced, proprioceptive resistance or opposition of one hand in pursuit of another hand is *paratonia.* The Pt is not necessarily rigid at rest. The Ex feels the paratonia as a slight stiffening of the Pt's limb in response to the contact when the Ex attempts to move the Pt's extremity.

    c. Clinical significance of paratonia. Paratonia occurs in dementia, often in combination with abulia and gait apraxia (described later). Some otherwise normal persons who cannot relax completely for testing muscle tone show a paratonia-like resistance to passive movement of their parts by the Ex.

E. *Summary of spasticity and rigidity*

See frame D.1

1. Give an operational definition of clasp-knife spasticity. _____
_____
_____

See frame D.2

2. Give an operational definition of lead-pipe rigidity. _____
_____
_____
_____

☑ *Pyramidal*
☑ *Extrapyramidal*

3. Clasp-knife spasticity indicates a lesion of the ☐ pyramidal tract/ ☐ extrapyramidal tracts, while lead-pipe rigidity indicates a lesion of the ☐ pyramidal tract/ ☐ extrapyramidal tracts.

4. Check the signs which require a brisk stimulus to elicit:

☑ *a*

    a. ☐ Clasp-knife spasticity
    b. ☐ Lead-pipe rigidity

☑ *c*
☑ *d*

    c. ☐ Hyperactive muscle stretch reflex
    d. ☐ Clonus
    e. ☐ Paratonia

5. Why do the signs checked in frame 4 require a brisk stimulus to elicit them?
_____
_____

Ans: To activate a strong afferent volley from muscle spindles, in order to fire the LMNs before the spindles adjust to their new length.

TABLE 7-5 Clinical differentiation of spasticity and rigidity

Spasticity (A component of the pyramidal syndromes)	Rigidity (A component of the extrapyramidal syndromes)
Clasp-knife phenomenon, in hemiplegic, quadriplegic, monoplegic, or paraplegic distribution	Lead-pipe phenomenon, often with cogwheeling and tremor at rest. Usually in all four extremities but may have a "hemi" distribution
The examiner elicits the clasp-knife phenomenon, a catch-and-yield sensation, by a quick jerk of the resting extremity	The examiner elicits the lead-pipe resistance of rigidity by making a relatively slow movement of the patient's resting extremity
Clonus and hyperactive MSRs	No clonus; MSRs not necessarily altered
Extensor toe sign	Normal plantar reflexes
Tends to predominate in one set of muscles such as flexors of the upper extremity and the extensors of the knee and plantar flexors of the ankle	Tends to affect antagonistic pairs of muscles about equally
EMG shows no activity with the muscle at complete rest	EMG tends to show electrical activity with the muscle as relaxed as the patient can make it

F. Differentiation of spasticity and rigidity. Lesions may affect both pyramidal and extrapyramidal pathways, causing mixtures of spasticity and rigidity, especially in cerebral palsy. Usually the Ex can differentiate the two (Table 7-5).

REFERENCES FOR SPASTICITY AND RIGIDITY

Clemente CD: Neurophysiologic mechanisms and neuroanatomic substrates related to spasticity. *Neurology,* 1978; 28:40–45

Glenn MB, Whyte J: *The Practical Management of Spasticity in Children and Adults.* Beckenham, Lea & Febiger, 1990

Weisendanger M: *Pathophysiology of Muscle Tone.* Berlin, Springer Verlag, 1972

G. Hypotonia (flaccidity)
  1. *Definition.* Hypotonia is a decreased resistance the Ex feels when manipulating a Pt's resting joint. Hypotonic Pts generally show an increased range of joint movement, such as hyperextensible knees (genu recurvatum) or flaccid heel cords.
  2. *Causes of hypotonia* (Fig. 7-28)
  3. *Hypotonia from lesions at the level of the reflex arc or peripheral neuromuscular system.* Review Fig. 7-20.
       a. Interruption of afferent fibers in peripheral nerves or dorsal roots reduces muscle tone by removing the inflow of excitatory afferent impulses. In fact dorsal rhizotomy is done therapeutically to reduce muscle tone in some spastic Pts.
       b. Manifestly, section of *ventral* roots would cause hypotonia because no nerve impulses could reach the muscles. *Primary myopathies* cause hypotonia by reducing the ability of the muscles to respond to tonic nerve impulses.
  4. *Differentiation of peripheral causes for hypotonia.* As usual, clinical differ-

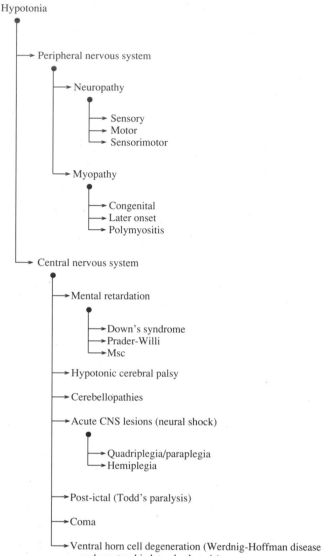

FIG. 7-28. Some common causes of hypotonia.

entiation depends on fitting the constellation of findings into a syndrome, as previously outlined in Table 7-3.

5. *Central causes of hypotonia* (Fig. 7-28)

   a. Although cerebral, cerebellar, and brainstem lesions sometimes cause hypotonia, the pathophysiology is elusive.

   b. Many congenital brain disorders, such as Down's syndrome and Prader-Willi syndrome, cause profound hypotonia. Pts with spastic cerebral palsy may present as hypotonic infants before spasticity evolves.

6. *Hypotonia from cerebral or spinal (neural) shock*

   a. *Definition.* Neural shock is a stage of hypotonic total paralysis and total areflexia that immediately follows acute, severe UMN lesions. Typically Pts with slowly evolving UMN lesions display hypertonia, hyperreflexia, and paralysis, in more or less parallel degree. The term *shock* in this context designates the disastrous disorganization of the acutely injured nervous system. Depending on the lesion site, the Ex may specify *cerebral* or *spinal* shock.

   b. *Diaschisis.* The concept of neural shock of the motor system merges with the general concept of diaschisis. After any acute lesion, the signs and symptoms often exceed what we can understand by the actual tracts interrupted or neurons destroyed. For example acute, strictly unilateral occipital lobe infarction, may result in complete (bilateral) cortical blindness for a period of hours or days, particularly if the Pt is somewhat obtunded. After that period, the Pt will show only the expected hemimanopia dictated by the unilateral destruction of the visual cortex. Von Monakow (1853–1930) named this distant impairment of function, beyond the confines of the acute lesion, *diaschisis* (Meyer, 1991).

   c. Causes of neural shock or diaschisis. Inciting lesions are large, acute and catastrophic, including trauma, spinal cord transection, or large brain infarcts or hemorrhages.

   d. If a Pt originally in a stage of neural shock begins to recover movement, the recovery usually parallels the emergence of the MSRs, spasticity, and clonus. In the chronic stage after an acute, large UMN lesion, as well as after most UMN lesions of slow onset, increased MSRs, clonus, and spasticity are present. Thus, the clinical signs of UMN lesions depend on

    (1) The rapidity of onset.
    (2) The size of the lesion.
    (3) The stage in the evolution of recovery of the CNS.

REFERENCES FOR DIASCHISIS

Meyer JS: Does diaschisis have clinical correlates? *Mayo Clin Proc* 1991; 66:430–432

  H. Range of Motion

   1. The Ex observes the range of motion during the Pt's active free movements of the extremities when testing muscle strength. When testing muscle tone, the Ex passively moves the Pt's relaxed parts through their entire normal range of motion. With hyperreflexia and spasticity, the range is reduced; with hypotonia, it is increased. For example, the Ex ordinarily can passively flex and extend the hand to approximately a 90-degree angle with the forearm. The foot normally dorsiflexes to nearly a 45-degree angle with the shin. A greater or lesser range of movement of these joints indicates hypertonia or hypotonia.

   2. If a joint shows a restricted range of movement, the Ex should continue to apply pressure, taking care not to elicit pain. The joint may then yield further. If it does not yield it is a *fixed* contracture of the joint. If it does yield it is a *dynamic* contracture.

   3. Record range of motion by degrees, using a goniometer or protractor when precise measurements are desired.

IX. Examination of the superficial reflexes (skin-muscle reflexes)

NOTE: Do the next part of the text at home, in order to test your own bare foot. Get a reflex hammer and a broken wooden tongue blade to use as stimulating objects.

  A. Superficial versus deep reflexes

   1. In addition to causing hyperactive MSRs, spasticity, and clonus, UMN lesions alter the *superficial reflexes.* Since stimulation of receptors deep to

the skin elicits the MSRs, the MSRs are classed with the *deep* reflexes. Stimulation of receptors in skin and mucous membranes elicit *superficial* reflexes or skin-muscle reflexes. By stimulating deep or superficial receptors with stimuli of appropriate quality and site (Vlach, 1989), the Ex can elicit a response from every muscle.

2. The superficial reflexes commonly elicited in the NE consist of
   a. Corneal reflex.
   b. Gag reflex.
   c. Abdominal skin-muscle reflexes.
   d. Anal wink and bulbocavernous reflexes.
   e. Plantar reflex.

B. *Standard method for eliciting plantar reflexes*
   1. Place the Pt supine with the limbs relaxed and symmetrically arranged, and with the knees straight or slightly flexed.
      a. Using the serrated, broken end of a tongue blade, a key, or the butt of a reflex hammer, the Ex strokes the *lateral* side of the sole (Fig. 7-29).

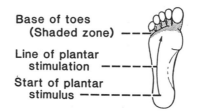

Base of toes
(Shaded zone)

Line of plantar
stimulation

Start of plantar
stimulus

FIG. 7-29. Sole of the right foot. The arrow marks the plantar stroke. Notice that it stops short of the shaded zone, the base of the toes.

      b. If the plantar stroke has the correct *length, velocity,* and *pressure,* the large toe normally *flexes.* After UMN interruption, the toe *extends,* a phenomenon called the *Babinski sign* (Joseph Babinski, 1857–1932) (Fig. 7-34).
   2. Since the sole is ticklish or sensitive, the Pt, especially if senile, demented, or paranoid may, view the act of plantar stimulation as unnecessary, ludicrous, or even hostile. Critique each of the following statements and check the best statement to insure the Pt's relaxation and cooperation.
      ☐ *a.* "Hold still while I tickle the bottom of your foot."
      ☐ *b.* "I am going to scratch the bottom of your foot. Hold it still."
      ☐ *c.* "Don't move your foot, I am going to stimulate your sole."
      ☐ *d.* "I am going to press gently on your foot. If it's unpleasant, tell me."
   3. Next, hold the Pt's ankle with one hand to keep the foot in place in order to control the pressure of the plantar stroke.
   4. Place the stimulus object at the Pt's *heel* and stroke it *slowly* along the sole (Fig. 7-29). The object is moved along the ☐ medial margin/ ☐ lateral margin/ ☐ center of the foot.
   5. *Characteristics of the plantar stimulus*
      a. Length is only one of the significant variables of the plantar stimulus. Figure 7-29 shows that the plantar stroke stops short of the base of the toes. Extending the stroke to the base of the toes produces unpredictable toe movements.

☑ *d*

☑ *Lateral margin*

b. Another variable is the amount of *pressure* applied.

c. A third variable of the plantar stroke is its *velocity.*

d. Hence, the three important variables of the plantar stroke are the _____, _____, and _____.

Length; pressure; velocity

6. *Self-demonstration of the plantar reflex*

a. Test your own foot and if available, another person's. Try different velocities, pressures, and lengths, always stopping the stroke short of the base of the toes.

b. In applying the plantar stimulus to yourself, what errors in positioning did you have to make? _____.

Ans: All of them! Your leg was flexed, many of your muscles were contracting, and you had a bent trunk and asymmetrical posture. Reread frame B.1 if you missed.

c. By stroking your own foot, you will learn to apply the plantar stroke with slight pressure. Pts with sensory neuropathy, who have extremely tender soles (hyperesthesia), find the slightest plantar stimulus intolerable. Thus, always begin with very slight pressure, or even apply the stroke first to the *lateral* aspect of the foot (Chaddock maneuver, Fig. 7-35*B*), which is less sensitive than the sole.

C. *The criterion for success in eliciting a reflex*

1. A reflex, by definition, consists of a relatively invariant response to a specified stimulus. Reproducibility is the goal in eliciting any reflex, either toe flexion or extension in the case of the plantar reflex. If no response or inconstant responses occur, your stimulus is probably wrong. Try again.

a. Consider *length* first. Having already started at the heel you can't get much more length there. You must avoid the base of the toes. What remains is to swing the stroke across the ball of the foot.

b. If you fail to get reproducible responses after varying length, next vary the velocity of the stroke.

c. If varying the length and velocity of the stroke and using gentle pressure fails, next increase the pressure. What consideration limits the amount of pressure you should apply? _____.

Ans: The Pt's comfort.

2. By what criterion do you know that you have applied the correct plantar stimulus? _____.

Ans: Reproducibility of toe movement, either flexion or extension.

D. *Summary of the standard method for plantar stimulation*

1. Write a statement to forewarn the Pt before a plantar stimulus. _____.

Ans: Well, would your statement put you at ease?

2. Describe the correct position of the Pt for the plantar stimulus? _____.

Ans: Supine, relaxed, all body parts symmetrical, legs extended or knees slightly flexed.

3. Why stop short of the base of the toes with the plantar stroke? _____.

Ans: It produces unpredictable toe movements.

4. If you obtain no response or variable responses, what is the most likely explanation? _____

_____

Ans: The stimulus was improper in respect to length, velocity, or pressure.

E. *Anatomy of the plantar reflex arc*

1. The *reflexogenous zone* is the zone from which a reflex can be elicited. The reflexogenous zone for the normal plantar reflex is usually restricted to the first sacral dermatome (S-1). Study the area of the S-1 dermatome and its relation to lumbar dermatomes 4 to 5 (L-4 to L-5) in Fig. 7-30.

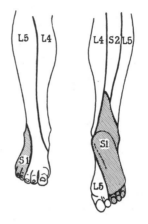

FIG. 7-30. Dermatomes of the foot.

2. Cover Fig. 7-30 and shade in the S-1 dermatome in Fig. 7-31.

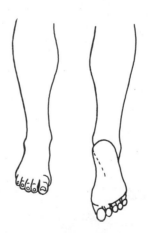

FIG. 7-31. Blank for shading the S-1 dermatome.

Ans: See Fig. 7-30

3. Clinical analysis of any reflex requires "thinking through" the reflex arc. According to first principles of thinking through a reflex arc, we begin at the _____.

Receptor

4. Since the skin contains the receptor nerve endings, the plantar reflex is classed as a ☐ superficial/ ☐ deep reflex.

☑ *Superficial*

5. Learn Fig. 7-32 and then answer frames a to f.

   a. The reflexogenous zone for the plantar reflex is the _____ dermatome.

S-1

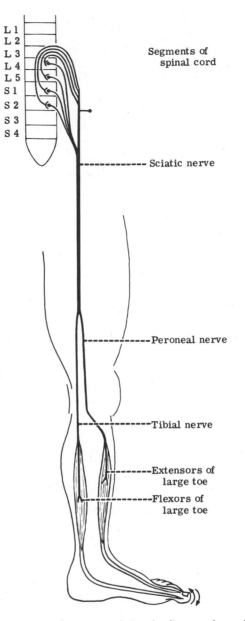

FIG. 7-32. Reflex arc for the plantar reflexes. For simplicity, the diagram shows the flexor hallucis brevis in the calf rather than in the foot.

Sciatic

Lumbar (L-4 to L-5)
Sacral (S-1 to S-2)

Tibial
Peroneal

Sciatic

Tibial

b. The *afferent* nerve is the *tibial* nerve. It is a branch of the _____ nerve.

c. Mediating the plantar reflex are the 4th and 5th segments of the _____ level of the spinal cord and the 1st and 2d segments of the _____ level.

d. The sciatic nerve divides into two large branches just proximal to the knee. The branch to the toe *flexors* is the _____ nerve, and the branch to the *extensors* is the _____ nerve.

e. The major nerve which divides into tibial and peroneal branches is the _____ nerve.

f. What nerve, if cut, would interrupt both the *afferent* and *efferent* arc of the normal plantar response, leaving the toe extensor muscles innervated? _____

F. *Physiology of the plantar stimulus*

1. *Pain and the plantar reflex.* The plantar stimulus results in a noxious feeling of tickling, pressure, and pain. The plantar stimulus is thought to act mainly through the *pain* receptors in the skin. However, one cannot safely infer from the subjective component of the reflex precisely which receptors, in fact, elicited the response, since the stimulus activates several types of afferent endings.

2. *Summation and the plantar reflex*

   a. Figure 7-33 shows the oscilloscopic patterns of electrical shocks applied to a Pt's nerve. The brief shock in Fig. 7-33*A* did not elicit a response. Increasing only the *duration* of the shock elicited a response (Fig. 7-33*B*).

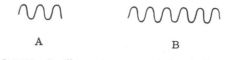

A   B

FIG. 7-33. Oscilloscopic pattern of electrical stimuli.

   b. A stimulus that requires increasing application to elicit a response is said to *summate* or to undergo *summation.* A certain minimum number of afferent impulses has to add up or summate to fire the LMNs to the muscles. When, as in Fig. 7-33, a stimulus increases over time, we say that *temporal summation* has occurred.

   c. Suppose a person fails to feel movement when an object moves a distance of 500 μm across the skin. Then, while keeping the time the same, the Ex moves the object 1000 μm, and the person does feel movement. The response occurs because the object acts on an increased area of skin. This exemplifies ☐ spatial/ ☐ temporal summation.

   ☑ *Spatial*

3. When the Ex elicits a plantar reflex, the toe may not move until the object reaches the instep or ball of the foot. This delay in the response indicates that some type of summation has occurred.

   a. The fact that moving the object from the heel to the instep requires a finite amount of time suggests that _____ summation is necessary.

   Temporal

   b. The fact that the moving object stimulated successively more receptors also suggests that _____ summation may have occurred.

   Spatial

4. Thus, to get the muscles of the toes to contract, the central excitatory state of the motoneurons was increased both by _____ and _____ summation.

   Temporal
   Spatial

G. *The role of agonist-antagonist contraction in the plantar reflex*

1. Reflexes differ greatly with respect to the required adequate stimulus and in the complexity and number of muscles acting. The relatively simple MSR involves the contraction of only one muscle, or even only one part of one muscle. In some reflexes, the action of the prime mover, the *agonist,* is opposed by simultaneous contraction of the *antagonist.* In other reflexes, the contraction of the antagonist is inhibited.

2. In the normal plantar reflex, we know that the toe flexors contract because we can see the toe flex. The question is whether the toe extensor muscles co-contract in opposition to the flexors and are simply overpowered by the flexors, or whether the toe extensors contract at all. What pathologic conditions or laboratory experiments would prove that the toe extensor and

flexor muscles contract simultaneously in the plantar reflex? If you cannot think of a way to solve the problem try one of the hints below.

   a. Begin by "thinking through" the reflex arc, Fig. 7-32. Would a lesion, or procaine injected at a particular site, help answer the question?

   b. How would you detect extensor muscle contractions even if the toe moved in the direction of the flexors?

   c. Could you use electromyography?

3. *Answers to frame 2*

   a. The clinically minded investigator would look for Pts in whom the flexor muscles of the toe were paralyzed, leaving the afferent impulses from the sole intact. Such a situation might be realized by interruption of the motor branch of the nerve to the flexor muscles, a muscle injury, or by a disease such as anterior poliomyelitis which might happen to destroy the LMNs supplying the flexors, leaving all *afferent* axons from the sole and *efferent* axons to the extensors intact.

   b. The laboratory-minded investigator would make simultaneous electromyographic recordings from the flexors and extensors during the application of the the plantar stimulus.

   c. Landau and Clare (1959) concluded that both flexors and extensors of the toe contract simultaneously in response to a plantar stimulus, with the outcome a mechanical competition between these muscles, but Van Gijn (1977) disagrees. At the spinal cord level, however, some integrative mechanism must fight out whether flexion or extension will occur.

H. Normal variations and flexion synergy in response to a plantar stimulus

  1. *Flexion synergy*

   a. *Some* normal persons will show little or no toe or leg movement after a plantar stimulus.

   b. *Most* normal persons tend to withdraw their foot from a plantar stimulus, as well as flexing their great toe. The withdrawal movement, like the response to stepping on a tack, consists of dorsiflexion of the ankle, and flexion of the knee and hip, a *flexion synergy* (Walshe, 1956; Van Gijn, 1978). The tensor fasciae latae, hamstrings, and tibialis anterior muscles visibly and palpably contract during this flexion synergy. Watch for these actions as you apply the plantar stimulus.

  2. The small toes may fan, but this does not constitute a consistent or clinically important part of the plantar reflex (Van Gijn, 1977).

I. Pathologic variations in the plantar reflexes

  1. After interruption of the UMNs to the lumbosacral cord, the great toe extends instead of flexing, which is called an *extensor* plantar response, *extensor* toe sign, or *Babinski* sign (Fig. 7-34*A*).

  2. For best communication simply state that the Pt has a *flexor plantar response* or an *extensor plantar response,* whichever is found. If you report a Babinski sign don't redundantly say that the Pt has a positive Babinski sign. There is no negative Babinski sign. The sign, dorsiflexion of the toe, is either present or not.

  3. The flexor synergy which withdraws the leg of a normal person after a plantar stimulus usually becomes more prominent and stereotyped when an extensor toe sign is present (Fig. 7-34*B*).

  4. Some Pts voluntarily extend or wiggle the big toe, making the response unreadable. After admonishing the Pt to relax, try again. A struggling child or some Pts with involuntary movement disorders or cerebral palsy may

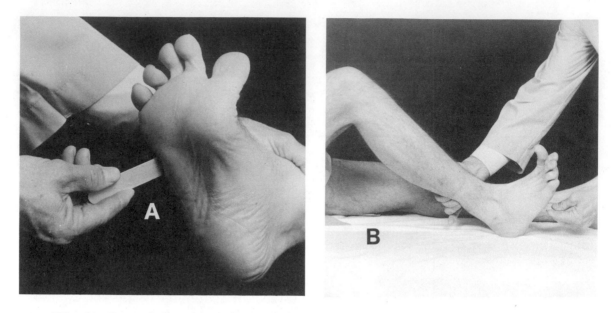

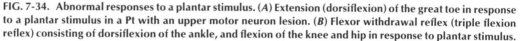

FIG. 7-34. Abnormal responses to a plantar stimulus. (*A*) Extension (dorsiflexion) of the great toe in response to a plantar stimulus in a Pt with an upper motor neuron lesion. (*B*) Flexor withdrawal reflex (triple flexion reflex) consisting of dorsiflexion of the ankle, and flexion of the knee and hip in response to plantar stimulus.

inadvertently or spontaneously dorsiflex the great toe and may hold it tonically extended. To best identify a true extensor toe sign, carefully notice the relation of the toe extension and the flexion synergy to the plantar stimulus. With a true extensor toe sign, the toe usually begins to extend only *after* the plantar stroke has moved a few centimeters along the sole to produce spatial and temporal summation. The toe remains tonically extended as the stroke continues and then promptly returns to the neutral position after release of the stroke. *Thus, the Ex must confirm that the toe movement is indeed related to, provoked by, and dependent on the plantar stimulus, and that any flexion of the leg displays a similar correlation.* To qualify as a reflex, the response should show a "machine-like fatality," to use Sherrington's words. Any other relation of the toe or leg movement to the plantar stimulus, or an inconstant relation, falls under suspicion of a false response.

5. Clinicians interpret the extensor toe response as a sign of *anatomic* or *pathophysiologic* interruption of the pyramidal tract (Van Gijn, 1977; Walshe, 1956). No other hypothesis fits the facts as well. However, some Pts, particularly with spinal cord lesions, may have extensor toe signs without anatomic evidence of pyramidal tract interruption (Nathan and Smith, 1955). Reversible pathophysiologic conditions that result in transient extensor toe signs, with or without the other features of the UMN syndrome, include toxic-metabolic coma, postictal hemiparesis after epileptic seizures (Todd's paralysis), trauma with concussion or contusion, transient ischemic attacks, and hemiplegic migraine. The Pt's prompt and full recovery provides the proof of a transient pathophysiological state rather than anatomic interruption of the pyramidal pathway (Walshe, 1956).

J. The plantar responses in infants

1. In normal young infants the toe response varies, depending on the pressure of the stimulus. Very slight pressure, merely a caress, elicits toe extension, but stronger pressure elicits plantar flexion. Strong plantar pressure elicits a *plantar grasp reflex* which competes with toe extension. The response elicited, extension or flexion, depends on the stimulus imposed.

2. Hence, the extension of the great toe, while pathologic in older Pts, does not convict the infant of a pyramidal lesion. In general, the more mature the infant and the more constant the extensor response, the greater the likelihood of an UMN lesion.
3. Contrast the clinical significance of an extensor toe response in infants and older subjects. _____

_____

_____

Ans: Normal infants variably show extensor or flexor toe responses, depending on the pressure of the stimulus. In older subjects, consistent extensor responses indicate an UMN lesion.

    K. *Changes in the stimulus dimensions and reflexogenous zone for the plantar reflex after UMN lesions*
1. To elicit a plantar response requires a fairly selective combination of site, length, velocity, and pressure of the stimulus. The usual reflexogenous zone for the plantar reflexes, either normal or pathologic, is the _____ dermatome. Draw a foot, shade this dermatome, and check against Fig. 7-30.

S-1

2. In Pts with severe structural lesions, such as complete spinal cord transection, the extensor toe sign and leg withdrawal lose all local signature or local specificity. Almost any stimulus of any part of the skin caudal to the level of the lesion results in toe extension, with a strong flexor synergy or flexor spasms.
3. *Additional maneuvers for eliciting superficial toe reflexes*
    a. The standard method is stimulation of the lateral aspect of the sole. Many other eponymic maneuvers elicit toe movement from superficial stimuli. Since many of the maneuvers apply the stimulus outside of the S-1 dermatome, the usual reflexogenous zone, they are in general less effective than stimuli within the S-1 dermatome. In the normal person, these stimuli do not usually cause toe flexion, but after UMN lesions, they tend to elicit toe extension just as with Babinski's maneuver (Fig. 7-35).
    b. The multitude of eponyms implies that the maneuvers represent different phenomena, but physiologically, as stimuli, the maneuvers betray a unifying simplicity. Do the maneuvers of Fig. 7-35 on yourself and a partner, paying attention to the stimulus properties of each maneuver. Can you define the common features of the stimuli? _____

_____

Ans: In each maneuver, the stimulus acts over a certain interval of time, stimulates more than one point of skin, and causes a noxious or uncomfortable sensation. We can infer that it is a spatially and temporally summated, noxious superficial stimulus which elicits the plantar response (Roby-Brami et al, 1989).

    c. From this information, you can now discover new signs yourself. Run your thumbnail down your shin: you have now discovered a new sign. Squeeze on a corn (a very effective way to get an extensor toe response) and you have another sign, and so on. Thus, it is not useful to consider the various maneuvers as different entities. The response from the S-1 dermatome is the most constant and useful. If stimulation of the S-1 dermatome produces a convincing, reproducible response, the other maneuvers are superfluous. Sometimes if the toe response to plantar stimulation alone is equivocal, doing another maneuver, such as the

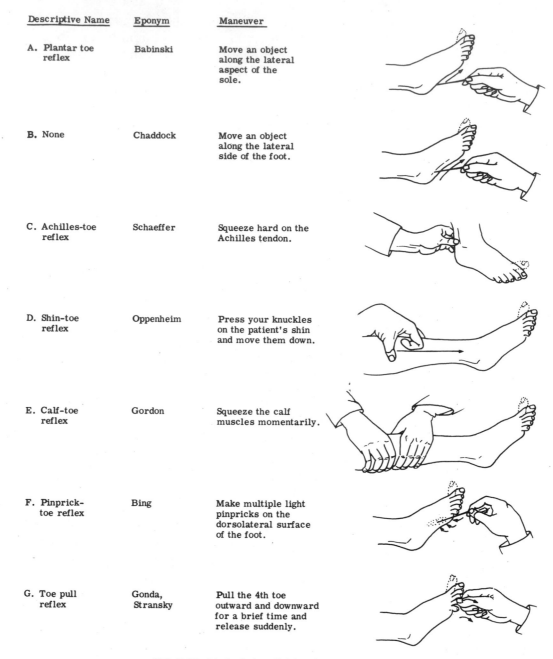

Descriptive Name	Eponym	Maneuver
A. Plantar toe reflex	Babinski	Move an object along the lateral aspect of the sole.
B. None	Chaddock	Move an object along the lateral side of the foot.
C. Achilles-toe reflex	Schaeffer	Squeeze hard on the Achilles tendon.
D. Shin-toe reflex	Oppenheim	Press your knuckles on the patient's shin and move them down.
E. Calf-toe reflex	Gordon	Squeeze the calf muscles momentarily.
F. Pinprick-toe reflex	Bing	Make multiple light pinpricks on the dorsolateral surface of the foot.
G. Toe pull reflex	Gonda, Stransky	Pull the 4th toe outward and downward for a brief time and release suddenly.

FIG. 7-35. Methods for eliciting the extensor toe sign.

Oppenheim or Gordon, simultaneously with the plantar stimulus may enhance toe dorsiflexion.

d. If you must know all of the eponyms to feel educated try this mnemonic: B is for Babinski, stimulate the *bottom* of the foot; C is for Chaddock, stimulate the *side;* G is for Gordon, *grip* the calf; O is for Oppenheim's *on* the shin maneuver; S is for Schaeffer, *squeeze* the Achilles tendon (Fig. 7-35).

REFERENCES FOR THE BABINSKI SIGN

Babinski JP: Sur le reflexe cutane plantaire dans certains affections organiques du system nerveux central. *Compt Rendu Soc Biol* 1896; 48:207–208

Landau W, Clare M: The plantar reflex in man, with special reference to some conditions where the extensor response is unexpectedly absent. *Brain* 1959; 82:321–355

Nathan P, Smith M: The Babinski response: A review and new observations. *J Neurol Neurosurg Psychiatry* 1955; 18:250–259

Roby-Brami A, Ghenassia JR, Bussel B: Electrophysical study of the Babinski sign in paraplegic patients. *J Neurol Neurosurg Psychiatry* 1989; 52:1390–1397

Van Gijn J: *The Plantar Reflex: A Historical, Clinical, and Electromyographic Study*. Meppel, The Netherlands, Krips Repro, 1977

Van Gijn F: The Babinski sign and the pyramidal syndrome. *J Neurol Neurosurg Psychiatry* 1978; 41:865–873

Vlach V: Evolution of skin reflexes in the first years of life. *Devel Med Child Neurol* 1989; 31:196–205

Walshe FMR: The Babinski plantar response, its forms and its physiological and pathological significance. *Brain* 1956; 79:529–556

L. *Explanations for the otherwise puzzling absence of extensor toe signs in patients who have UMN lesions, or, how to avoid being fooled*

1. *Analysis of a Pt*

   A 24-year-old man struck his head on the bottom of a swimming pool when he dove in. His head had been forced sharply backward. Examination shortly after his neck injury disclosed complete paralysis and areflexia for superficial and deep reflexes and complete anesthesia caudal to C-5. Breathing was solely diaphragmatic.

   a. Such a phase of complete paralysis, hypotonia, and areflexia after an acute, severe spinal cord injury is called _____ shock.

   Spinal

   b. Within 8 days, his MSRs returned and became very hyperactive. Extensor toe signs appeared and sensation started to return. Within 15 days after injury, the full UMN syndrome was present, and some weak voluntary movements returned. Eight weeks after the injury he was able to move all extremities. Six months after the injury, he had slight hyperreflexia of the left leg and a suggestive extensor toe sign on the left, but otherwise he seemed normal.

   c. The Pt had suffered a contusion of the spinal cord which had temporarily interrupted all impulse transmission through the lesion site. After recovery, he still had residual signs indicating permanent destruction of some UMN axons on the left side of the cord.

   d. Thus one reason for absence of an extensor toe sign after UMN lesions is the stage of spinal or cerebral (neural) shock.

2. *Compression damage to the common peroneal nerve*

   a. Compression neuropathy of the common peroneal nerve may account for absence of a Babinski sign by interrupting the innervation of the toe extensor muscles. Pts paralyzed from any cause, UMN or LMN, may suffer from compression damage to the common peroneal nerve because the paralyzed leg may rest in outward rotation, in the same position, for long periods of time. The nerve then gets compressed between the fibular head and the bed surface or bed rail. The common peroneal nerve usually gets compressed where it runs obliquely downward across the fibula (Fig. 7-36).

   b. Feel the head of your fibula. Move your fingertip a half a centimeter or so distally. Pressing fairly hard, move your fingertip back and forth across the fibula. As the nerve angles downward and forward, you should be able to feel it slip back and forth under your fingertip.

3. *Common peroneal palsy and foot drop*

   a. Damage to the common peroneal nerve causes a foot drop because it

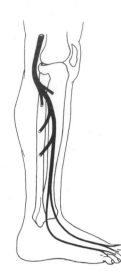

FIG. 7-36. Distribution of the common peroneal nerve. Notice how it courses superficial to the fibula, where it is exposed to injury.

supplies all foot and toe extensors. The Pt cannot dorsiflex the foot, and the toes will drag when the Pt walks. If the Pt recovers from UMN paralysis, it is tragic if a remaining peroneal palsy precludes a satisfactory gait. The physician has to insure proper measures to protect the peroneal nerve, ulnar nerve, and other nerves of paralyzed Pts and when applying casts for fractures.

b. *Crossed knee peroneal palsy.* The superficial position of the nerve accounts for a common cause of foot drop, the so-called "crossed knee palsy." The Pt compresses the nerve when sitting with one knee crossed over the other. Cross your legs and notice how the peroneal nerve may be entrapped between the fibula and the lateral condyle and patella of the opposite knee.

4. Give two basically different reasons for the absence of an extensor toe sign after an undoubted UMN lesion. _____

_____

Ans: (1) Spinal or cerebral shock. (2) A lesion of the reflex arc, such as peroneal nerve injury, loss of afferent impulses, etc.

5. Even after exclusion of all of the foregoing alternative explanations, some Pts with UMN lesions will fail to show one or more of the features of the UMN syndrome. Then we have to hide behind the mask of "biologic variability." But don't use that disguise as a substitute for careful analysis of all of the possible pathogenic factors.

REFERENCE FOR PERONEAL NEUROPATHY

Sourkes M, Stewart JD: Common peroneal neuropathy: A study of selective motor and sensory involvement. *Neurology,* 1991; 41:1029–1033.

M. *Technique for eliciting the superficial abdominal and cremasteric reflexes*
1. Stroking the skin of the abdominal quadrants or thighs elicits the superficial abdominal and cremasteric reflexes (Fig. 7-37).
2. Using a broken tongue blade, a key, or the blunt end of a reflex hammer, practice obtaining the superficial abdominal reflexes on yourself and a partner. The partner may sit or recline. You may be unable to obtain the reflex on yourself, but by trying, you will learn two important things:

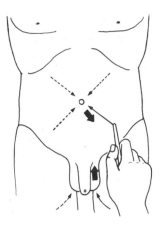

FIG. 7-37. Method for eliciting the superficial abdominal and cremasteric reflexes. The thin arrows are the direction of the examiner's stroke. The thick are the direction of the response.

a. The stimulus is somewhat unpleasant.

b. Excessive tension in the abdominal muscles obscures the abdominal skin-muscle reflexes. Since you will have to flex or raise your head, you may tense your muscles too much. On the other hand, a slight degree of abdominal tension may reinforce the response.

3. The normal response to abdominal skin stimulation is twitching of the umbilicus ☐ toward/ ☐ away from the quadrant stimulated.

4. The normal response to thigh stimulation is ☐ elevation/ ☐ depression of the ☐ ipsilateral/ ☐ contralateral/ ☐ both testicles. (Females do not display this reflex.)

5. The abdominal stimulus has the same properties as the plantar stimulus. If perceived by the Pt, the stimulus is felt as _____, and it requires _____ and _____ summation.

6. Therefore in deference to the Pt's comfort, apply the first abdominal stimulus gently.

7. *Effect of UMN lesions on the abdominal and cremasteric reflexes.* These superficial reflexes *disappear* after UMN lesions.

8. *Natural history of the abdominal and cremasteric reflexes*

a. You may find it difficult to elicit abdominal reflexes in normal young infants. The individual, whether infant or adult, has to relax to tolerate the somewhat uncomfortable or tickling sensation produced. Abdominal tension obscures the response. As the infant matures, the abdominal reflexes appear.

b. In normal elderly or obese Pts, or in multiparous women with lax abdomens, the abdominal reflex is often absent.

c. In the acute phase of an UMN lesion, the abdominal and cremasteric reflexes are usually absent. Later they may recover. If the brain lesion occurs early in life, these reflexes regularly return, as in cerebral palsy.

9. What two normal features of the superficial reflexes in young infants would indicate UMN interruption in a more mature patient? _____

_____.

Ans: Extensor toe responses and absence of abdominal reflexes.

N. Anal wink (S-2, S-3, S-4) and bulbocavernous reflexes (S-3, S-4)

1. Pricking the skin around the anus causes a quick, twitchlike constriction of the anal sphincter, the so-called anal wink. The anal reflex is the first to return after spinal shock (Pedersen et al, 1978).

✓ *Toward*

✓ *Elevation*
✓ *Ipsilateral*

Unpleasant (noxious)
Spatial; temporal

2. Pricking the glans penis causes reflex contraction of the bulbocavernosus muscle, detected by pressing a (gloved) finger against the Pt's perineum. The pinprick may also elicit an anal wink.

3. These tests are not part of the routine NE. Include them to investigate symptoms such as incontinence or impotence that suggest a lesion of the lumbosacral cord, cauda equina, or lumbosacral plexus. EMG studies of the anal sphincter and anal wink reflex are also helpful (Pedersen et al, 1978).

REFERENCE FOR ANAL REFLEXES

Pedersen E, Harving H, Klemar B et al: Human anal reflexes. *J Neurol Neurosurg Psychiatry* 1978; 48:813–818

O. *Recording the reflexes*
1. A stick figure conveniently displays several reflexes routinely elicited (Fig. 7-38). Record the MSRs as 0 to 4+; the toe response with an up or down arrow; the abdominal and cremasteric reflexes with a 0 if absent, ± if equivocal or barely present, and + if normally active.

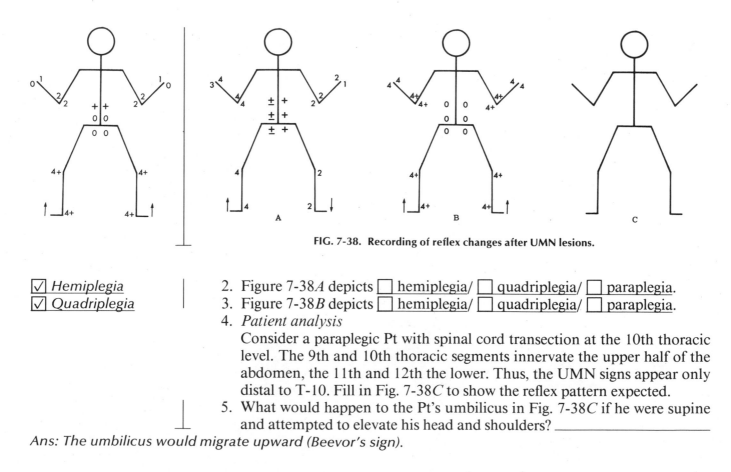

FIG. 7-38. Recording of reflex changes after UMN lesions.

☑ *Hemiplegia*
☑ *Quadriplegia*

2. Figure 7-38*A* depicts ☐ hemiplegia/ ☐ quadriplegia/ ☐ paraplegia.
3. Figure 7-38*B* depicts ☐ hemiplegia/ ☐ quadriplegia/ ☐ paraplegia.
4. *Patient analysis*
   Consider a paraplegic Pt with spinal cord transection at the 10th thoracic level. The 9th and 10th thoracic segments innervate the upper half of the abdomen, the 11th and 12th the lower. Thus, the UMN signs appear only distal to T-10. Fill in Fig. 7-38*C* to show the reflex pattern expected.
5. What would happen to the Pt's umbilicus in Fig. 7-38*C* if he were supine and attempted to elevate his head and shoulders? _____

Ans: *The umbilicus would migrate upward (Beevor's sign).*

X. Summary of the standard "textbook" syndromes of UMN and LMN lesions and their variations

A. *Complete Table 7-6 to summarize the typical findings in a Pt with a chronic UMN lesion.*

UMN	LMN
✓	
	✓
✓	
	✓
	✓
✓	
	✓
✓	
✓	
	✓
✓	*
✓	

TABLE 7-6 Clinical syndrome of UMN and LMN lesions

1 UMN	2 LMN	3 Characteristic
		Paralyzes movements in hemiplegic, quadriplegic, or paraplegic distribution, not individual muscles
		Paralyzes individual muscles or sets of muscles in root or peripheral nerve distributions
		Atrophy of disuse only (late and slight)
		Atrophy of denervation (early and severe)
		Fasciculations and fibrillations
		Hyperactive MSRs
		Hypoactive or absent MSRs
		Clonus
		Clasp-knife spasticity
		Hypotonia
	*	Absent abdominal-cremasteric reflexes
		Extensor toe sign

*Note: Direct disease of the LMNs to the effector muscles abolishes these reflexes, but disease confined to other LMNs does not.

B. *Clinical variations in the pyramidal (UMN) syndrome.* The level of the lesion along the course of the pyramidal tract (Fig. 2-15) determines the distribution of the weakness and other UMN signs. For the effect on the gait, see the gait essay at the end of Chap. 8.

1. *Standard hemiplegic distribution.* Unilateral interruption of the pyramidal tract at any level from the cortex to the caudal level of the pons causes weakness of the the contralateral side of the body, from the lower facial muscles on down (Fig. 6-5*B*). The arm is weaker than the leg and the finger movements are weakest of all. The degree of paralysis depends on how many of the million or so axons of the pyramidal tract (DeMyer, 1959) the lesion interrupts.

2. *Double hemiplegia.* The lesion interrupts both pyramidal tracts rostral to the medulla. The lower part of the face is affected bilaterally as are all four extremities. The Pt also shows *pseudobulbar palsy.*

3. *Pseudobulbar palsy.* Bilateral interruption of the corticobulbar component of the pyramidal tract, at cerebral or brainstem levels, causes weakness of the oropharyngeal muscles with dysphagia, dysarthria, and spastic dysphonia. In direct contrast to the loss of volitional control of the bulbar muscles, the Pt is emotionally labile and shows exaggerated smiling and crying responses.

4. *Spastic diplegia.* Bilateral pre- or perinatal cerebral lesions may result in a bilateral pyramidal syndrome with the legs more affected than the arms, and the bulbar muscles relatively spared. This reverses the arm-leg gradient of the weakness of double hemiplegia. Spastic diplegics often display involuntary movements, such as athetosis.

5. *Locked-in syndrome.* Bilateral interruption of the pyramidal tracts in the basis pontis or cerebral peduncules causes UMN paralysis of all volitional movements except vertical eye movements. The Pts remain conscious and not demented but are "locked-in" to themselves by the paralysis. See Chap. 12.

6. *Quadriplegia (tetraplegia).* Bilateral interruption of the pyramidal tracts in the caudal medulla or cervical region paralyzes the volitional movements of the trunk and all four extremities, with loss of volitional bladder and bowel control and of volitional control of breathing. The lesion spares those corticobulbar fibers to the face and bulbar muscles which depart rostral to the medullary level (Ropper et al, 1979; Chokroverty et al, 1975).

7. *Paraplegia.* Bilateral interruption of the pyramidal tracts caudal to the cervical region spares the arms but causes UMN paralysis of the legs, with loss of bladder and bowel control.

8. *Monoplegia.* A small lesion of the motor cortex or internal capsule, where the pyramidal fibers have a discrete somatotopic arrangement, may cause contralateral weakness of only one arm or one leg. Interruption of the pyramidal tract on one side of the thoracic spinal cord causes monoplegia of the ipsilateral leg.

C. *Paralysis and sensory deficits immediately after acute spinal cord transection*

1. Spinal cord transection at the medullocervical junction or at segments C-1 to C-3 (Fig. 2-5) results in complete apnea, complete quadriplegia, and complete anesthesia caudal to the lesion. The Pt dies of hypoxia within minutes unless given artificial respiration. The blood pressure also drops because interruption of the reticulospinal tracts stops the downflow of vasoconstrictor tone to the preganglionic sympathetic neurons in the intermediolateral column of the spinal cord. The sensorimotor deficits affect only the trunk and legs if the lesion is caudal to T-1 (paraplegia).

2. During the stage of spinal shock, the Pt loses all somatomotor and most visceromotor responses caudal to the level of the lesion. The Pt shows flaccid paralysis of somatic muscles and sphincters, and flaccid (atonic) bladder and bowel paralysis, with incontinence. All superficial and deep reflexes and most autonomic reflexes are abolished. If any visceral-related function remains it is usually anal sphincter tone.

3. Gradually the classical UMN signs of increased MSRs, spasticity, and extensor toe signs will appear, as well as reflex emptying of the bladder and bowel. In contrast, slowly evolving spinal cord compression results in spastic paralysis from the start. The Pt does not go through a phase of spinal shock.

4. After the phase of spinal shock, the transected spinal cord, isolated from the brain, can mediate simple reflexes, such as MSRs and flexor withdrawal responses to pain. It can also mediate reflex sweating, piloerection, micturition, defecation, and ejaculation (although the Pt feels no sensation), but it cannot produce respiratory drive, respiratory related reflexes, like coughing, sneezing, and hiccoughing which require coordination of bulbar and spinal muscles, nor any volitional, goal-directed movements. In other words, the spinal cord, when separated from the brain, can reflexly twitch some muscles, sweat, and ejaculate, and reflexly eliminate urine and feces, but the isolated spinal cord cannot breathe or move muscles voluntarily. These actions require intact reticulospinal and corticospinal tracts from the brain.

D. *Pt analysis*
1. *Medical history.* This 57-year-old man awakened one morning unable to move his right side and with double vision. He noticed mild numbness and tingling of his right side. When he called to his wife, he noticed that his speech was slurred. He had been diabetic and hypertensive for many years.
2. *Physical findings.* The Pt was conscious, cooperative, and intact mentally. He could not abduct his left eye. He had mild dysarthria. He had severe weakness of the right extremities, including the lower part of his face. His right extremities were flaccid and somewhat hyporeflexic. He had a flexor plantar response on the left but little response at all on the right. He was somewhat less responsive to pain and touch on the right side.
3. *Lesion localization*
    a. Before continuing with the text, you may want to try to reach your own conclusions as to where and what the lesion is. It may help you to review the brainstem cross sections, Figs. 2-15 to 2-18, page 54.
    b. In localizing a single lesion to explain the Pt's findings, we first of all assemble the data that require explanation. The weakness, in a hemiplegic distribution, indicates interruption of the pyramidal tract in the acute stage, when the reflexes may be temporarily reduced or absent. The slight sensory findings suggest some involvement of a sensory pathway. The inability to abduct the left eye indicates a VIth nerve palsy. Therefore the Ex should "think circuitry" by visualizing the course of the pyramidal tract to try to locate a site where it comes into anatomic relation with a somatosensory pathway and the VIth cranial nerve.

☑ Pons; ☑ left (Fig. 2-16)

    c. The association of a LMN VIth nerve palsy on the *left* and hemiplegia of the *right* extremities suggests a lesion in the basis of the ☐ mesencephalon/ ☐ pons/ ☐ medulla on the ☐ right/ ☐ left side.
    d. Magnetic resonance imaging (MRI) scans showed the evolution of a cavitating infarct in the basis pontis near the pontomedullary junction, where the VIth nerve runs on the lateral margin of the pyramidal tract before exiting at the pontomedullary junction. At this level of the neuraxis, the pathway for somatic sensation via the medial lemniscus has already crossed the midline. Review Fig. 2-16, page 54, to see how a single pontine lesion could explain the left VIth nerve palsy, right-sided pyramidal tract signs, and right-sided sensory findings. The Pt has the classical localizing findings of a brainstem lesion, a cranial nerve palsy on one side and long tract signs on the other (Fig. 6-15).
    e. What normal findings in our Pt would indicate that the dorsal part of the pontine tegmentum is intact? _____

    Hint: again review Fig. 2-16, page 54, to see what structures would have caused clinical signs if they had been destroyed. For example, does he show a medial longitudinal fasciculus (MLF) syndrome?

Ans: Normal facial movements and no MLF syndrome.

    f. Since the Pt's hemiparesis included his face, the lesion in the caudal end of the basis pontis destroyed the corticobulbar axons to the VIIth nerve nucleus. What does this fact tell you about how far the corticobulbar UMN fibers to the face accompany the rest of the pyramidal tract? ____
    _____

Ans: The corticobulbar fibers must accompany the other pyramidal tract fibers to at least the caudal end of the pons before departing for the VIIth nerve nucleus in the pontine tegmentum. Lesions of the pyramidal tract at the medullary level usually spare the UMN facial fibers, since they have already left the tract (Ropper et al, 1979).

5. *Clinical course.* After several days the MSRs on the right began to be hyperactive and spasticity, clonus, and a classical extensor toe sign appeared. The Pt did not regain any useful movements of his arm or fingers and could only walk when his leg was supported by a brace. His right VIth nerve palsy also remained but the sensory loss disappeared, indicating only a transient ischemia of the medial lemniscus.

REFERENCES FOR THE PYRAMIDAL TRACT

Chokroverty S, Rubino F, and Haller C: Pure motor hemiplegia due to pyramidal infarction. *Arch Neurol* 1975; 32:647–648

DeMyer W: Number of axons and myelin sheaths in adult human medullary pyramids. *Neurology* 1959; 9:42–47

Jagiella WM, Sung JH: Bilateral infarction of the medullary pyramids in humans. *Neurology* 1989; 39:21–24

Lenn NJ, Freinkel AJ: Facial sparing as a feature of prenatal-onset hemiparesis. *Pediatr Neurol* 1989; 5:291–295

Nyberg-Hansen R, Rinvik E: Some comments on the pyramidal tract with special reference to its individual variations in man. *Acta Neurol Scand* 1963; 39:1–30

Paulsen GW, Yates AJ, Paltan-Ortiz JD: Does infarction of the medullary pyramid lead to spasticity? *Arch Neurol* 1986; 43:93–95

Ropper AH, Fisher CM, Kleinman GM: Pyramidal infarction in the medulla: A cause of pure motor hemiplegia sparing the face. *Neurology* 1979; 29:91–95

Walshe F: On the role of the pyramidal system in willed movements. *Brain* 1947; 70:329–354

XI. The concept of deficit and release phenomena after lesions of the motor and sensory pathways

Upon this gifted age, in its dark hour,
Rains from the sky a meteoric shower
Of facts . . . they lie unquestioned, uncombined,
Wisdom enough to leech us of our ill
Is daily spun, but there exists no loom
To weave it into fabric; . . .

Edna St. Vincent Millay (1892–1950)

A. *The theory of deficit and release phenomena.* By this time, the litany of positive and negative effects of neurologic lesions will surely have perplexed the student. Fortunately we can weave these effects into a dichotomous theory of *deficit* and *release* phenomena.

1. *Deficit phenomena* are sensorimotor functions that are lost after a neurologic lesion, e.g., loss of movement or loss of vision.

2. *Release phenomena* are sensorimotor functions that become increased or first emerge after a neurologic lesion. The release phenomenon may be an exaggeration of a normal action, e.g., hyperactive MSRs, or a new response, e.g., the change in the behavior of the large toe from flexion to extension (Babinski sign).

B. *Deficit and release phenomena after UMN (pyramidal) lesions*
1. Review the components of the UMN syndrome (Table 7-6) and list the deficit and release phenomena seen in the classical or chronic stage.
    a. Deficit phenomena: _____

        _____.

    b. Release phenomena: _____

        _____.

Ans: Deficit: paresis or paralysis, mild disuse atrophy, absence of abdominal and cremasteric reflexes, which may however return.
    Release: hyperactive MSRs, clonus, spasticity, and an extensor toe sign.

2. The extensor toe sign would be classed as a ☐ deficit/ ☐ release phenomenon because _____

    _____.

Ans: ☑ *Release phenomenon, because it is a new behavior or response not present before the UMN lesion and which is unmasked or released by the UMN lesion.*

☑ *Deficit*
☑ *Release*

3. In the acute phase after pyramidal tract interruption, particularly after spinal cord transection, the Pt may show only ☐ deficit/ ☐ release phenomena and no ☐ deficit/ ☐ release phenomena.

C. *Pathophysiology of release phenomena*
1. Release phenomena appear because the lesion has interrupted connections that presumably inhibited or suppressed the overactive function and because some intact pathway positively drives the overactivity.
2. Whether interruption of the pyramidal tract alone accounts for all of the release phenomena of the UMN syndrome remains in some question, but the clinician will make few errors in localization by assuming that pyramidal tract interruption is a necessary and sufficient condition for the full UMN syndrome to appear. Undoubtedly however, involvement of other sensory and motor pathways will condition the expression and degree of the various components of the UMN syndrome.

D. *Deficit and release phenomena after LMN lesions.* If we forsake a procrustean obstinacy, we can extend the deficit-release concept to the peripheral nervous system and even the sensory pathways.
1. *Deficit* phenomena after LMN lesions consist of
    a. Paresis or paralysis of individual muscles, in a segmental or peripheral nerve distribution
    b. Decreased or absent MSRs
    c. Denervation atrophy (early and severe atrophy)
2. *Release* phenomena after LMN lesions consist of
    a. Fasciculations
    b. Fibrillations
3. In the case of fasciculations, the disease of the LMN "releases" the depolarization mechanism of its own neuronal membrane, allowing the motor unit to fire randomly. In the case of fibrillations, the denervation results in a release of the depolarization mechanism of the individual muscle fibers, allowing them to fire randomly.

E. *Deficit phenomena after interruption of autonomic motor axons*
1. Paralysis and atony of smooth muscle, abolishing peristalsis, propulsion, and emptying

2. Vasomotor paralysis, with vasodilation, orthostatic hypotension, and impotence
3. Anhidrosis
4. Trophic changes, consisting of hair loss, atrophy of skin, and dystrophy of nails

F. *Autonomic release or irritative phenomena after peripheral nerve lesions.* In certain instances lesions of peripheral nerves (or spinal cord lesions) release autonomic signs of *hyperhidrosis* or *vasoconstriction,* rather than anhidrosis and vasodilation (see causalgia in Chap. 10).

G. *Deficit and release phenomena after lesions of the basal motor nuclei (see section L, page 272)*

XII. Involuntary movement disorders

A. *Introduction to the concept of voluntary and involuntary movements and the notion of free will*
1. We experience ourselves as having free will. This experience leads us to classify behaviors intuitively as *voluntary* and *involuntary.* But then we must puzzle over behaviors like breathing, bladder and bowel emptying, and postural reflexes that straddle the voluntary-involuntary dichotomy. For example, you can freely will yourself to hold your breath for a period of time, but ultimately you simply have to breathe. You have no choice. The physiologic imperative to act overpowers the will. Mental Pts often experience their behaviors and even their very thoughts as involuntary or directed by external forces. Thus, Pts come to the physician because they do, indeed, have behaviors and thoughts that they cannot willfully control.
2. By virtue of operational definitions and observation of the pattern of movements, we can identify certain movements and behaviors that we can all agree qualify as involuntary.

B. *Working definition of voluntary and involuntary movements*
1. A *voluntary* movement is one that the standard normal person can start or stop at the person's own command or an observer's command.
2. An *involuntary* movement is one that the standard normal person cannot stop at the person's own or an observer's command.
   a. As strictly construed by neurologists, involuntary movements mean those patterns of muscle contractions (tremors and other movement sequences) caused by identifiable structural or biochemical lesions in the circuitry of the basal motor nuclei, reticular formation, and cerebellum.
   b. Broadly construed the concept of involuntary movements can also include the gamut of all muscle fiber contractions of peripheral as well as cortical origin, thus ranging from fibrillations to epileptic seizures.

C. *Clinical operations for identifying voluntary and involuntary movements*
Disease produces patterns of involuntary movements, recognizable from the history and inspection. The operations for clinical diagnosis of involuntary movements are these:
1. Find out when the movements started, what conditions trigger or alleviate the movements, their relation to sleep and emotion, and their evolution over time. In other words, what is the history?

2. Describe the pattern of the movements, their distribution, rate, amplitude, and force. In other words, what are the physical findings? Inspection is pivotal, allowing recognition without recourse to the Pt's testimony, in most cases. To see is to diagnose, because most involuntary movements fall into stereotyped, identifiable patterns (Fig. 14-3).

D. *Some normal involuntary movements*

1. *Physiologic synkinesias* (syn = with; kinesis = motion). A synkinesia is an involuntary or automatic movement that accompanies a voluntary movement. Close your eyes voluntarily and your eyeballs automatically roll up (Bell's phenomenon). Walk and your arms swing. Lean forward and your leg muscles automatically brace. Use these examples to identify other synkinesias (hint: what about convergence?) The degree of volition in the synkinesias varies. You can't stop Bell's phenomenon, but you can stop your arms from swinging when walking.

2. *Myoclonic jerks*

   a. Myoclonic jerks are sudden, shocklike twitches of individual muscles or sets of muscles. A myoclonic twitch may appear in a single muscle, such as the biceps, perhaps after unaccustomed work. Or a more widespread startle response may cause an upright jerk of the head as the person falls asleep. A sudden discharge in the reticular activating system of the brainstem causes the lightning, myoclonic jerk of the head and the sudden restoration of consciousness.

   b. Epileptic myoclonic jerks, often refractory to treatment, occur in many serious diseases of the CNS. What is *physiologic* under one circumstance is *pathologic* under another.

   c. Myoclonic jerks are separate from fasciculations. Define a fasciculation.

   _____

   _____

   _____

Ans: *A fasciculation is a twitch of a small part of a muscle due to random discharge of a LMN and its fascicle of muscle fibers (a motor unit discharge).*

Myoclonic

Fasciculation

   d. A twitch of a whole muscle or groups of muscles is called a _____ jerk, while a twitch of a single fascicle of muscle is called a _____.

3. *Benign fasciculations*

   a. Fasciculations appear in some normal persons, particularly after exercise. If the person has no weakness or other signs of LMN disease, the diagnosis is *benign fasciculations.* Twitching of an eyelid is a benign fasciculation.

   b. What clinical and EMG findings would differentiate pathologic from benign fasciculations? _____

   _____

   _____

Ans: *If LMN disease causes the fasciculations, the Ex should find the full syndrome of LMN disease: weakness, hypo- or areflexia, hypotonia, and denervation atrophy, as supported by EMG evidence of fibrillations and giant polyphasic motor units along with the fasciculations.*

4. *Physiologic tremor.* See next section.

E. *Tremors*

1. *Definition.* Tremors are rhythmic, more or less regular oscillations of a body part. The part oscillates usually around a fixed point and in one plane.

Several phenomena, such as clonus, shivering, and nystagmus, although more or less meeting this definition, are generally excluded from a discussion of tremor per se.

2. *Clinical characteristics of tremor.* Tremors differ in distribution, rate, amplitude, relation to rest or movement, and in their relation to sleep and emotion, in their response to drugs, and in their pathogenesis or lesion site (Elble and Koller, 1990).

    a. *Distribution.* Tremors most commonly affect the hands, jaw, tongue, and head, but may affect the trunk or legs.

    b. *Rate.* Tremors vary in rate between 3 and 12 cycles per second (cps).

    c. *Amplitude.* Tremors vary from barely perceptible to gross.

    d. *Relation of tremors to movement, posture, or rest.* Tremors occur under four conditions, thus classifying tremors into four types.

        (1) Tremor while the part is at rest: resting tremor.

        (2) Tremor while the part is making a voluntary movement: intention or ataxic tremor.

        (3) Tremor while the part is sustaining a volitional posture: postural tremor.

        (4) Tremor which increases as the part reaches an endpoint, such as finger to nose: terminal or endpoint tremor.

    e. *Response of tremors to sleep and emotion.* Like virtually all involuntary movements, tremors generally dampen or disappear during tranquility and cease during sleep. Likewise anxiety and emotional tension generally increase tremors and other involuntary movements.

    f. *Response of tremors to drugs.* Specific drugs may increase or decrease tremor, e.g., alcohol and propanolol decrease physiologic or essential tremor, while adrenalin increases such tremors. Anticholinergic drugs or dopamine decrease the rest tremor of parkinsonism.

    g. *Lesion site for tremors.* No single "tremorogenic" center exists. Tremors generally arise from disruption of the feedback circuits of the basal motor nuclei (Fig. 2-30), brainstem tegmentum, and the cerebellum.

    h. *Brief clinical classification of tremors* (Fig. 7-39)

3. *Physiologic tremor and its pathologic variations*

    a. *Self-demonstration of physiologic tremor.* Insert a large sheet of paper between your index finger and the adjacent finger, and hold your arm straight out in front of you. The rustling of the paper demonstrates *physiologic tremor*. The tremor has a frequency of about 10 cps.

    b. Physiologic tremor is generally low in amplitude, relatively rapid (6–13 cps), and is most evident when sustaining a posture, as when holding the arms extended, or during movements. It varies from 6 cps in childhood, to 8 to 13 cps in adulthood, and back to around 6 cps in senility.

    c. Physiologic tremor arises from a combination of neurally mediated oscillations and the ballistic effects of respiratory and cardiac actions (ballistocardiogram). Thus, it has both *neurologic* and *mechanical* origins.

    d. *Emotional tremor* is possibly an exacerbation of physiologic tremor. It occurs at rest, but it worsens during volitional movement: witness the quavering knees and voice of the novice orator. From personal experience you know that emotional tremor is ☐ rapid/ ☐ very slow and of ☐ very great/ ☐ relatively low amplitude.

    e. *Familial or essential tremor* is similar in frequency to physiologic tremor, about 10 cps, but of greater amplitude. The lesion site is unknown (Rajput et al, 1991). It affects the hands predominantly, but

☑ *Rapid*
☑ *Relatively low*

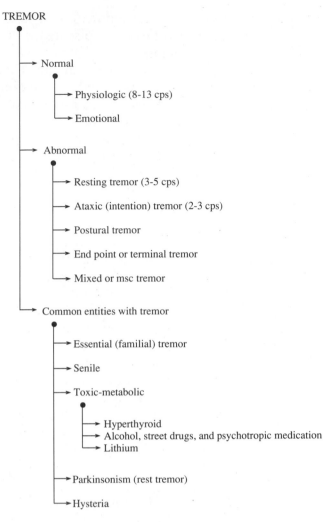

FIG. 7-39. Brief classification of tremors.

may affect the head and bulbar muscles (Lou and Jankovic, 1991). It usually follows an autosomal dominant hereditary pattern.

    f. Senile tremor has a frequency of about 6 to 10 cps. Senile and familial tremor merge in their clinical manifestations, but senile tremor, while frequently familial, may result from nonfamilial lesions of aging.

4. *Parkinsonian tremor and parkinsonism.* Parkinsonian tremor has a frequency of 3 to 6 cps and low to moderate amplitude. It appears when the part is at rest and increases during emotional tension, but disappears or dampens during intentional movement. Drum your fingertips on the table, timing 25 beats per 5 seconds, to observe two features of this tremor: moderate frequency and relatively low amplitude. Typically affecting the hands and digits, the rustling of the thumb against the pads of the fingers resembles pill-rolling; hence it is called a *pill-rolling tremor.* The cause of parkinsonism is degeneration of the dopaminergic axons that run from the substantia nigra of the midbrain to the striatum.

    a. Parkinsonian tremor differs from emotional tremor by ☐ increasing/ ☐ decreasing during volitional movement, and resembles other involuntary movements by ☐ increasing/ ☐ decreasing during emotional stress.

    b. The resting tremor of parkinsonism, a hyperkinesia, contrasts with a reduction in the overall mobility of the Pt, called *bradykinesia.* Para-

☑ *Decreasing*
☑ *Increasing*

doxically, an irresistible need to move, a physiologic imperative called *akathisia,* also plagues the Pt, requiring abrupt, restless shifts of position against the bradykinetic background. In a given Pt, one or more of the signs may predominate. Thus one Pt displays mainly tremor and the next mainly rigidity (Duvoisin, 1990). The basic motor signs of parkinsonism include a quatrain of:

(1) Resting tremor

(2) Lead-pipe rigidity, often with "a cog wheeling," ratchet-like yielding due to the superimposition of the beats of the tremor

(3) Overall bradykinesia

(4) Akathisia.

    c. Derivative signs of the rigidity of the laryngeal muscles are loss of inflections of the voice resulting in a monotonous tone, "plateau speech," and words running together (Caekebeke et al, 1991). Rigidity of the facial muscles results in an absence of emotional expression, a "masked face."

    d. Oculogyric crises are spasms of upward deviation of the eyes, or eyes and head (Clough et al, 1983; Onuaguluchi, 1961). Common in parkinsonism, oculogyric crises may occur in other disorders of the basal motor nuclei. Summarize for yourself the motor manifestations of parkinsonism.

5. *Intention (ataxic) tremor* is a somewhat irregular tremor of low to moderate amplitude that appears during intentional movements. At rest, the hand remains still, but upon movement, as when the Pt brings the finger to touch the nose, mild to moderate deviations detour the part from a straight line.

6. *Postural or position maintenance tremor* occurs during the maintenance of an intentional posture, such as holding the head up, the trunk erect, or the hands outstretched. When extended in front of the Pt, the hands show a regular, rhythmic tremor of several cycles per second. If the Pt brings the finger in to touch his nose, the tremor may dampen or intention tremor may appear. As the finger approaches the nose and the Pt attempts to stop the finger to maintain a position, the tremor reappears or heightens as an endpoint or terminal tremor. When the finger actually touches the nose, the tremor may dampen. When the Pt returns the hands to his lap, at rest, the tremor disappears. *Intention* and *postural tremor* appear in various degrees and combinations. They implicate a lesion of the cerebellum or its efferent pathways. The combination of a rest tremor, intention tremor, and postural tremor constitutes so-called *rubral tremor,* implying a lesion of the dentatorubral or dentatothalamic tract (Berkovic and Bladin, 1984; Samie et al, 1990).

7. *Mixed and miscellaneous types of tremors.* A number of tremors, as with hyperthyroidism, lithium administration, delirium, and drug overdosage or withdrawal (including alcohol), share features of one or more of the foregoing types of tremors or may be an enhancement of physiologic tremor. Psychogenic tremors have inconsistent, complicated patterns and change in intensity with circumstances (Koller et al, 1989).

    F. The kymographic records of tremors

     1. From these kymographic recordings, identify the type of tremor and the pathophysiologic basis:

      a. The Pt is sitting quietly in a chair. An accelerometer attached to a hand records this tremor (Fig. 7-40).

      b. The rate of the tremor is about _____ cps.

      c. Since the tremor occurs at rest but disappears during intentional movement, it is classified as a ☐ rest/ ☐ intention/ ☐ postural tremor.

5 or 6

☑ *Rest tremor*

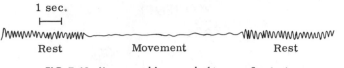

Rest   Movement   Rest

FIG. 7-40. Kymographic record of tremor. See text.

Parkinsonism

    d. This type of tremor signifies a lesion of the extrapyramidal pathways and is characteristic of the disorder called _____ (eponym).

2. The next Pt was sitting quietly, holding her arms extended in front, at shoulder level. Only a faint instability appeared. Figure 7-41 shows the tremor that occurred when the Pt attempted to touch her index finger to her nose. After she reached her nose, she showed very little tremor.

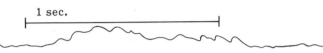

Arms out-   Moving finger in to touch nose   At rest on nose
stretched

FIG. 7-41. Kymographic record of tremor. See text.

Intention (ataxic)
  tremor
☑ *Cerebellar*

    a. The tremor in Fig. 7-37 is called _____ tremor.

    b. It signifies a lesion of the ☐ pyramidal/ ☐ basal ganglia/ ☐ cerebellar pathways.

3. The next Pt had no tremor when sitting still, but when she held her arms straight out, a tremor appeared (Fig. 7-42).

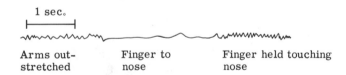

Arms out-   Finger to   Finger held touching
stretched   nose   nose

FIG. 7-42. Kymographic record of tremor. See text.

☑ *Postural tremor*
Cerebellum

☑ *Parkinsonian*

    a. After she reached her nose, the tremor was accentuated. The tremor shown in the initial and last part of Fig. 7-38 is called ☐ resting/ ☐ physiological/ ☐ postural tremor.
    b. It signifies a lesion of the _____ or its efferent pathways.
    c. Since it dampens during movement, postural tremor is like ☑ parkinsonian/ ☑ intention/ ☑ essential tremor.
    d. Give the full clinical characteristics of parkinsonian tremor. _____

_____

_____

Ans: Parkinsonian tremor appears at rest, has a low amplitude and a regular
   frequency of 5 cps, disappears during intentional movement, and increases
   during emotional stress.

    G. *Review of tremors.* Before proceeding with the text, review the tremorous hyperkinesias by actually *acting them out* (Figs. 7-40 to 7-42). If necessary organize your own table or differential diagnostic dendrogram.

REFERENCES FOR TREMOR

Berkovic SF, Bladin PF: Rubral tremor: clinical features and treatment of three cases. *Clin Exp Neurol* 1984; 20:119–128

Caekebeke JFV, Jennekens-Schinkel A, van der Linden ME et al: The interpretation of dysprosody in patients with Parkinson's disease. *J Neurol Neurosurg Psychiatry* 1991; 54:145–148

Clough CG, Plaitakis A, Yahr MD: Oculogyric crises and Parkinsonism. *Arch Neurol* 1983; 40:36–37

Duvoisin RC: *Parkinson's Disease* (3d ed). New York, Raven, 1990

Elble RJ, Koller WO, *Tremor (Johns Hopkins Series in Contemporary Medicine and Public Health)* Baltimore, Johns Hopkins University Press, 1990

Koller W, Lang A, Vetere-Overfield B et al: Psychogenic tremors. *Neurology* 1989; 39:1094–1099

Lou JS, Jankovic J: Essential tremor: Clinical correlates in 350 patients. *Neurology* 1991; 41:234–238

Onuaguluchi G: Crises in post-encephalitic Parkinsonism. *Brain* 1961; 84:395–414

Rajput AH, Rozdilsky B, Ang L et al: Clinicopathologic observations in essential tremor: Report of six cases. *Neurology* 1991; 41:1422–1424

Samie MR, Selhorst JB, Koller WC: Post-traumatic midbrain tremors. *Neurology,* 1990; 40:62–66.

H. *Nontremorous types of hyperkinesias* (Chokroverty, 1990; Klawans et al, 1988; Lang and Weiner, 1992).

   1. *Chorea* refers to incessant, random, moderately quick movements—a grimace, elevation of a finger or arm, a misstep when walking, an interruption when speaking. Overall, chorea resembles the "fidgets." One part or another of the body is flickering into motion all of the time. The movements resemble a choreographer working out the movements for a dance, or, perhaps better described, they simulate fragments of normal movements. For instance, at one time or another, after starting to make an inappropriate movement (perhaps reaching up to pick your nose), you may have suddenly decided to arrest it midway. Or after starting such a movement, you may have diverted it to brushing back your hair. Nevertheless, an observer can perceive the stoppage or the diversion in the continuity of the initial movement.

   2. *Athetosis* refers to slow, writhing movements of the fingers and extremities. If severe, athetosis affects speech and some proximal movements. These movements come and go and generally do not hold the part in a fixed posture. Athetosis often accompanies or follows partial interruption of the pyramidal tracts, particularly in cerebral palsy Pts with spastic quadriplegia or diplegia. The quick random fidgety movements called _____ contrast with the slow writhing distal movements called _____ .

Chorea
Athetosis

   3. *Dystonia* refers to prolonged, slow, alternating contraction and relaxation of agonists and antagonists. The prolonged muscular contractions hold the part in one position for periods of time, and may lead to pretzel-like body positions with fixed scoliosis and fixed contractures of joints.

      a. *Focal dystonia,* such as spasmodic torticollis and writer's cramp, may affect more or less restricted muscular groups (DeMyer, 1977).

      b. The sustained postural deviations of dystonia differ from the quick movements of chorea and the slower writhing, mainly distal movements called _____ .

Athetosis

      c. Although dystonia is traditionally classed as an extrapyramidal movement disorder, the lesion site and pathophysiology of the hereditary form are unknown (Zeman and Dyken, 1968). Dystonia can result from known lesions of the basal motor nuclei (Zeman and Whitlock, 1968).

4. *Hemiballismus* refers to violent flinging movements of one half of the body. *Ballista* means to throw, as in ballistics. The Pt's arm thrashes about as if it were trying to fling away a handful of snakes. Hemiballismus usually appears abruptly in elderly hypertensive Pts. The lesion is predictable. A peculiar, sharply delimited hemorrhage destroys the contralateral subthalamic nucleus of Luys or its immediate surrounding pathways. This almond-sized and almond-shaped diencephalic nucleus belongs to the basal motor nuclei.

5. *Tics* are quick, lightning-fast, stereotyped movements of face, tongue, or upper extremities (Jankovic and Tolosa, 1988). In contrast to the preceding hyperkinesias, the sequence of movements is identical each time if the Pt has only one type of tic. However the Pt may have multiple different kinds of tics. All of us display minor tics: wrinkling of the forehead, followed by blinking the eyes, or hitching up the trousers, or a shrug of the shoulder. Athletes display a number of tic-like maneuvers, as when a basketball player prepares to shoot a free throw, or a tennis player prepares to serve. Tics increase during emotional stress. Although mostly of low amplitude, tics, when violent, may throw the Pt to the floor, thus resembling an exaggerated startle response called *hyperexplexia.* Some tics are regarded as psychogenic, but an organic syndrome (syndrome of Gilles de la Tourette) consists of multiple tics that change from time to time; the involuntary production of sounds, such as squawks, barks, or howls; the utterance of expletives; and obsessive-compulsive, often abrasive, personality traits (Shapiro et al, 1988; Trimble, 1989). Of the movement disorders discussed, tics, being quick, and usually of low to moderate amplitude, most closely resemble ☐ chorea/ ☐ athetosis/ ☐ hemiballismus, but they differ from the other hyperkinesias in being ☐ purely random/ ☐ very stereotyped in pattern.

☑ *Chorea*
☑ *Very stereotyped*

6. *Duration of the patterned hyperkinesias.* Dystonia, athetosis, and chorea represent way stations along a continuum of involuntary movements, not necessarily discrete entities. They differ perhaps more in their speed than in any other way. Tics and chorea rank fastest, each individual movement measured in a second or even less, a little faster than myoclonic jerks (but sometimes hard to distinguish from them). Next comes athetosis, lasting just a little longer, in seconds. Then comes dystonia, which lasts many seconds to minutes, or even longer, as in spasmodic torticollis, a form of dystonia in which the head remains deviated for long periods of time. As an oversimplified 1, 2, 3 mnemonic, think of each individual tic as less than a second, choreiform movements as lasting 1 second, athetosis as 1 to 3 seconds, and dystonia as longer than 3 seconds. Hemiballismus differs from chorea in its more violent amplitude and in being more commonly unilateral.

I. *Drug-induced extrapyramidal movement syndromes and the tardive dyskinesias.* Various tranquilizers, antipsychotics, and antidepressant drugs alter the balance of neurotransmitters in the basal motor circuits (Yassa et al, 1990). These chemical lesions mimic the effect of anatomic lesions, producing hypo- and hyperkinesias, ranging from parkinsonism to dystonia, but typically causing Meig's syndrome, which consists predominately of facial, oral, buccal, and pharyngeal movements with dysphonia and dysphagia (Lang and Weiner, 1992). Unfortunately, tardive dyskinesia may be permanent and very resistant to therapy.

J. *Akathisia, restless legs, and hyperactivity*

1. *Akathisia.* The Pt displays motor unrest manifested by continual shifting of positions and sometimes by restlessly walking about. When questioned, the Pts often report an actual feeling in their muscles of an urge to move. Akathisia appears typically in Parkinson's disease and also in other diseases of the basal motor nuclei.

2. *Restless legs syndrome (Ekbom's syndrome; Ekbom, 1960).* When attempting to rest or sleep, these Pts feel an irresistible urge, a necessity, to move their legs around. No force of will can hold the legs still against the pathophysiologic imperative, and the aimless, incessant wandering of the legs prevents the onset of sleep. Exhaustive exercise or some drugs, such as antihistamines, may induce restless legs.

3. *The hyperactive child.* Hyperactive children display incessant, rapidly changing motor activity, often starting in infancy. Their driven, inappropriate, and usually annoying activity consists of fidgeting, pushing, pulling, banging, rummaging, clamoring, whining, and running. The hyperactivity continues with little regard for other people, or danger, and responds but little to reward and punishment. Rather than a standard, stereotyped pattern like athetosis or dystonia, the disorder consists of the sheer quantity of activity. Usually these children are so clamorous that my secretary can diagnose them by the noise they make as they clatter down the long hall to my office. By stretching the imagination, we might think of restless legs as a localized type of akathisia, and of childhood hyperactivity as its generalized childhood counterpart. No specific known brain lesion underlies this common hyperkinesia, but most hyperkinetic children have other subtle or overt evidence of brain damage or frank mental retardation. The foregoing syndromes of drivenness border on a variety of cursive states such as compulsive walking or running and cursive epilepsy.

4. *Self-mutilation.* The Pt compulsively inflicts self-injury by biting, scratching, or pounding, in spite of all punishments or rewards. While generally seen in mentally retarded Pts, some individuals with normal intelligence scratch, bite fingernails, pick their nose or lips or otherwise injure themselves compulsively (neurodermatitis) in response to some pathophysiologic imperative that overcomes willpower. Smoking with its intermittent irritation of the lungs may fall into the same category. The Pt scratches, as it were, the respiratory mucosa.

K. *Epilepsy* is any change in the mental, motor, or sensory state of the Pt caused by abnormal hypersynchronous discharge of neurons. Epileptic involuntary motor activity may consist of tonic or clonic spasms and myoclonic jerks that affect all or part of the body, or of complex automatisms with laughter and cursive states during psychomotor seizures. If epilepsy causes the abnormal motor activity, the Pt will usually lose consciousness and have amnesia for the episode, and the EEG usually shows epileptiform activity (See Chap. 13).

L. *The concept of deficit and release phenomena after lesions of the basal motor connections (For general discussion see Section XI, page 262 of this chapter)*

1. *Deficit phenomena* include overall bradykinesia, difficulty in walking, masked facies, and loss of voice inflection.

2. *Release phenomena* include a form of hypertonia called lead-pipe rigidity, tremor (generally tremor of the part at rest), akathisia, and patterned hyperkinesias such as tics, chorea, athetosis, dystonia, and hemiballismus.

How the other syndromes of excessive behavior relate to this scheme is uncertain.

M. *Rating scales for involuntary movements.* Various rating scales such as the AIMS (Abnormal Involuntory Movement Scale) scale enable the Ex to quantify various involuntary movements to determine the degree of disability, to follow the course of the disease, and to identify the effects of treatment (Marsden and Schachter, 1981).

N. *Avoiding pitfalls (pratfalls) in distinguishing psychogenic and organic motility disturbances*
   1. Hysterical movement disorders or malingering may imitate organic movement disorders. See Chap. 13.
   2. Anxiety or emotional tension makes virtually all hyperkinesias worse, but they dampen or disappear when the Pt is relaxed or asleep. Only a few abnormal involuntary movements occur during sleep: sleep myoclonus, palatal myoclonus (actually palatal tremor), somnambulism, and some epileptic seizures.
   3. During the evolution of one illness, the form of the hyperkinesias or the degree of hypo- or hypertonia may change. Hence, what starts as a flaccid hemiparesis may end as spastic hemiparesis. Simple athetosis may end as dystonia or so-called *tension athetosis,* in which the harder the Pt tries to make a voluntary movement, the more the part goes into an athetoid or dystonic spasm. Torsion dystonia and tension athetosis are classic examples of pathophysiologic imperatives that determine the behavior of the muscles rather than the Pt's "will."
   4. Frequent causes today of hypokinetic or hyperkinetic motility disturbances are psychotrophic medications, alcohol, and street drugs. Consider drugs in the differential diagnosis of tremors or any other movement disorder of new onset.
   5. Mothers of hyperactive children invariably appear distraught, depressed, and defeated by their inability to cope with their child. Usually the child's hyperactivity discloses itself by the slap-dash, frenetic way the child executes the Ex's requests. If, however, the child appears calm during the period of examination, as a few will, the Ex may mistakenly conclude that the mother is "overanxious." The usual problem is an underanxious physician, not an overanxious mother. Thus the immediate inspection of the Pt, which serves so well to recognize the standard hyperkinesias of extrapyramidal origin, may on some occasions fail in recognizing the hyperactive child if the observation period is too brief. On the next visit, detain the child in the waiting room for a considerable period before the appointment. Then, after the child has demolished your decor, scattered the toys all over the reception room (without actually playing with any), has exasperated your other Pts, and driven your receptionist mad, you will understand the mother's plight.

O. *Patient analysis.*
   The Pt is a mentally normal 47-year-old woman who was born with mild spastic cerebral palsy. Her motor disorder has not changed over the decades since childhood. For the serial photographs, she was requested to extend her arms out in front of her and to hold them as still as possible. Similar movements appear when she is at rest or walking. The movements have a slow rate and low

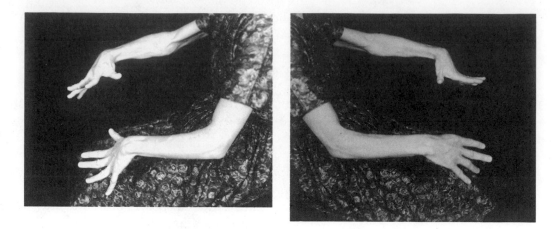

FIG. 7-43. Action sequence of involuntary movements.

Athetosis

to moderate force and amplitude. The movements in Fig. 7-43 would best be classified as _____.

P. *A summary of involuntary movements (hyperkinesias) by operational definition*

1. For clinical diagnosis, I have defined hyperkinesias broadly to include *any* extra muscular activity of peripheral or central origin, caused by a lesion of the nervous system.
2. For the clinical characteristics in *a* to *s*, write down the proper descriptive diagnosis in the blank to the right. Where possible, act out the motility disorder described.

Fibrillations

    a. Spontaneous random contractions of denervated muscle fibers, detected by EMG.

    a. _____

Fasciculations

    b. Spontaneous random twitches of small parts of muscles, detected by clinical inspection and EMG.

    b. _____

Myoclonic jerks

    c. Sudden spontaneous contraction of a muscle or group of muscles, which may simulate a startle reaction.

    c. _____

Tics

    d. Spontaneous stereotyped sequence of muscular contractions, seen most prominently in facial muscles in patients with obsessive-compulsive personality traits.

    d. _____

Epilepsy

    e. Spontaneous tonic or clonic jerking of the body, often accompanied by loss of consciousness.

    e. _____

Chorea

    f. Spontaneous, quick movements, simulating fragments of normal movements, usually most prominent in extremities.

    f. _____

Athetosis

    g. Spontaneous, writhing movements of fingers and extremities, sometimes involving face and axial muscles.

    g. _____

Dystonia

    h. Spontaneous, long-sustained deviations of appendicular and axial parts, with alternating agonist-antagonist contractions, that may ultimately lead to fixed deformities.

    h. _____

Hemiballismus	*i.* More or less incessant (during waking hours) wild, flinging movements of one-half of the body, seen usually in elderly hypertensive patients.	*i.* _____
Oculogyric crisis	*j.* Spontaneous upward deviation of the eyes and head, seen usually with rest tremor and lead-pipe rigidity.	*j.* _____
Restless legs syndrome of Ekbom	*k.* Irresistible wandering of the legs when the patient tries to rest.	*k.* _____
Hyperkinetic child	*l.* Incessant, driven, usually annoying or aggressive behavior in a child.	*l.* _____
Parkinsonian (rest) tremor	*m.* A tremor at rest of 6 cps which dampens or disappears on intentional movement.	*m.* _____
Intention (ataxic) tremor	*n.* Irregular tremor of a movement in progress, but no tremor at rest.	*n.* _____
Postural tremor	*o.* Rapid tremor of an outstretched hand, which dampens when a movement is in progress and reappears when a new posture is held.	*o.* _____
Familial tremor	*p.* A 10 cps tremor of the hands which often has an autosomal dominant hereditary pattern.	*p.* _____
Senile tremor	*q.* An 8 cps tremor of the head, or head and hands, occurring in an elderly patient.	*q.* _____
Tardive dyskinesia (Meige's syndrome)	*r.* A therapy-resistant hyperkinesia usually with predominant face, lip, and tongue movements that appear after prolonged ingestion of psychotropic medications.	*r.* _____
Akathisia	*s.* A state of motor unrest in a parkinsonian Pt, characterized by irresistible restless movements and shifting of postures.	*s.* _____

REFERENCES FOR INVOLUNTARY MOVEMENTS

Aron AM, Carter S: Sydenham's chorea, in Goldensohn ES, Appel SH (eds): *Scientific Approaches to Clinical Neurology.* Philadelphia, Lea & Febiger, 1977

Chokroverty S: *Movement Disorders.* Great Neck, NY, PMA Pub. Corp., 1990

DeMyer W: Spasmodic torticollis, status marmoratus and status dysmyelinatus, in Goldensohn ES, Appel SH (eds): *Scientific Approaches to Clinical Neurology.* Philadelphia, Lea & Febiger, 1977

Cohen DJ, Bruun RD, Leckman JF: *Tourette's Syndrome and Tic Disorders.* New York, Wiley, 1988

Ekbom K: Restless legs syndrome. *Neurology* 1960;10:868–873

Fahn S, Marsden D, Calne DB (eds): *Dystonia 2.* (vol. 50: *Advances in Neurology*). New York, Raven, 1988

Jankovic J, Tolosa E: *Facial Dyskinesias.* (vol. 49: *Advances in Neurology*). New York, Raven, 1988

Klawans HL, Goetz CG, Tanner CM: *Common Movement Disorders.* New York, Raven, 1988

Lang AE, Weiner W: *Drug-induced Movement Disorders.* Mount Kisco, NY, Futura Publishing, 1992

Marsden CD, Schachter M: Assessment of extrapyramidal disorders. *J Clin Pharmacol* 1981;11:129–151

Shapiro AK, Shapiro SE, Young JG, Feinberg TW: *Gilles de la Tourette Syndrome* (2d ed). New York, Raven, 1988

Trimble M: Psychopathology and movement disorders: a new perspective on the Gilles de la Tourette syndrome. *J Neurol Neurosurg Psychiatry* 1989;52(Suppl):90–95

Yassa R, Nair NPV, Iskandar H et al: Factors in the development of severe forms of tardive dyskinesia. *Am J Psychiat* 1990;147:1156–1163

Zeman W, Dyken P: Dystonia musculorum deformans, in Vinken, P.J., Bruyn, GH (eds): *Diseases of the Basal Ganglia* (vol 6: *Handbook of Clinical Neurology*). Amsterdam, Elsevier, 1968

Zeman W, Whitlock C: Symptomatic dystonias, in Vinken PJ, Bruyn GH (eds): *Diseases of the Basal Ganglia.* (vol. 6: *Handbook of Clinical Neurology*). Amsterdam, Elsevier, 1968

Editorial comment on the neurologic examination and free will

The dichotomy into voluntary and involuntary movements facilitates the bedside diagnosis of classical involuntary movement syndromes, but many physicians (and most laymen) uncritically extend the concept of volition, i.e. free will, beyond that practical purpose to encompass criminology, social failure, and the ultimate issue of blame and moral responsibility for behavior.

In defining behavior in Chap. 1 as consisting of adjusting the length of muscle fibers and secreting substances, I avoided any question of cause or origin. Let us agree that you can contract your quadriceps muscle voluntarily, i.e., in response to your own command or an Ex's command. Similarly we can agree that the quadriceps muscle contracts involuntarily in response to stretch. We can also agree that pathophysiologic forces beyond the Pt's will cause the quadriceps muscle to contract in the restless legs syndrome or chorea. Then what causes the muscles to contract in compulsions such as stealing, fire-setting, drug-seeking, or even serial murder? Do pathophysiologic imperatives drive only the tics of Tourette's syndrome, but not the urgent compulsions and abrasive behaviors of many such patients? Do pathophysiologic imperatives command only the chorea of Sydenham's chorea but not the emotionality and regressive outbursts that often accompany it?

Not too long ago, our forefathers punished Pts who had involuntary movements, such as chorea, by imprisonment in stocks or by execution for allowing themselves (by free will) to be possessed of demons and devils. Our understanding of brain disease has advanced beyond that barbaric stage, yet we still condemn, prosecute, punish, and execute people whose behavior we do not understand. Physicians aid and abet the process when they mount the witness stand to argue whether some outcast who has dismembered a child or assassinated a president acted in response to free will. In fact, the very act committed may offer the best evidence that the accused could not, at the particular instant of the crime, control his impulses. After the disputations of physicians, whose opinions predictably differ when hired by the prosecution or the defense, the judge tries to fix responsibility and blame. Then the judge metes out punishment proportional to the degree of willfullness, presumably to deter the criminal, or other individuals whose will might, in similar circumstances, weaken. On a philosophical plane, Tolstoy in *War and Peace* and Clarence Darrow in his defense plea in the Leopold–Loeb murder trial provocatively explore the role of free will versus determinism, but like all opinion-renderers, they offer debating points, not scientific data.

The neuroscientist might propose that *all,* or better, *each* behavior derives from laws or determinants as inevitable and binding as those governing reflexes. In fact we can almost state that if we understand the neurophysiological determinants of a particular behavior, such as a muscle stretch reflex or a tonic neck reflex, we regard it as involuntary, but if we do not understand the neurophysiologic determinants of a behavior, such as a person rioting, we regard it as voluntary. If we could only understand what drives the neurons to act when a person commits a crime, or when entrapped in a neurotic web . . . if we could only understand what causes the electrical currents to surge through the brain's circuits, the ebb and flow across synaptic clefts of the excitatory and inhibitory neurohumors that trip the delicate balance between repose and aggression. Perhaps then we might rightly identify those behaviors that derive from pathophysiologic imperatives that nullify or at least modify free will. If we could translate motivation into neuronal properties, we could see why your free will directs you to turn left instead of right as you walk out the door. The experience of a free will, then, would become an artifact of consciousness, rather than a mystical energizing force for behavior.

For physicians the productive question is not what is wrong with the Pt's will, but what is wrong with the Pt's brain? Could depression be the turning on and off of genes, not a deficiency of will? Does the presence or absence of a few hundred neurons in one tiny hypothalamic nucleus determine sexual orientation (Le Vay, 1991)? Is homosexuality a biological resultant or a choice? Do homosexuals "choose" or "prefer" the same-sex pelvis over the opposite-sex pelvis, independent of the anatomicochemical state of their brain, and, therefore, are they blameworthy and responsible for "unchoosing" it? Does the 95 percent of grossly obese Pts who regain their weight after losing it constitute a group of moral degenerates who merely lack willpower, or does their hypothalamic appetitostat determine their feeding behavior with the fatality of the next dawn?

You can sit in your armchair debating free will forever, and condemning persons whose behaviors you disapprove of or do not understand. Or you can ask whether the presumed defect of will might reflect a defect in the very circuitry of the brain; what deviations might exist in the neurohumoral balances and chemistry; whether the life experiences may have shaped the very synapses and circuitry of the person's brain; and how such anatomic, chemical, and environmental factors might cloud the brain's perceptions, and whether they might lead to pathophysiological imperatives that nullify free will. Could the behavior result from a brain deviation subtler than Babinski signs and beyond detection by the routine mental status examination?

Such questions impel you to get out of your chair to investigate, to hypothesize, and to devise scientific tests of your opinions. For goodness' sake, closet yourself with an actively hallucinating schizophrenic Pt before naively accepting the free will theory of behavior. Then try it with the next less obviously mentally ill Pt, and the next, until you reach the starting point of all knowledge, the appreciation of what you don't know, and in fact can't know. We can never settle these questions by recourse to jurisprudence, strident polemics, political agendas, or preconceptions, but only by open-mindedly starting at the Pt's bedside, by formulating testable hypotheses, with humility and grace, "Well, I am unsure about the origin or correlates of this behavior, but I suppose that if such and such is so, then such and such is likely to result. That is what I will test."

> . . . *there are in fact two things, science and opinion; the former begets knowledge, the latter ignorance.* **Hippocrates** (fifth century B.C.)

Having said all of that, let us also admit that commitment, choice, and dedication, i.e., free will and moral considerations, do, in the right circumstances, alter behavior. To try to answer the questions of science does not obviate or replace personal effort and moral decisions. Although biology may determine whether you are homosexual or heterosexual, you still must choose as to how you display or utilize your genitalia and as to what you allow to be inserted into your orifices. But the physician has to recognize when the person requires appropriate medical management—not moral condemnation and exhortation to try harder. Not only does force of will fail to improve many behaviors, but many behaviors manifestly get worse the harder the Pt willfully tries to control them, for example, tics, tension athetosis, dystonia, and the aphasic Pt or stutterer struggling to will out a few words. In what circumstances does simply urging the Pt to try harder hasten the downward spiral of failure, depression, despair, and more failure, and become medically counterproductive and therefore contraindicated?

In summary, I would propose that free will originates in, derives from, and operates through the brain. The more deviant and impaired the brain, the more deviant and impaired the will and the behavior. This is the brain-behavior equation. Physicians find that Pts benefit most from appropriate medical management, not condemnation, exhortation, and moral flagellation. When disease dictates deviant behavior, the Pt is first and foremost a victim, not a willing perpetrator. Think on these things. They add the flavor, the spice to neurology.

REFERENCES FOR FREE WILL

Darrow C: *Attorney for the Damned,* edited by Arthur Weinberg. New York, Simon and Schuster, 1957

Le Vay S: A difference in hypothalamic structure between heterosexual and homosexual men. *Science* 1991; 253:1034–1037

Learning Objectives for Chapter Seven

I. Inspection of body contours, postures, and gait

Describe the initial steps in appraising the Pt's motor system, prior to formal testing of individual parts and muscles (section VI.A of the Summarized Neurologic Examination).

II. Principles of strength testing

1. Explain which option offers the best test of muscle strength: a movement that the Ex can very easily overcome, a movement the Ex can just about match, or a movement that is much stronger than the Ex's.
2. Relate the strength of a muscle to its length (length-strength law) as applied to clinical testing.
3. Demonstrate how to use the length-strength law to minimize the strength of a very strong muscle or to maximize the strength of a weak one so that their strengths more closely match the Ex's arm and hand strength.
4. Describe which movements at the jaw, neck, trunk, shoulder, elbow, wrist, fingers, hip, knee, and ankle are the strongest, and explain how the quadrupedal posture (Fig. 7-2) and the concept of postural antigravity muscles provides an easy way to remember the relative strength of these movements.
5. Explain why the dorsiflexors of the foot are not classed as antigravity muscles, even though they lift the foot against gravity in walking.
6. State the principle for remembering which movements or positions of a normal person the Ex can just about match with hand and arm opposition and which the Ex cannot even begin to overcome.

III. The sequence and technique to test for muscular weakness

1. Demonstrate how to test the strength of the muscles acting at the shoulders, elbows, wrist, and hand joints.
**2. Describe the three actions required to abduct (elevate) the arm from the side to a vertical position.
**3. Name the muscles which hold the scapula to the thoracic wall.
4. Demonstrate how to match finger strength with the Pt's, finger to finger (Fig. 7-3).
5. Demonstrate how to test the strength of the Pt's grip, and explain the concept of the functional position of the hand.
6. Demonstrate how to test the strength of the abdominal muscles.
7. Describe the results of the umbilical migration test (Beevor's sign) in a Pt who has a transverse spinal cord lesion at the 10th thoracic level.
8. Demonstrate how to test the strength of the muscles of the back, and those acting at the hip, knee, ankle, and foot joints. Describe the relative strength of the agonist-antagonist actions at these joints.
9. Demonstrate the entire screening examination for muscle strength (exclusive of cranial nerves), (section VI.C of the Summarized Neurologic Examination).
10. Describe quantitative scales for recording the strength examination in the clinical record.

IV. Results of direct percussion of the muscles

1. Define and describe percussion irritability of muscle, percussion myoedema, and percussion myotonia. State

whether these are normal or pathologic and, if pathologic, what they may indicate.

2. Demonstrate how to elicit myotonic aftercontraction of muscle.

3. Describe the difference in the response of normal, denervated, and myopathic muscle to direct percussion.

V. Examination of muscle stretch reflexes

1. Name the receptor for the MSR.
2. Draw a diagram showing the innervation of the muscle spindle and of the regular muscle fibers (Fig. 7-4).
3. Describe the response of the muscle spindles to lengthening or shortening of the muscle.
4. Explain why only a quick stretch of a muscle elicits a MSR.
5. Contrast the effect of section of the efferent nerve to a muscle on percussion irritability and the MSR.
6. Explain why the Ex percusses tendons, not the muscle itself to elicit the MSRs.
7. Describe and demonstrate the proper technique for eliciting a MSR with a percussion hammer, differentiating between *swinging* the hammer and *pecking* with the hammer (Fig. 7-5).
8. Demonstrate the sequence used to elicit the MSRs in the routine neurologic examination (Figs. 7-6 to 7-18).
9. Demonstrate how to prevent hurting the Pt in eliciting the brachioradialis reflex.
10. Describe the procedure to go through when you fail to obtain a MSR on your first attempt.
11. Describe two methods of reinforcing a MSR.
12. Explain why the traditional term "deep tendon reflex" is a misnomer for a MSR.
13. By means of a stick figure, record typical MSR responses as elicited from a normal person and give the normal range of the grading system (Fig. 7-19 and Table 7-2).
14. Explain why a right-left comparison of the magnitude of MSRs is more informative than the absolute value assigned to the response.

VI. Clinical and electromyographic signs accompanying areflexia and hyporeflexia from interruption of the reflex arc

1. Describe how to "think through" the reflex arc (Fig. 7-20) to analyze hyporeflexia or areflexia.
2. Describe the major differences in the sensory and motor findings when the lesion interrupts only the afferent or only the efferent limb of the reflex arc.
3. Explain the difference between *disuse* atrophy of muscle, *denervation* atrophy, and *myopathic* atrophy.
4. Define so as to distinguish *atrophy, aplasia,* and *hypoplasia* of muscle.
5. Define a motor unit (Fig. 7-21).
6. Define a fasciculation and its clinical expression.
7. Define wallerian degeneration (Fig. 7-23).
8. Define a fibrillation and describe how it is detected.

9. Differentiate the pathophysiology of fasciculations and fibrillations.
10. Describe the pathogenesis and detection of giant polyphasic motor units.
11. Describe how various combinations of sensory loss, areflexia, hypotonia, fasciculations, fibrillations, and percussion mytonia localize the lesion to the dorsal root, LMN, peripheral nerve, or muscle (Table 7-3).
12. Describe the relative time of appearance of weakness, areflexia, atrophy, and fibrillations after the acute onset of a LMN lesion (Table 7-4).

VII. Clinical analysis of hyperactive muscle stretch reflexes (MSRs) and clonus

1. Outline the common causes for hyperreflexia (Fig. 7-24).
2. Describe the difference in the effect of UMN and LMN lesions on the magnitude of MSRs.
3. Demonstrate how to elicit clonus and discuss its clinical implication (Fig. 7-25).
4. Explain why the Ex must make a very brisk initial movement to elicit clonus.
5. Distinguish between nonpathologic and pathologic clonus.

VIII. Disorders of muscle tone: hypertonia and hypotonia

1. Give an operational definition of muscle tone.
2. Give operational definitions of spasticity and rigidity, and demonstrate how to elicit them (Fig. 7-27 and Table 7-5).
3. Describe the difference in the pathways implicated in causing spasticity and rigidity.
4. Describe the difference in the speed of the movements required to elicit spasticity and rigidity.
5. Describe and demonstrate how to elicit the cogwheel phenomenon.
6. Describe some disorders of the PNS and CNS that may cause hypotonia (Fig. 7-28).
7. Define neural shock (diaschisis, cerebral or spinal shock) and describe what that state implies about the severity and rapidity of onset of the UMN lesion.
8. Contrast the usual motor signs of neural shock with the usual motor signs of a chronic UMN lesion.
9. Describe how to test and record the range of motion of the joints.

IX. Examination of the superficial reflexes (skin-muscle reflexes)

1. Describe the difference in the location of the receptors for superficial and deep reflexes.
2. Recite the superficial reflexes elicited in the standard NE (mnemonic hint: recite them in rostrocaudal order).
3. Recite a sentence to prepare the Pt for a plantar stimulus.
4. Demonstrate how to elicit the plantar reflex by stimulation of the sole (Fig. 7-29), and describe the usual movement of the great toe in a normal person.

5. Name the three physiologically significant variables in the stroke used to elicit the plantar reflex.

6. Explain why the Ex applies very slight pressure for the first stimulus to elicit a plantar reflex.

7. State the endpoint criterion for having properly elicited the plantar reflex.

8. Describe the position of the Pt for eliciting plantar responses.

9. State the dermatome stimulated by the Babinski maneuver and describe the afferent and efferent arc of the plantar reflex, naming the nerves, spinal cord segments, and muscle groups involved (Figs. 7-30 and 7-32).

10. State the two types of summation required to elicit a plantar response.

11. Describe the lower extremity movements that usually accompany plantar flexion of the great toe after a plantar stimulus in a normal person.

**12. Describe ways to investigate whether the plantar response should be judged as a balance between agonist-antagonist muscle contraction or merely an agonist contraction.

13. Describe the response of the great toe to a plantar stimulus in a Pt who has a UMN lesion (Fig. 7-34*A*). Give two names for it.

14. Describe the additional movements of the lower extremity that usually accompany an extensor plantar response (Fig. 7-34*B*).

15. Describe how to discriminate a true extensor toe sign from other causes for extension (dorsiflexion) of the great toe.

17. State what tract is interrupted when an extensor toe sign is present.

18. Name several transient pathophysiologic states in which an extensor toe sign or other features of the UMN syndrome may appear without actual anatomical interruption of the pyramidal tract.

19. State several different reasons why a Pt with an undoubted UMN lesion may not show an extensor toe sign.

20. State the nerve that is usually involved and the usual site of the lesion in a Pt with a foot drop.

21. Demonstrate how to palpate the common peroneal nerve (Fig. 7-36).

22. Describe crossed knee palsy.

23. Describe what may happen to the size of the receptive zone for the extensor toe sign after spinal cord transection. Describe what usually happens to the flexion synergy of the lower extremities in such patients.

**24. Demonstrate several methods in addition to the standard plantar stimulus for eliciting an extensor toe sign. State the common physiological properties of the stimulus for most of these maneuvers (Fig. 7-35).

25. Describe the characteristic differences in the plantar response of infants as contrasted to more mature individuals.

26. Demonstrate how to elicit the abdominal and cremasteric reflexes and describe the normal responses (Fig. 7-37).

27. State the physiologic properties shared by the stimulus that produces the abdominal-cremasteric and plantar reflexes.

28. Describe the characteristic changes in the abdominal-cremasteric reflexes in the acute and chronic stages of UMN lesions.

29. State some instances in which absence of the superficial abdominal reflexes does not necessarily implicate UMN interruption.

30. Describe how to elicit the anal wink and bulbocavernous reflexes, and state what level of the spinal cord mediates these reflexes.

31. Show on a stick figure how to record the typical deep and superficial reflex responses in a normal person, a hemiplegic Pt, and a paraplegic Pt with a chronic lesion at T-10 (Fig. 7-38).

32. Describe what would happen to the umbilicus when a supine Pt with a T-10 level spinal cord lesion attempts to elevate his head.

X. Summary of the standard "textbook" syndromes of UMN and LMN lesions and their variations

1. Recite the clinical signs produced by a slowly evolving or chronic UMN.

2. Contrast the UMN syndrome with the LMN syndrome (Table 7-6).

3. Define so as to differentiate the following clinical terms for syndromes caused by UMN lesions at various sites: hemiplegia, double hemiplegia, pseudobulbar palsy, spastic diplegia, locked-in syndrome, quadriplegia (tetraplegia), paraplegia, and monoplegia.

4. Describe the motor, sensory, and autonomic changes that follow acute spinal cord transection at C-1.

5. Describe the effects of spinal shock on the deep and superficial reflexes, both visceral and somatic.

XI. The concept of deficit and release phenomena after lesions of the motor and sensory pathways

1. Define deficit and release phenomena and classify the signs of acute and chronic UMN lesions as one or the other.

2. Apply the concept of deficit and release phenomena to the clinical features of LMN lesions.

3. Apply the concept of deficit and release phenomena to the clinical features of autonomic dysfunction after lesions of the peripheral nervous system (mnemonic hint: effect on sweating, and vasoconstrictor tone).

XII. Involuntary movement disorders

1. Give an operational definition of voluntary and involuntary movements.

2. Describe some normal involuntary movements or physiologic synkinesias.

3. Describe Bell's phenomenon.

4. Define myoclonic jerks and describe one circumstance in which a myoclonic jerk is normal.
5. Distinguish myoclonic jerks from fasciculations.
6. State which abnormal clinical or EMG findings would distinguish pathologic from benign fasciculations.
7. Show how to demonstrate your own physiologic tremor.
8. Give the clinical characteristics of parkinsonian tremor.
9. List the major motor disabilities disclosed by the neurologic examination in parkinsonism.
10. Describe the effects of parkinsonism on facial expression and speech.
11. Define or describe pill-rolling tremor, lead-pipe rigidity, cogwheeling, akathisia, and oculogyric crisis.
12. Describe the distinguishing clinical characteristics of familial tremor, parkinsonian tremor, intention tremor, postural tremor, and terminal tremor, and mime these tremors yourself.
13. Describe the site of the lesion or the system affected for parkinsonian tremor, intention (ataxic) tremor, postural tremor and terminal tremor; or combinations of rest, intention, and postural (rubral) tremor.
14. Define and mime chorea, athetosis, and dystonia, and rank the speed of the movements.
15. Describe one type of focal dystonia.
16. Describe hemiballismus and state the usual site of the lesion.
17. Define a tic and name a syndrome consisting of multiple tics and urgent personality traits.
18. Applying the basic definitions of deficit and release phenomena, classify the signs of lesions of the basal motor nuclei.
20. Give examples of overactive or driven behavior that derive from pathophysiologic imperatives that transcend the Pt's will.
21. State how the hyperactivity in the hyperactive child syndrome differs from the standard extrapyramidal hyperkinesias.
22. Describe the effect of pyramidal tract section on voluntary movements and most abnormal involuntary movements of extrapyramidal origin (page 80).
23. Explain why a brief period of observation of a child in the examining room may lead the doctor to erroneously distrust the history given by the mother of a hyperactive child.
24. Describe the usual effects of emotional tension and tranquility or sleep on most involuntary movements.
25. Discuss the difficulties in deciding which determinants, free will, pathophysiologic imperatives, or unconscious motivations cause any particular behavior.

XIII. Summary of the somatic motor system examination

Demonstrate the motor examination, commencing with the initial inspection for gait, posture, tremors and abnormal movements; followed by palpation, strength testing, and muscle tone; and proceeding through the deep reflexes, percussion, and superficial reflexes.

Chapter Eight

Examination for Cerebellar Dysfunction

But how great was his apprehension, when he farther understood, that [the force of parturition] acting upon the very vertex of the head, not only injured the brain itself, or cerebrum,—but that it necessarily squeezed and propelled the cerebrum towards the cerebellum, which was the immediate seat of the understanding!—Angels and ministers of grace defend us! cried my father,—can any soul withstand this shock?—No wonder the intellectual web is so rent and tattered as we see it; and that so many of our best heads are no better than a puzzled skein of silk,—all perplexity,—all confusion within-side.

Laurence Sterne (1713–1768), *The Life and Opinions of Tristam Shandy Gentleman*

I. Introduction to the function of the cerebellum

A. *What the cerebellum does not do.* Laurence Sterne correctly satirized the speculative neurophysiology of his time, which localized "the immediate seat of the understanding" to the cerebellum.

   1. The cerebellum has no clinically evident role in mental processes, consciousness, emotion, homeostasis, or autonomic functions.
   2. The cerebellum has no clinically evident role in the conscious appreciation of sensation, despite massive sensory connections (Macklis and Macklis, 1992).

B. *What the cerebellum does do.* To the clinician, the major role of the cerebellum is to adjust the rate, regularity, and force of willed muscular contractions (Holmes, 1939). In a word, we might say to *coordinate* willful muscular contractions.

   1. We would err if we attributed all coordination to the cerebellum, or all incoordination to cerebellar lesions. As Hughlings Jackson (1834–1911) stated, "It will not suffice . . . to speak of coordination as a separate 'faculty.' Coordination is the function of the whole and every part of the nervous system." Although visual, tactile, auditory, pyramidal, and extrapyramidal circuits all contribute afferents to the cerebellum, coordination preeminently requires proprioceptive input.

*The light vertical rule on the left side of the text sets off an answer column. Cover the answers with a card until you have responded to the text. Then after each response, slide the card down to check your answer.

The heavy vertical rule or asterisk denotes optional material.

2. The proprioceptors transmit positional information from the muscles, the joints, and the vestibular system. Proprioceptors inform the cerebellum about joint position and the length of, and tension on, muscles: in other words what the muscles are doing at any instant. The brain decides where to move to, i.e., what it wants the muscles to do. From this information, the cerebellum coordinates the range, velocity, and strength of contractions to produce steady volitional movements and steady volitional postures. Thus as the crucial test for cerebellar dysfunction, examine the patient (Pt) for incoordination of volitional movements and for incoordination of volitional postures.

3. Now, if you understand the role of the cerebellum, you can answer this question: could you test a paralyzed or comatose Pt for cerebellar dysfunction? ☐ Yes/ ☐ No. Explain: _____

_____

Ans: ☑ *No. A comatose or paralyzed Pt makes no willed movements and maintains no willed postures.*

II. Anatomy of the cerebellum

A. *The three cerebellar lobes*
   NOTE ON NOMENCLATURE: The cerebellum, more than any other part of the CNS, suffers from too many names for its bumps and crevices. Angevine et al (1961) list 24 different nomenclatures, in which authors may use the same names for different subdivisions. This text uses Larsell's (1972) terms.
   1. The cerebellum is subdivided *transversely* into three lobes, and *longitudinally* into three parts, one midline vermis uniting two hemispheres. Learn Fig. 8-1.

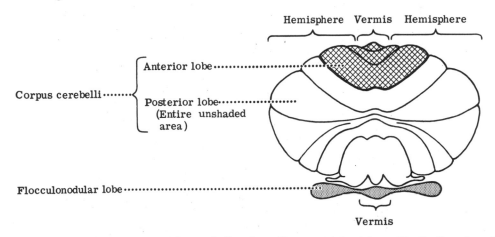

FIG. 8-1. Schematic dorsal view of the cerebellum (Larsell's nomenclature). In reality, the flocculonodular lobe is rolled under, out of sight, when the cerebellum is viewed dorsally (Fig. 8-2).

   2. In contrast to the schematic depiction of lobes in Fig. 8-1, Fig. 8-2 shows the flocculonodular lobe rolled under in its true position. Label the lobes.

B. *Cerebellar phylogenesis*
   1. You will understand the clinical syndromes of the cerebellum best by starting where the cerebellum started, with its phylogenesis. The cerebellum evolved out of the vestibular nuclei. Its vestibular origin condemns it to straddle forever the vestibular nerves and nuclei, at the pontomedullary

A. Anterior

B. Posterior

C. Flocculonodular

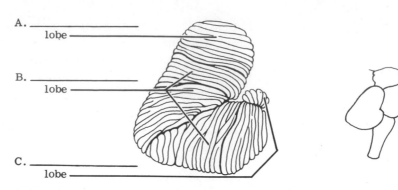

A. _____
    lobe _____

B. _____
    lobe _____

C. _____
    lobe _____

FIG. 8-2. Right lateral view of the cerebellum, showing the rolled-under position of the flocculonodular lobe. The insert (right) shows the relation of the cerebellum to the brainstem. Label the lobes at *A* to *C*.

junction, and to retain forever its connections with the vestibular system—the law of original innervation.

2. Vestibular proprioceptors provide information about the movement of the head and its position in relation to the pull of gravity. Having no limbs, primitive animals require only a small nubbin of cerebellum to coordinate the axial muscles which position the eyes, head, and trunk. This nubbin of vestibulocerebellum is the *flocculonodular lobe* (Fig. 8-1).

3. All higher animals retain the vestibulocerebellar connections and their axial functions, but the budding limbs impress new roles on the cerebellum; it must now coordinate axial (trunk) and appendicular (limb) muscles. The emergence of the vertical bipedal from the quadripedal posture places particular demands on gait coordination. A second portion of the cerebellum evolves to receive most of the proprioceptive input from limbs and trunk, the *anterior lobe* (Fig. 8-1).

4. The third and newest cerebellar lobe expands in equal measure with the cerebrum, motor cortex, pyramidal tract, pontine basis, and inferior olivary nuclei. The corticopontocerebellar and olivocerebellar pathways send the most conspicuous inputs to this newest part, the *posterior lobe* (Fig. 8-1).

5. To recapitulate: we recognize three lobes of the cerebellum, the *anterior, posterior,* and *flocculonodular,* based on phylogenesis and the major source of afferent connections. Complete Table 8-1.

6. Lesions of each of the lobes cause different clinical syndromes. From the clinical findings the examiner (Ex) can predict the location and often the type of lesion (Table 8-4).

C. *The three pairs of cerebellar peduncles and the pathways they convey*

1. Three pairs of peduncles anchor the cerebellum to the pons. These thick stalks convey only and all afferent and efferent cerebellar nerve fibers (DeMyer, 1988). Transection of the peduncles allows the cerebellum to fall free, exposing their cut surfaces (Fig. 8-3).

Flocculonodular
Anterior

Posterior

TABLE 8-1 Some major afferent pathways to the lobes of the cerebellum	
Major afferent source	Lobe
Vestibular system	_____ lobe (archicerebellum)
Spinocerebellar tracts (from trunk and extremities)	_____ lobe (paleocerebellum)
Corticopontocerebellar tracts	_____ lobe (neocerebellum)

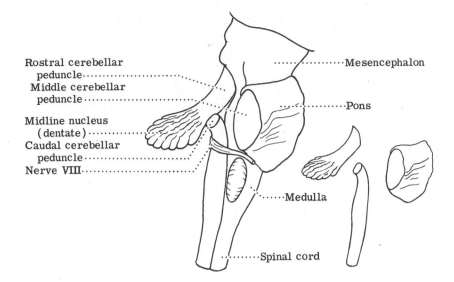

Rostral cerebellar peduncle

Middle cerebellar peduncle

Midline nucleus (dentate)

Caudal cerebellar peduncle

Nerve VIII

Mesencephalon

Pons

Medulla

Spinal cord

FIG. 8-3. Right lateral view of the brainstem to show the cerebellar peduncles. The insert at the right is an exploded view of the peduncles.

☑ *Pons*

2. The three pairs of peduncles anchor the cerebellum to only one division of the brainstem, the ☐ mesencephalon/ ☐ pons/ ☐ medulla. Therefore, all afferent and efferent cerebellar fibers pass through the pons and through one of the peduncles.

3. The *middle peduncle,* the simplest peduncle in composition, conveys almost exclusively corticopontocerebellar fibers. Remember it by the *L* mnemonic: *l*argest, *l*ateralest, *l*atest, and simp*l*est. It is the *l*argest by far of the cerebellar peduncles, conveys the *l*argest pathway to the cerebellum (from the cerebrum, the *l*argest part of the brain), constitutes the *l*ateral bulk of the pons (the largest division of the brainstem), is the *l*atest to develop phylogenetically, simp*l*est in composition, and ends in the *l*argest lobe of the cerebellum, the _____ lobe.

Posterior

4. The *inferior* cerebellar peduncle's composition is predicted by its neighbors, the spinal cord, medulla, and vestibular nerve. Thus it conveys spinocerebellar, medullocerebellar (including olivocerebellar), and vestibulocerebellar and cerebellovestibular pathways.

5. The *superior* cerebellar peduncle dives forward and ventrally into the pons. It aims the major efferent cerebellar pathway, the *brachium conjunctivum,* towards the red nucleus and thalamus (Fig. 8-3). For the priggish neuro-anatomist, we will recall and profess that whereas the *dorsal* spinocerebellar tract veers directly into the cerebellum via the inferior peduncle, the *ventral* spinocerebellar tract ventures rostrally to enter via the superior peduncle—but the latter fact has no particular clinical value. More importantly, *both* spinocerebellar tracts end in the anterior lobe, mainly in the vermis. These tracts convey proprioceptive information to the anterior lobe from the muscles of the trunk and extremities.

D. *Recapitulation of the cerebellar peduncles*

Posterior

Middle

1. In activating muscles for voluntary movements, the cerebrum informs the cerebellum via the corticopontocerebellar pathway, which ends mainly in the _____ lobe.

2. The corticopontocerebellar pathway runs in the _____ peduncle.

Superior (rostral)

Inferior (caudal)

Flocculonodular

3. The major efferent peduncle, containing the brachium conjunctivum, is the _____ peduncle.
4. Medullary, vestibular, and many spinocerebellar afferents enter the cerebellum via the _____ peduncle.
5. Recall that the lobe which arose out of the vestibular system and retains strong vestibular connections throughout its phylogenetic history is the _____ lobe.
6. Of the three cranial nerves attached along the pontomedullary sulcus, the most dorsal one, closest to the inferior peduncle, is number _____ and the most ventral one is number _____.

Ans: VIII; VI. Review Fig. 2-22 if you missed.

E. *Circuits of the cerebellum*
1. *Intrinsic cerebellar circuits.* All afferent fibers ascend through the cerebellar white matter to influence ultimately the large Purkinje neurons of the cerebellar cortex. The Purkinje axons afford the only way out of the cerebellar cortex. They descend through the cerebellar white matter, the vast majority synapsing on the deep nuclei of the cerebellum, and a small minority synapsing on the vestibular nuclei. The deep nuclei sit in the roof of the 4th ventricle. Learn Fig. 8-4.

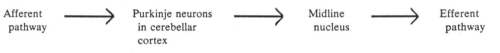

FIG. 8-4. Flow of impulses through the cerebellum.

2. *Extrinsic cerebellar circuits:* the cortico-ponto-cerebello-thalamo-cortico-bulbo-spinal circuit
    a. Well, yes, instead of inventing such a word, I could just introduce a law: *cerebral hemisphere lesions cause contralateral motor signs, whereas in direct contrast, cerebellar hemisphere lesions cause ipsilateral signs,* if that's all you want to know. It's more elegant, if more demanding, to learn the actual circuit that underlies the correlation between lesion site and clinical signs. Learning it will cause no harm and has practical value, as you can verify at your next opportunity: by deliberately thinking through this circuit as a volitional, cerebral act, you can inhibit impending orgasm, a reflex act, and prolong copulation (of course, for the same purpose, some people, instead of thinking circuitry, just recite poetry or work math problems).
        Study Fig. 8-5 this way:
        (1) Learn the labeled structures.
        (2) Starting at the frontal motor cortex, trace a motor impulse from the motor cortex down to the cerebellar cortex, back to the motor cortex, and down the pyramidal tract.
        (3) Using a colored pencil, draw the circuit on the other half of Fig. 8-5.

    ☑ *Contralateral*

    b. By means of the single pyramidal decussation, one cerebral hemisphere controls volitional movements on the ☐ ipsilateral/ ☐ contralateral side of the body.
    c. By means of double crossing pathways in conjunction with the pyramidal decussation, one cerebellar hemisphere ultimately coordinates movements on the ☐ contralateral/ ☐ ipsilateral side of the body.

    ☑ *Ipsilateral*

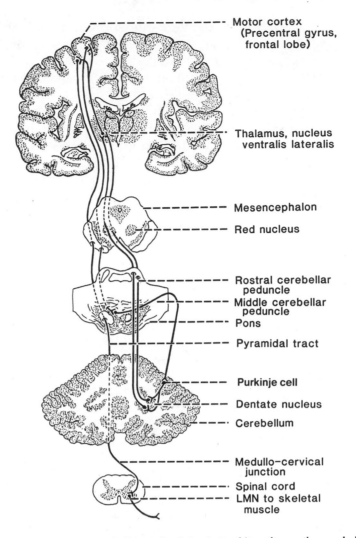

FIG. 8-5. Diagram of the cerebro-cerebello-cerebral circuit. By this pathway, the cerebellum coordinates volitional movement by feeding back information to the cerebral motor cortex to influence its commands to the LMNs via the pyramidal tract. Start at the motor cortex and trace through the circuit. Notice that the cerebro-cerebello-cerebral circuit double-crosses the midline and that the pyramidal crossing brings the influence of one cerebellar hemisphere back to the same side.

☑ *Ipsilateral*

Hence a lesion of one cerebellar hemisphere causes incoordinated movements on the ☐ ipsilateral/ ☐ contralateral side.

III. Clinical signs of cerebellar dysfunction

A. *Incoordination (ataxia) as the key cerebellar dysfunction*
Clinically, cerebellar lesions manifest as incoordination of volitional movements or of volitionally maintained postures. As a model to understand cerebellar dysfunction, consider drunkenness. Depressant drugs such as alcohol and barbiturates preferentially poison vestibulocerebellar neurons. If you have ever been or seen an inebriated person, you will understand the syndrome immediately. A drunken person cannot coordinate any volitional muscular contractions. Thus, the person sways when standing, reels when walking, slurs words when talking, and has jerky eye movements when looking. The limbs are loose and floppy. If we apply technical terms to these features, as is the habit of physicians, we define the cerebellar syndrome.

1. The incoordination of intentional movements is called *intention tremor, dystaxia,* or *ataxia* (taxis = ordering or arranging in rank and file, as taxonomy).
2. The slurred speech, is called *dysarthria,* like any neurogenic disturbance of voice articulation.
3. The oscillating eye movements are called *nystagmus.*
4. The floppiness of the extremities is called *hypotonia.*
5. List the four major clinical signs of the cerebellar syndrome: _____, _____, _____, and _____.

Ans: Dystaxia, dysarthria, nystagmus, hypotonia.

B. *Clinical tests for dystaxia of station (stance) and gait*
1. Inspect the Pt for swaying when standing, which involves volitional posture, and for dystaxia of gait, which involves volitional movements. The unsteady stance and reeling gait of the drunken person need no wordy description. To compensate for unsteadiness of stance and gait, the cerebellar Pt assumes a *broad-based stance* and *broad-based gait,* just as a toddler does before gaining coordination, or an elderly Pt does after losing some. To challenge the Pt's coordination and overcome the compensatory broad-base, the Ex asks the Pt to stand with the feet together. Similarly, to expose gait incoordination, use a test known to every policeman: ask the Pt to step along a straight line, placing the heel of one foot directly in front of the toe of the other, so-called *tandem* walking. Now stand up and try this test yourself. You will find that to balance on a narrow base when walking takes no little ability.

☑ *On*

See next frame

2. To judge broad-based gaits, you must know where the heels fall in relation to the midline when a normal person walks. First, just for fun, guess where the medial margins of the heels fall in relation to the midline sagittal plane: ☐ on/ ☐ 2.5 cm off/ ☐ 3 to 5 cm off/ ☐ more than 5 cm off.
   a. To remember this point forever, try this test: stand up, and walk at a normal pace in a straight line. Hitch up your garments so that you can note the exact placement of your heels. Where do they fall in relation to the midline? _____ _____
   b. Unless you have huge thighs, the medial margin of your heels fell exactly on the line. Verify this the next time you watch someone walk, or, just as instructive, note the neat, precise tightrope placement of a dog's hind feet.
   c. Next stretch a string in a straight line and walk along it with your midline directly over the strand. Notice again where your heels fall and that even slight displacement of your heels off of the midline will introduce a waddle in your gait.
3. To the original four signs of cerebellar dysfunction, we can add a swaying, broad-based stance and gait. State the original four signs: _____, _____, _____, and _____.

Ans: Dystaxia, dysarthria, hypotonia, and nystagmus.

C. *Clinical tests for arm dystaxia*
1. Finger-to-nose test
   a. Ask the Pt to extend the arms straight out in front. Inspect the arms for wavering, indicating incoordination during this volitionally maintained posture, and for frank, rhythmic postural tremor. Then instruct the Pt to place his index finger on the tip of his nose. To enlist the Pt's best effort, say, "Move your finger in slowly and place the tip of your finger exactly on the tip of your nose. Don't miss." Inspect for intention tremor

(dystaxia) of the movement in progress, and how precisely the Pt can touch the tip of his nose. If uncertain of the result, have the Pt alternately touch his nose, your finger, and his nose several times.

Postural (position maintenance)

   b. If the Pt has a tremor of the outstretched hands it is called a _____ tremor.

   c. Postural tremor indicates a lesion of the superior cerebellar peduncle (brachium conjunctivum), which runs to the thalamus and thence relays modulating influences to the cerebral cortex.

   d. If the Pt maintains the posture of the outstretched arms well but has tremor during the finger-to-nose movement, it is called _____ tremor.

Ans: Intention or ataxic tremor, or simply ataxia.

☑ *Ipsilateral*

   e. Dystaxia of the right hand implicates a lesion of the ☐ ipsilateral/ ☐ contralateral cerebellar hemisphere.

Terminal or endpoint

   f. A tremor which is exaggerated as the finger approaches the nose or is reaching the target, is called _____ tremor.

  2. *Dysmetria.* The dystaxic Pt, in seeking a specific endpoint, such as the nose on the finger-to-nose test, frequently *under*shoots or *over*shoots the target because of incoordination of the agonists and antagonists that produce the movement. Such an error in metering distance, we call *dysmetria.*

  3. *The rapid-alternating-movements tests for dystaxia-dysmetria (dysdiadochokinesia)*

   a. The Pt holds out the hands and pronates and supinates them as rapidly as possible. Test the hands separately and together. The dystaxic hand overshoots one time, undershoots the next, and is slower than normal. See Fig. 8-6.

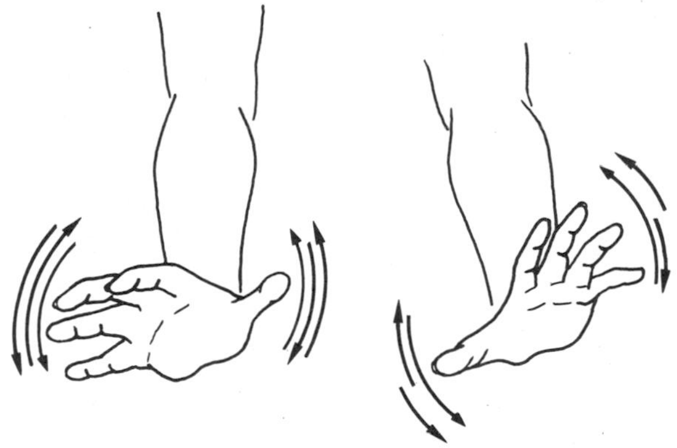

FIG. 8-6. Pronation-supination test for dystaxia-dysmetria of the hands. Notice the even excursions of the normal right hand, and the uneven excursions of the ataxic left hand.

   b. A subtler and therefore superior method is the *thigh-slapping test.* Test each hand separately. First demonstrate the action to the Pt by lightly slapping your own thigh, alternating first with the palm and then with the back of the hand, as rapidly and rhythmically as possible, making an audible sound with each slap. Instruct the Pt to make actions that *sound* exactly like yours. The Ex sees *and* hears the dysrhythmia of the ataxic hand (Fig. 8-7).

   c. The technical term for dystaxia-dysmetria of rapid alternating, movements, *dysdiadokokinesia,* is a lovely dactylic trimeter. *This is the forest primeval: dys dǐ ǎ dó kǒ kǐ né šǐ ǎ."* This term describes nothing qual-

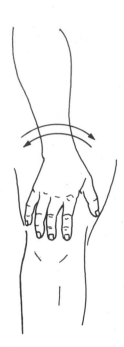

FIG. 8-7. Thigh-slapping test for dystaxia-dysmetria. The cerebellar patient slaps irregularly, and turns the hand too much or too little in alternately slapping the front and the back of the hand on the thigh.

itatively different. It means only incoordination of muscular contractions during rapid alternating movements.

D. *Clinical tests for leg dystaxia:* the heel-to-shin and heel-tapping tests
   1. The *heel-to-shin test* for dystaxia supplements gait testing. The Pt is supine or sitting. Instruct the Pt to place one heel precisely on the opposite knee and run the heel in a straight line precisely down the shin.
   2. For the *heel-tapping test,* ask the Pt to place one heel over the other shin and to tap the shin with the heel as rapidly as possible on one spot. The cerebellar Pt misses the spot (dysmetria) and taps dysrhythmically (dysdiadokokinesia).
   3. Try these tests yourself. Again, such simple tasks offer a considerable challenge. Does your leg waver *any* as you do the tests?

E. *Clinical demonstration of hypotonia*
   1. Muscle tone is operationally defined as _____
   _____
   _____.

Ans: The muscular resistance the Ex feels when moving the Pt's resting extremity.

   2. *Inspection for hypotonia*
      a. At rest, the hypotonic Pt assumes floppy postures, and joint positions uncomfortable for a normal subject—rag-doll or dumped-in-a-heap postures. In a normal person, muscle tone helps to limit joint excursions.
      b. When walking, the hypotonic Pt presents a floppy, saggy, loose-jointed appearance. The arms fail to swing properly, the knees may bend backward slightly (genu recurvatum), the head and trunk bob—a rag-doll gait, as seen in drunkenness.
   3. *Pendulous or hypotonic muscle stretch reflexes (MSRs) in cerebellar Pts.* The MSRs, once elicited in the cerebellar Pt, fail to check normally; this is best seen with the quadriceps femoris reflex. The Pt sits with the legs

swinging freely over a table edge. After the quadriceps MSR is elicited, the leg normally stops swinging after one or two excursions. The cerebellar Pt's leg swings to-and-fro several times, like a pendulum, without the normal checking of the excursions by muscle tone. Paradoxically, pendular reflexes also occur after pyramidal tract lesions, which usually cause some degree of spasticity and hyperreflexia. The explanation for this paradox is unclear.

4. Three methods for detecting hypotonia are_____

_____

_____.

Ans: *Passive movement of the Pt's extremities by the Ex, inspection for rag-doll postures and a rag-doll gait, and pendular reflexes.*

    F. *Overshooting and checking tests of the arms*

      1. The cerebellar Pt has difficulty in maintaining a posture or position against a sudden, unexpected displacement. Have the Pt stand with eyes closed and arms outstretched.

      2. Tell the Pt, "I am going to bump your arms. Hold them still. Don't let me move them." The Ex strikes the back of the Pt's wrist a sharp blow, strong enough to displace the arm. The normal subject's arm returns quickly to its initial position. The cerebellar Pt's arm oscillates back and forth; it *overshoots* several times (Fig. 8-8).

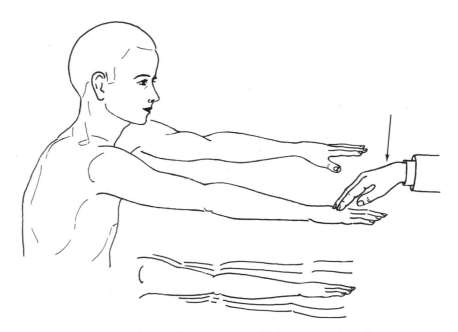

FIG. 8-8. Wrist-slapping test for abnormal overshooting oscillations after sudden displacement of a part that is maintaining a volitional posture. The thin arrow shows the direction of the examiner's blow, which displaces the part.

      3. The *arm-pulling* test also demonstrates overshooting.

        a. The Ex pulls hard against the Pt's flexed arm. When the Ex suddenly releases the Pt's arm, the cerebellar Pt fails to check the arm's flight (Fig. 8-9).

        b. Precaution: notice in Fig. 8-9 how the Ex places an arm to protect the Pt's face in case the Pt's arm fails to check and overshoots.

        c. Angel (1977) points out that neurologists have erroneously called the overshooting phenomenon the rebound sign of Gordon Holmes.

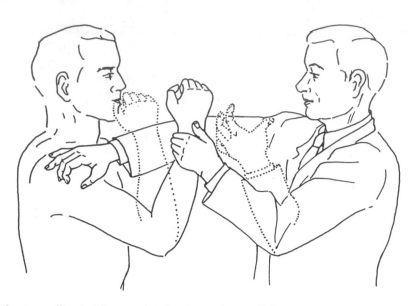

FIG. 8-9. The arm-pulling test for overshooting. It tests how well the cerebellum functions to check movement and to maintain a given posture after a sudden release of tension on a muscle that is voluntarily contracting.

G. *The effect of cerebellar lesions on eye movements*

Lesions of the eye, cerebellum, and vestibular system may cause nystagmus. The nystagmus may reflect interruption of the vestibular pathways via the flocculonodular lobe and fastigial nucleus, or in the pontine tegmentum (Hood et al, 1973; Carlow and Bicknell, 1978). Acute unilateral destructive lesions regularly cause a particular nystagmus with the slow component towards a null or resting point (Holmes, 1917; Holmes, 1939); see the nystagmus dendrogram, Fig. 5-5. Cerebellar nystagmus occurs preeminently during fixation, i.e., during volitional use of the eyes. Other disturbances of ocular movements include jerky rather than smooth pursuit, slowness in initiating eye movements, and skew deviation (Bogousslavsky and Meienberg, 1987; Glaser, 1990; Pierrot-Deseilligny et al, 1990).

H. *The effect of cerebellar lesions on speech*

The cerebellar Pt has slurred speech or *dysarthria* and *scanning speech,* in which the voice varies from a low volume to a high volume as if scanning from peak to peak. Tremulousness, analogous to postural tremor may also occur (Ackerman and Ziegler, 1991). The Pt may initiate speech slowly and may speak too loudly.

I. *Effect of cerebellar lesions on strength and endurance*

The cerebellar Pt may experience mild *asthenia,* that is, weakness and fatigability, although formal strength testing by dynamometry shows only some slight decrease in the maximum force of contraction. The pathway that connects the cerebellar cortex with the cerebral motor cortex may explain the symptom (Fig. 8-5). Stimulation of the cerebellar cortex in the experimental animal *increases* the sensitivity of the cerebral motor cortex to stimulation. Interruption of the cerebellocerebral pathway *decreases* the sensitivity of the motor cortex to stimulation. Apparently cerebellar impulses facilitate discharge of the cerebral motor cortex. Lacking this facilitation, the cerebellar Pt might not muster full discharge of upper motor neurons (UMNs).

J. *Decomposition of movement.* Numerous tests may demonstrate the basic cerebellar deficits of dystaxia, hypotonia, and overshooting. In *decomposition of movement,* the Pt performs a movement as though it were decomposed "by the numbers." When moving the arm from his side to touch his nose, the Pt does so in two stages.

1. Movement *one* consists of lifting the arm to the level of the nose.
2. Movement *two* then consists of bringing the fingertip to the nose, the two movements producing a long, inefficient trajectory. The normal person performs both movements simultaneously, to produce the optimal and most efficient movement trajectory. Gordon Holmes (1876–1965) summarized decomposition of movement among other cerebellar tests in a classic article that you might enjoy reading (1939).

K. *Summary of clinical tests for cerebellar dysfunction.* Complete Table 8-2 and practice the cerebellar tests on a normal person, in the order listed in Table 8-2.

L. *As a review,* before learning some specific cerebellar syndromes, draw the cerebro-ponto-cerebello-dentato-rubro-thalamo-cortico-spinal circuit in Fig. 8-10. Compare your drawing with Fig. 8-5.

TABLE 8-2 Tests for cerebellar dysfunction	
Abnormality	Method of examination
Gait dystaxia	*Free walking for broad-based gait and tandem walking*
Nystagmus	*Inspect and have patient follow your finger through fields of gaze*
Arm dystaxia and irregular alternating movements	*Finger-to-nose: pronation-supination test, thigh-slapping test*
Overshooting	*Wrist-slapping test and arm-pulling test*
Leg dystaxia (other than gait)	*Heel-to-knee test; shin-tapping test*
Hypotonia	*Inspection for rag doll postures and rag doll gait; passive movement of extremities; pendular quadriceps reflexes*

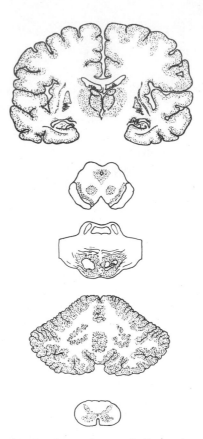

FIG. 8-10. **Blank for drawing the cerebro-cerebello-cerebro-pyramidal pathway.**

IV. Analysis of Pts and the four cerebellar syndromes

A. *Patient 1*

1. *Medical history.* This 62-year-old woman awakened, and, on arising, fell to the left. She became dizzy, vomited, and struggled back into bed. When she called to her husband, he noticed slurring of her speech. Hypertensive for many years, she had suffered a myocardial infarct at the age of 60.

2. *Physical findings.* The Pt was conscious, cooperative, and intact mentally. She was mildly dysarthric. She had a bidirectional nystagmus, with the slow movement toward a null point a little to the right of center. The nystagmus increased on looking to the left. She had slight ptosis of the left eyelid and miosis on the left. The corneal reflex was reduced on the left. Otherwise the cranial nerves functioned normally. She could not walk unless supported. She had equal strength on the two sides, but less muscle tone on the left. She had severe dystaxia on finger-to-nose and heel-to-knee testing on the left side only. She had left-sided dysdiadochokinesia. Her left arm overshot. Her left quadriceps femoris reflex was pendular. Plantar stimulation on both sides produced plantar flexion of the large toes. Pain and temperature discrimination were reduced on the right side of the body and in the right extremities.

3. *Lesion localization in Pt 1*

   a. Before continuing in the text, try to diagnose the location of the lesion. First review the brainstem cross sections in Figs. 2-15 to 2-18.

   b. In seeking a single lesion or at least a single pathologic process, first of all assemble the clinical data that require explanation (Table 8-3).

   c. The left-sided dystaxia and other cerebellar signs implicate a lesion of the ☐ vermis/ ☐ right/ <u>left</u> cerebellar hemisphere.

☑ *Left*

TABLE 8-3 Localizing Findings in Patient 1.
Collate with Fig. 10-17, page 375.

Clinical symptom or sign	Localizing significance
Left-sided cerebellar signs, bidirectional nystagmus, dysarthria, and unsteady gait	All indictive of, or compatible with, left cerebellar hemisphere lesion
Dizziness and vomiting	Vestibular connections in pontomedullary tegmentum
Ptosis and miosis on the left	Descending autonomic pathway in dorsolateral medullary tegmentum
Decreased left corneal reflex	Descending root of CN V in dorsolateral medullary tegmentum
Reduced pain and temperature sensation on the right side	Spinothalamic tract ascending in lateral medullary tegmentum
Bidirectional nystagmus with null point just off midline	Acute cerebellar hemisphere lesion

    d. Review the nystagmus dendrograms, Figs. 5-4 and 5-5, and state whether the Pt's nystagmus helps to localize the lesion and if so to where.

    Ans: Yes. Left cerebellar hemisphere.

4. *Noncerebellar findings in Patient 1*

Since cerebellar lesions do not impair sensation or autonomic functions, damage at another site must have caused the left-sided ptosis and miosis (Horner's syndrome), the reduced left corneal reflex and the right-sided sensory loss.

5. *Clinicopathologic correlation in Patient 1*

    a. Magnetic resonance imaging (MRI) showed infarction of the lateral aspect of the medulla on the left and of the left cerebellar hemisphere. The lateral wedge of medullary tissue that was infarcted conveys (Fig. 2-15 to 2-18, and especially see Fig. 10-17*A*):

        (1) The autonomic fibers that descend from the hypothalamus to the intermediolateral cell column of T-1 and T-2, accounting for the Horner's syndrome.

        (2) The ipsilateral descending root of cranial nerve V that mediates the corneal reflex (Fig. 10-2).

        (3) The crossed, ascending spinothalamic tract for pain and temperature.

    b. The vertigo and vomiting reflect interruption of the vestibular connections with the medullary reticular formation.

    c. To assign the cerebellar and medullary findings to one cause requires knowledge of the arterial supply of the posterior fossa. One artery, the *posterior inferior cerebellar artery* (PICA), irrigates the lateral medullary wedge and the overlying cerebellum. Because of the Pt's hypertension, the probable diagnosis is a *PICA syndrome,* i.e., ischemia or frank infarction in the distribution of PICA. PICA arises from the vertebral artery and irrigates the lateral aspect of the medulla and cerebellar hemisphere with blood, the two vertebral arteries unite to form the basilar artery that irrigates the pons and rostral brainstem. Notice how the history, general physical findings, and knowledge of neuroanatomy, blood supply, and probable pathogenesis converge to make the diagnosis.

    d. If we set aside the medullary signs, Patient 1 had the typical *cerebellar hemisphere syndrome* (essentially the posterior lobe syndrome), consisting of the full panoply of cerebellar signs (Table 8-4) *ipsilateral* to the lesion and a particular type of bidirectional nystagmus. Figure 8-11*A*

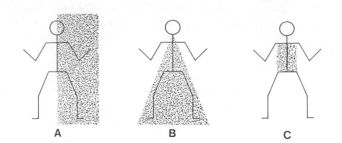

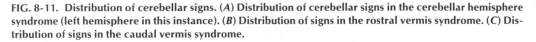

FIG. 8-11. Distribution of cerebellar signs. (*A*) Distribution of cerebellar signs in the cerebellar hemisphere syndrome (left hemisphere in this instance). (*B*) Distribution of signs in the rostral vermis syndrome. (*C*) Distribution of signs in the caudal vermis syndrome.

shows the unilateral distribution of signs in the cerebellar hemisphere syndrome.

e. The cerebellar hemisphere syndrome follows any acute cerebellar hemisphere lesion: infarct, abscess, trauma, hemorrhage, neoplasm, or demyelinating disease.

f. Summarize the neurologic signs of a PICA syndrome.

Ipsilaterally: _____

Contralaterally: _____.

Ans: Ipsilaterally, a reduced corneal reflex, Horner's syndrome, and cerebellar hemisphere signs. Contralaterally, loss of pain and temperature sensation.

B. *Patient 2*

1. *History.* This 48-year-old man had drunk alcohol excessively for 13 years, resulting in numerous hospitalizations for drunkenness, convulsions, and delirium tremens. For three years his gait had become increasingly unsteady, to the degree that his family thought he was drunk, even when he was sober. He stopped drinking 3 days prior to the examination.

2. *Physical Examination.* The Pt was malnourished and unkempt but sober. He was disoriented as to time and date. The cranial nerves functioned normally. He had no nystagmus or dysarthria. Although, generally somewhat tremulous, his finger-to-nose, alternating-movements, and overshoot tests of the arms were normal bilaterally. He had moderate truncal unsteadiness when sitting or standing. He had an unsteady, broad-based gait and could not tandem walk. His heel-to-shin movements were dystaxic. His quadriceps femoris reflexes were pendular. See Fig. 8-12.

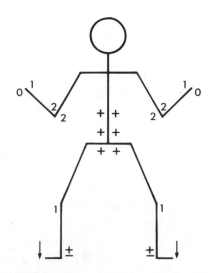

FIG. 8-12. Reflex stick figure of patient 2.

3. *Course of Patient 2.* Five days after hospitalization, the Pt began to display severe delirium tremens with hyperthermia and convulsions. He died from irreversible hyperthermia. At autopsy, a sagittal cut through the vermis of the cerebellum showed severe atrophy of all of the folia of the rostral part of the vermis. Microscopically the rostral part of the vermis and adjacent anterior lobe cortex showed severe depletion of neurons.

4. *Clinicopathologic correlation in Patient 2*

   a. Which panel in Fig. 8-11 shows the distribution of cerebellar signs in Patient 2? ☐ A/ ☐ B/ ☐ C.

   b. The rostral vermis and adjacent cortex belong to which lobe of the cerebellum? ☐ anterior/ ☐ posterior/ ☐ flocculonodular.

   c. The rostral part of the vermis receives proprioceptive information from the legs and trunk via the _____ tracts.

   d. The clinical picture of classical cerebellar signs in the legs, mild truncal dystaxia, minimal or no arm dystaxia, and absence of dysarthria or nystagmus predicts atrophy limited to the rostral part of the vermis, as shown by Patient 2 (Victor et al, 1959). Most common in severe alcoholism and malnutrition, it presents the closest approximation to an *anterior cerebellar lobe syndrome* found in humans. The extensor hypertonus seen in experimental animals only rarely occurs in humans (Ringel and Culbertson, 1988). What permits antemortem prediction of the lesion is the gradient of cerebellar signs: the cerebellar signs are *least* severe in the ☐ cranial nerve musculature/ ☐ arms/ ☐ trunk/ ☐ legs and *most* severe in the ☐ cranial nerve musculature/ ☐ arms/ ☐ trunk and legs.

C. *Patient 3*

1. *History.* This 6-year-old boy had trouble walking for 3 months, with increasing headaches and vomiting. Formerly very active, he no longer ran or played.

2. *Physical examination*

   a. Cranial nerve examination showed questionable papilledema. He had faint nystagmus in the extreme field of gaze to each side, with a quick component in the direction of gaze. When his eyes were returned slightly toward the midline, the nystagmus disappeared. He walked with an unsteady gait, and he could not tandem walk. At times he veered to the right, at others to the left. With the boy reclining in bed, formal cerebellar testing showed no definite abnormalities on finger-to-nose or heel-to-knee testing, or on the rapid-alternating-movements and overshoot tests. However, he had an unsteady trunk in any vertical position—thus when sitting, standing, or walking. In other words he had predominately an *axial* or *truncal ataxia*. Sensation was normal. Figure 8-13 shows the reflex pattern.

   b. MRI examination showed a posterior fossa tumor and enlargement of the aqueduct, 3d, and lateral ventricles, indicating obstructive hydrocephalus (Fig. 1-17*B*). Posterior fossa craniotomy disclosed a medulloblastoma involving the flocculonodular lobe and posterior vermis, filling the 4th ventricle.

3. *Clinicopathologic correlation in Patient 3*

   a. From the nystagmus dendrograms, identify the type of nystagmus (Figs. 5-4 and 5-5): _____.

   b. *Pseudonystagmus* usually has no pathologic significance and was not clearly related to the neoplasm. The equivocal extensor toe signs and

---

☑ *B*

☑ *Anterior*

Spinocerebellar

☐ *Cranial nerve musculature*

☐ *Trunk and Legs*

Pseudonystagmus

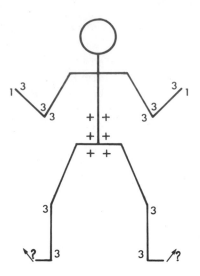

FIG. 8-13. Reflex stick figure of patient 3.

vomiting probably reflect compression of the medulla and the increased intracranial pressure. Since the skull sutures had split, the boy had no florid papilledema, as would be expected with an obstructed 4th ventricle.

c. The critical clinical feature in this 6-year-old boy was a nearly pure syndrome of *postural disequilibrium* or *truncal ataxia* whenever he had to maintain an erect posture, either sitting or standing. However, formal cerebellar tests with the Pt reclining were very nearly normal. It is tempting to suggest that the postural disturbance was caused by disruption of vestibulocerebellar and cerebellovestibular connections, that he had a *flocculonodular lobe syndrome* of dystaxia of the axial muscles. But we schematize too much. "The facile gates of hell are too slightly barred." (Milton). The large size of the neoplasm and distorted posterior fossa anatomy silence further speculation.

d. Which panel in Fig. 8-11 shows the distribution of cerebellar signs in Patient 3? ☐ A/ ☐ B/ ☐ C.

☑ C

D. *Summary of the four syndromes of the cerebellum*

1. Since the nodule of the flocculonodular lobe is in the caudal part of the vermis, we can contrast the *caudal vermis syndrome* of Patient 3 with the *rostral vermis syndrome* of Patient 2, and the *cerebellar hemisphere syndrome* of Patient 1. Then if we recognize a *pancerebellar syndrome* caused by any agent affecting the cerebellum bilaterally, we see that the first step in diagnosing cerebellar lesions is to classify, if possible, the Pt's deficits into one of the four cerebellar syndromes, as follows:

Rostral vermis (anterior lobe)

a. Dystaxia predominantly in the legs, sparing the cranial nerve musculature, is the _____ syndrome.

Caudal vermis (flocculonodular lobe)

b. Dystaxia or disequilibrium of stance and gait (axial dystaxia) with little or no extremity dystaxia is the _____ syndrome.

Hemisphere (posterior lobe)

c. Lateralized cerebellar signs limited to one half of the body is the cerebellar _____ syndrome.

Pancerebellar

d. Cerebellar signs bilaterally in all musculature, cranial, axial, and appendicular, is the _____ syndrome.

2. *Tabular summary of the four cerebellar syndromes.* Study the clinical characteristics listed in columns A and B of Table 8-4, and from these characteristics complete columns C and D.

TABLE 8-4 Cerebellar syndromes								
A	B						C	D
Distribution of deficits	Dysarthria	Arm overshoot	Hypotonia	Dystaxia of:			Clinical syndrome of:	Lobe(s) most affected
				Arms	Gait and trunk	Legs	Nystagmus		
1.	+	+	+	+	+	+	Bidirectional, coarser to side of lesion; fast component to sides of gaze		
2.	0	±	+	±	+	+	0		
3.	0	0	±	0	+	±	variable		
4.	+	+	+	+	+	+	+ (variable type)		

Ans:

C	D
1. Cerebellar hemisphere syndrome	Mainly posterior, variably anterior lobe
2. Rostral vermis syndrome	Anterior lobe
3. Caudal vermis syndrome	Flocculonodular and posterior lobe
4. Pancerebellar syndrome	All lobes

3. Run down each of the subcolumns under B in Table 8-4 to see an important bonus from displaying the data in tabular form. The only column with a strong plus for each of the four cerebellar syndromes is the gait dystaxia column. Gait incoordination is the one ubiquitous cerebellar sign, common to all four cerebellar syndromes. The upright posture and gait demand integration of the entire sensory and motor system by the cerebrum and cerebellum. Hence, gait testing is the most efficient clinical test for cerebellar dysfunction, as well as for many other neurologic deficits.

E. *Etiologic implications of the four cerebellar syndromes*
   1. Earlier I stated that by identifying the cerebellar syndrome, the Ex could predict the probable lesion. The *rostral vermis syndrome* results from alcoholism-nutritional deficiency. The *caudal vermis* syndrome implies a midline cerebellar neoplasm, usually a medulloblastoma, ependymoma, or astrocytoma. The *cerebellar hemisphere syndrome* comes from an acute destructive lesion, most likely an infarct, hemorrhage, neoplasm, abscess, or trauma. The *pancerebellar syndrome* requires a lesion which affects the entire cerebellum and, therefore, it usually results from toxic-metabolic, demyelinating, or heredofamilial degenerative diseases. Thus, by identifying the cerebellar syndrome, the Ex defines or delimits the diagnostic probabilities, which in turn leads to the most effective diagnostic procedures.
   2. The pancerebellar syndrome presents the most difficult differential diagnosis, because the causative agents span the ocean of possibilities from heredofamilial diseases to the toxic effects of drugs. Intermittent pancerebellar signs suggest a metabolic disorder with intermittent flare-ups, disclosed by measuring aminoacids and organic acids, or a demyelinating disorder, such as multiple sclerosis. The fairly common vascular syndromes that affect the distribution of only one cerebellar artery are relatively easy to diagnose (Amarenco, 1991).

V. Summary of the clinical examination for cerebellar dysfunction

Rehearsal time again! Can you give the commands, make the observations, and do the tests for cerebellar dysfunction? Start with gait testing and do section VI. H, of the Summarized Neurologic Examination. Remember that you have already tested muscle tone and elicited the MSRs, which would have disclosed pendular reflexes and hypotonia.

REFERENCES FOR CEREBELLAR DYSFUNCTION

Ackerman H, Ziegler W: Cerebellar voice tremor: an acoustic analysis. *J Neurol Neurosurg Psychiatry* 1991;54:74–76

Amarenco P: The spectrum of cerebellar infarctions. *Neurology* 1991;41:973–979

Angel RW: The rebound phenomenon of Gordon Holmes. *Arch Neurol* 1977;34:250

Angevine J Jr, Mancall E, Yakovlev P: *The Human Cerebellum. An Atlas of Gross Topography in Serial Sections.* Boston, Little, Brown & Co, 1961

Bougousslavsky J, Meienberg O: Eye-movement disorders in brainstem and cerebellar stroke. *Arch Neurol* 1987;44:141–148

Brown SH, Hefter H, Mertens M, Freund H-J: Disturbances in human arm movement trajectory due to mild cerebellar dysfunction. *J Neurol Neurosurg Psychiatry* 1990;53:306–313

Carlow TJ, Bicknell JM: Abnormal ocular motility with brainstem and cerebellar disorders, In: Burde RM, Karp JS, eds. *International Ophthalmology Clinics: The Efferent Visual System and the Orbit.* 1978;18(1):37–56

DeMyer W: *Neuroanatomy.* New York, John Wiley & Sons, 1988

Glaser JS: *Neuro-ophthalmology* (2d ed). Philadelphia, Lippincott, 1990.

Holmes G: The symptoms of acute cerebellar injuries due to gunshot injuries. *Brain* 1917;40:461–535

Holmes G: The cerebellum of man. *Brain* 1939;62:1–30

Hood JD, Kayan A, Leech J: Rebound nystagmus. *Brain* 1973;96:507–526

Kark RAP, Rosenberg RN, Schut LF (eds). *The Inherited Ataxias: Biochemical, Viral and Pathological Studies* (vol 21: *Advances in Neurology*).

Larsell O, Jansen J: *The Comparative Anatomy and Histology of the Cerebellum. The Human Cerebellum, Cerebellar Connections, and Cerebellar Cortex.* Minneapolis, University of Minnesota Press, 1972

Macklis RM, Macklis JD: Historical and phrenologic reflections on the nonmotor functions of the cerebellum: Love under the tent? *Neurology,* 1992; 42:928–932.

Pierrot-Deseilligny C, Amarenco P, Roullet E, Marteau R: Vermal infarct with pursuit eye movement disorders. *J Neurol Neurosurg Psychiatry* 1990;53:519–521

Ringel RA, Culberson JL: Extensor tone disinhibition from an infarction within the midline anterior cerebellar lobe. *J Neurol Neurosurg Psychiatry* 1988;51:1597–1599

Victor M, Adams R, Mancall E: A restricted form of cerebellar degeneration occurring in alcoholic patients. *Arch Neurol* 1959;1:579–688

VI. An essay on testing station (standing) and gait (walking)

A. *Importance of the station and gait examination*

If given just one chance to make the diagnosis, most neurologists would choose the most important single part of the neurologic examination: watching the Pt arise, stand, and walk. First notice how the Pt arises and the steadiness of the vertical posture. Then ask the Pt to walk freely back and forth. As the Pt walks, look for irregular strides, a heel-toe foot action, unsteadiness, a wide-based gait, an overplay of involuntary movements, and lack of arm-swinging. Notice whether the Pt turns by stepping around freely or rotates on the spot, en bloc, with tiny steps (see Parkinsonian gait and marche à petits pas, below). Next, test triceps surae strength and balance by having the Pt walk on the balls of the feet, and then on the heels. Next request tandem walking (heel-to-toe down a straight line). Finally, request a deep knee-bend. Ask a child to run and hop. Throughout, note how well the Pt comprehends and executes the commands. Retarded, demented, psychotic, and passive-aggressive or oppositional Pts require constant coaxing.

If the Pt arises, stands, and walks completely normally, then, in all probability, the Pt's *motor* system is completely intact. If the Pt's motor system is completely intact then, in all probability, the *sensory* system is completely intact. If the Pt follows all commands promptly and well, with no confusion or hesitancy, then in all probability the Pt's *mental* state and sensorium are intact. With *motor, sensory,* and *mental* functions intact, then in all probability, the Pt's nervous system is intact. Of course, you must still complete the entire neurologic examination to confirm these initial inferences. A normal gait requires the integrity of vast circuits of the PNS and CNS: circuits that underlie the willing of movements, and the antigravity, supporting, and righting reflexes; circuits that coordinate the rate, regularity, and force of the muscular contractions; circuits that generate reciprocal limb actions (Pearson, 1976); and circuits that mediate touch, proprioception, and vision (Hagard and Wolff, 1991). Most disorders of the muscles, nerves, spinal cord, cerebellum, brainstem, basal ganglia, or cerebrum impair the gait, and in a characteristic way. Thus, the features of the gait disorder suggest the lesion location and probable cause.

B. *Developmental gaits*

Gait examination begins with the genetically preprogrammed *automatic or reflex stepping* of the neonate. If the Ex holds the neonate vertically, with its feet contacting the bed surface, the infant reflexly lifts its legs alternately and steps. Volitional trunk control and volitional standing then replace automatic stepping, leading to *cruising,* in which the infant takes steps when holding on to a couch or when steadied by a parent. Then, at about one year the infant walks freely, with a *toddler's gait,* featured by a broad base, short, jerky, irregular steps, a semiflexed posture of the arms, and frequent falls. Finally the toddler, now a child, develops a normal *mature gait,* with a narrow-based, heel-toe stride, contrabody movement, and reciprocal swinging of the arms (Woollacott et al, 1989).

C. *Neuromuscular gaits*

Let us start with the neuromuscular system and work up to cerebral lesions. If you wish to learn the most from this essay, I strongly recommend that you get up and act out the gaits described. If an infant has a *clubfoot gait,* the gait depends on which of a variety of valgus-varus deformities exists. With tibial torsion the infant has an *in-toed* or *pigeon-toed gait.* Many clubfoot deformities correct themselves. Most myopathies (the muscular dystrophies and the polymyositides) weaken the proximal muscles of the shoulders, back, and hips. Because of weak paraspinal muscles, the myopathic Pt shows a characteristic, usually sway-backed, waddle, a *lordotic waddling gait,* resembling the *pride of pregnancy gait* of the third trimester. Because of the weak proximal muscles, the myopathic Pt has trouble when getting up on, or down from, the examining table, or when standing up from a sitting or a reclining position. In so arising, the myopathic Pt may display *Gower's sign,* the bracing of the arms against the thighs to push the weak trunk erect.

The next Pt's toes do not clear the floor because of paralysis of foot dorsiflexion, causing a *toe-drop* or *foot-drop gait.* In compensation, the Pt jerks the knee high, flipping the foot up into dorsiflexion, and slaps the foot down. With either unilateral or bilateral foot-drop gait, the sound of the slapping feet alone permits the Ex to suspect the diagnosis, without even seeing the Pt. Unilateral foot-drop suggests a unilateral, perhaps mechanical or compressive neuropathy of the common peroneal nerve, frequently from a crossed-knee palsy. A *bilateral foot-drop* or *steppage gait* suggests a symmetrical distal peripheral neuropathy of toxic, metabolic, or heredofamilial type, as in alcoholic neuropathy or Charcot-Marie-Tooth's progressive peroneal atrophy.

A tibial, as contrasted to a peroneal, nerve palsy causes a *heel-drop gait.* The Pt can dorsiflex the foot, but not plantarflex it. A complete sciatic palsy causes a *flail-foot gait* in which the Pt can neither dorsi- nor plantarflex the foot. Now you see why the Ex asks the Pt to walk both on the toes *and* heels. These actions test all of the muscles innervated by the sciatic nerve, as well as testing proprioception and balance.

This 4-year-old boy, striding on the balls of his feet, without a definite heel strike has a *toe-walking gait.* Tight heel cords limit dorsiflexion of the foot to about 90 degrees. Such a gait occurs in Duchenne's muscular dystrophy, in spastic diplegia, and in autistic or other retarded children. The toe-walking child who moves along jauntily, runs, skips, and hops normally, with no hint of neuropsychiatric abnormality, has none of these serious disorders and no handicap, merely an idiosyncratic, often familial, gait pattern.

D. *Sensory gaits*

The next Pt has a *painful sole* or *hyperesthetic gait.* The Pt sets the foot down gingerly, bears as little weight on it as possible, and limps off the foot as soon as possible, wincing and hunching the shoulders. If the pain is unilateral, suspect Morton's metatarsalgia, a painful neuroma of an interdigital nerve, or gout. If bilateral, as when a person walks barefooted on a hot pavement, suspect hyperesthesia of both soles, common in painful distal peripheral neuropathies, usually metabolic, toxic, or alcoholic-nutritional in origin.

The next Pt has a *radicular pain gait* or *antalgic gait.* The Pt complains of extreme pain radiating into the big toe, caused, in all probability, by a herniated intervertebral disc compressing the L-5 nerve root. Coughing, or straight leg-raising, shoots pain into the foot (Chap. 12). To arise from a chair, the Pt pushes up with the arms and has a stiff back, with a completely flat lumbar curve. When standing, the Pt does not put weight on the painful leg. The Achilles tendon feels soft as compared to the weight-bearing leg. When walking, the Pt places little weight on the painful leg and takes stiff, slow, short strides with no heel strike, to avoid painful jarring. Often the Pt's trunk tilts slightly to the side opposite the pain.

Even the upper extremity neuropathies may cause a characteristic gait disorder. If the Pt's transverse carpal ligament compresses the median nerve, causing a carpal tunnel syndrome, excruciating pain in the hand typically awakens the Pt at night. Night after night, the Pt gets up and paces the bedroom flipping or shaking the hand in an effort to gain some relief, the *nocturnal flipping-hand gait,* a nearly pathognomonic gait. Autistic and other retarded children show a variety of *flipping-hand gaits* as repetitive, self-stimulating mannerisms.

A tabetic, dorsal column, or sensory ataxic gait resembles a double foot-drop or steppage gait but has its own unique signature. In tabes dorsalis, syphilitic infection causes degeneration of dorsal roots and dorsal columns of the spinal cord. Lacking position sense, the Pt lifts the knees too high and slaps the feet down, placing them irregularly because of sensory ataxia. The Pt simply does not know where the legs are. When in bed, the Pt literally has to peek under the covers to locate the feet and legs. To compensate for the lack of position sense, the tabetic Pt must use visual cues in order to stand. Eye closure removes the visual cues that compensate for the absence of position sense. The Pt then sways and falls over, thus failing the Romberg test (Chap. 10), which the cerebellar Pt passes. The Ex differentiates the steppage gait of dorsal column disease from the double foot-drop gait of peroneal palsy by the presence of normal dorsiflexor power, irregular foot placement due to the sensory ataxia, the absence of position and vibration sense in the legs, absence of MSRs, and by the abnormal Romberg test. The presence of Argyll Robertson pupils and a positive serologic test for syphilis (Table 4-5) separates tabes dorsalis from other dorsal column diseases such as the subacute combined degeneration of pernicious anemia or the spinocerebellar degenerations. The experienced Ex will not confuse any of the gaits in this entire essay with the slow, deliberate, searching steps of the blind Pt, the *blind person's gait.*

E. *Cerebellar ataxic gaits*

Cerebellar lesions cause dystaxia of volitional movements and of volitionally maintained postures, hence a reeling gait. If you have ever been or seen an inebriated person, you know the syndrome exactly. A unilateral cerebellar lesion causes only *ipsi*lateral cerebellar signs, most likely from neoplasm, infarct, or demyelinating disease. After an acute cerebellar lesion, the Pt frequently veers or falls in one direction (lateropulsion, anteropulsion, or retropulsion). Bilateral cerebellar signs, thus a pancerebellar syndrome, imply a toxic, metabolic, or heredofamilial disorder; or multiple sclerosis, if combined with other exacerbating and remitting signs. Relatively pure dystaxia of the legs and gait, with little or no dystaxia of the arms, and no dysarthria or nystagmus, suggests a rostral vermis syndrome, most commonly secondary to alcoholism. Relatively pure truncal ataxia suggests a flocculonodular lobe or caudal vermis lesion, generally a 4th ventricle tumor (Table 8-4).

F. *Spastic gaits*

With a *hemiplegic gait,* the Pt circumducts a leg, dragging the toe, placing the ball down without a heel strike, with the ipsilateral arm held in partial flexion or, more rarely, flaccidly at the side. The weakness of hemiplegia affects the hand and arm more than the leg. The lesion is most likely an infarct, tumor, or trauma. The next Pt walks with stiff legs, not clearing the floor with either foot, the exact opposite of the Pt with a high steppage gait. This Pt gives the appearance of wading through water because she must work against the spastic opposition of her own muscles, as if walking in a viscid environment of molasses instead of air. Her knees tend to rub together in a scissoring action. She has a *spastic gait.* If the Pt has a *spastic diplegic gait* from diplegic cerebral palsy, she has small, short legs in contrast to normally developed chest, shoulders, and arms. In spastic diplegia, in direct contrast to double hemiplegia, the Pt has severe spasticity in her legs, minimal spasticity in her arms, and little or no deficit in speaking or swallowing, whereas the double hemiplegic has pseudobulbar palsy and more arm weakness than leg. The spastic diplegic's knees may remain bent when walking, the spastic diplegic *crouch gait* (Tylkowski and Howell, 1991). A pure spastic or *paraplegic gait,* with no sensory deficits, coming on after infancy, suggests a pure corticospinal tract disorder, such as familial spastic paraplegia. If in addition to spasticity, the disease impairs the dorsal columns or cerebellum, the Pt will have a wider-based unsteady gait and takes irregular steps—the *spastic-ataxic gait,* suggesting a spinocerebellar degeneration or multiple sclerosis.

G. *Basal ganglia gaits*

This elderly Pt with the shuffling, short steps, who does not lift the feet from the floor, has the *marche à petits pas* (the march of small steps) (Sudarsky, 1990). When the Pt tries to speak, progress ceases, leading to the somewhat pejorative, but expressive, colloquialism, "He can't walk and chew gum [in this case walk and talk] at the same time." Many of the elderly Pts in a nursing home display this type of gait. The lesion frequently consists of *status lacunaire,* multiple small cavitations in the basal ganglia from arteriosclerosis. This next Pt, with a *parkinsonian gait,* arises and walks slowly with short steps, lacks any arm swing, turns en bloc like a statue rotating on a pedestal, and has a tremor at rest which disappears during intentional movement. It results from degeneration of the substantia nigra or from neuroleptic medication. If the Ex (after a forewarning) shoves the Pt, the Pt will move forward or backward on tiny steps of increasing speed and decreasing length, as if chasing the center of gravity, and may fall over, a *festinating gait.* Pts with the marche à petits pas often also turn en bloc and festinate. When the Pt with a *choreiform gait* walks, the play of finger and arm movements increases, or may even appear clearly for the first time. Random missteps mar the evenness of the strides, as the choreiform twitches supervene. A family history of chorea and dementia establishes Huntington's chorea. A history of rheumatic fever and a fussy personality signify Sydenham's chorea. When the athetoid Pt walks, the slow writhing movements of fingers and arms tend to increase. A combination of athetosis with moderate spastic diplegia or double hemiplegia, a *spastic-athetoid gait,* usually signifies status marmoratus (état marbre) of the basal ganglia and thalamus, secondary to perinatal hypoxia. Dystonia may first manifest in a child, say of 9 years of age, by an intermittent inturning of the foot that impedes walking, an *equinovarus dystonic gait.* In the later stages dystonic truncal contortions and tortipelvis may cause the trunk to incline strongly forward. The Pt may take giant uneven strides, exhibiting flexions or rise and fall of the trunk, the dystonic *dromedary gait,* imitating the ungainly gait of a dromedary camel. It looks for all of the world like histrionics but the Pt has dystonia musculorum deformans, a hereditary organic disorder. Pts with involuntary movement disorders can sometimes walk backwards or dance better than they can walk forwards.

H. Cerebral gaits

The next Pt, an elderly woman, has difficulty initiating the sequence of movements to rise, stand, or walk. When lying down she makes fairly normal leg movements. When trying to arise from the chair, she will rock up and down several times in order to rise, or when commencing to walk, she will make several efforts to move the feet, in both cases appearing somewhat puzzled, as if searching for lost motor engrams, or the right buttons to press to start progressing. The effort to progress may only result in stepping on the same spot as if trying to free the feet from thick, sticky mud, the *dancing bear gait.* If she does progress, her feet cling to the floor as if magnetized. This Pt has an *apraxic gait,* usually from severe bilateral cerebral disease, most likely Alzheimer's disease, multi-infarct dementia, or senility. Elderly Pts may display a mixed gait disorder with apraxia, marche à petits pas, and some parkinsonian features.

I. Psychiatric gaits

To fully appreciate the *astasia-abasia* (astasia = not standing; abasia = not walking) of the hysteric Pt, the new physician will have to witness it (Lempert et al, 1991; Keane, 1989). The Pt tilts, gyrates, and undulates all over the place, unwittingly proving by not falling during the marvelous demonstration of agility, that strength, balance, coordination, and sensation have to be intact. Do not mistake some of the bizarre involuntary movement disorders, particular the dromedary gait of dystonia, for hysteria. To learn how other mental illnesses affect the gait, just watch any group of Pts in a psychiatric hospital as they walk along to the cafeteria. Hardly a single Pt steps out with a perfectly normal gait. This Pt, hopelessly moving along, sighing, shoulders sagging, head down looking at the floor, obviously suffers from depression (Sloman, 1982). That one over there wringing her hands and wrinkling her brow has an agitated depression. That unkempt middle-aged man, walks with small irregular, wincing steps placed gingerly on a wide base. His spindly arms and legs contrast with a disproportionate, pregnancylike fullness of the abdomen. His alcoholism has caused ascites, a rostral vermis syndrome, and a painful sensory neuropathy with hyperesthetic soles. That young adult Pt with a mild parkinsonian gait is probably a schizophrenic taking large doses of neuroleptic medication. That young woman, gesticulating as if conversing as she walks along, is a schizophrenic, attending to her hallucinations. She is underdosed, or her medication has not yet taken hold. That next grim-looking Pt, walking cautiously and peering around suspiciously, suffers from severe paranoid schizophrenia. That child, running helter-skelter, bumping into people and objects, giggling inappropriately, has an attention deficit disorder with hyperactivity. The teenager who, of inner necessity, steps on every crack, pats every door, and suddenly halts his progression to whirl around and utter expletives, suffers from the disabling compulsions of severe Tourette's syndrome. That aged Pt with silvery white hair, confusion of purpose and direction, and marche à petits pas has, as you now know, organic dementia, most likely caused by senility or Alzheimer's disease. Thus does the gait disclose the mental as well as the neurologic status of the Pt.

J. *The gait as an expression of biological sexual orientation*
That the gait of heterosexual females and males differs, not only in pelvic contour and undulation, but also in style requires no further comment. But notice this next young man, with rather dainty steps, swishy hips, and exaggerated wrist movements characteristic of the effeminate male homosexual (see the Whitman quotation at the beginning of Chap. 7). Then notice the gait of the next person, dressed in khaki fatigues and boots, marching along with determined, masculine strides, with no hip undulation, chin vigorously thrust forward, short, cropped hair and no makeup. It takes some looking to determine her sex, decided, at the last moment, by the absence of any hint of a beard. She has the determined gait of the aggressive type of lesbian. The gait, whether of toddlers, of senile persons, or of heterosexual males and females and some homosexuals, is characteristic of and diagnostic of the biologic state of the individual's brain. The gait, as related to sexual orientation, thus often reflects another of the structural and functional biological differences demonstrated to exist along the male-female continuum (Kimura, 1992).

Gentle reader, if I have overdone the gait examination a little, forgive me. If not quite the whole neurologic examination, nothing else discloses so much so quickly.

REFERENCES FOR GAIT ANALYSIS

Brown JK, Rodda J, Walsh EG, Wright GW: Neurophysiology of lower-limb function in hemiplegic children. *Dev Med Child Neurol* 1991;33:1037–1047

Gage JR: *Gait Analysis in Cerebral Palsy.* New York, Cambridge University Press, 1991

Hagard J, Wolff PH (eds): *The Development of Timing Control and Temporal Organization in Coordinated Action.* Amsterdam, Elsevier, 1991

Keane JR: Hysterical gait disorders. *Neurology* 1989;39:586–589

Lempert S, Brandt S, Dieterich M, Huppert D: How to identify psychogenic disorders of stance and gait. *J Neurol* 1991;238:140–146

Pearson K: The control of walking. *Sci Am* 1976;235:72–86

Sloman L, Berridge M, Homatidis S et al: Gait patterns of depressed patients and normal subjects. *Am J Psych* 1982;139:94–96

Sudarsky L: Geriatrics: gait disorders in the elderly. *New Engl J Med* 1990;322:1441–1446

Tylkowski CM, Howell VL: Crouch gait in cerebral palsy. *Internat Pediat* 1991;6:153–160

Vilensky JA, Damasio AR, Maurer RG: Gait disturbances in patients with autistic behavior. *Arch Neurol* 1981;38:646–649

Woollacott MH, Connolly K. Shumway-Cook A: *Development of Posture and Gait Across the Life Span.* Columbia, SC, University of South Carolina Press, 1989

I. The function of the cerebellum

1. State as briefly as possible the role of the cerebellum in movement as inferred from clinical observations.
2. Explain why you cannot test for cerebellar dysfunction in a comatose or paralyzed patient.
3. Explain the importance of proprioceptive input to the cerebellum.

II. The anatomy of the cerebellum

1. Name the three lobes of the cerebellum according to Larsell, and state the major source of afferent fibers to each one (Table 8-1).
2. Make a schematic dorsal view drawing of the cerebellum showing its division into Larsell's three lobes and into the vermis and hemispheres (Fig. 8-1).
*3. Give the phylogenetic name for the three lobes of the cerebellum (Table 8-1).
4. Name the three pairs of peduncles of the cerebellum. State where they attach the cerebellum to the brainstem and their anatomical relation to each other (Fig. 8-3).
5. Describe the major afferent and efferent fibers conveyed through each of the three cerebellar peduncles.
6. State which lobe of the cerebellum anatomically and phylogenetically has the closest relation to the vestibular nerve.
7. Describe the general plan of the flow of impulses through the cerebellum, beginning with the afferent pathway (Fig. 8-4).
*8. Name the cerebellar neuron that provides the final common pathway out of the cerebellar cortex.
9. Diagram the cortico-cerebello-cortical circuit, beginning with one cerebral motor cortex (Fig. 8-5).
10. Describe the decussations underlying the aphorism: "Cerebral hemisphere lesions cause contralateral motor signs, whereas cerebellar hemisphere lesions cause ipsilateral motor signs."

III. Clinical signs of cerebellar dysfunction

1. Describe the characteristic changes in the gait of a Pt with a cerebellar lesion.
2. Describe where the medial edge of the heels falls when a normal person walks a straight line.
3. Demonstrate how to test for dystaxia of the upper extremities (Table 8-2).
4. Define dysmetria and dysdiadochokinesia and describe how to test for them (Figs. 8-6 and 8-7).
5. Explain why the thigh-slapping test for dysdiadochokinesia is superior to the free hand test (Fig. 8-7).
6. Describe the overshooting (often called rebound) test of the upper extremities (Figs. 8-8 and 8-9) and how to protect the Pt's face during the test.
7. Describe the clinical manifestations of hypotonia in a Pt with cerebellar dysfunction (Table 8-2).

8. Describe in principle the clinical effect of cerebellar lesions on eye movements, speech, strength, and endurance.
*9. Describe the characteristic nystagmus of an acute unilateral destructive lesion of a cerebellar hemisphere (Fig. 5-5).
*10. Describe decomposition of movement and how the Pt might manifest it.

IV. Analysis of Pts and the four cerebellar syndromes

1. Describe (or shade on stick figures) the distribution of cerebellar signs in a cerebellar hemisphere lesion, rostral (superior) vermis lesion, caudal (inferior) vermis lesion, and pancerebellar lesions. Relate these syndromes to the cerebellar lobes involved (Table 8-4).
2. Explain why gait testing is the single most important test for cerebellar dysfunction.
3. Describe how the classification of the Pt's cerebellar syndrome into one of the four types, e.g., hemispheric, rostral vermis, caudal vermis, or pancerebellar, suggests the cause or lesion type responsible.

V. Summary of the clinical examination for cerebellar dysfunction

Demonstrate in an orderly sequence how to test a Pt for cerebellar dysfunction (Table 8-2).

VI. An essay on testing station (standing) and gait (walking)

1. Describe the station and gait examination and what the Ex looks for when a Pt walks.
2. Describe the inferences that the Ex can make about the function of the nervous system if the Pt does all of the station and gait tests perfectly.

Note: Describe and act out the following features observed in testing station and gait, and where appropriate describe the pathophysiology or lesion.

3. *Developmental gaits.* Automatic stepping of the newborn, cruising, toddler's gait, and normal mature gait.
4. *Neuromuscular gaits.* Lordotic waddling (myopathic) gait, pride-of-pregnancy gait, Gower's sign, unilateral and bilateral foot-drop or steppage gait, heel-drop gait, flail-foot gait, and toe-walking gait.
5. *Sensory gaits.* Hyperesthetic gait, radicular pain or antalgic gait, nocturnal flipping-hand gait in an adult and a flipping-hand gait in a retarded child, a sensory ataxia or tabetic gait, and a blind person's gait. Explain why a Pt with degeneration of dorsal columns sways and falls over upon closing the eyes (Romberg test) but a Pt with cerebellar lesion does not.
6. *Cerebellar ataxic gaits.* Cerebellar hemisphere versus rostral and caudal vermis lesion gaits.

7. *Spastic gaits.* Hemiplegic gait, spastic diplegic gait, crouch gait, paraplegic gait and spastic-ataxic gait.

8. *Basal ganglia gaits.* Marche à petit pas, parkinsonian gait, festinating gait, en bloc or pedestal turning, choreiform gait, spastic-athetoid gait, equinovarus dystonic gait, dromedary or tortipelvis dystonic gait.

9. *Cerebral gaits.* Dancing bear and apraxic gait.

10. *Psychiatric gaits.* Astasia-abasia, gaits of depression and agitated depression, schizophrenic gaits, Tourette's syndrome gait, and hyperactive child gait.

Chapter Nine

Examination of the Special Senses

And there I stood, a man grown, shaking in the sunshine with that old boyish emotion brought back to me by an odour! Often and often have I known this strange rekindling of dead fires. And I have thought how, if our senses were really perfect, we might lose nothing out of our lives: neither sights, nor sounds, nor emotions . . .
                                                    Ray Stannard Baker

I. The senses

A. *Sensation and subjectivity*

The possibility for sensation begins when a chemical or physical change stimulates the receptor endings of sensory neurons and alters the flow of impulses in the sensory pathways. The impulses in the sensory pathways then lead to a state of mind that we call a sensation, whether of pain, touch, sight, or whatever. Nothing is more real to the patient (Pt) than the experience of a sensation, such as pain, nor less real to the observer. Although thc Pt can judge the degrees of sensation, even scale a sensation like pain from 0–10, no one else can verify the sensation nor measure it objectively in grams, centimeters, or seconds, the classical units of the physical sciences. Nevertheless, by carefully eliciting the Pt's history, the examiner (Ex) can recognize and diagnose various sensory syndromes, such as migraine or nerve root compression, with about the same degree of certainty as motor syndromes.

B. *Classifications of sensation*
   1. Aristotle recognized five primary senses:
      a. Sight
      b. Sound
      c. Smell
      d. Taste
      e. Touch
   2. Tradition also recognizes *special* and *general* senses. The special senses are sight, sound, taste, smell, and equilibrium. The general sensations are the rest.

*The light vertical rule on the left side of the text sets off an answer column. Cover the answers with a card until you have responded to the text. Then, after each response, slide the card down to check your answer.

The heavy vertical rule or asterisk denotes optional material.

3. Modern classifications of sensation adopt the views of Charles Sherrington (1857–1952). Depending on the origin of the stimulus and the location of the receptor tips of the axons, whether in superficial or deep structures, Sherrington recognized *exteroception, proprioception,* and *interoception.*

   a. *Exteroceptor* tips are located near the external body surfaces. They mediate stimuli that originate from sources external to the body and that impinge on the body's external surfaces. These stimuli produce sight, sound, smell, taste, and superficial cutaneous sensation. Superficial skin sensations consist of:

      (1) Touch
      (2) Superficial pain
      (3) Temperature
      (4) Itching and tickling

   b. *Proprioceptor* axonal tips are located beneath body surfaces. They mediate stimuli that originate from receptors in muscles, joints, and the vestibular labyrinth. (Chapter 10 gives a fuller definition of proprioception.) Proprioceptive sensations consist of:

      (1) Position
      (2) Movement
      (3) Vibration
      (4) Pressure (weight)
      (5) Deep pain
      (6) Equilibrium (vestibular sensation)

   c. *Interceptor* axonal tips are located in the viscera and vessels. They mediate:

      (1) Visceral and vascular pain
      (2) Stretch or distension of the viscera

4. To avoid memorizing sensory classifications, think systematically. Simply sort through your own senses. Start rostrally with the mouth, nose, eyes, ears, skin, and so on over the exteroceptors of the body. Then visualize the body in 3D, and you will encounter first the deep sensations of the proprioceptors, and finally the interoceptors.

C. *The concept of sensory modalities*

   1. No one ever confuses the stench of carrion with a taste of honey, or a pinprick with a sound. Each different, each *unique* sensation not resolvable into a more elementary sensation is called a *primary sensory modality.* Ay, but there is the rub, in defining "unique," "resolve," and "elementary."

   2. *Operations to disclose primary sensory modalities*
      Stick yourself with a pin: there, that is pain, one modality. Stroke yourself with a piece of cotton: there, that is touch, another modality.

   3. *Operation to disclose multimodal sensations*
      With your eyes closed, grasp any object from your pocket or purse, say a quarter. You will recognize it as metal and a coin by a combination of touch, texture, weight and size (pressure), proprioception (how far your fingers open and close to encompass it), and even to some degree by its slightly cold feel. We can, I think, agree that sight does not resolve into elementary modalities of sound and taste, but the perception of a coin in your hand resolves, at least in part, into touch, position sense, and other primary exteroceptive and proprioceptive modalities. Multimodal sensations include:

      a. Form, size, and texture
      b. Weight

      c. Two-point discrimination

      d. Wetness

D. *Implications of the theory of modality specificity*

  1. The neurologist could yield the modality issue to the philosopher except for one thing: the pathways of the nervous system provide for modality separation. In fact, we might even suggest defining a modality as any sensation that the nervous system represents by a unique pathway, but then that forces us into negative definitions. What is sight? It is that sensation lost after cutting both optic nerves. We return to relying on our own intuitive, private experience, to separate modalities.

  2. Since special senses have unique receptors, investigators have sought unique receptors for all modalities. Carried to its extreme, the theory of modality specificity requires unique receptors, unique peripheral axons, unique pathways through cord, brainstem, and thalamus, and unique cortical receptive areas. Apart from some controversy about the specificity of skin receptors, the theory of modality specific pathways proves sound enough for the clinician to use it to localize lesions.

  3. By testing all sensations, the Ex tests the integrity of a large volume of neural tissue. Add the volume of tissue assayed by testing motor pathways, and the Ex has tested the integrity of the spinal cord, the brainstem, the cerebellum, and much of the diencephalon and cerebral hemispheres. The more pathways that function normally, the more the Ex can exclude neurologic disease. The more pathways that function abnormally, the more the Ex can predict the size, location, and type of the lesion.

E. *Basic principles of sensory physiology,* summarized from the doctrine of specific nerve energies of Johannes Müller (1801–1858)

  1. *Sensation is an awareness of the state of nerve impulses in the sensory neural pathways.* We only know the external world by the changes that occur in the state of impulses in our receptor pathways.

  2. *Stimulation of a sensory nerve by any means, electrical, mechanical, or chemical, causes only the type of sensation ordinarily mediated by the nerve.* A blow on the eye causes a sensation of light; not taste, but light.

  3. *The same stimulus applied to different sensory organs causes only the sensation appropriate to the organ.* Put a stimulating electrode on the cochlea and you *hear.* Put the same electrode on the skin and you *feel.*

II. Smell (olfaction): Ist cranial nerve

A. *Olfactory receptor and nerve*

  1. Study Figs. 9-1 and 9-2.

  2. Mucus covers the olfactory nerve endings. Any odiferous agent must first dissolve in the mucus, which acts as the first censor for smell. Colds or allergic rhinitis impair olfaction by mechanical reduction of air flow, and by excessive mucus secretion.

  3. Olfactory impulses travel centrally past the ganglion cells. The ganglion cells are ☐ external to/ ☐ within/ ☐ internal to the cribriform plate.

  4. Axons from the olfactory ganglion cells form *olfactory nerve* filaments. The filaments perforate the cribriform plate and attached dura. The olfactory axons then cross the subarachnoid space to synapse on the olfactory bulbs. Viruses may gain access to the subarachnoid space or brain via the olfactory nerve filaments and cause encephalitis (Twomey et al, 1979).

☑ *External to*

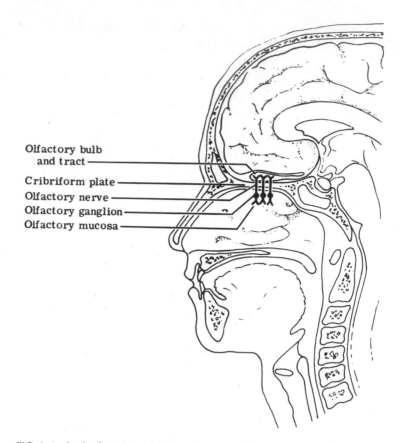

Olfactory bulb
and tract
Cribriform plate
Olfactory nerve
Olfactory ganglion
Olfactory mucosa

FIG. 9-1. Sagittal section of the head to show olfactory nerve, bulb, and tract.

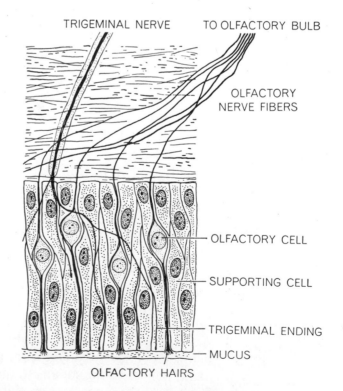

TRIGEMINAL NERVE   TO OLFACTORY BULB

OLFACTORY
NERVE FIBERS

OLFACTORY CELL

SUPPORTING CELL

TRIGEMINAL ENDING

MUCUS

OLFACTORY HAIRS

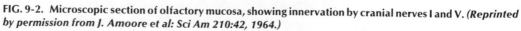

FIG. 9-2. Microscopic section of olfactory mucosa, showing innervation by cranial nerves I and V. (*Reprinted by permission from J. Amoore et al: Sci Am 210:42, 1964.*)

B. *Olfactory-related consequences of head injuries*

1. Head injuries may cause the delicate olfactory nerve filaments to shear off (Jafek et al, 1989) and may also result in cribiform plate fracture. The Pt loses the sense of smell, a condition called *anosmia* (Getchel et al, 1991). If the wafer-thin cribriform plate fractures, the meninges may rupture initially or later when the Pt coughs, causing a fistula that allows cerebrospinal fluid (CSF) to gush into the nose. During physiologic fluctuations in intracranial pressure, fluid then refluxes back through the fistula into the subarachnoid space, introducing nasal bacteria and causing meningitis. Therefore, consider a CSF fistula in the differential diagnosis of a runny nose (rhinorrhea) (Schechter and Henkin, 1974). Suspect such a fistula whenever a Pt, usually one with a history of head injury, has a runny nose and anosmia but does not have a cold or allergic rhinitis (Brisman et al, 1970). The fistula may require surgical closure (Allen et al, 1972).

2. To differentiate a CSF leak from nasal mucus or allergic rhinorrhea, stain a drop for eosinophiles and measure the glucose. CSF has greater than 30 mg/dl of free glucose, whereas mucus has less than 30 mg/dl. Final proof of the presence of a fistula depends on CT tomography, metricimide cisternography, or demonstration of radioactivity in the nasal cavity after injection of a radionuclide tracer into the CSF by lumbar puncture (Fig. 9-3).

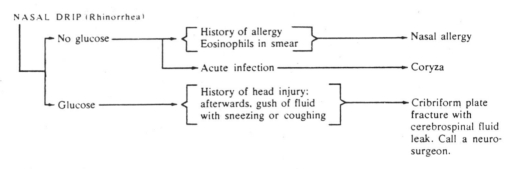

FIG. 9-3. Microdendrogram for nasal drip (reference only).

3. Some complications of a head injury are:

Anosmia

a. Loss of smell, a condition called _____.

Subarachnoid
Meningitis

b. The formation of a fistula between the nasal cavity and the _____ space.

c. A potentially lethal complication of such a fistula is _____.

C. *Central olfactory pathways:* The concept of a rhinencephalon

1. After receiving the synapses from the primary olfactory axons, the olfactory bulbs send secondary pathways to the adjacent basal frontotemporal junction (basal forebrain). Tertiary pathways then disperse through a bewildering array of circuits in the basal forebrain that are not directly accessible to clinical testing. Taken together the olfactory bulbs and tracts and their immediate central connections constitute the *rhinencephalon.* At one evolutionary stage, the cerebrum consisted mostly of rhinencephalon. Ontogenetically and phylogenetically our own brain retains the primitive rhinencephalic ground plan (Fig. 9-4).

2. The sense of smell originally served the two fundamental functions of *feeding* and *mating.* These two visceral drives and their attendant visceral emotions were originally localized in the rhinencephalon before extending to those parts of the forebrain, essentially the limbic lobe, that evolved most

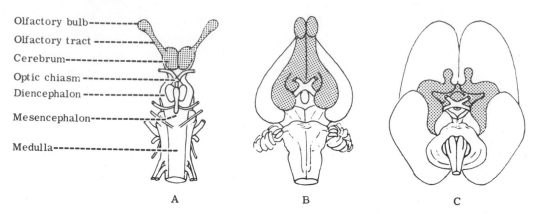

Olfactory bulb
Olfactory tract
Cerebrum
Optic chiasm
Diencephalon
Mesencephalon
Medulla

A   B   C

FIG. 9-4. Ventral view of shark (*A*), rabbit (*B*), and human fetal brain (*C*). The rhinencephalon (shaded) comprises most of the shark brain. Notice in the rabbit and human brain that the nonrhinencephalic cortex (unshaded) which began as patches on the cerebral wall of primitive animals has overgrown to dwarf the rhinencephalon. Nevertheless the rhinencephalon set its imprint forever on the form and function of the human brain.

directly from the olfactory ground plan. These forebrain regions remain the "seats" of emotion and affective experience. Humans no longer exude the natural musks and pheromones, but we assiduously replace them with perfumes and colognes. In any event, smell remains as the most evocative of sensations. Here, eavesdrop on Ray Stannard Baker's thoughts again, as he set out on his farm one morning, a century ago, to dig a ditch:

Of all hours of the day there is none like the early morning for downright good odours—the morning before eating. Fresh from sleep and unclogged with food a man's senses cut like knives. The whole world comes in upon him. A still morning is best, for the mists and moisture seem to retain the odours which they have distilled through the night. Upon a breezy morning one is likely to get a single predominant odour when the wind comes through the orchard, but upon a perfectly still morning, it is wonderful how the odours arrange themselves in upright strata, so that one walking passes through them as from room to room in a marvellous temple of fragrance. . . .

So it was this morning. As I walked along the margin of my field I was conscious, at first, coming within the shadows of the wood, of the cool, heavy aroma which one associates with the night: as of moist woods and earth mould. The penetrating scent of the night remains long after the sights and sounds of it have disappeared. In sunny spots I had the fragrance of the open cornfield, the aromatic breath of the brown earth, giving curiously the sense of fecundity—a warm, generous odour of daylight and sunshine. Down the field, toward the corner, cutting in sharply as though a door opened (or a page turned to another lyric), came the cloying, sweet fragrance of wild crab-apple blossoms, almost tropical in their richness, and below that, as I came to my work, the thin acrid smell of the marsh, the place of the rushes and the flags and the frogs. . . .

So I walked this morning, not hearing not seeing, but smelling. Without desiring to stir up strife among the peaceful senses, there is this further marvel of the sense of smell. No other possesses such an aftercall. Sight preserves pictures: the complete view of the aspect of objects, but it is photographic and external. Hearing deals in echoes, but the sense of smell, while saving no vision of a place or a person, will re-create in a way almost miraculous the inner emotion of a particular time or place. . . .

Only a short time ago I passed an open doorway in the town. I was busy with errands, my mind fully engaged, but suddenly I caught an odour from somewhere within the building I was passing. I stopped! It was as if in that moment I lost twenty years of my life. I was a boy again, living and feeling a particular instant at the time of my father's death. Every emotion of that occasion, not recalled in years, returned to me sharply and clearly as though I experienced it for the first time. . . .

And there I stood, a man grown, shaking in the sunshine with that old boyish emotion brought back to me by an odour! And I have thought how, if our sense were really perfect, we might lose nothing out of our lives: neither sights, nor sounds, nor emotions. . . . **Ray Stannard Baker**

3. *Déjà vu and déjà pensée*
   The uncus, the medial-most gyrus of the temporal lobe, contains a cortical receptive area for smell. Uncal lesions cause olfactory hallucinations, usually of very disagreeable odors. One of my Pts tore down his bedroom walls because of the conviction that he smelled a dead animal entrapped within them. Each time the odor came powerfully to him, he also experienced a peculiar feeling of familiarity, of something happening that had all happened before (just as Baker described). Autopsy showed a metastatic bronchogenic carcinoma in his uncus. The feeling of familiarity, as if something had all happened before, is called *déjà vu* (previously or already seen) or *déjà pensée* (previously or already thought). Although we each experience this sense of undue familiarity from time to time, when a Pt reports it in association with an olfactory hallucination, suspect a medial temporal lobe lesion. Get a magnetic resonance imaging (MRI) scan.

D. *The olfactory stimulus*

I; V (Fig. 9-2)
I

1. The two cranial nerves that supply sensory fibers to the olfactory epithelium are numbers _____ and _____. Of these, only cranial nerve number _____ serves olfaction.
2. As a general law in testing any sensation, the Ex isolates the chosen modality from all other modalities. Otherwise the Ex does not know which sensory pathway caused the response. To test *only* the sense of smell, should the Ex use an irritating substance like ammonia or an aromatic substance like coffee? ☐ ammonia/ ☐ coffee.

☑ *Coffee*

3. Ammonia irritates all receptors of a mucus membrane. Even the conjunctiva reacts to (smells as it were) ammonia. To test smell, use a vial of coffee grounds. Should the vial be ☐ opaque or ☐ clear. Why? _____
_____.

Ans: ☑ *Opaque. The Ex wishes to test smell, not vision.*

4. Although not part of the routine neurologic examination (NE), the University of Pennsylvania Smell Identification Test (UPSIT; available through Sensonics, Inc., Haddonfield NJ) provides a battery for testing olfaction (Jafek et al, 1989; Schiffman, 1983).

E. *Technique for testing olfaction*
1. Successful sensory testing depends on Ex–Pt communication. Say to the Pt, "Close your eyes and try to identify this odor."
2. Compress *one* of the Pt's nostrils and hold the vial in front of the *other*. Ask the Pt to sniff, and allow a moment for the Pt to answer as to whether an odor is present and what it is.
3. For the second trial, compress the opposite nostril and this time do *not* present the stimulus. Withholding the stimulus tests the Pt's suggestibility and attentiveness. The Ex must include such safeguards in all sensory testing.
4. The third time, present the stimulus to the untested nostril.

F. *Clinical analysis of anosmia*

1. To analyze anosmia systematically, start at the receptor. What initial barrier must any aromatic agent in the inspired air pass through before it stimulates olfactory receptors? _____.

Ans: *Mucus coating of the olfactory nerve endings.*

    a. The most frequent causes of anosmia in younger individuals are the *common cold* and *allergic rhinitis,* smoking, and head trauma.

    b. Sadly, the sensitivity of all sensation decreases with aging. Sight, hearing, vibration sense: they all diminish. Hence age-related decay of the metabolic machinery of the neurons commonly causes anosmia in the elderly. Anosmia also occurs in dementia and motor neuron diseases (Elian, 1991; Schiffman, 1983).

2. Next, consider lesions of the olfactory bulbs and tracts. While rare, the most significant are meningeal neoplasms—classically, olfactory groove meningiomas—that compress the olfactory bulbs and tracts. The olfactory bulbs and tracts may fail to evaginate (arhinencephaly), resulting in congenital, lifelong anosmia (DeMyer, 1987; Louis et al, 1992).

3. Lesions of the olfactory cortex rarely if ever cause anosmia. If the lesion irritates the cortex which elaborates olfactory impulses into conscious appreciation, mainly the _____ of the temporal lobe, the Pt experiences hallucinations of disagreeable odors and another peculiar symptom called _____ or _____.

Uncus

Déjà pensée; déjà vu

4. Figure 9-5 reviews the differential diagnosis of anosmia.

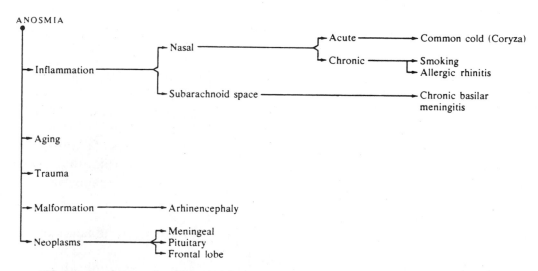

FIG. 9-5. Dendrogram for differential diagnosis of common causes of anosmia (reference only).

5. What is the explanation for nasal drip caused by sneezing or coughing?

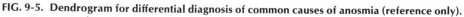

_____

Ans: *The venous system transmits the pressure from coughing or sneezing intracranially, forcing CSF out of a cribriform plate fistula.*

6. The Pt with anosmia may complain mainly of loss of taste, since taste and smell are so intimately linked. For the Pt's experience of anosmia, read Birnberg (1988).

REFERENCES FOR ANOSMIA

Allen M Jr, Gammal T, Ihnen M, Cowan M: Fistula detection in cerebrospinal fluid leakage. *J Neurol Neurosurg Psychiatry* 1972;35:664–668

Baker RS (David Grayson, pseudonym): *Adventures in Contentment.* New York, Grosset, 1907

Birnberg JR: Living with a lack of taste. *Newsweek.* March 21, 1988, p. 10

Brisman R, Hughes JEO, Mount LA: Cerebrospinal fluid rhinorrhea. *Arch Neurol* 1970;22:245–252

DeMyer W: Holoprosencephaly (cyclopia-arhinencephaly), in Vinken PJ, Bruyn GW, Klawans HL (eds): *Malformations,* vol. 6, *Handbooks of Clinical Neurology.* Amsterdam, Elsevier Science Publishers, 1987

Elian M. Olfactory impairment in motor neuron disease: a pilot study. *J Neurol Neurosurg Psychiatry* 1991;54:927–928

Getchel TV, Bartoshuk LM, Doty RL, Snow JB (eds): *Smell and Taste in Health and Disease.* New York, Raven Press, 1991

Jafek BW, Eller PM, Esses BA, Moran DT: Post-traumatic anosmia: ultrastructural correlates. *Arch Neurol* 1989;46:300–306

Louis DN, Arriagada PV, Hyman BT, Hedley-Whyte EJ: Olfactory dysgenesis or hypoplasia: a variant in the arhinencephaly spectrum. *Neurology* 1992;42:179–182

Schechter PJ, Henkin RI: Abnormalities of taste and smell after head trauma. *J Neurol Neurosurg Psychiatry* 1974;37:802–810

Schiffman SS: Taste and smell in disease. Part I. *N Engl J Med* 1983;308:1275–1279

Schiffman SS: Taste and smell in disease. Part II. *New Engl J Med* 1983;308:1337–1342

Twomey JA, Barker CM, Robinson G, Howell DA: Olfactory mucosa in herpes simplex encephalitis. *J Neurol Neurosurg Psychiatry* 1979;42:983–987

III. Taste or gustation, and loss of taste (ageusia)

A. *Receptors.* The epithelium of the tongue and tonsillar pillars contains taste buds. As in olfaction, the chemical agents that stimulate taste must first dissolve in a liquid, the saliva (Cagan, 1989). The loss of taste is called *ageusia.* Often the Pt who complains of ageusia actually has anosmia, since taste and smell complement each other in producing flavor and full gustatory sensation (Schiffman, 1983; Clee and Burrow, 1983; Finger and Silver, 1987).pbc

B. *Innervation of taste receptors*

1. The taste buds of the anterior two-thirds of the tongue are innervated by. . . . What cranial nerve was it? Well, if you have forgotten, start at number I and sort through them:

I; II

Cranial nerve number _____ smells, _____ sees.

III; IV; VI

Cranial nerves, _____, _____, _____, and _____ rotate the eyeball.

V

_____ chews and feels the front of the head.

_____ moves the facial muscles, tears, salivates, and _____.

Ans: VII; tastes. (Should you review Tables 2-5 and 2-6?)

2. The Ex only tests taste on the anterior two-thirds of the tongue, the area innervated by VII. The taste buds on the posterior third of the tongue and tonsillar pillars are inconvenient to test. Learn Fig. 9-6.

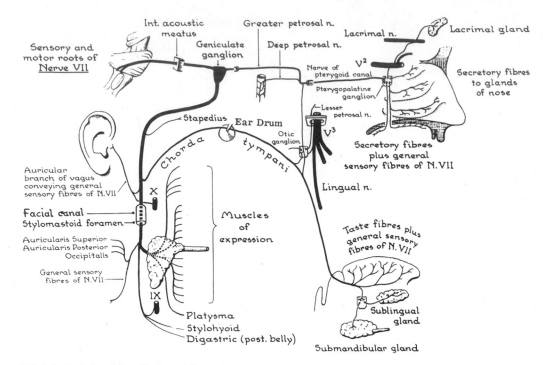

FIG. 9-6. Peripheral distribution of the VIIth cranial nerve. *(Modified from J.C.B. Grant: An Atlas of Anatomy, 5th ed, Baltimore, Williams & Wilkins, 1962).*

C. *Review of the VIIth cranial nerve*

Pontomedullary

1. The VIIth nerve attaches to the brainstem at the _____ sulcus.
2. In ventrodorsal order, the cranial nerves attaching at the pontomedullary sulcus are _____.

Ans: VI, VII, VIII (Review Fig. 2-21 if you erred.)

VIII

3. VII enters the internal auditory meatus in company with cranial nerve _____.

Geniculate

4. The *primary* neurons for taste are located in the only ganglion on cranial nerve VII, the _____ ganglion.
5. The name *geniculate* ganglion comes from the kneelike downward bend of the VIIth nerve after it clears the ganglion and heads for the stylomastoid foramen (Fig. 9-6).

D. *Central pathways for taste.* Lesions of the central taste pathways rarely cause isolated loss of taste. The brainstem pathway ascends to the thalamus homo-laterally, without decussation. Gustatory sensation is probably represented in the insular cortex (island of Reil) and adjacent parietal operculum (area 43 of Brodmann). Irritative lesions in this region may cause gustatory hallucinations (Bornstein, 1940; Penfield and Jasper, 1954).

E. *Technique of testing for loss of taste (ageusia)*
1. The stimulus is any salty, sweet, sour, or bitter substance. Salt, sugar, or quinine are suitable. Conceal salt or sugar. The Pt who sees a white crystalline substance will almost automatically guess either salt or sugar.
2. *Communication with the patient*
   a. Tell the Pt, "I want to place something on your tongue for you to taste. Stick out your tongue and keep it out. When you recognize the taste, hold up your hand."

b. Place a few crystals of your test material on the right or left half of the tongue and massage them around with the well-moistened cotton tip of an applicator stick. Take care to confine the stimulus to one half of the tongue. Do not allow the Pt to return the tongue to the mouth because the saliva will diffuse the taste stimulus beyond the area selected for testing. Salt and sugar are best perceived near the tip of the tongue but avoid the tip itself. If the tongue is dry moisten it slightly. Allow 15 to 20 seconds for the substance to dissolve and for the Pt to respond. Some normal subjects will not perceive sugar. Test again with salt.

c. After the Pt rinses his mouth, test the opposite side of the tongue with the same or a different substance. For routine clinical purposes you need try only one substance to test for ageusia. Although not part of the routine NE, taste can be measured by impregnated paper discs and also by galvanic currents.

d. Test your own sense of taste as described.

e. The main indications for testing taste are a complaint of loss of taste or the presence of a VIIth cranial nerve palsy. Taste is the only clinically testable sensation mediated by cranial nerve VII. Commonly, Pts may lose taste or have a perversion of taste, dysgeusia, in association with various medications, systemic illness, cancer, and endocrinopathies (Schiffman, 1983).

F. *Clinical analysis of taste testing in facial palsy*

1. *Pt protocol:* A 26-year-old woman awoke one morning with her face "drawn to the side." Examination disclosed that on the left side she could not wrinkle her forehead, close her eye, pull back the corner of her mouth, or wrinkle the skin of her neck. She moved the right side of her face normally. Her complaint of "drawing" of her face was due to the unopposed pull of the intact right-sided facial muscles, which pulled her lips to the right when she spoke or smiled (as the Pt in Fig. 6-5*A*). The remainder of the examination was completely normal, including taste sensation and hearing.

2. Let us work through the clinical data to see how they lead us to conclude *where* and *what* the VIIth nerve lesion is.

    a. In analyzing a motor deficit, consider first of all its distribution. Does it match a *central* (pyramidal tract) or upper motor neuron (UMN) distribution? Does it match a *root* or peripheral *nerve* or myopathic distribution?

    b. Which distribution does the motor deficit of the present Pt match? ☐ UMN/ ☐ peripheral nerve/ ☐ myopathic.

    ☑ *Peripheral nerve*

    c. The paralysis involves the muscles of a single nerve, cranial nerve _____.

    VII

    d. The distribution of the paralysis in the field of a single nerve excludes a neuromyal junction disorder or myopathy; these are widespread disorders, not limited to a single nerve.

    e. Since interruption of a single nerve explains the paralysis, the disorder consists of a ☐ mononeuropathy/ ☐ polyneuropathy/ ☐ myopathy.

    ☑ *Mononeuropathy*

3. Having identified a mononeuropathy of the VIIth nerve, we still have to specify the location of the lesion along the course of the nerve. In analyzing a sensory disturbance or a reflex arc, we invoked the principle of starting at the _____, in order to trace along the entire pathway of the nerve impulses.

Receptor

4. Where should you start in order to trace along the course of the impulses in a motor nerve? _____
_____.

Ans: At the nucleus or cell body of the LMNs.

☑ *Tegmentum;*
☑ *pons*

5. The VIIth nerve nucleus is located in the ☐ tectum/ ☐ tegmentum/ ☐ basis of the ☐ midbrain/ ☐ pons/ ☐ medulla.

6. Because of the close packing of tracts and nuclei, a brainstem lesion would rarely affect only one cranial nerve nucleus. Signs indicating involvement of structures neighboring on the facial nucleus, would result from:
   a. Interruption of lemniscal, cerebellar, or VIIIth nerve pathways.
   b. Involvement of adjacent nuclei or nerves. In addition to VII, the cranial nerve motor nuclei in the pons are _____.

Ans: V, VI (Fig. 2-16. Notice the relation of the intraaxial course of the axons of VII to the VIth nucleus.)

☑ *Outside*

7. The Pt had no signs implicating structures in the vicinity of the VIIth nerve nucleus in the central nervous system (CNS); therefore, the lesion is most likely located ☐ inside/ ☐ outside the brainstem.

8. After leaving the pontomedullary sulcus of the brainstem and before entering the internal auditory meatus, the VIIth nerve must cross the _____ space.

Subarachnoid

9. The subarachnoid space between the cerebellum and the brainstem is called the *cerebellopontine angle.* A lesion here, such as a neoplasm, would interrupt not only cranial nerve VII, but also cranial nerve _____.

VIII

10. As the neoplasm enlarged, it would affect in addition to cranial nerves VII and VIII, cranial nerves _____.

Ans: V and VI (and possibly IX, X, and XII)

VIII

11. If the lesion occupied the internal auditory meatus, what other cranial nerve should it affect besides VII? _____

12. If the lesion interrupted the VIIth nerve trunk somewhere between its point of exit from the brainstem and the geniculate ganglion, the Pt should have lost _____ sensation on the anterior two-thirds of the tongue; however, the Pt did *not* have ageusia.

Taste (Fig. 9-6)

Stapedius

13. VII innervates one muscle in the middle ear, the _____ muscle. Contraction of this muscle dampens the vibration of the ossicles, protecting the inner ear from excessively loud sounds. After stapedius muscle paralysis, the Pt experiences sounds as uncomfortably loud, a symptom called *hyperacusis.*

14. Since the Pt retained taste and had no hyperacusis, the VIIth nerve lesion must be ☐ distal to/ ☐ proximal to/ ☐ within the middle ear.

Ans: ☑ Distal to. (Should you review Fig. 9-6?)

15. If distal to the middle ear, the lesion might be in the facial canal, but the deep location of the canal in the temporal bone bars direct clinical examination. If a lesion interrupted the VIIth nerve after its exit from the stylomastoid foramen, the Ex should find pain or swelling in the parotid region, as from an inflammatory or neoplastic mass, but the Pt had no parotid mass.

Neuromyal (neuromuscular)

16. The next link in a motor nerve comes at the terminal tips of its axons, where the axons contact their effector muscles, a region called the _____ junction.

17. Explain why the Pt's lesion is not at the neuromyal junction or in the muscle itself. _____
_____
_____.

Ans: Neuromyal junction lesions or myopathies are diffuse disorders and generally are not confined to a single nerve distribution.

⊥   18. Make a line across Fig. 9-6 at the most likely site of the Pt's lesion.

Ans: Your line should cross the facial canal distal to the chorda tympani nerve but proximal to the stylomastoid foramen.

19. The Pt had "idiopathic facial paralysis" (Bell's palsy), a common mononeuropathy of the VIIth nerve (Adour and Wingerd, 1974; Graham and House, 1982). The lesion is usually due to inflammation, frequently caused by viruses or *Borrelia burgdorferi* (Roberg et al, 1991). It compresses and sometimes completely transects the axons and may occur at various sites along the facial nerve. The Pt recovered good facial function by six weeks after onset.

20. This Pt shows how testing taste helps to localize lesions along the course of the VIIth nerve. Unless the Pt's symptoms and signs implicate taste, smell, or the VIIth nerve, the Ex may omit taste testing; but make the omission by discretion, not through carelessness.

REFERENCES FOR TASTE TESTING AND BELL'S PALSY

Adour KK, Wingerd J: Idiopathic facial paralysis (Bell's palsy): factors affecting severity and outcome in 446 patients. *Neurology* 1974;24:1112–1116

Birnberg JR: Living with a lack of taste. *Newsweek*. March 21, 1988, p 10

Bornstein W: Cortical representation of taste in man and monkey. I: Functional and anatomical relations of taste, olfaction, and somatic sensibility. *Yale J Biol Med* 1940;12:719–736

Bornstein W: Cortical representation of taste in man and monkey. II: The localization of the cortical taste area in man and a method of measuring impairment of taste in man. *Yale J Biol Med* 1940;13:133–156

Cagan RH (ed): *Neural Mechanisms in Taste*. Boca Raton, FL, CRC Press, 1989

Clee MD, Burrow L: Taste and smell in disease (letter to editor). *N Engl J Med* 1983;309:1062

Finger TE, Silver WL (eds): *Neurobiology of Taste and Smell*. New York, Wiley-Interscience, 1987

Graham MD, House WF (eds): *Disorders of the Facial Nerve*. New York, Raven, 1982

Noda S, Hiromatsu K, Umezaki H, et al: Hypergeusia as the presenting symptom of a posterior fossa lesion. *J Neurol Neurosurg Psychiatry* 1989;52:804–805

Penfield W, Jasper HH: *Epilepsy and the Functional Anatomy of the Human Brain*. Boston, Little, Brown & Co, 1954

Roberg M, Ernerudh J, Forsberg P: Acute peripheral facial palsy: CSF findings and etiology. *Acta Neurol Scand* 1991;83:55–60

Schiffman SS: Taste and smell in disease. Part I. *N Engl J Med* 1983;308:1275–1279

Schiffman SS: Taste and smell in disease. Part II. *N Engl J Med* 1983;308:1337–1342

IV. Hearing

The specialist told him: "Fine let's leave it at that.
The treatment is done: you're deaf. That's how
It is you have quite lost your hearing."
And he understood only too well, not having heard.
Tristan Corbiere (1845–1875)

A. *Cranial nerve VIII.* Cranial nerve VIII consists of a *cochlear* (auditory) and a *vestibular* division. Each division has its own specialized receptors, its own bundle within the trunk of VIII, and separate brainstem nuclei and central pathways.

B. *Anatomy of the cochlear division of VIII*
1. The cochlear division mediates hearing, doing that and nothing else. It detects sound vibrations between 20 cps and 20,000 cps. By its design, the ear is the most exquisitely sensitive vibration detector in the human body.
2. *Receptor for hearing.* The cochlea contains the receptor (the organ of Corti) and the cochlear (spiral) ganglion that originates the cochlear division of VIII. Learn Fig. 9-7.

A. Mesencephalon

B. Pons

C. Pontomedullary junction (and superior olivary nucleus)

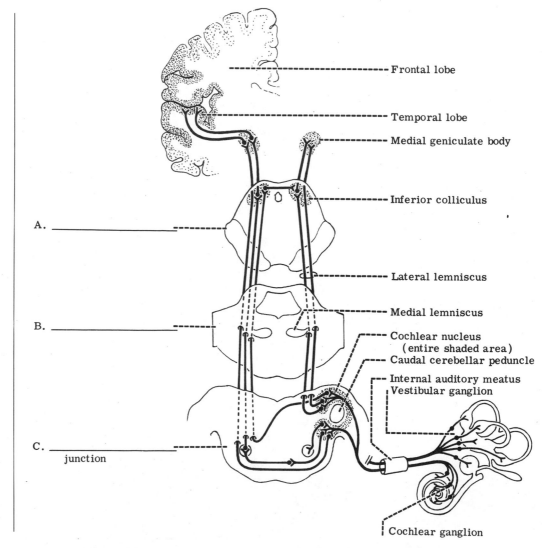

A. _____

B. _____

C. _____
   junction

Frontal lobe

Temporal lobe

Medial geniculate body

Inferior colliculus

Lateral lemniscus

Medial lemniscus

Cochlear nucleus (entire shaded area)

Caudal cerebellar peduncle

Internal auditory meatus
Vestibular ganglion

Cochlear ganglion

FIG. 9-7. Diagram of the cochlear (auditory) pathway. At *A*, *B*, and *C* label the subdivisions of the brainstem.

☑ *Primary*

VII
Pontomedullary

3. The cochlear ganglion contains the ☐ primary/ ☐ secondary/ ☐ tertiary neuron for hearing.
4. *Peripheral course of the cochlear nerve.* The cochlear and vestibular divisions of VIII run through the internal auditory canal, accompanied by cranial nerve number _____. VII and VIII attach to the brainstem at the _____ sulcus.

5. *Central connections of cochlear nerve (Fig. 9-7)*

a. Upon penetrating the brainstem, the cochlear axons synapse at the _____ nuclei.

b. These nuclei drape around the _____ cerebellar peduncle.

c. In the auditory pathway, the cochlear nuclei contain the ☐ primary/ ☐ secondary/ ☐ tertiary neuron.

d. In ascending through the brainstem, the auditory pathway disperses about equally ipsilaterally and bilaterally. Therefore, if a Pt has a profound unilateral hearing loss the lesion most likely would affect ☐ a central pathway/ ☐ an auditory nerve.

e. The name of the auditory pathway through the brainstem is the lateral _____, through which axons run to the _____ _____ body.

f. Neurons of the medial geniculate body relay to the superior surface of the _____ lobe.

g. Would a unilateral temporal lobe lesion cause complete deafness in either ear? ☐ Yes/ ☐ No. Explain: _____ _____.

Cochlear
Caudal (inferior)

☑ *Secondary*

☑ *An auditory nerve*

Lemniscus; medial
geniculate

Temporal

Ans: ☑ *No. A unilateral central lesion does not cause unilateral deafness since the brainstem pathways disperse about equally to both hemispheres.*

i. Whenever you test a Pt's hearing, "think through" the auditory pathway, naming the structures en route.

C. *Symptoms of cochlear nerve lesions.* The most common symptoms are deafness and tinnitus. Tinnitus is a persistent or intermittent hyperacusis consisting of a buzzing or ringing sound (Marion, 1991). Do not confuse tinnitus with vascular bruits which may be audible to the Pt, as well as to the Ex's stethoscope. The most common causes of impaired hearing and tinnitus are aging (presbyacusis), drugs such as aspirin and some antibiotics, viral infections, recurrent otitis media, hereditary cochlear degenerations, and chronic exposure to loud sound.

D. *The threshold or sensitivity concept.* In testing olfaction and taste, the Ex merely seeks a *"Yes"* or *"No"* answer and does not fractionate the stimulus to test the threshold. For the best test of a muscle, the Ex requires the Pt to exert the maximum strength. For the best test of a sensory system the Ex determines not the maximum stimulus it can withstand but the minimum stimulus it can detect, in other words its sensitivity.

E. *Technique for screening hearing*

1. Determine whether the Pt can hear the telephone and hears normal conversational voice and whispering.

2. Do otoscopy to insure that the external auditory canals are open and that the eardrums are normal. In analyzing hearing deficits, the Ex has to decide whether the Pt has a mechanical impediment to conduction of sound or has a nerve lesion. Otoscopy discloses some obvious mechanical impediments such as damaged eardrums, wax, or foreign bodies in the external auditory canal, but it does not disclose others, such as immobility of the ossicles (otosclerosis). The otologist measures the mechanical conductive ability of the eardrum and ossicles with impedanceaudiometry and tympanometry (Bierman and Donaldson, 1970; Jaffe, 1977).

3. Rub your fingers together beside one of the Pt's ears and then the other.

4. Present a vibrating tuning fork to each ear and ask the Pt to compare the loudness. To present the most uniform sound, hold the fork prongs *perpendicular,* not parallel, to the Pt's ear. Forks with a frequency of 512 cps up to 2000 cps match the frequencies most important for speech perception, but they do not vibrate very long. Neurologists compromise by using a fork of either 126 cps or 256 cps (middle C) that also serves to test vibration sense in the digits.

5. To semiquantitate the tests, move the fork from one ear to the other and ask the Pt to compare the loudness of the sound in the two ears. Also compare the distance from the ear at which you hear the sound with the distance at which the Pt hears it.

6. *Masking the opposite ear.* When the Ex tests one ear, the sound vibrations may travel through air or the skull bone, resulting in detection by the opposite ear, even though the ear directly tested is impaired. To improve test reliability, mask the opposite ear by rubbing a piece of paper over it or rustling your fingers beside it as you present the tuning fork to the other ear. Alternatively, the Ex can insert a stethoscope in the Pt's ears and apply the vibrating tuning fork to the diaphragm. The Ex can then direct the sound to both ears or only to one by compressing the tubing at the Y of the stethoscope with a hemostat (Arbit, 1977).

7. *The air–bone conduction test of Rinne* compares the efficiency of the conduction of sound vibrations by bone and by air.

   a. Hold a faintly vibrating tuning fork on your mastoid process. Just after the sound disappears, hold the fork beside your ear. Can you again hear the sound? ☐ Yes/ ☐ No. Normally air conduction is ☐ more/ ☐ less efficient than bone.

   ☑ *Yes;* ☑ *more*

   b. If you press your fingertip in your ear while holding a tuning fork beside it, you know that that will block the sound, but try this: place the fork against your mastoid and as you listen to the sound, press your finger hard into your ear to occlude the canal. What happens to the sound? _____.

   Gets louder

   c. This test shows that while a mechanical impediment in the auditory canal causes an apparent ☐ increase/ ☐ decrease in air conduction, it also causes an apparent ☐ increase/ ☐ decrease in bone conduction.

   ☑ *Decrease*
   ☑ *Increase*

   d. If anything impedes the conduction of sound vibrations through the external auditory canal or ossicles of the middle ear, the Pt has a *conduction* hearing loss. Contrarily, reduction of hearing by a lesion of the organ of Corti or of the auditory nerve is called a *neurosensory* loss. Notice that a *conduction* loss of hearing refers to *mechanical* conduction of sound vibrations through the external and middle ear, not to conduction of nerve impulses through the VIIIth nerve. Loss of hearing from an VIIIth nerve lesion is called a ☐ conduction/ ☐ neurosensory loss.

   ☑ *Neurosensory*

   e. Upon application of the tuning fork to the mastoid process, the bone mechanically transmits vibration to the inner ear to excite auditory impulses, bypassing the conduction channels of the external and the middle ear. Bone conduction tests the integrity of the nerve even though something blocks mechanical conduction of sound vibration through the normal channels. Characteristically, neurosensory hearing losses cause a decrease in the hearing for high frequencies via air conduction and a decrease in bone conduction as well. In other words nerve lesions block hearing by either channel, air, or bone, whereas mechanical lesions block only the sounds transmitted through the ☐ air/ ☐ bone.

   ☑ *Air*

f. Clinical analysis of the air–bone conduction test of Rinne

(1) A Pt hears better with the fork applied to his mastoid process than with it in the air beside his ear. The best inference is:

☐ (a) The Pt is normal.

☐ (b) The Pt must have a lesion of the organ of Corti.

☐ (c) The Pt has a conduction lesion: a mechanical impediment such as wax in his auditory canal, a damaged drum, or immobility of the ossicles.

✓ *(c)*

☐ (d) The Pt has a neurosensory lesion in the organ of Corti or in the auditory nerve.

(2) If the test had shown reduced hearing both for air and bone conduction of sound, the best inference is: ☐ (a)/ ☐ (b)/ ☐ (c)/ ☐ (d).

✓ *(d)*

8. *The sound-lateralizing test of Weber.*

   a. The test consists of placing a vibrating tuning fork on the middle of the forehead or the vertex of the skull. Try this test yourself. The sound seems to come from _____.

Ans: The center (if you are normal).

   b. Is the sound equally loud in both ears? ☐ Yes/ ☐ No

Ans: ✓ *Yes (if you are normal).*

   c. With the vibrating fork in place on the vertex of your head, press your fingertip in one ear and then the other. What happens to the sound? ___

_____.

Ans: Lateralizes to the occluded side.

   d. The normal person hears the vertex vibration equally in both ears. If a mechanical impediment blocks sound conduction in one ear, the vertex sound localizes to ☐ the same/ ☐ the opposite/ ☐ neither side.

✓ *The same*

   e. If the Pt has an auditory nerve lesion on one side, the vertex vibration sounds loudest on the ☐ same/ ☐ opposite/ ☐ neither side.

✓ *Opposite*

   f. Only a consistent lateralization to one side is considered significant.

F. *Analysis of Pts for conduction versus neurosensory hearing loss*

   1. This Pt showed an increased auditory threshold to finger rustling on the left; the vertex test lateralized to the left, and bone transmission was better than air transmission. These findings most likely indicate:

      ☐ (a) A normal Pt.

      ☐ (b) A mechanical impediment, a *conduction* lesion.

      ☐ (c) An auditory nerve or cochlear lesion, a *neurosensory* lesion.

      ☐ (d) Temporal lobe lesion.

✓ *(b)*

      ☐ (e) Insufficient data to reach a conclusion.

   2. This next Pt showed an increased auditory threshold to the tuning fork on the left; bone and air transmission of sound were reduced on the left, and the vertex test lateralized to the right. Which of the previous inferences applies to this Pt?

✓ *(c)*

      ☐ (a)/ ☐ (b)/ ☐ (c)/ ☐ (d)/ ☐ (e)

G. *Testing the auditopalpebral reflex or startle response to sound.* Standing just behind the Pt's line of sight, make a loud, unexpected sound such as a hand clap. Observe the Pt for blinking or a startle response. A response indicates an intact auditory pathway. No response means deafness, or that the Pt ignored the stimulus. Use the auditopalpebral reflex to test auditory function in non-cooperative, hysterical, or malingering Pts or infants. Always ask a mother whether her infant shows an alerting response to sound.

Simultaneous
(double, bilateral).

H. *Auditory tests for cerebral dysfunction*
1. In testing visual fields, we found that some Pts could not detect visual stimuli from both sides. This test is called _____ stimulation.
2. Similarly the Ex can present simultaneous auditory stimuli, if the previous tests have demonstrated intact auditory pathways (Heilmann, 1971). Hold one hand beside each of the Pt's ears. Gently rub your fingers together, first on one side then the other, and have the Pt point to the side from which the stimulus comes. Then rub the fingers of both hands to see whether the Pt identifies the simultaneous stimuli. You may also snap your fingers, if you can make the sound equally loud on both sides. Consider only a consistent inattention to sound from one side significant. Repeat the test several times, randomly alternating single and simultaneous stimuli. Pts with large right cerebral hemisphere lesions tend to suppress sound from the left side (see also Chap. 11).
3. The Ex can test sound localization by presenting rustling fingers in the anterior or posterior quadrants of the right and left sides, with the Pt's eyes closed (Klingon and Bontecou, 1966).

I. *Laboratory tests for auditory dysfunction*
1. If the foregoing screening tests suggest loss of hearing, refer the Pt for electronic tests. These may include pure tone audiometry, speech discrimination batteries, and the von Bekesy loudness descrimination test. Brainstem auditory evoked responses (BAER or BSER) do not require conscious responses, and objectively test for the integrity of the auditory pathways in conscious or unconscious Pts, as discussed under Electroneurodiagnosis in Chap. 13.
2. The commonest causes of delayed speech are mental retardation and deafness. Always investigate every infant or young child thoroughly with bedside and electronic tests if the child does not appear to hear, or has delayed speech.

J. *Rehearsal time.* Do all of the foregoing hearing tests as outlined in Section V,C,3 of the Summarized Neurologic Examination.

REFERENCES FOR AUDITORY TESTING

Arbit E: A sensitive bedside hearing test. *Ann Neurol* 1977;2:250–251
Bierman PW, Donaldson J: The evaluation of middle ear functions in children. *Am J Dis Child* 1970;120:233–236
Heilman K, et al: Auditory inattention. *Arch Neurol* 1971;24:323–325
Jaffe BF (ed): *Hearing Loss in Children: A Comprehensive Text.* Baltimore, University Park Press, 1977
Klingon G, Bontecou D: Localization in auditory space. *Neurology* 1966;16:879–886
Marion MS, Cevette MJ: Tinnitus. *Mayo Clin Proc* 1991;66:614–620

V. The vestibular system: vertigo and its postural compensations

A. *Dizziness and vertigo*
1. Among the commonest symptoms that plague humankind are headaches, backaches, dizziness, fatigability, and blackout spells, and if I had to list the

most difficult symptoms to diagnose, I would answer "Headaches, back-aches, dizziness, fatigability, and blackout spells."

2. In the Pt's lexicon, dizziness may mean giddiness, light-headedness, unsteadiness, vertigo or spinning, and so on. When the Pt complains of dizziness, ask for a more specific description, "Describe how you feel different when you have the dizziness," echoing the Pt's own words to avoid prejudicing the answer. Later ask the Pt to compare the sensation to that produced by a merry-go-round. If strictly defined, vertigo excludes the multitude of less specific symptoms encompassed by dizziness (Rubin and Brookler, 1991). *Vertigo means a specific sense of dysequilibrium as though the person or the world were spinning around or undergoing a swerving or tilting movement.* True vertigo implies a disorder of the vestibular receptors, their nerves, or central connections (Barber, 1974; Glasscock et al, 1990).

3. Several afferent avenues provide stabilizing information for a sense of equilibrium: vision, proprioception (vestibular and dorsal column), and cutaneous touch and pressure. Vertigo occurs whenever the major senses provide conflicting information. The vestibular system sends in impulses at the rate of 100 impulses per second from each side (Barber, 1974). The brain accustoms itself to the balanced input. With rotation, the input from one side increases and that from the other decreases, thus magnifying the discrepancy between the two sides. The brain interprets the information as movement. If disease causes an imbalance in the vestibular input, the brain interprets it as movement, in conflict with other senses that signal no movement. A person standing at the top of the Empire State Building or the Grand Canyon who suddenly glances down will feel vertiginous, because of the loss of the sense of stereoscopy that signals distance. Even diplopia causes vertigo because of the mismatch of information from the two eyes. Which image is the person to believe? When you walk in the dark and put out your hand to touch a wall, you instinctively confirm the role of cutaneous sensation in the sense of balance.

4. *Self-induction of vertigo.* To appreciate how vertigo affects the Pt, try this experiment. Since it may cause you to fall, follow the instructions carefully.

   a. Place a penny on the floor about 40 cm to 50 cm from a bed or a fully cushioned easy chair (to receive you in case you fall).

   b. Stand directly over the penny, with it between your feet and with the receptacle to your *right*.

   c. Flex your neck to stare at the penny, and while staring at the penny, turn around to your *right* fairly rapidly for six complete turns. Stop with your right side toward the receptacle. At the end of the six turns try to stand erect, look ahead, and hold your arms straight out. Record these observations:

      (1) In which direction do you experience an illusion of movement? ☐ to the right/ ☐ to the left?

Ans: ☑ *To the left. Most persons feel as if they were spinning to the left, but some may experience another type of movement.*

☑ *To the right*

      (2) Which way do you tend to fall? ☐ to the right/ ☐ to the left?

      (3) Which way do your outstretched arms tend to deviate? ☐ to the

☑ *To the right*

      right/ ☐ to the left.

   d. Repeat the rotation experiment, but this time rotate to the *left*. The direc-

☑ *Right*

☑ *Left*

      tion of vertigo is to the ☐ right/ ☐ left, and the direction of falling and arm deviation is to the ☐ right/ ☐ left.

   e. We can now generalize that when the vertigo is felt in one direction, the

☑ *Opposite*

      falling and arm deviation are in the ☐ same/ ☐ opposite direction.

f. The vertigo comes from the conflict or mismatch of sensory information when you stop rotating: the fluid in the semicircular canals continues to rotate because of inertia, signalling movement, but the other proprioceptors and vision signal no movement (Brandt and Daroff, 1980). What you have experienced is, of course, motion sickness.

g. During vestibular vertigo, eyelid closure increases the Pt's postural instability by removing the compensatory information from vision, just as when the Pt has dorsal column disease (Romberg test). Thus darkness or deprivation of vision makes Pts with vestibular or dorsal column disease worse, but does not have much effect on cerebellar ataxia, an important point in taking the history (Barber, 1974).

B. *The signs and symptoms of vestibular dysfunction*
   1. Acute transection of a vestibular nerve causes the full syndrome of vestibular dysfunction.
      a. The *symptoms* consist of intense constant vertigo to the opposite side of the lesion, nausea, oscillopsia, and anxiety. The Pt refuses to stand or walk and resists any change in position because it aggravates the symptoms. Nystagmus causes the oscillopsia.
      b. The *signs* consist of falling and past-pointing to the side of the lesion, jerk nystagmus with the slow phase to the side of the lesion, and autonomic dysfunction: vomiting, pallor, sweating, and hypotension. The hypotension may lead to syncope.
      c. A common disorder, Ménière's disease presents both vestibular and cochlear symptoms, consisting of paroxysmal vertigo, tinnitus, and fluctuating hearing loss. Some Pts also suffer hypotensive syncope.
   2. Bilateral, symmetrical vestibular disease may produce only unsteadiness of the gait and vertical balance, without the vertigo or vegetative symptoms. Vision and dorsal columns compensate for the loss of vestibular function.

C. *Physiology of the peripheral vestibular system*
   1. *Vestibular receptors.* The membranous labyrinth of the internal ear contains the end organs that initiate vestibular impulses. Each of the three semicircular canals contain an *ampullary crista.* The utricle and saccule each contain a *macula.* Head movements and the pull of gravity stimulate these vestibular receptors (Glasscock et al, 1990).
      a. The cristae of the semicircular canals detect fast angular accelerations or rotations of the head in the plane of the canal. Figures 9-8 and 9-9 show the planes of the semicircular canals.
      b. In tilting your head downward while spinning around the penny, you placed the horizontal canal more nearly ☐ horizontal/ ☐ vertical.
   2. The *maculae* of the *sacculae* respond to linear acceleration in the lateral and vertical planes. The otoliths of the *macula* of the *utricle,* a gravity-operated receptor, respond to linear acceleration and to slow tilting, acting as an "out-of-position" or tilt receptor. The vestibular system counterrolls the eyes against the direction of head movement and mediates postural reflexes that maintain verticality when the person sits, stands, and walks. In spite of some uncertainty, we will assume that interruption of the vestibular connections that orient the vertical posture causes the caudal vermis syndrome of the cerebellum. In summary, the vestibular receptors initiate three functions:
      a. They detect head movement and the inclination of the head with respect to the pull of gravity, which leads to a vertical posture and a sense of balance.

☑ *Horizontal*

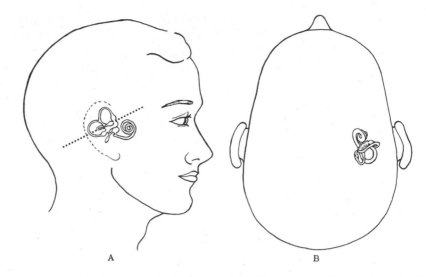

FIG. 9-8. Orientation of the labyrinth. The size of the labyrinth is exaggerated for clarity of the drawing. (*A*) Lateral view of right labyrinth. Notice that the plane (dotted line) of the "horizontal" semicircular canal angles 30 degrees upwards. (*B*) Superior view of the labyrinth.

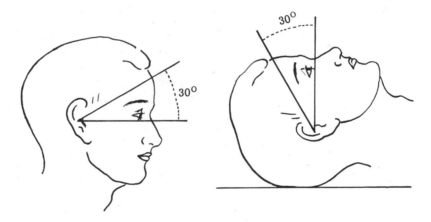

FIG. 9-9. Inclination of the horizontal canal with the patient erect, and supine.

> *b.* They counterroll the eyes against the direction of head movement, thus keeping the eyes on the visual target when the head moves, e.g., if the head turns to the right, the vestibular system counterrolls the eyes to the left.
>
> *c.* They control the tone in the antigravity muscles. Through the pathways described below the vestibular system mediates major postural reflexes, namely, the symmetric and asymmetric tonic neck reflex (Fig. 5-2), head- and trunk-righting reflexes, positive supporting reflexes, and decerebrate rigidity (Fig. 12-13).

D. *Vestibular pathways*

1. The vestibular ganglion is in the internal auditory canal (Fig. 9-7). Hence the primary vestibular neurons, like the primary cochlear neurons of VIII, sit very close to their place of duty. So does the sensory ganglion for cranial nerve number _____.

2. The primary vestibular neurons synapse at the vestibular nuclei, located at the _____ junction of the brainstem.

Ans: Pontomedullary. (Review Fig. 2-23, if necessary.)

☑ *Secondary*

3. The vestibular nuclei contain the ☐ primary/ ☐ secondary/ ☐ tertiary neurons in the vestibular pathway.

4. *The central pathways for the signs of vestibular stimulation*
   a. Since the major ocular sign of vestibular stimulation is nystagmus, strong vestibular pathways run to the nuclei of cranial nerves III, IV, and VI. The pathway linking the vestibular system with cranial nerve nuclei III, IV, and VI is the _____.

Ans: Medial longitudinal fasciculus or MLF (Fig. 2-31).

   b. Extensive connections between the vestibular system and the dorsal motor nucleus of the vagus and the pontomedullary reticular formation mediate the autonomic signs of vestibular dysfunction.
   c. Since the vestibular system coordinates head and eye movements with trunk and limb movements, the vestibular nuclei have strong descending pathways to the spinal cord via the MLF and vestibulospinal tracts (Zilstorff-Pederson and Peitersen, 1963). These tracts along with reticulospinal tracts mediate the postural reflexes listed in section C.2.c above. Should you recite these reflexes?

5. *The pathways for the symptoms of vestibular stimulation.* The fact that vestibular impulses influence consciousness implies a pathway to a thalamic nucleus and a cortical receptive area. A priori, the vestibular cortex should associate with the auditory cortex in the superior temporal gyrus. Attempts to locate such a vertiginous center by electrical stimulation of the brain in conscious Pts have proven indecisive. Many epileptic Pts complain of dizziness before their attacks, but few describe true vertigo.

6. *Summary.* Vestibular impulses which arrive at the vestibular nuclei can box the compass, and disperse to every major subdivision of the nervous system: the cerebrum, the brainstem, the cerebellum, and the spinal cord.

Vestibulospinal

   a. If they go caudally to the spinal cord, they descend via the MLF and the _____ tract.

Caudal (inferior)

   b. If they go dorsally to the flocculonodular lobe of the cerebellum, they travel via the _____ cerebellar peduncle.

MLF

   c. If they go rostrally to nuclei for the ocular muscles they travel via the _____.
   d. If they go into the reticular formation the impulses go via many short circuits of bewildering complexity.
   e. If they go to the thalamus and cortex, the course is uncertain. Presumably they ascend ipsilaterally and contralaterally to the thalamus and thence to the temporal lobe cortex adjacent to the auditory area.

E. *Review of clinical features of vestibular dysfunction*
   1. Recall that the response to vestibular stimulation is subjective and objective. The subjective responses, the *symptoms*, are _____

Ans: Vertigo, nausea, anxiety, oscillopsia, and exacerbation of these symptoms upon moving or changing position.

   2. The objective responses, the *signs*, are _____

Ans: Nystagmus, falling or postural deviation, sweating, pallor, vomiting, and hypotension.

F. *Physiology of nystagmus from caloric irrigation of the external auditory canals*
   1. The inertia or flow of fluid within the semicircular canals due to head rotation provides the normal stimulus. Syringing the external auditory canal with warm or cold water induces convection currents in the fluid in the *hor-*

izontal semicircular canal, the one closest by. Cooled fluid falls and heated fluid rises. Since these convection effects are weak, the Ex places the horizontal canal in the vertical plane to add the effect of gravity to the convection currents. Refer to Fig. 9-9 to answer these questions:

30

☐ *60;* ☑ *backward*

    a. For a *reclining* Pt, tilt the head _____ degrees forward to get the horizontal canal vertical.

    b. For a *sitting* Pt, tilt the head ☐ degrees ☐ forward/ ☐ backward to get the horizontal canal vertical.

2. *Characteristics of vestibular-induced nystagmus*

☑ *Jerk*

    a. The nystagmus has a fast and a slow phase. It is therefore a ☐ jerk/ ☐ pendular nystagmus.

    b. While observing the nystagmus, have the Pt's eyes pursue your finger as you move it from side to side. The nystagmus increases in amplitude when the Pt looks in the direction of the fast component because the volitional saccade adds to the kickback saccade.

3. *Nomenclature note.* Naming the direction of vestibular induced nystagmus presents a problem. The slow deviation of the eyes is the specific *vestibulo-ocular reflex* that initiates the nystagmus. A compensatory saccade then jerks the eyes back towards the midline, recentering the eyes for another deviation by the vestibular stimulus. Coma or anatomic interruption of the frontotegmental pathway may abolish the kickback saccade, even though the deviation phase remains. The well-known COWS mnemonic (*c*old-*o*pposite/*w*arm-*s*ame) misleadingly names the direction of the nystagmus for direction of the fast component: after *c*old irrigation the fast phase is to the *o*pposite side, and after *w*arm water to the *s*ame side, as the ear irrigated.

    The term vestibulo-ocular reflex (VOR) means the slow deviation of the eyes induced by head rotation (counterrolling) or caloric irrigation. The semicircular canals are the essential receptor in both of these cases. The deviation of the eyes after head rotation is called the oculocephalic reflex or doll's eye test.

G. *Indications for caloric irrigation.* Because of discomfort, the time required, and because the Ex has to interpret the results in relation to symptoms, exclude caloric irrigation from the routine NE. Do caloric irrigation if the history or examination indicate dizziness, vertigo, auditory dysfunction, or the recent onset of nystagmus. Chapter 12 discusses its use in coma, and Chap. 13 discusses objective recording of caloric or induced nystagmus by electronystagmography.

H. *Technique for caloric irrigation*

1. *Forewarn and position the Pt.* Because caloric testing causes discomfort, courtesy requires the Ex to forewarn the Pt; but mentioning the expected symptoms voids the objectivity and validity of the test. Therefore, say this: "I am going to rinse out your ear. It's somewhat uncomfortable, but I'll help you manage it all right." Since vertigo may cause the Pt to fall, place the Pt in a sitting or reclining position.

2. *Do otoscopy.* Exclude a mechanical impediment or perforated eardrum. A perforated eardrum might allow water into the middle ear, causing pain and infection. Remove excessive wax that may preclude adequate heat conduction.

3. *Place spectacles on the Pt that have strong positive lenses (Frenzel lenses).* (These can be purchased cheaply in a dime store.) The lenses serve

two purposes. They magnify the Pt's eyes, making any nystagmus easier to see, and they impair fixation by blurring vision. Fixation inhibits induced nystagmus. Thus, the glasses increase the likelihood of eliciting nystagmus, and make it easier to study if it occurs (Cohen, 1976; Tschang and Harrison, 1971).

4. *Irrigate the ear with warm or cold water.* Fill a 50-cc syringe with water at a temperature of 7° above or below the normal 37° of body temperature (30° or 44°). Gently instill the 50 cc of water through a short rubber tube into the external auditory canal over a timed period of 45 seconds. Hold an emesis basin or a towel next to the Pt's ear to prevent wetting the Pt (and also for emergency service if the Pt should vomit). Barber (1974) advocates instilling only 2 cc of ice water. Tilt the Pt's head to the opposite side and hold the water in the canal for a timed 20 seconds. After 20 seconds, place the horizontal canal vertical.

5. *Observe the Pt's responses*
   a. At the end of irrigation, ask the Pt to direct the gaze more or less ahead and hold the arms straight out. The Ex observes for:
      (1) Nystagmus. Record the duration and direction.
      (2) Postural deviation and past-pointing. To test for past-pointing, have the Pt elevate an arm and try to bring it down on your finger which you hold directly in front of the Pt.
   b. Finally the Ex asks whether the caloric irrigation reproduced the original sensation of movement, and asks about the direction of any vertigo. Pts with vertigo and postural deviations may report confusing directionality, depending on whether they are attending to their vertigo or their body tilt. Normal individuals likewise respond somewhat variably to caloric irrigation. Some Pts show little or no response from either ear. Determine whether irrigation of the two ears produces any consistent difference. Thus, a strong normal response from the right ear with little or no response from the left indicates a lesion of the vestibular end organ, nerve, or immediate central connections on the left.

6. To gain a profound and enduring sympathy for your vertiginous Pts, submit to caloric irrigation yourself. Get a partner and follow the foregoing instructions. To make all of the observations, you may have to irrigate more than once. Use the right ear and ice water and compare your observations with the answers to section V.A.4 above.

I. *Summary of the results of caloric irrigation*
   1. If the vertigo goes in one direction, to the right or to the left, the slow deviation phase of the nystagmus, the truncal tilt, arm deviation, and past-pointing go to the opposite side.
   2. Since the vertigo causes the Pt to feel movement or rotation in one direction, the postural deviations can all be regarded as reflex overcompensation for the erroneous information coming from the artificially stimulated horizontal canal. In other words the Pt compensates for the feeling of moving to the left, by leaning and past-pointing to the right. In relation to the vertigo, the Pt compensates by postural deviations that go in the ☐ same/ ☐ opposite direction.

☑ *Opposite*

J. *Summary of vestibular testing*
   1. The symptoms are _____

   _____.

Ans: Vertigo, nausea, anxiety, oscillopsia, and a resistance to moving around.

2. The signs of labyrinthine disease are _____
_____.

Ans: Nystagmus, postural deviation and falling, vomiting, hypotension, pallor, and sweating.

3. What precautions does the Ex take before doing the caloric irrigation test?
_____
_____
_____

Ans: Counsel the Pt, do otoscopy, have the Pt sitting or reclining, tilt the horizontal canal to the vertical plane, and protect the Pt against wetting.

4. Describe the nystagmus to be expected after irrigating the left ear of a normal person with cold water:_____
_____
_____
_____

Ans: Horizontal jerk nystagmus with the slow phase to the left and rapid phase to the right.

5. State the law that relates the postural deviations to the direction of the vertigo. _____
_____.

Ans: The posture deviates in the direction opposite to that of the vertigo, as if compensating for it.

6. Now can you put it all together? Fig. 9-10 shows a person at the height of a strong vestibular response. Reason out which ear was irrigated with cold water. ☐ right/ ☐ left.

☑ *Right*

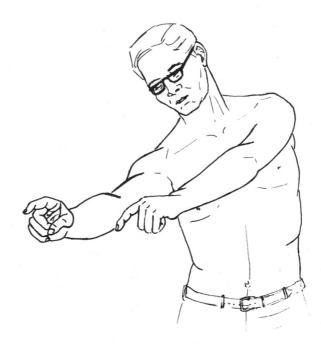

FIG. 9-10. Postural deviation after one ear was irrigated with cold water. The patient was sitting upright with his head tilted 60 degrees backward during irrigation.

K. *Positional nystagmus and vertigo*

1. *Introduction.* Whenever a Pt complains of dizziness, the Ex should ask about the effect of changes in posture. Dizziness when first standing up, a phenomenon you have all experienced, suggests orthostatic hypotension.

However, disease of the labyrinth or its central connections may cause true vertigo after changes of position, such as turning over in bed (Jannetta et al, 1984; Harrison and Ozahinoglu, 1972). Positional nystagmus provides an objective sign of organic disease of the labyrinthine system.

2. *Technique to test for positional nystagmus and vertigo.* Occlude visual fixation by Frenzel lenses. The Ex drops the Pt's head back over the edge of a table (Fig. 9-11). Start by laying the Pt's head straight back; then return the Pt to the erect position, and lay the Pt down with the head turned to the right; repeat to the left. Try both fast and slow changes from the initial vertical position. After laying the Pt's head back, look for nystagmus for one minute before considering the test negative. The Ex may also turn the Pt's head to the sides, or flex and extend it. At the end of any such positional tests, inquire whether the maneuver reproduced the Pt's sensation of dizziness, but do not suggest that it should have.

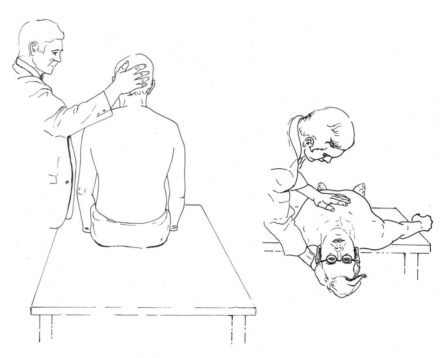

FIG. 9-11. Method for eliciting positional vertigo and nystagmus.

L. *Hyperventilation and dizziness*
   1. *Indications for hyperventilation.* Hyperventilation causes dizziness and may occur in panic attacks. It may provoke fainting (hyperventilation syncope), and epileptic seizures, particularly petit mal attacks. Have the Pt hyperventilate whenever the history suggests any of these possibilities.
   2. *Technique for hyperventilation.* Since the Pt may faint, have the Pt sit or recline during the test. Ask the Pt to breathe as deep and as fast as possible for three full minutes by the clock. Throughout the test, keep encouraging the Pt to breathe hard: "Come on now. We are racing up a mountain." At the end, ask how the test made the Pt feel and whether it matched the original symptoms. Try this test yourself.
   3. *Normal results.* The Pt feels light-headed and somewhat faint and may experience tingling in the perioral region and extremities. Carpopedal spasm may also occur.

TABLE 9-1 Clinical tests for workup of patient with dizziness or vertigo

Tests for vestibular dysfunction
   Inquire about the circumstances of onset of vertiginous attacks and the
      necessity of remaining still to avoid vertigo
   Inspect the gait and posture for tilting and unsteadiness
   Inspect the eyes for nystagmus
   Caloric irrigation of the ear
   Whirling
      Direct whirling of infant
      Rotating (Barany) chair
   Tilt tests for postural vertigo and nystagmus
   Doll's eye maneuver for counterrolling of the eyes (see Chap. 12)
   Romberg test (increased swaying with vestibular or dorsal column disease,
      but not cerebellar)
Nonvestibular tests
   Reclining/standing blood pressure for orthostatic hypotension
   Valsalva maneuver
   Hyperventilation for 3 minutes
   Carotid sinus stimulation

M. Summary of clinical tests for workup of the Pt with dizziness (Table 9-1). See also Drachman and Hart, 1972; Doig, 1972; and Hughes and Drachman 1977.

BIBLIOGRAPHY FOR DIZZINESS AND VERTIGO

Dizziness and vertigo

Barber HO. Diagnostic techniques in vertigo: *J Vertigo* 1974;1:1–16

Brandt T, Daroff RB: The multisensory physiological and pathological vertigo syndromes. *Ann Neurol* 1980;7:195–203

Cohen B: Use of Frenzel glasses in diagnosis of lesions of the vestibular system. *J Vertigo* 1976;2:1–10

Doig J: Auditory and vestibular function and dysfunction, in Critchley M (ed): *Scientific Foundations of Neurology.* Philadelphia, F A Davis, 1972

Drachman A, Hart C: An approach to the dizzy patient. *Neurology* 1972;22:323–334

Froehling DA, Silverstein MC, Mohr DN, et al: Benign positional vertigo: incidence and prognosis in a population based study in Olmstead County, Minnesota. *Mayo Clin Proc* 1991;66:596–601

Glasscock ME, Cueva RA, Thedinger BA: *Handbook of Vertigo.* New York, Thieme Medical Publishers, 1990

Harrison M, Ozahinoglu C: Positional vertigo: aetiology and clinical significance. *Brain* 1972;75:369–372

Hughes JR, Drachman DA: Dizziness, epilepsy, and the EEG. *Dis Nerv Syst* 1977;38:431–435

Jannetta PJ, Moller MB, Moller AR: Disabling positional vertigo. *N Eng J Med* 1984;310:1700–1706

Rubin W, Brookler KH: *Dizziness: Etiologic Approach to Management.* New York, Thieme Medical Publishers, 1991

Tschang H, Harrison M: Note on the value of Frenzel's glasses for the recognition and qualitative evaluation of spontaneous nystagmus. *J Neurol Neurosurg Psychiatry* 1971;34:362–366

Zilstorff-Pederson K, Peitersen E: Vestibulospinal reflexes. *Arch Otolaryngol* 1963;77:237–242

I. The senses

1. Enumerate the sensations mediated by exteroceptors, proprioceptors, and interoceptors.
2. Describe how to use your own body to systematically enumerate the special and general senses to avoid formally memorizing them.
3. Define a sensory modality and distinguish between a unimodal and multimodal sensation.
4. Summarize the principles of sensory physiology as stated in Johannes Müller's doctrine of specific nerve energies.

II. Smell (olfaction): Ist cranial nerve

1. On a sagittal diagram of the head, draw the primary olfactory neurons, showing their receptor endings and central synapses (Fig. 9-1).
2. Name the two sensory nerves of the nasal mucosa (Fig. 9-2).
3. Name the bony plate perforated by the olfactory axons.
4. Give the technical term for loss of the sense of smell.
5. Explain why sneezing or coughing may cause a gush of fluid into the nose of a person who has had a head injury.
6. State a potentially lethal complication of a CSF fistula.
7. Name two clinical manifestations of a cribriform plate fracture.
8. Define the rhinencephalon.
9. Explain the evolutionary significance of the rhinencephalon and the original biological importance of the senses of smell and taste (Fig. 9-3).
10. Define *déjà pensée* and *déjà vu.* Explain their clinical significance and localizing value.
11. Name appropriate aromatic substances for testing the sense of smell and explain why avoiding an irritating substance is necessary.
12. Demonstrate how to test the sense of smell.
13. Explain how to monitor the Pt's suggestibility and reliability in testing the sense of smell.
14. Describe some common conditions that cause reduction in, or loss of, the sense of smell (Fig. 9-5).
15. Describe how to "think through" the pathway for the sense of smell in analyzing the causes for anosmia.

III. Taste or gustation, and loss of taste (ageusia)

1. State which cranial nerve innervates the taste buds of the anterior two-thirds of the tongue.
2. Name and locate the ganglion that contains the perikarya of the primary neurons for the sense of taste.
**3. State the presumed location of the cortical taste center and contrast it with the presumed cortical center for smell.
4. Name two readily available substances for routine clinical testing of taste.

5. Describe and demonstrate how to test for loss of taste (ageusia).
6. List the muscles, glands, and special sense mediated by cranial nerve VII.
7. Diagram the VIIth cranial nerve, and describe the difference in the clinical signs when the nerve is interrupted at various sites along its course (Fig. 9-6).
8. Name the clinical symptom of stapedius muscle paralysis.
9. Describe how taste testing aids in localizing the site of a lesion along the course of the VIIth nerve.
10. Describe some neighborhood signs indicating that a lesion has affected the nucleus or intraaxial course of the VIIth nerve rather than its peripheral or extraaxial course.
11. Discuss the clinical indications for taste testing. Describe the circumstances when you may omit it.

IV. Hearing

1. Trace the auditory pathway from receptor to cerebral cortex, naming the way stations (Fig. 9-7).
2. Explain whether unilateral deafness implicates a lesion of the peripheral nervous system or the CNS.
3. Describe the symptoms of lesions of the cochlear division of cranial nerve VIII.
4. Explain why threshold testing with minimal stimuli provides a better test of sensory systems than the maximal testing used in the strength examination.
5. Describe and demonstrate how to screen a Pt's hearing and how to make the bedside tests semiquantitative.
6. Describe how to mask hearing from the opposite ear when presenting a sound to one ear.
7. Describe and demonstrate how to do the air–bone conduction test of Rinne and state the result in a normal person.
8. Explain the importance of otoscopic inspection of the external auditory canal in interpreting hearing tests.
9. Describe and demonstrate how to do the sound lateralizing test of Weber. Describe the result in a normal person.
10. Describe a simple test on yourself to remember the effect of mechanical impediments to hearing on the Weber sound lateralizing test.
11. Explain the difference between a conductive and a neurosensory hearing loss and describe how to differentiate the two with bedside tests, including tuning fork tests.
12. Deduce the probable type of hearing loss, given various patterns of results on the bedside hearing tests (Section IV.F, page 325.)
13. Describe how to elicit and interpret the auditopalpebral reflex as a crude test of hearing in an infant or uncooperative patient.
14. Describe how to test the auditory system for inatten-

tion to bilateral simultaneous stimuli, and for sound localization.

15. Give the name of an electronic test for the integrity of the auditory pathways that does not require a cooperative or even a conscious patient.

16. State in principle the kind of information derived from an audiogram and BAER test and give the full name for the BAER acronym.

17. Demonstrate how to do the several bedside tests that screen hearing (see Section V.C.3 of the Summarized Neurologic Examination).

V. The vestibular system: vertigo and its postural compensations

1. Define the terms dizziness and vertigo.

2. Describe the various senses that contribute to the overall sense of balance and equilibrium.

3. State the direction the person will experience postrotatory vertigo after rotating to the *left*.

4. Describe the symptoms and signs that follow acute interruption of the of vestibular division of VIII.

5. State the adequate stimulus for the neurons of the semicircular canals (cristae).

6. State in a general way the adequate stimulus for the macula of the utricle and saccule.

7. Enumerate the major normal functions of the vestibular system.

8. Name some postural reflexes mediated through the vestibular system and the spinal pathway that mediates them.

9. Name the brainstem pathway by which axons from the vestibular nuclei reach the nuclei of cranial nerves III, IV, and VI.

10. Discuss the dispersion of pathways from the vestibular nuclei mentioning, in principle, their destinations.

11. Explain, in terms of the physics involved, why hot or cold water irrigation stimulates the semicircular canals, and how the angle of inclination of the horizontal canal affects the process.

12. Describe how to make the horizontal canal vertical when the Pt is sitting or prone (Fig. 9-9).

13. Describe the type of nystagmus produced by vestibular stimulation and describe the effect of eye movement on it.

14. Describe the convention for naming the direction of a jerk-type nystagmus. State which is the vestibular-induced phase and which is the compensatory or kickback phase and relate this to the COWS mnemonic.

15. State the clinical indications for caloric irrigation, and explain why it is not a necessary part of the routine screening examination.

16. Describe how to prepare the Pt for caloric irrigation, emotionally and physically, and recite the instructions to the Pt prior to the caloric irrigation test.

17. Explain why the Ex must inspect the external auditory canal before instilling fluid.

18. Explain why the Pt should wear Frenzel (strong positive) lenses during caloric irrigation.

19. Describe and demonstrate two alternative caloric irrigation tests. State the water temperature and the amount of water to use.

20. Describe the normal result from cold caloric irrigation of the right ear (Fig. 9-10).

21. Describe when and how to test for positional vertigo and nystagmus (Fig. 9-11).

22. Describe the indications for and how to do the hyperventilation test and the normal result.

23. Recite the battery of bedside tests, vestibular and otherwise, for the workup of the Pt presenting with dizziness or vertigo (Table 9-1).

Chapter Ten

Examination of the General Somatic Senses

Nature, indeed has had a triple end in view in the distribution of nerves: she wished to give sensibility to organs of perception, movement to organs of locomotion, and to all others the faculty of recognizing the experience of injury.

Galen (A.D. 130–200)

I. Introduction to testing general somatic sensations

A. Special and general senses

Sight, smell, taste, hearing, and equilibrium constitute *special* senses. Touch, pain, temperature, position, and vibration constitute the *general* senses routinely tested. Unique receptors and unique central pathways mediate each of the special senses. Some skin receptors and somatosensory pathways serve only one general sensory modality, but other receptors are polymodal. Hence, the text will not attempt to specify the skin receptors for general sensation.

B. General principles in testing all somatic sensations

1. Because sensory testing tires both the patient (Pt) and the examiner (Ex), do the tests in the form of a game or contest. "Let's see how light a touch you can feel." Sometimes the Ex should defer part of the sensory examination for another day and certainly should recheck any doubtful results.
2. The Ex should demonstrate and describe the tests and generally should call for "Yes" or "No" responses. Then the Ex does the actual testing. Have the Pt close the eyes, to avoid visual clues and to place full reliance on the skin stimuli.
3. Continually compare homologous areas of the right and left sides and compare normal and any suspected abnormal areas. The skin areas differ greatly in sensitivity to stimuli. The highly sensitive skin of the face and armpits contrasts with the horny skin of palms and soles. Hairy skin perceives tickling and touch better than glabrous skin. The forehead is the most sensitive area for temperature discrimination. Cold skin loses sensitivity. Ensure a warm skin before testing the Pt.
4. The Ex must understand the difference in dermatomal and peripheral nerve

*The light vertical rule on the left side of the text sets off an answer column. Cover the answers with a card until you have responded to the text. Then, after each response, slide the card down to check your answer.

The heavy vertical rule or asterisk denotes optional material.

distributions in order to test for sensory loss competently (Figs. 2-10 and 2-11).

C. *Positive and negative sensory phenomena after lesions of central and peripheral sensory pathways*

Sensory lesions cause either positive phenomena, with too much sensation, i.e., pain and tingling, or negative or deficit phenomena, with too little sensation.

1. *Nomenclature for deficits in superficial sensation*

   a. Since *esthesia* = touch or feeling, *hypesthesia* = partial loss of touch, and *anesthesia* = total loss.

   b. Since *therm* = heat, *thermhypesthesia* = partial loss of temperature sensation, and *thermanesthesia* = total loss.

   c. Since *algesia* = pain, *hypalgesia* = partial loss of pain sensation, and *analgesia* = total loss.

2. *Positive or irritative phenomena after interruption of peripheral or central sensory pathways*

   a. Disease of afferent nerve fibers may cause excessive sensation (Nashold and Ovelmen-Levitt, 1991). Because of lowering of the sensory threshold light touch, or merely air blowing on the skin, may result in extreme discomfort. *Hyperesthesia, hyperalgesia,* and *hyperthermesthesia* describe an oversensitivity to what should be ordinary stimuli of touch, pain, and temperature. *Hyperpathia* (anesthesia dolorosa) refers to an extreme oversensitivity to pain, but often with a raised threshold. *Neuralgia* means multiple, very severe, electric shocklike pains that radiate into a specific root or nerve distribution. Examples include trigeminal neuralgia (Fromm and Sessle, 1991; Stookey and Ransohoff, 1959); occipital, or glossopharyngeal neuralgia (Bohm and Strang, 1962); and pre- or postherpetic neuralgia (Gilden et al, 1991). The neuralgia may or may not alter the sensory threshold, but testing is always difficult because of the intense pain and the presence of trigger points that, if touched, elicit the pain. *Causalgia* describes a constant, intense, unbearable, burning, relentless hyperesthesia-hyperalgesia that may follow injury to the fibers of a peripheral nerve (Sunderland, 1978).

   b. Many Pts experience uncomfortable sensations of numbness, tingling, or pins and needles, or burning pain short of neuralgia or causalgia. They are called *paresthesias* when such sensations accompany a normal external stimulus to the skin, or *dysesthesias* when they occur spontaneously without any obvious external stimulus (Wartenberg, 1953). (Unfortunately, as happens too often in medicine, some authors use these terms in exactly the opposite sense.) You will notice paresthesias and dysesthesias if you study your own sensations when recovering from a local anesthetic for a dental procedure or after having sat too hard on your own sciatic nerve, causing it to "go to sleep."

   c. *Irritative or positive phenomena of sensory cranial nerves*

      (1) Cranial nerve I: hyperosmia.

      (2) Cranial nerve II: flashes of light, scintillating scotomas (phosphenes or seeing stars).

      (3) Cranial nerves V and IX: trigeminal and glossopharyngeal neuralgia.

      (4) Cranial nerve VII: hypergeusia (increased sense of taste).

      (5) Cranial VIII: tinnitus, hyperacusis, diplacusis (auditory division), vertigo (vestibular division).

    d. Mechanisms of such hyperesthesias might include:
- (1) Excessive firing of diseased axons because of destabilization of their membranes.
- (2) Changes in the sensitivity of receptors or of central conducting mechanisms.
- (3) A discrepancy or imbalance of the sensory information conveyed when disease affects the ratio of impulses delivered by fibers of different diameters, resulting in imbalanced input.
- (4) Cross talk or short circuiting of impulses in demyelinated axons.

II. Examination of somatosensory functions of cranial nerve V

A. Functions of the afferents from cranial nerve V

    1. *Sensory domain of V.* The Vth cranial nerve mediates all general sensory modalities for the face; teeth; mucous membranes of the nose, cheeks, tongue, and sinuses; and proprioception from the ocular, facial, and chewing muscles. It conveys *no* special sensory fibers. With a single scimitar blow, let us slice the face off from the head, along the line shown in Fig. 10-1, creating the mask of Trigeminus.

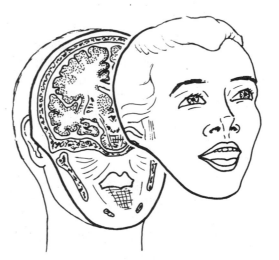

FIG. 10-1. The mask of Trigeminus. Obtain it by a single slice through the head with a scimitar. The mask that falls away is no ordinary Halloween mask. It has three dimensions. It contains all of the territory, both motor and sensory, innervated by the Vth nerve: skin, chewing muscles and their proprioceptors, mucous membranes, and the dura mater. Only the cerebrum itself has no nerve supply. Notice that the angle of the mandible is spared, left behind with the head: see also the face in Fig. 10-2 to fix this fact permanently in your mind.

    2. To best appreciate the function of afferents from V, let us observe a newborn baby as it roots for a nipple, sucks, chews, swallows, protrudes its tongue, blinks, and sneezes. Stimuli acting through V initiate all of these reflexes. Then, too, you will understand the rooting reflex and something about the descending root of V by observing the very first cutaneous reflex that the human fetus exhibits: the turning of the head in response to stimulation of the upper lip. This appears when the fetus reaches the 8th week of gestation, and just after the axons of the descending root of V grow down into the cervical region to make this reflex possible. To further understand the descending connections of V, consider the rat, a nocturnal animal with

weak eyes, as it feels its way along a totally dark passage, by touching its whiskers against the wall, an action which provides afferent information to orient the head, neck and body. Then, consider the autonomic responses: lacrimation from corneal irritation, salivation from mechanical stimulation of the oral mucosa (as opposed to taste), and pupillodilation and bradycardia or tachycardia from pain. Then, think of the role of V in sinus pain and toothache, not to mention headache in general.

B. Neuroanatomy of cranial nerve V

1. From Fig. 10-2 learn the three divisions of the *tri*geminal nerve, their facial skin areas, and central connections. The text discusses the mesencephalic nucleus of V later.

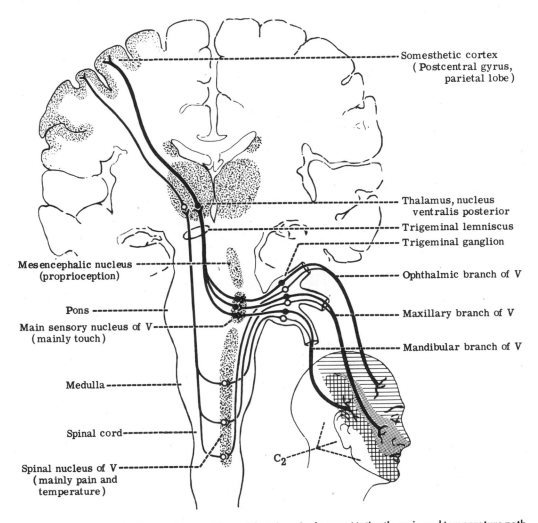

FIG. 10-2. Peripheral and central connections of the trigeminal nerve. Notice the pain and temperature pathway descending to the spinal cord. Compare the posterior margin of the line of facial innervation with Fig. 10-1.

2. V receives its name *trigeminal* because of its three large sensory divisions, the _____, _____, and _____ divisions.

Ans: Ophthalmic; maxillary; mandibular.

3. The three sensory branches funnel into a single root that attaches to the ☐ mesencephalon/ ☐ pons/ ☐ medulla.

✓ *Pons*

☑ *Primary*

Dorsal root

I and VIII

4. The sensory ganglion of V, the trigeminal (semilunar, gasserian) ganglion, contains the ☐ primary/ ☐ secondary/ ☐ tertiary neuron of the sensory pathway from the face.

5. The trigeminal ganglion corresponds to the _____ _____ ganglia of the spinal nerves.

6. The primary ganglia for the special senses that are very near their end organs belong to cranial nerves numbers _____. (If you don't recall the answer readily, how should you systematize your approach?) _____.

Ans: Start at cranial nerve I and sort through them one by one.

☑ *Secondary*

7. The trigeminal *nuclei* (*nuclei,* not ganglia) contain the ☐ primary/ ☐ secondary/ ☐ tertiary neuron of the trigeminal pathway.

8. Where is the tertiary neuron? _____.

Ans: Thalamus (diencephalon). Review Fig. 10-2 if you missed.

9. The mesencephalic nucleus of V violates the rule that the primary neuron of a sensory pathway is outside of the central nervous system (CNS). It consists of primary neurons within the neuraxis—a unique fact but of no clinical use. The mesencephalic portion of V probably mediates proprioception; the pontine and rostral medullary portion mediates *touch,* and the spinal nucleus mediates *pain* and *temperature* (Humphrey, 1969). Thus, in rostrocaudal order, the functions mediated by the three portions of the sensory nucleus of V are _____, _____, _____, and _____.

Ans: Proprioception; touch; pain; temperature.

10. Taken all together, trigeminal sensory fibers and nuclei extend from the rostral part of the cervical region of the spinal cord into the mesencephalon (Fig. 10-2).

C. *Technique for testing touch in the Vth nerve area*

1. *Instruction to the Pt.* Ask the Pt to say "Touch" in response to each touch by a wisp of cotton. After the Pt closes his eyes, lightly brush each area of the three sensory divisions of V with a wisp of cotton. Touch alternate areas and sides of the face randomly. Also vary the time between touches to keep the Pt from getting into a rhythm of answering without actually attending to the stimulus.

2. The reason for using a wisp of cotton is to avoid a rigid test object that will cause pressure. What principle of sensory testing would that violate? _____.

Ans: Principle of testing a single modality at a time.

3. After the Pt has responded several times, how would you test the Pt's reliability and attentiveness? _____.

Ans: Occasionally withhold the stimulus and ask whether the Pt felt something. Recall that in testing smell, the Ex also withheld the stimulus at times.

4. As a general rule, if you suspect a sensory loss in any area, based on the history, commence all forms of sensory testing in a normal area, to give the Pt the experience of the normal sensation for comparison with any abnormal region. Then, start in the middle of the abnormal area and continually ask the Pt to make comparisons between normal and abnormal areas and between the right and left sides.

D. *The corneal reflex*

1. *Anatomy of the corneal reflex arc*

   a. The corneal reflex consists of closure of the both eyelids in response to touching one cornea. It is entirely distinct from the corneal light reflection test described earlier.

   Ophthalmic

   b. The afferent arc of the corneal reflex travels through the _____ division of V.

   Orbicularis oculi
   VII

   c. The muscle that closes the eyelid is the _____ _____, innervated by cranial nerve number _____.

   d. The corneal reflex thus tests the integrity of two cranial nerves, (afferent) _____ and (efferent) _____.

   V; VII

2. *Instructing the Pt for the corneal reflex.* Tell the Pt, "I am going to just touch your eyeball very lightly." Use a free piece of cotton, rolled to a fine point. Do not use cotton attached to a stick (Q tip). Avoid sticks around the eyes. A demented, retarded, or delirious Pt may flinch against the tip of the stick and injure an eye. Instruct the Pt to look to one side and a little up. Gently hold the lids apart to avoid stimulating the eyelashes. Bring in a wisp of cotton from the lateral side, to touch the lateral side of the cornea of the *adducted* eye. *Bring the cotton directly in from the side to avoid entering the field of vision.* That would cause a visually mediated flinch reflex, not a corneal blink reflex. In Fig. 10-3, make an X on the exact spot to stimulate the cornea without entering the Pt's field of vision.

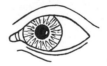

FIG. 10-3. Blank to mark the site for stimulation of the cornea to elicit the corneal reflex.

3. *Clinical interpretation of the corneal reflex.* Most normal individuals display a corneal reflex. Exceptions include some aged or postcataract surgery Pts. If no response occurs, do not conclude that the V–VII arc is interrupted, until you have checked for a contact lens. Acute hemispheric lesions may abolish the corneal reflex on the contralateral side for hours or days as a deficit or "shock" phenomenon (Ross, 1972). As with the gag reflex, in the absence of symptoms, the Ex may elect to eliminate the corneal reflex from the screening neurologic examination (NE) (Chapter 14, Table 14-1).

4. *The corneomandibular reflex* consists of a twitch of the jaw to the opposite side, along with eyelid closure, after stimulation of one cornea. It appears contralaterally after a hemispheric lesion and bilaterally in coma (Guberman, 1982).

5. *The glabellar blink reflex* consists of bilateral contraction of the orbicularis oculi muscles in response to percussion of the glabella with the fingertip or percussion hammer, or to electrical stimulation of the supraorbital branch of the trigeminal nerve. Electrical stimulation with electromyogram (EMG) recording provides an objective, quantitative method of measuring the afferent and efferent arcs of this V–VIIth cranial nerve reflex (Fine et al, 1992; Kimura, 1989). Various lesions of the afferent and efferent arc reduce the blink response. It disappears on the side of an acute hemiplegia and disappears bilaterally in coma.

E. *Technique for testing temperature discrimination*
1. *Instruction to the Pt.* State, "I want to see how well you can tell warm from cool. Please close your eyes, and I will place something on your cheek. Tell me whether it is warm or cool."
2. *Tuning fork versus finger test.* Apply the metal shaft of a tuning fork to the side of the Pt's cheek for a few seconds and then remove it and apply the side of your little finger to the same spot. Ask the Pt whether each is cool or warm (Fig. 10-4).

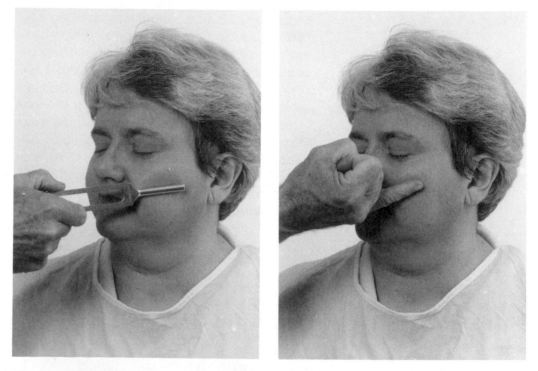

FIG. 10-4. Randomly touch the tuning fork shaft and your little finger to test temperature discrimination over the face and dorsum of the hands and feet.

   a. Use the fork first because it will feel colder than the finger feels warm, immediately establishing communication. The Pt will attend to the temperature and not to texture or size.
   b. Randomly alternate the finger and tuning fork as you proceed over the three trigeminal sensory areas and then over the dorsum of both hands and both feet.
3. *Warm and cold tube test.* Fill one tube with warm water and one with cold. Test the hot tube on yourself first to insure that it will not scald. Avoid extremes of temperature. You want to test temperature *discrimination,* not how much heat or cold the Pt can withstand.
4. Because pain *and* temperature share peripheral receptors and pathways in the spinal tract of V and in the spinothalamic tract, disease generally affects both modalities. For screening purposes, testing one tests both. *Always test temperature discrimination first, not pain.* If the Pt discriminates temperature normally, and the history does not suggest neurologic disease, you do not need to prick every Pt with a pin to test pain. No one relishes a pinprick, especially about the face. If you approach (attack) a young child with a pin first, you will already have ended the entire sensory examination. Yet even an intelligent 3-year-old child will play the temperature game. Finally by

testing temperature sensation, you avoid leaving a trail of pinpricks across the skin, oozing blood, a matter of some importance in this AIDS era.

F. *Testing pain perception.* If the history suggests a sensory disorder, test pain sensation over the face after testing temperature discrimination. See section III.C of this chapter.

G. *Differentiation of hysterical and organic loss of facial sensation*
   1. Draw a line across the head in Fig. 10-5 to show the exact dividing line between the part of the head innervated by V and the cervical dermatomes. Compare with Fig. 10-2 to see how exact your line is.

Compare your drawing with Fig. 10-2

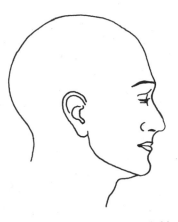

FIG. 10-5. **Blank to draw in the sensory innervation field of the trigeminal nerve.**

   2. Now shade and label the parts of the face supplied by each of the three major sensory branches of V. Check with Fig. 10-2.
   3. Does V innervate the skin over the angle of the mandible? If you included it in your drawing above, check Fig. 10-2 again. You missed a point of considerable clinical value. Organic sensory loss of facial sensation from trigeminal nerve lesions spares the angle of the mandible, while hysterical loss of facial sensation includes it. Review Fig. 2-10 and Fig. 10-2 to recall where cranial nerve V abuts on spinal nerve root C-2. Comparison of hysterical and organic sensory losses leads to a useful general law: *hysterical Pts lose sensation according to their mental image of the body parts; organic Pts lose sensation according to the wiring diagram of the nervous system.* As a further example, in hysteria the loss of arm sensation usually cuts off sharply at the shoulder because that agrees with one's mental image of an arm, but it does not agree with the actual anatomic distribution of peripheral nerves, nerve roots, or their central pathways (Chap. 14).
   4. Therefore, in hysterical sensory loss of facial sensation the angle of the mandible is ☐ spared/ ☐ affected, whereas in organic loss of affected facial sensation due to a Vth nerve lesion, the angle of the mandible is ☐ spared/ ☐ affected.

☑ *Affected*

☑ *Spared*

H. *Analyze this patient*
   1. This 76-year-old woman complains of severe pain in her face, starting 4 months ago and gradually worsening. She describes very brief, shocklike episodes of unbearable pain which run from the side of her cheek down to the tip of her jaw, on the right side only. She has become irascible and

impossible to live with according to her husband. Because eating triggers the pain, she has lost 18 pounds. The NE discloses normal motor and sensory functions of the cranial nerves, except that she will not allow the Ex to test sensation over the right lower jaw because touching the right lower lip triggers excruciating shocks of pain.

2. In analyzing a sensory complaint, the Ex must determine its nature and whether its distribution conforms to an anatomic pattern or to the person's mental image of the body and hence is psychogenic. The term which best matches the Pt's sensory disorder is (review the descriptors in section I.C.2a before answering): ☐ hyperesthesia/, ☐ hyperalgesia/ ☐ causalgia/ ☐ neuralgia.

Ans: ☑ *Neuralgia. (While some of the terms more or less apply, the best is neuralgia.)*

3. Does the location of the sensory disorder match:
   ☐ *a.* The distribution of a central pathway.
   ☐ *b.* The distribution of a dermatome.
   ☑ *c.* The distribution of a peripheral nerve or nerve branch.
   ☐ *d.* A nonanatomic distribution, which, in combination with the Pt's obvious personality change, indicates a psychogenic disorder.
4. What peripheral nerve area does the Pt's pain correspond to? _____.

Ans: Mandibular division of V on the right.

5. This Pt had no other abnormalities either on general physical examination or on radiographic examination of the skull with a basilar view to show the foramina of exit of V. She had *trigeminal neuralgia* (tic douloureux), a very typical idiopathic neuropathy which causes excruciating shocklike single pains in one or more of the branches of the trigeminal nerve (Fromm and Sessle, 1991; Stookey and Ransohoff, 1959). Typically the pain erupts spontaneously and also after touching a "trigger point" on the cheek or the inside of the mouth.

I. *Summary of the tests for the sensory functions of the cranial nerves.* Get a partner and rehearse sections V, steps C and D, of the Summarized Neurologic Examination.

REFERENCES FOR SOMATOSENSORY TESTING OF THE FACE

Bohm E, Strang R: Glossopharyngeal neuralgia. *Brain* 1962;85:371–388

Fine EJ, Sentz L, Soria E: The history of the blink reflex. *Neurology* 1992;42:882

Fromm GH, Sessle BJ: *Trigeminal Neuralgia: Current Concepts Regarding Pathogenesis and Treatment.* London, Butterworth-Heinemann, 1991

Gilden DH, Dueland AN, Cohrs R et al: Preherpetic neuralgia. *Neurology* 1991;41:1215–1218

Guberman A: Clinical significance of the corneomandibular reflex. *Arch Neurol* 1982;39:578–581

Humphrey T: The central relations of the trigeminal nerve, in Kahn EA, Crosby EA, Schneider RC, Taren JA (eds): *Correlative Neurosurgery* (2d ed). Springfield, Charles C Thomas, 1969

Kimura J: *Electrodiagnosis of Diseases of Nerve and Muscle* (2d ed). Philadelphia, FA Davis, 1989

Nashold BS, Ovelman-Levitt JO: *Deafferentation pain syndromes* (vol. 19: *Advances in pain research and therapy*). New York, Raven 1991

Ross R: Corneal reflex in hemisphere disease. *J Neurol Neurosurg Psychiatry* 1972;35:877–880

Stookey B, Ransohoff J: *Trigeminal Neuralgia: Its History and Treatment.* Springfield, Charles C Thomas, 1959

Sunderland S: *Nerves and Nerve Injuries* (2d ed). Edinburgh, Churchill-Livingstone, 1978

Wartenberg R: *Diagnostic Tests in Neurology: A Selection for Office Use.* Chicago, Year Book Publishers, 1953

III. Testing somatosensory functions of the body and extremities

A. *Testing touch sensation*

1. Test touch over the rest of the body exactly as described for the face. For screening purposes test only the dorsum of the hands and feet, in addition to the face. To explore suspected sensory loss, test each area as carefully as required by the history. Review Fig. 2-10 to see why the Ex moves the touch stimulus *up and down* the trunk to discover a dermatomal loss or spinal cord sensory level, but would move it *around* the limbs.

2. Review the anatomy of touch in Chapter 2, section VIII. B, pages 70–76.

    a. Recall that touch impulses ascend to the somesthetic cortex by two spinal pathways: one in the _____ _____ of the cord and the other in _____ _____ .

Ans: Dorsal columns (fasciculi gracilis and cuneatus); the ventrolateral quadrant (spinothalamic tract or spinal lemniscus).

    b. The dorsal column pathway decussates at the _____ junction, while the spinothalamic tract decussates at the _____ .

Ans: Cervicomedullary; level of entry of the dorsal root.

☑ *Pain and temperature*

Spinal

3. The pathway for touch in the ventrolateral columns most closely resembles the pathway for ☐ pain and temperature/ ☐ vibration and position sense.

    a. These two tracts, the ventral and lateral spinothalamic tracts, unite to form the _____ lemniscus.

    b. All lemnisci unite in the brainstem to travel to the thalamus as one with the medial lemniscus (DeMyer, 1988). Complete Table 10-1.

4. Interruption of the rostral part of the medial lemniscus or its thalamic termination in the posterior nucleus ventralis can lead to contralateral hemianesthesia (Fisher, 1978).

B. *Testing temperature sensation from the body and extremities*

Proceed exactly as described for the face. Test temperature discrimination first. Use the tuning fork versus finger or warm and cold tube tests described above in section II.E.

1. Trigeminal

2. Lateral

3. Medial

4. Spinal

TABLE 10-1 Origin and name of the lemnisci	
Site of origin of axons	Name of lemniscus
Trigeminal sensory nuclei	
VIIIth nerve nuclei	
Dorsal column nuclei	
Dorsal horn nuclei	

C. *Testing pain sensation from the body and extremities*

1. *Use of a pin.* Use a straight pin, with one blunt end and one sharp end. By alternating ends of the pin, the Ex monitors the Pt's attentiveness and reliability. Hold the shaft of the pin lightly between thumb and index finger to allow it to slip a little, thus applying the stimulus with the same pressure. Make about three successive pricks for each stimulus because not all individual pricks will hit a pain-sensitive spot. *Always discard the pin after use.* Never use it again. I don't know how many angels can dance on the point of a pin but several diseases can: syphilis, infectious hepatitis, and AIDS, for starters.

2. *Instructions for the Pt.* Demonstrate what you plan to do by lightly touching the Pt with the sharp and the dull end of a pin. Ask the Pt to respond "Sharp" or "Dull." Then have the Pt shut the eyes to prevent visual cueing. Start with a *normal* area to establish communication, so that the Pt knows what to expect. Test the face, and dorsum of the hands and feet. Avoid the horny skin of the palms and soles. Recall again the differing sensitivities of various skin areas.

3. *Pain in neonates and fetuses.* The custom of doing procedures such as circumcision on newborn infants without the use of anesthetics, as if they felt no pain, has been called into question (Anand and Hickey, 1987). Certainly newborns and even fetuses show the behavioral responses associated with pain: crying, agitation, and autonomic responses. Absence of crying after painful stimuli below a certain dermatomal level, with prompt crying when stimulated above the level by cold or pain provides a reliable way of detecting spinal cord transection in a neonate or young infant.

4. *Relation of pain and temperature sensation to types of axons*

    a. Prick yourself with a pin. After a pinprick you will experience two types of pain. The first, a sharp, bright localized "fast" pain is mediated by small myelinated fibers of the A group. This pain is thought to ascend mainly through the classical lateral spinothalamic pain and temperature pathway. Small myelinated axons (IA gamma fibers) also mediate cold sensation (Willis, 1985; Willis and Coggeshall, 1991; Yarnitsky and Ochoa, 1991).

    b. Unmyelinated C fibers mediate the second type of pain, an afterglow of dull, diffuse, stinging, and burning pain. This pain is thought to ascend through diffuse polysynaptic pathways, rather than solely in the classical spinothalamic pathway, and to have strong connections with the reticular formation and ultimately the limbic system (Casey, 1991; Gordon, 1977). The small, unmyelinated axons (C fibers) also convey warm sensations.

    c. Quantitative or automated methods for testing touch, pain, and temperature are available, but are not in routine use (Beecher, 1959; Dyck et al, 1993; Hannsson et al, 1991; Navarro and Kennedy, 1991; Smith et al, 1991; Yarnitsky and Ochoa, 1991).

5. *Anatomy of the temperature and pain pathways from the body and extremities*

    a. Learn Fig. 10-6.

    b. Review Fig. 2-12*A* and *B*.

    c. Draw and verbally trace a nerve impulse for pain and temperature sensation from the skin on the lateral side of the foot to the cerebral cortex. Start by naming the dermatome: _____
    _____
    _____

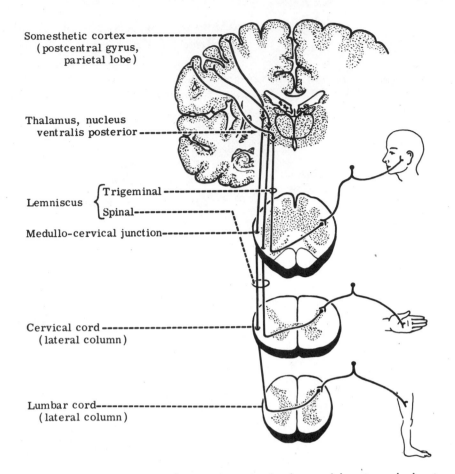

Somesthetic cortex
(postcentral gyrus,
parietal lobe)

Thalamus, nucleus
ventralis posterior

Lemniscus { Trigeminal
Spinal

Medullo-cervical junction

Cervical cord
(lateral column)

Lumbar cord
(lateral column)

FIG. 10-6. Pathway for pain and temperature sensation from periphery to cerebral cortex.

Ans: S1 dermatome receptor to peripheral branch of dorsal root axon to central branch to secondary neuron in dorsal horn. Secondary axon crosses, ascends in spinal lemniscus to tertiary neuron in n. ventralis posterior of thalamus. N. ventralis posterior relays to somesthetic cortex in postcentral gyrus of parietal lobe.

6. The pain and temperature axons from the foot, trunk, and hand synapse on secondary neurons at, or within one or two segments of, their level of entry into the spinal cord, but the axons from the face descend through the brainstem to reach their secondary neuron. Review Figs. 10-2 and 10-6.

   a. The descent of the axons from the face permits the secondary nucleus that relays pain and temperature sensation to be continuous from the medulla to the last sacral segment. The order of representation of parts in this continuous long columnar nucleus is face, neck, arm, trunk, lower extremity, and sacral region. The technical name for this nucleus is the *substantia gelatinosa of Rolando,* but you need remember only its location in the tip of the dorsal horn and its function in relaying temperature and pain sensations.

   b. If you wanted to abolish only pain and temperature sensation without abolishing touch, you would make a cut in the ☐ ventrolateral/ ☐ dorsal column to interrupt the _____ _____ tract.

   c. Neurosurgeons make just such a cut in the ventrolateral column of the spinal cord to relieve Pts of intractable pain, an operation known as

☑ *Ventrolateral*
Lateral spinothalamic

cordotomy (Guybels and Sweet, 1988). Would this cut eliminate touch sensation? ☐ Yes/ ☐ No. Explain _____

Ans: ☑ *No. Touch impulses reach the thalamus by two pathways, ventral and dorsal columns. Section of only one pathway does not eliminate touch sensation.*

7. In addition to the foregoing classical spinothalamic pathway (Keele, 1957), a multisynaptic pain pathway also ascends from the face, body, and extremities to reach the thalamus and conscious appreciation (Gordon, 1977; Willis, 1985; Willis and Coggeshall, 1991).

8. *Delayed pain and deep pain perception.* If the history and examination suggest a sensory disturbance, proceed as follows to test the extremities, but do not use these tests on the face:

    a. *Delayed pain.* Pinch the dorsum of the Pt's foot briskly between the finger nails of your thumb and index finger. The normal person feels pain almost immediately. A delayed response indicates an abnormality in sensory conduction.

    b. *Deep pain.* Test by squeezing very hard on an Achilles tendon or a muscle, or by compressing very hard over a bony surface. Classical causes of delayed pain are tabes dorsalis and other diseases that interrupt dorsal roots and dorsal columns.

9. *Location of trigger points.* Palpate along nerves and muscles for pain and trigger points in examining the Pt with any acute or chronic pain syndrome.

10. *Referred pain.* The site at which the Pt feels the pain may be distant from the site of the lesion. Thus cardiac pain is referred down the left arm. The pain from a carpal tunnel syndrome, with median nerve compression at the wrist may be felt proximally in the arm, as well as in the expected distribution of the median nerve distally. This phenomenon is called referred pain (Casey, 1991; Gordon, 1977; Hockaday and Whitty, 1967).

11. Some have remarked that the function of the internist or the surgical consultant is to do the rectal exam (and discover that a metastatic prostatic carcinoma has caused the Pt's baffling weight loss and back pain). Physicians habitually neglect the same things, such as the rectal examination, and temperature and pain testing. As a neurologist, my function sometimes is to do the temperature and pain testing that no one else has done, and frequently it pays off.

REFERENCES FOR SOMATOSENSORY TESTING OF THE BODY AND EXTREMITIES

Anand KJS, Hickey PR: Pain and its effects in the human neonate and fetus. *N Eng J Med* 1987;317:1321–1329

Beecher H: *Measurement of Subjective Responses: Quantitative Effects of Drugs.* New York, Oxford University Press, 1959

Casey KL (ed): *Pain and Central Nervous System Disease: The Central Pain Syndromes.* New York, Raven, 1991

DeMyer U: *Neuroanatomy.* Baltimore, Williams & Wilkins, 1988

Dyck PJ, Thomas PK, Lambert EH, et al (eds): *Peripheral Neuropathy* (3d ed). Philadelphia, Saunders, 1993

Fisher CM: Thalamic pure sensory stroke: a pathologic study. *Neurology* 1978;28:1141–1144

Gordon G (ed): Somatic and visceral sensory mechanisms. *Br Med J* 1977;33:89–182

Guybels JM, Sweet WH: *Neurosurgical Treatment of Chronic Pain* (vol 11: *Pain and Headache*). New York, S Karger, 1988

Hansson P, Lindblom U, Lindstrom P: Graded assessment and classification of impaired temperature sensibility in patients with diabetic polyneuropathy. *J Neurol Neurosurg Psychiatry* 1991;54:527

Hockaday J, Whitty C: Patterns of referred pain in the normal subject. *Brain* 1967;90:481–496

Keele K: *Anatomies of Pain.* Springfield, Charles C Thomas, 1957

Navarro X, Kennedy WR: Evaluation of thermal and pain sensitivity in type I diabetic patients. *J Neurol Neurosurg Psychiatry* 1991;54:60–64

Smith SJM, Ali Z, Fowler CJ: Cutaneous thermal thresholds in patients with burning feet. *J Neurol Neurosurg Psychiatry* 1991;54:877–881

Willis WD Jr: *The Pain System. The Neural Basis of Nociceptive Transmission in the Mammalian Nervous System* (vol 8: *Pain and Headache*). New York, S Karger, 1985

Willis WD, Coggeshall RE: *Sensory Mechanisms of the Spinal Cord* (2d ed). New York, Plenum, 1991

Yarnitsky D, Ochoa JL: Warm and cold specific somatosensory systems: psychophysical thresholds, reaction times and peripheral conduction velocities. *Brain* 1991;114:1819–1826

IV. Pain in the back, shooting down the leg: the sciatica syndrome

A. *Pt analysis.* Consider this characteristic Pt with the commonest back and leg pain of neurologic origin (Rothman and Simeone, 1992; Seimon, 1990). For some time, in fact off and on for several years, this 34-year-old man has suffered from lumbosacral backache. A few days ago when straightening up, he felt a pop in his back, and since then he has had severe, sharp radiating pain into his right foot along its lateral aspect into the little toe. Movement or coughing exacerbates the pain. He sits rigidly in his chair, his trunk slightly tilted forward. When arising, he pushes himself erect with his arms. He stands with most of his weight on his unaffected left leg, holding the knee of the right leg slightly bent. You can confirm the uneven weight distribution by placing your hand around his ankle with your thumb on his Achilles tendon. By squeezing firmly with your thumb, the tendon on the non–weight-bearing leg yields. His lumbar spine is virtually straight, rather than showing the normal concavity. Palpation discloses paravertebral muscle spasm. The triceps surae reflex on the right side is reduced. He has weakness of plantar flexion on the right, as shown when he tries to rise onto the ball of his right foot, as compared to the left. His right calf measures 1.8 cm less than the left.

B. *Identifying the origins of radiating pain.* An accurate description of where the pain radiates often identifies the affected nerve, or the nerve root in a nerve root compression syndrome (Frymoyer, 1988; Mulder and Dale, 1991). Since the Pt has motor and sensory findings, the lesion cannot be limited to one of the small superficial cutaneous nerves of the lateral aspect of the foot. Review Figs. 2-10 and 2-11.

1. If the Pt complains that the pain radiates into the little toe or along the *lateral* side of the foot you would suspect the _____ nerve root.

Ans: S-1. Review Fig. 2-10, if you erred.

2. If the Pt complains of pain radiating along the medial side of the foot or into the great toe, you would suspect the _____ nerve root.

Ans: L-5. Review Fig. 2-10, if you erred.

3. What evidence does the history and physical examination provide that the weakness is due to an UMN or LMN lesion? _____

Ans: The evidence for a LMN lesion is weakness, atrophy, and a decreased MSR at the ankle (decreased triceps surae reflex).

4. What would an EMG of the muscles innervated by the S-1 nerve root show? _____.

Ans: Fibrillations, giant motor unit potentials, and possibly fasciculations.

C. *Leg-raising tests for nerve root compression.* While the foregoing clinical data already point to the diagnosis of a nerve root compression syndrome, the leg-raising tests help to confirm it. Two in number, the tests consist of the *straight-knee leg-raising test* (Laseague's sign) and the *bent-knee leg-raising test* (Kernig's sign).

1. *Technique of the straight-knee leg-raising test for pain (Laseague's sign)*

a. The Pt lies supine with the legs relaxed. Grasp the calf or heel of the affected limb and elevate it gently as far as possible, flexing the hip but keeping the knee straight (Fig. 10-7).

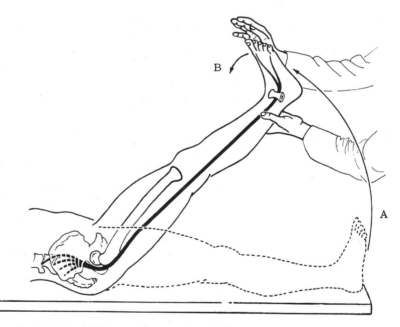

FIG. 10-7. Straight-knee leg-raising test. (*A*) The Ex elevates the leg. (*B*) The Ex then dorsiflexes the foot. Both maneuvers stretch the sciatic nerve and elicit pain if the nerve roots are inflamed, compressed, or imprisoned by a mechanical lesion.

b. Normally the Ex can elevate the Pt's thigh to about 90 degrees. The Pt with nerve root compression winces with pain and flexes the knee at some point less than 90 degrees. Then, if the Ex holds the leg just short of the position of pain, gentle dorsiflexion of the foot produces another twinge of pain—the pain, as before, shooting into the foot. The same maneuvers on the unaffected limb may produce nearly a normal range of movement, without pain, or may produce pain down the affected limb, the *crossed, straight leg-raising sign* that is nearly pathognomonic of a herniated disc (Frymoyer, 1988; Hudgins, 1977).

2. *Explanation of the pain and limitation of leg elevation*

    a. Elevation of the lower extremity with the knee straight stretches the sciatic nerve. We might appropriately call it the *sciatic nerve stretching test.* As the nerve stretches, it pulls against any impediment to free movement. The resultant pain causes hamstring muscle spasm, flexing of the knee, and splinting against further extension, stretch, and pain. The commonest impediment by far is a ruptured intervertebral disc, which impinges on the nerve root (Fig. 10-8).

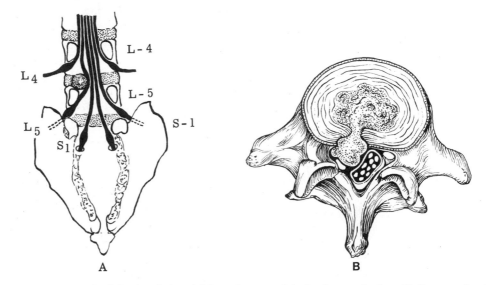

FIG. 10-8. Intervertebral disc herniation. (*A*) Dorsal aspect of the lumbosacral spine with the neural arches of the vertebrae and dura mater removed. Nerve roots labeled on the left side, vertebral bodies on the right. Notice how the nerve roots relate to the intervertebral discs and to their point of exit from the vertebral canal. The L-4 to L-5 disc has herniated, impinging on nerve root L-5. (*B*) Transverse section of vertebrae L-5, as seen from above, showing disc herniation. The dural sac containing the cauda equina remains intact.

    b. Explain why the Pt tended to flex his knee as you reached the end point of excursion in the straight-knee leg-raising test? _____ .

Ans: Flexion relaxes tension on the sciatic nerve.

    c. When you held the limb just short of maximum permissible elevation, why did dorsiflexion of the foot elicit a twinge of pain? _____

Ans: Foot dorsiflexion placed tension on the sciatic nerve, impinging it on the
    herniated disc.

    d. We can understand all the postural and movement limitations in this nerve root compression syndrome as protecting against pain: the splinting of the back by paravertebral muscle spasm to prevent movement, the flexing of the knee which relaxes tension on the sciatic nerve, and the limitation of straight leg-raising. To prove this theory, we can do this: with the Pt supine, set him up, leaving his legs flat against the bed. This action again stretches the sciatic nerve. What do you predict that the Pt

Flex it

        will do with the affected lower extremity to avoid pain? _____ .

3. *The bent-knee leg-raising test (Kernig's sign).* With the Pt supine as for the straight-knee leg-raising test, flex the limb at the hip while keeping the knee flexed. When the thigh reaches the vertical position, gently, *gently*

straighten the knee. The Pt will wince with pain, and reflex hamstring spasm will prevent further straightening of the knee.

4. Xavier, Mc Danal and Kissin (1989) suggest that antidromic activation of peripheral pain receptors, rather than simple mechanical impingement, may cause the pain of sciatica.

REFERENCES FOR BACK PAIN AND RADIATING LEG PAIN

Frymoyer JW: Back pain and sciatica. *N Engl J Med* 1988;318:291–300

Hudgins WR: The cross-straight leg raising test. *N Engl J Med* 1977;297:1127

Mulder DW, Dale AJD: Spinal cord tumors and discs, in Joynt RJ (ed): *Clinical Neurology.* Philadelphia, Lippincott, 1991

Rothman RH, Simeone LP: *The Spine* (3d ed). Philadelphia, Saunders, 1992

Seimon LP: *Low Back Pain. Clinical Diagnosis and Management* (2d ed), New York, Demos, 1990

Xavier A V, Mc Danal J, Kissin J: Mechanism of pain caused by nerve-root tension test in patients with sciatica. *Neurology* 1989;39:601–602.

V. Proprioception, position, and vibration sense: the dorsal column or deep modalities

A. *Definition of proprioception.* The term *proprioception* comes from *proprius* = one's own, and *capio* = to take or capture; therefore, literally to take or capture one's own. The term refers to the capturing, by receptors within the depth of one's own body, of the movements of one's own body parts. The body parts which move, and whose movements its proprioceptive system captures, consist of one's own muscles and joints, i.e., the skeletomuscular apparatus, and one's vestibular fluid and otoliths. Formally defined, *proprioception is the sense of movement, of position, and of skeletomuscular tension provided by deep mechanical receptors in muscles, joints, connective tissue, and the vestibular system.* Along with vision and touch it provides a sense of equilibrium. Charles Sherrington (1859–1952), to whom we owe the concept, put it this way:

We arrived earlier at the notion that the field of reception which extends through the depth of each segment is differentiated from the surface field by two main characters. One of these was that while many agents which act on the body surface are excluded from the deep field as stimuli, an agency which does act there is mass, with all its mechanical consequences, such as weight, mechanical inertia, etc., giving rise to pressures, strains, etc., and that the receptors of this field are adapted for these as stimuli. The other character of the stimulations in this field we held to be that the stimuli are given in much greater measure than in the surface field of reception, by actions of the organism itself, especially by mass movements of its parts. . . . In many forms of animals, e.g., in vertebrates, there lies in one of the leading segments a receptor-organ (the labyrinth) derived from the extero-ceptive field of the remaining segments. This receptive organ, like those of the proprio-ceptive field, is adapted to mechanical stimuli. It consists of two selective parts, both endowed with low receptive threshold and with refined selective differentiation. One part, the otolith organ, is adapted to react to changes in the incidence and degree of pressure exerted on its nerve-endings by a little weight of higher specific gravity than the fluid otherwise filling the organ. The other part, the semicircular canals, reacts to minute mass movements of fluid contained within it. These two parts constitute the labyrinth. . . . This system as a whole may be embraced within the one term "proprio-ceptive." (Charles Sherrington, The Integrative Action of the Nervous System. Yale University Press, New Haven, reprint, 1952.)

B. *Anatomy of skeletomuscular proprioception*
1. Review the pathway through the dorsal columns in Fig. 10-9.

Compare your answers with Fig. 10-6.

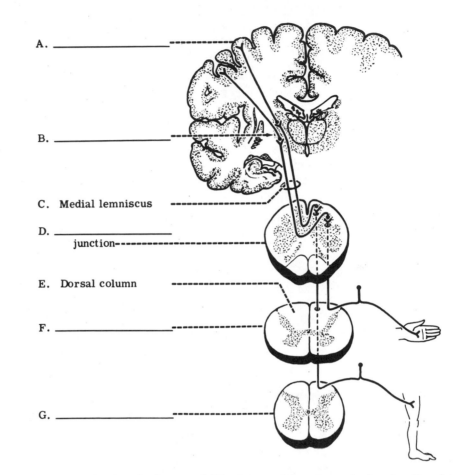

A. _____

B. _____

C. Medial lemniscus

D. _____
 junction ----

E. Dorsal column

F. _____

G. _____

FIG. 10-9. Pathway for dorsal column modalities from periphery to cerebral cortex. Complete labels *A* through *G*.

2. A variety of receptors in the connective tissue of joints and tendons mediate proprioception. The muscle spindles would, a priori, seem ideal to mediate a sense of movement, but no pathway from them to the somesthetic cortex has been found. The primary skeletomuscular proprioceptive neurons, like all primary somatic sensory neurons, are located in the _____.

Ans: Dorsal root ganglia.

3. Cranial nerve VIII has two ganglia which are homologous to dorsal root ganglia, the _____ ganglion and the _____ ganglion.

Cochlear; Vestibular

4. The axons ascending in the dorsal columns are from ☐ primary/ ☐ secondary/ ☐ tertiary neurons.

☑ Primary

5. Fig. 10-9 shows that the processes of dorsal root ganglion cells extend from the toe to the dorsal column nuclei, the remarkable distance of 170 cm in man, the astonishing distance of 450 cm in a giraffe, and the incredible distance of 2000 cm in the blue whale.

☑ *Medial*

6. The axons from the foot ascend ☐ lateral to/ ☐ intermingled with/ ☐ medial to those from the arm.

   Nomenclature note. Anatomists call the *leg dorsal column* the fasciculus gracilis or column of Goll and the *arm dorsal column* the fasciculus cuneatus or column of Burdach. I prefer the terms *arm dorsal column* and *leg dorsal column* rather than fasciculus gracilis and cuneatus, which you will forget two weeks after you lay aside the text. The sensory homunculus in the dorsal columns is a headless man sitting with his rump on the dorsal median septum. The head gets added to the homunculus as the trigeminal lemniscus joins the medial lemniscus. Review Fig. 2-12*B*.

7. At what level of the neuraxis is the secondary neuron of the dorsal column pathway? _____ .

Ans: At the medullocervical junction.

Lemniscus
Medial

8. The decussating axons are secondary axons conveying impulses to the thalamus, impulses destined to affect consciousness. The tract they form is called a _____ (general term).

9. The particular name of this lemniscus is the _____ lemniscus.

10. The medial lemniscus terminates in a thalamic nucleus called the nucleus _____ .

Ans: Ventralis posterior.

Postcentral
Parietal

11. From the nucleus ventralis posterior the pathway for the dorsal column modalities goes to the somesthetic cortex in the _____ gyrus of the _____ lobe.

12. Try the whole thing at once. Wiggle your toe and think through the pathway to the cortex by which you know your toe has wiggled. Can you draw the pathway (Fig. 10-9)?

C. *The general concept of dorsal column modalities or deep sensations*

1. The dorsal columns mediate many sensations besides position and movement. In general, these sensations all depend on receptors deeply placed in the dermis and the connective tissue of the joints, tendons, and muscles. These deep receptors are attuned, as Sherrington said, to mass, inertia, pressure, and movement. Since distance is inherent in the concept of movement, we have the ingredients of classical Newtonian mechanics. The proprioceptive or proprioceptive-related discriminatory sensations mediated by the dorsal columns are:

   a. Sense of position or statognosia
   b. Sense of movement of joints and of body (kinesthesia)
   c. Two-point discrimination
   d. Sense of pressure
   e. Texture
   f. Localization of touch
   g. Sense of weight
   h. Sense of numbers or letters written on the skin or graphesthesia

2. The association of these sensations as basically mechanical stimuli may seem more rational after these considerations:

   a. Vibration is easy to associate with proprioception as mediated by mechanical receptors. Recall that the cochlea, a receptor exquisitely specialized for detecting vibration, developed as the phylogenetic kin of the vestibular apparatus, a receptor exquisitely specialized for detecting position and motion. Vibration sense is merely the detection of fast changes in the pressure on and position of a minute portion of tissue, the eardrum being the most specialized example.

    b. The amount of pull on the joint and connective tissue proprioceptors leads to a sense of weight.

    c. To a large extent, discriminative touch, such as texture, depends on minute variations in the pressure upon any area of skin. You feel texture best when an object is moved across your skin, causing almost a slow vibration sense. Discrimination of characters written on the skin demands first of all the perception of the path traced by an object pressing on the skin, followed by comparison of the pattern with memory traces. Touch, itself, involves some mechanical displacement, some pressure. Two-point discrimination is the distance between two pressure points. Localization of a touch stimulus depends on comparing the location of a touch stimulus with the mental image of the body parts. It is essentially the problem of distance. In contrast with all these mechanical deformations of skin or joints that cause sensations conveyed by dorsal columns, an object that does not directly touch you, such as the sun 93,000,000 miles away, can burn you and cause pain. Ventrolateral column pathways mediate these temperature and pain sensations, not dorsal column pathways.

D. *Technique for testing position sense by digital movement*
   1. *Instruction to the Pt*
      a. With one hand, support the part to be tested and ask the Pt to remain completely relaxed. With the other hand, grasp the digit by its side and wiggle it up and down, stopping in one direction or the other randomly. Separate the digit being tested so that it does not touch other digits (Fig. 10-10).

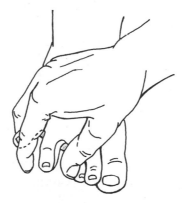

FIG. 10-10. Method of separating the digits to test position sense in the fourth toe. The Ex grasps the toe on the sides and randomly moves it up and down.

      b. While the Pt watches, stop the digit at one position or the other, and instruct the Pt to report whether the finger is "Up" or "Down." This step communicates what the Ex expects of the Pt. Then, for the actual testing, have the Pt close the eyes. Additionally, instruct the Pt not to move the digits at all. They should remain totally passive. Tell the Pt, "Let me do all of the moving." Test the digits of all four extremities.

      c. Take care not to apply different pressures or use a different tone of voice on the up or down movement. The Pt may attend to the wrong stimulus.

2. *Use of the fourth digits in testing position sense*
    a. When testing position sense, the novice instinctively grasps the thumb, index finger, or large toe; but using digits three and four presents the greatest challenge to and therefore the best test of the sense of position. Fig. 10-11 shows why.

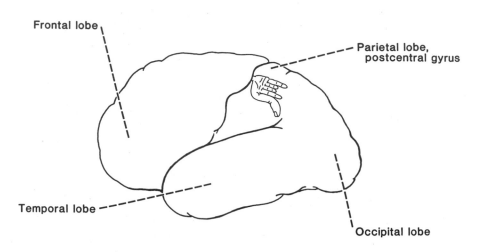

FIG. 10-11. Lateral view of left cerebral hemisphere. The right hand is projected onto the left postcentral gyrus to show the relative area devoted to each of the digits. The face projects to the area immediately inferior to the hand, the trunk and leg superior, just as the representation is in the precentral motor cortex (see Fig. 2-2C). In reality, the motor and sensory representations somewhat overlap the central sulcus.

    b. The first, second, and fifth digits of the hands and feet have the richest innervation and the largest cortical representation. Therefore, to interrupt position sense of these digits requires a relatively large lesion. Practice using digits three and four according to Fig. 10-10.
    c. When initial testing suggests loss of position sense, always test several digits several times. After understanding the test, the Pt should reply promptly and make no, *no,* errors. Occasionally the Pt will become bored, or carelessly reply one direction while meaning the other. A delay in responding means lack of attention or genuine loss of position sense. Immediate repetition and inquiry will disclose whether the error implies carelessness or disease.
3. If position sense is normal distally, it will be normal proximally. If abnormal at the digits, work proximally to test it at the wrist or ankle to establish the severity of the loss.

E. Position sense testing, probability theory, and all "Yes" or "No" sensory tests
    1. Pts with defective position sense often give an answer because they know a reply is expected, and they try to please the Ex. The Ex who does not understand probability theory misinterprets the responses of the Pt with mild or even complete position sense loss.
    2. Even with *no* position sense at all, what percent of the time would the Pt guess the correct direction when a digit is randomly placed up or down? ☐ 0 percent correct/ ☐ 25 percent/ ☐ 50 percent/ ☐ 75 percent.

☑ *50 percent*

    3. The situation exactly duplicates trying to call heads or tails in flipping a coin. The guesser wins 50 percent of the time, on the average.
    4. Next consider impaired but not absent position sense. The Pt responds correctly, sometimes because of chance and sometimes because of correct

perception of the position. The novice Ex may erroneously conclude that the Pts are unreliable, because they miss one time and then give several correct responses. If you are satisfied that the Pt has not simply made a careless error, recall the rule that the normal person makes _____ percent errors. If the Pt makes even a few noncareless errors, your best interpretation is that position sense is impaired; a few errors are not acceptable as normal. You still have to decide whether the Pt is malingering, hysterical, or has a neurologic disease, but you know certainly that something is amiss.

0

5. The next question is how to reduce the probability of getting the correct answer by chance. How could you accomplish this? _____
_____.

Ans: One method is to give three alternatives, up, down, and straight. Start by wiggling the finger up and down and then stop up, down, or in the neutral position; or you can move the digit medially or laterally.

6. By giving three alternatives instead of two, you reduce the chance of guessing the correct answer from one in two, to one in _____.

Three

7. Ordinarily *two*-alternative testing is easier and faster than *three*-alternative, and is reliable. Probability theory sets the minimum number of trials that should be made in *two*-alternative testing of position sense. As in flipping a coin, you will expect to call heads or tails correctly about one-half of the time. In mathematical notation ½ may be written as $(½)^1$. Now when you try to call the coin twice in a row, the probability of being right is $(½)^2$ or one in four. The probability of calling three in a row would be $(½)^-$ or 1 in _____.

$(½)^3 = 1$ *in 8*

8. Each time you try to stretch your luck one more time, the denominator ☐ halves/ ☐ doubles/ ☐ triples/ ☐ quadruples. Soon the odds against chance success are astronomic. Chance success becomes not impossible, but more and more improbable.

☑ *Doubles*

9. In testing position sense, the question is where to cut off the trials in order to have confidence that the Pt has not succeeded by chance alone, when in fact the Pt has no position sense. Statisticians agree that when the probability of an event is one in twenty or less, chance is an unlikely explanation. Thus, in testing position sense, where chance has a 50 percent success rate, the smallest number of trials the Pt must get right to make chance success unlikely is _____.

Ans: 5 trials $(½)^5 = ⅟_{32}$, which is less than the needed ⅟_{20} and therefore makes chance unlikely.

9. Some mental Pts reply exactly the opposite to each up or down position, ipso facto proving intact position sense. Even with no position sense, a Pt just guessing gets _____ percent right by chance.

50

10. *Final admonition.* In previous sensory tests, we have implicitly relied on statistical concepts. If we offer coffee as a smell stimulus to an anosmic Pt, some will reply because they expect to smell something. Then the question is, how many Pts with anosmia will report coffee when in fact they smell nothing? Since the probability of reporting coffee is less than one in twenty, chance is an unlikely explanation for a correct answer. The same consideration holds for taste. In testing pain, we have to consider probability, as well as the fact that some pinpricks do not stimulate pain endings. Hence the Pt may report no pain on a particular prick, although you stuck him. Moreover, pain thresholds vary considerably from Pt to Pt, and from age to age. These considerations lead to a general observation. As a teacher I find that medical students and residents often report that the history or

the sensory examination "was unreliable." What that generally means is that the student failed to communicate adequately with the Pt to derive the historical information or produce the test results that the Pt was actually capable of. Usually such a Pt has a different culture, diction, syntax, and English than the student is accustomed to. Nothing tests the skill of the Ex more than the sensory examination. Make a successful sensory examination a matter of personal pride. By practicing sensory testing on yourself and many other subjects, you will appreciate the variables and avoid coming to erroneous conclusions about the Pt's reliability. Practice testing position sense on a normal subject, using the *two-* and *three-*alternative methods and the third and fourth digits.

F. *Clinical testing of position sense by the swaying (Romberg) test*
   1. *Instructions to the Pt*
      Ask the Pt to stand with the heels together. Note whether the Pt sways. Then ask the Pt to close the eyes, and note whether the swaying increases. Stand behind the Pt with arms held up ready to catch the Pt, but do not touch the Pt.
   2. *Results of the Romberg swaying test*
      a. Normal subjects will sway slightly more with the eyes closed than with them open, but they never fall. Stand up and try this test yourself. Stand on both feet and then on one foot.
      b. Hysterical Pts may fall against a convenient support, such as a wall or the Ex, or they may bobble precariously without falling, ipso facto proving competent position sense.
      c. Pts with vestibulocerebellar disease may sway some with the eyes open. They will sway slightly more with the eyes closed, but usually do not fall unless they also have vertigo. Then the loss of visual orientation is critical.
      d. Pts with dorsal column lesions sway much more with eyes closed and may fall unless supported.
   3. *Interpreting the Romberg swaying test*
      a. Students misinterpret this test more than any other one, because they mistake it for a test of cerebellar function. As usual, the problem stems from failure to analyze the actual operations of the test. Let us see, in terms of the three operations of the test, why the Pt with dorsal column lesions performs poorly.
         (1) Operation one requires the Pt to stand with the feet together narrowing the base and increasing the stress on the balance mechanisms of the body.
         (2) Operation two requires the Pt to close the eyes, thus removing visual clues to spatial orientation and balance.
         (3) Operation three requires the Ex to judge whether the Pt sways more with eyes open or eyes closed.
      b. Hence a definition of the swaying (Romberg) test is that we compare the degree of swaying when the Pt is standing heels together, eyes open, with the degree of swaying after the eyes are closed. This is an ☐ operational/ ☐ interpretational definition.

☑ *Operational*

      c. The critical point in interpretation is that we test the competency of the proprioceptive system to provide cues for the erect posture when deprived of visual cues. Normally, an integrated sensorimotor complex—consisting of the proprioceptive system (including the vestibular apparatus, dorsal columns, and cerebellum), basal ganglia, visual system, and pyramidal tracts—maintains the standing posture. The critical afferent system, in the absence of vision, is the dorsal column proprioceptive system. We know this because dorsal column modality loss, as in tabes dorsalis, causes the most severe swaying with eyes closed.

    d. Why do you ask the Pt to close the eyes for the swaying test? _____

Ans: To deprive the Pt of visual cues for balance and to place the sole responsibility on the proprioceptive system, particularly in the dorsal columns of the spinal cord.

Tandem walking

    e. Which part of the gait examination utilizes the principle of narrowing the base, thus increasing the stress on balance? _____.

  4. *Hysteria and the swaying test*

    a. Hysterical Pts cause the most difficulty in interpreting the swaying test. Hysterical Pts often gyrate wildly, but they usually do not fall, thus proving that they have intact balance mechanisms.

    b. The Ex can often divert the hysterical Pt into performing well on the swaying test. Wait until later in the exam, after your first trials of the swaying test. Then have the Pt stand with the feet together, hands straight out in front and eyes open. Ask the Pt to alternately touch the finger to his nose with the right and left hand, as in ordinary cerebellar testing. While the Pt continues to repeat the finger-to-nose test, ask the Pt to close the eyes. Usually the Pt, now engrossed in the finger-to-nose task, will maintain the posture without swaying.

    c. Hysteria never manifests solely by a positive swaying test. A positive swaying test is only one element in a pattern of psychiatric findings. Nor is a positive swaying test ever the sole sign of dorsal column lesions. It is really only a second-best test for pathways tested more directly and specifically by digital position sense, vibration, and stereognosis.

G. *Cerebellar versus sensory dystaxia*

  1. Earlier, we stated that the cerebellum could coordinate the muscles only if it received the proper proprioceptive information. Loss of proprioceptive afferents via dorsal roots results in sensory dystaxia that has to be distinguished from cerebellar dystaxia.

  2. We might expect, in theory, that lesions of the corticopontine pathways might cause dystaxia. In practice, ataxia from corticopontine pathway lesions is rare or nonexistent, although a controversial form of ataxic hemiplegia has been advocated and refuted (Landau, 1988).

  3. The Romberg test shows that vision can substitute for proprioception. Hence, one aid in distinguishing sensory from cerebellar dystaxia is to have the Pt perform with eyes open and closed. Which type of dystaxia, sensory or cerebellar, would be much worse when the Pt's eyes were closed? ☐ sensory/ ☐ cerebellar. Explain: _____

Ans: ☑ Sensory. Since visual guidance substitutes for proprioceptive guidance, eye closure increases sensory dystaxia but not cerebellar.

  4. The most reliable differentiation of cerebellar and sensory dystaxia comes from the pattern of cerebellar signs on the one hand, and the pattern of sensory and reflex findings on the other. In Table 10-2 place plus signs in the appropriate column, if the clinical finding in column 1 is found in the type of dystaxia.

Sensory	Cerebellar
+	
+	
	+
+	+
+	
	+

TABLE 10-2 Differentiation of sensory and cerebellar dystaxia

Clinical finding	Sensory dystaxia	Cerebellar dystaxia
Loss of vibration and position sense		
Areflexia		
Nystagmus		
Hypotonia		
Dystaxia much worse with eyes closed		
Overshooting		

H. *Testing for loss of vibration sense (pallanesthesia)*
   1. *Instruction to the Pt and procedure*
      a. As usual, start with the Pt's eyes open until communication is established, and then do the test with the Pt's eyes closed.
      b. Hold a tuning fork (128 cps or 256 cps) by the round shaft and strike the tines a crisp blow against the ulnar side of your palm to set the fork vibrating. Apply the free end of the shaft to the Pt's fingernails and toenails. By pressing your finger against the pad of the Pt's digit and nail, you can feel the fork nearly as long as the Pt. Inquire, "Do you feel the buzz?"
      c. If the Pt cannot feel vibration at the nails for as long as you can, apply the fork to proximal bony prominences, the wrist or malleoli or elbow and knee.
   2. *Reliability monitoring in testing for pallanesthesia*
      a. How would you monitor the Pt's attentiveness and reliability in this test? _____

Ans: Sometimes apply the tuning fork when it is not vibrating.

      b. To do the foregoing reliability test, the Ex strikes the fork to set it into motion. Although the Pt's eyes are closed, the Pt may hear the strike and expect to feel vibration, but the Ex squeezes the vibrating tines *after* striking the fork, stopping its vibration, before applying the fork to the Pt. Strike your fork and squeeze its ends to familiarize yourself with this action.
   3. *Interpretation of vibration testing.* Aging increases the threshold to vibration and reduces the sensitivity, particularly in the feet (Calne and Pallis, 1966). Interruption of afferents from the peripheral nerves up through the thalamus reduces vibratory perception (Roland and Nielsen, 1980). At spinal levels, dorsal column pathways mediate vibration, but some evidence suggests that the pathway may also travel in the dorsal part of the lateral columns (Willis and Coggeshall, 1991).

I. *Alternative efficient tests for dorsal column dysfunction*
   1. *Directional scratch test*
      a. The Ex draws two transverse lines 2 cm apart across the distal shin and the dorsum of the hand.
      b. Using the tip of a tongue blade broken longitudinally, the Ex makes

2-cm long strokes between the two lines, randomly alternating between a proximal and distal direction.

c. Start with two practice trials with the Pt's eyes open to establish communication. Then, with the Pt's eyes closed, present 10 trials in random proximal–distal order. The normal person gets all 10 correct. If the Pt errs, increase the distance to 5 cm and to 10 cm to get a quantitative estimate of the deficit. Hankey and Edis (1989) claim that this test is better than the foregoing standard tests of position and vibration, and it correlates with abnormal evoked responses (Motoi et al, 1992).

2. *Depth-sense esthesiometry and two-point discrimination*
Testing two-point discrimination requires calipers and a table of normal values (Cope and Antony, 1992). Simple plastic devices may prove to be more sensitive and quicker than the traditional clinical methods (Renfrew, 1969).

J. *Review of somatosensory pathways*
1. Practice testing yourself and a companion with a cotton wisp, with a pin, and with a tuning fork for temperature (Fig. 10-4) and vibration sense, and then do the directional scratch test and test that position sense. As you test each modality, "think through" the pathway to the cerebral cortex. You must, in particular, review the location of the secondary neuron and the level of the decussation. To prove that you can "think through" these pathways, draw them (Figs. 2-27, 10-6, and 10-9).

2. Cortical lesions impair vibration, touch, pain, and temperature sensation to some extent, but less than infracortical lesions of the pathways (Adams and Burke, 1989). Some appreciation of these modalities may occur at thalamic or infracortical levels. Unilateral suprathalamic lesions do not increase the vibration threshold (Roland and Nielsen, 1980).

REFERENCES FOR DORSAL COLUMN MODALITIES

Adams RW, Burke D: Deficits of thermal sensation in patients with unilateral cerebral lesions. *Electroencephalogr Clin Neurophysiol* 1989;73:443–452

Calne D, Pallis C: Vibratory sense: a critical review. *Brain* 1966;89:723–746

Cope EB, Antony JH: Normal values for the two point discrimination test. *Ped Neurol* 1992;8:251–254

Hankey GJ, Edis RH: The utility of testing tactile perception of direction of scratch as a sensitive clinical sign of posterior column dysfunction in spinal cord disorders. *J Neurol Neurosurg Psychiatry* 1989;52:395–402

Kornhuber HH (ed): *The Somatosensory System* (2d ed). Stuttgart, Thieme, 1975

Landau W: Neuromythology, part III: ataxic hemiparesis: special deluxe stroke or standard brand? *Neurology* 1988;38:1799–1801

Motoi M, Matsumoto H, Kaneshige Y, Chiba S: A reappraisal of "direction of scratch" test: Using somotosensory evoked potentials and vibration perception. *J Neurol Neurosurg Psychiatry* 1992;55:509–510

Renfrew S: Fingertip sensation. A routine neurological test. *Lancet* 1969;1(591):396–397

Roland PE, Nielsen VK: Vibratory thresholds in the hands. *Arch Neurol* 1980;37:775–779

Schwartzman R, Bogdonoff M: Proprioception and vibration sensibility discrimination in the absence of the posterior columns. *Arch Neurol* 1969;20:349–353

Willis WD, Coggeshall RE: *Sensory Mechanisms of the Spinal Cord,* 2d ed. New York, Plenum, 1991

VI. The multimodal sensations, the gnosias or knowing sensations and the agnosias

A. *Introduction*

1. We can regard sensations as requiring two stages of cortical activity.

   a. The first stage occurs in the primary cortical receptive areas which register the sensory impulses relayed through the thalamus.

   b. For the next stage the brain has to elaborate the meaning or significance of the sensory impulses that shuttle into the primary sensory cortex. The mind must recognize these impulses, compare them with stored memories, and finally integrate them into the value system of the individual to adjudicate their significance, to know whether to act on them or ignore them. For example, to know a dime placed in your hand in the dark, you have to recognize its disclike form, its weight, its size and texture, its metallic nature, and finally its significance as money.

2. The part of the parietal lobe behind the primary sensory cortex of the postcentral gyrus acts as the association area for the process of "knowing" the symbolic significance or meaning of somatic sensation. The association areas for sight and sound occupy the zones adjacent to their primary sensory receptive areas in the occipital and temporal lobes. These zones meet and become confluent at the parietooccipitotemporal junction, a region called the *posterior parasylvian area*. Locate this area in Fig. 10-12.

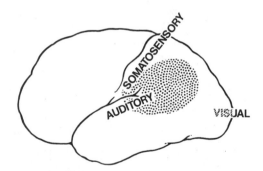

FIG. 10-12. Lateral view of the left cerebral hemisphere. The posterior parasylvian area is shaded. The figure also shows sometosensory, auditory, and visual receptive aareas.

B. *The gnosias, the terminology of knowing*

1. Clinicians have devised a nomenclature of sensation, based on the presumption that the elaboration of sensation into its ultimate meaning depends on the association cortex (Critchley, 1966). The sensations that require a high degree of cortical integration, that require a great deal of knowing, we call *gnosias*. Knowledge and gnosia are etymologically related: dia*gnosis* is literally through knowing (*dia* = through as in diarrhea; *gnosis* = know); pro*gnosis* is knowing beforehand (*pro* = before; *gnosis* = knowing).

Statognosia or statognosis
Station knowing

2. The sense of position (station) or awareness of posture is called stato _____.

3. Literally, *statognosia* means _____ _____.

4. Sense of form is called stereo _____. Literally, it means _____.

Ans: *Stereognosia; form knowing.*

Topognosia

5. Sense of localization of a skin stimulus is topo-_____.

Graphognosia

6. The *graphic* sense of numbers or letters written on the skin is _____.

7. Sense of awareness of a bodily defect is named by using the root *nos* for disease. Hence, nosology is the science of disease classification, and the sense of awareness of disease is _____.

Nosognosia

8. Give the medical meaning of these roots:

Position or station
    a. Stato- means _____.

Form
    b. Stereo- means _____.

Place
    c. Topo- means _____.

Writing
    d. Grapho- means _____.

Disease
    e. Noso- means _____.

C. *The agnosias, the terminology of not knowing*

An
A
Not knowing

1. The negating prefix to designate lack or absence of, is _____ before a vowel, or _____ before a consonant. Hence agnosia literally means _____.

2. To designate a gnostic defect due to a lesion in the association cortex or its circuits, we negate the term for the normal sensation:

Astatognosia
    a. Loss of position sense, loss of statognosia, becomes _____.

Astereognosia
    b. Loss of form sense is _____.

Atopognosia
    c. Loss of cutaneous localization is _____.

Agraphognosia
    d. Loss of graphic sense is _____.

Anosognosia
    e. Loss of disease awareness is _____.

    f. Alternatively, the word could be stereoagnosia, topagnosia, etc., to describe the same thing.

D. *How to designate whether the lesion that causes loss of sensation is in the sensory pathway or the association circuit*

1. Lesions may interfere with the knowing of sensory stimuli in two ways: by interrupting the sensory pathways from receptor to primary sensory cortex, or by interrupting the association cortex or its circuits with the thalamus and hippocampus.

    a. If the lesion destroys the receptor, the sensory pathway through nerve or neuraxis, or the primary receptive cortex, the impulses cannot reach the association cortex for interpretation. The Pt does not know, because the association cortex does not receive adequate information. We return to one of Muller's laws: all we know of the external world is a change of state in impulses in one of our afferent pathways (Chapter 9).

    b. If the lesion destroys the association cortex or its circuits with the thalamus or hippocampus, the Pt does not know, because of inability to appreciate the significance or meaning of the impulses which reach the primary cortex.

Hypesthesia

2. If, for example, a peripheral nerve or the spinal cord is cut, the complete loss of sensation is called anesthesia. If sensation is merely reduced it is called _____.

3. Similarly, complete lack of pain sensation is _____gesia, reduced pain sensation is _____ and excessive pain sensation is _____.

Ans: Analgesia; hypalgesia; hyperalgesia.

4. If a lesion causes loss of position sense because of a lesion in the pathway between receptor and primary sensory cortex, the sensory loss is called *statanesthesia* or *astatesthesia.* If it is lost because of a lesion of the association

Astatognosia or
statagnosia

cortex or its connections with primary sensory cortex, it is called _____
_____.

5. Loss of hearing because of VIIIth nerve interruption is called ☐ deafness/
☐ auditory agnosia.

☑ *Deafness*

6. What would auditory agnosia mean? _____
_____.

Ans: Inability to understand the meaning of sounds.

7. If a lesion in the optic pathways or calcarine cortex causes hemianopsia, the
Pt is said to have ☐ blindness/ ☐ visual agnosia in that field of vision.

☑ *Blindness*

8. Explain why we say the Pt in 7 is blind, rather than having visual agnosia.
_____
_____
_____.

Ans: Since the lesion is in the optic pathway or calcarine cortex, not in the
association cortex, the primary impulses for vision cannot get to the
association cortex for interpretation. It is improper to diagnose agnosia if
impulses fail to reach the association cortex.

9. You might suppose that astereognosia would be used to mean complete
lack of form perception and hypostereognosia would be used to mean
diminished form perception, as in anesthesia and hypesthesia. But not even
neurologists like such cumbersome terms as hypostereognosia, and in practice the prefixes *a* or *an* mean either absent or diminished gnostic sensation.
Since we do not find a heightened sense of gnosia, as in *hyperesthesia,* the
prefix *hyper* is not used with gnosias.

E. *Testing for astereognosia and tactile agnosia*

1. With the Pt's eyes closed, the Ex places various common objects in the Pt's
hand. The Ex instructs the Pt to feel the object and identify it. If the Pt's
hand is paralyzed, the Ex may move the item over the fingers to substitute
for the Pt's active finger movement.

2. The best items are keys, safety pins, paper clips, and a series of coins, such
as a penny, dime, nickle, and quarter. The penny and dime are especially
hard to distinguish, and the normal person may miss occasionally. Caselli
(1991) separates tactile gnosia or full recognition of objects placed in the
hand from simple form perception, that is, distinguishing a cone from a pyramid, which he calls stereognosis.

3. Stereognosis and tactile gnosia require intact touch, position sense, and
finally synthesis of the primary modalities into the concept of key, coin, or
pin. Hence, all pathways of the primary modalities from the receptor to the
parietal cortex must be intact. If you place the object in the Pt's right hand
you are testing the ☐ left/ ☐ right parietal lobe.

☑ *Left*

4. If the Pt has lost the sense of form because of a lesion in the periphery, spinal
cord, brainstem, or thalamus, the term *astereognosia* is incorrect. The correct term is stereo_____.

Stereoanesthesia

5. The term *agnosia* is correct only if the lesion is in the ☐ nerve/ ☐ spinal
cord/ ☐ brainstem/ ☐ thalamus/ ☐ association cortex.

☑ *Association cortex*

6. If a Pt has lost position sense because of a spinal cord lesion, the sensory
deficit is called _____.

Statanesthesia

F. *Testing for distortions of the body scheme: somatoagnosia, topagnosia, and*
autotopagnosia

1. *Definition.* The brain visualizes one's anatomic configuration, boundaries,
postures, and body parts in a grand gestalt called the *body scheme* (soma-

tognosia). Several synonyms or near synonyms encompass the concept of somatognosia or its antonym somatagnosia. *Topagnosia* is the inability to localize skin stimuli. *Autotopagnosia* is the inability to locate, recognize, and orient one's body parts. Thus lesions can interfere with the neural processing or representation of the body scheme, giving rise to a variety of body scheme agnosias. Even a puppy knows self from nonself, but the normal body scheme, such as finger localization (finger gnosia) and right-left orientation, only becomes formally testable in 5- to 6-year-old children, and thus follows a definite developmental sequence (Benton, 1959; Reed, 1967). Neuropsychiatric disorders may cause a variety of body scheme delusions. In anorexia nervosa the person perceives herself as too fat, no matter how emaciated she actually becomes. As so often happens in neurology, such neuropsychiatric diseases merge imperceptibly with purely psychiatric disorders in which the person may erroneously perceive a part of his/her body as imperfect such as the nose, breasts, or genitalia. These delusions may make the Pt seek unwarranted recontouring by plastic surgery. The Ex must recognize psychiatric as well as neurologic distortions of the body scheme and must not simply accede to the Pt's requests for interventional surgery or medication. Otherwise, as in anorexia nervosa or the surgical Munchausen syndrome (as the Pt's multiscarred belly attests), the Pt may end up as a pathetic caricature of the desired result.

2. *Method of testing for tactile finger agnosia and right-left disorientation*
   a. Work out a system of finger identification with the Pt (Poeck and Orgass, 1969). Number the fingers 1 to 5 on each hand, beginning with the thumb; then with the Pt's eyes closed, the Ex randomly touches digits on the right or left hand and asks the Pt to identify the finger and whether it is the right or left hand. If the Pt seems to have right-left disorientation, give further commands, such as "Touch your right hand to your left ear," to verify the deficit.
   b. Test for autotopagnosia also, by placing a part in one position and asking the Pt to duplicate the position with the opposite extremity, with the eyes closed. For example, the Ex elevates the Pt's arm to a position on one side, asks the Pt to hold it there, and then requires the Pt to duplicate the position with the opposite extremity. The peripheral pathways for position sense have to be intact to make this a test for autotopagnosia.

3. *Localizing value of agnosias.* Agnosias signify lesions of the association areas which extend from the primary sensory receptive areas. For the somatagnosias, the relevant association area is the posterior parasylvian area. Lesions of the left posterior parasylvian area cause bilateral finger agnosia and right-left disorientation (see Gerstmann's syndrome in Chap. 11).

4. *Two-point discrimination.* Discrimination of two points from one when the skin is touched with the tips of calipers is a cortical function closely allied to topognosia. Since two-point discrimination varies with the part of the body tested and the age of the Pt, it requires a chart of normal values. While too time-consuming for the screening NE, it may confirm questionable parietal lobe sensory deficits suggested by the screening tests.

G. *Testing for agraphognosia (agraphesthesia)*
   1. With the Pt's eyes closed, the Ex traces numbers between 1 and 10, or letters, on the skin of the palm or fingertips, using any blunt tip, such as the cap end of a ball-point pen (Bender et al, 1982).
      a. The normal person rarely misses the stimulus. The uneducated person,

or one unpracticed in numbers, may have some difficulty in the absence of a brain lesion.

☑ *Right parietal*

  b. In testing for agraphognosia in the left hand, you test the ☐ right/ ☐ left _____ lobe of the brain.
2. For a Pt unable to recognize letters written on the skin, and whose lesion had destroyed sensory pathways in the brainstem or spinal cord, the correct term would be _____.

Graphanesthesia

3. Bender et al (1982) propose that the same pathway from periphery to somatosensory cortex that detects the direction of movement of a stimulus across the skin also mediates graphognosia.

H. *Testing for anosognosia*
 1. *Definition.* Josef Babinski (1857–1932) introduced the term *anosognosia* to describe a Pt who had left hemiplegia and left-sided sensory loss but who was unaware of his neurologic deficit. Although also applied in a general sense, the term anosognosia is perhaps best restricted to the original use of Babinski. While highly characteristic on the left side after right parietal lobe lesions, it can occur with left parietal lesions, particularly in the acute phase of a lesion (Stone et al, 1991).
 2. *Clinical testing for anosognosia*
  Most Pts with enduring anosognosia have large right hemisphere lesions, persistent left-sided hemiplegia and hemispatial inattention, and often mental impairment (Levine et al, 1991). If you ask whether the Pt can move the left arm, the Pt will reply, "Yes," even though it is completely hemiplegic. The most dramatic test for anosognosia is this: stand on the left side of the Pt's bed and place the hemiplegic arm on the bed, alongside of the Pt. Lay your own left arm across the Pt's waist. Ask the Pt to reach over and pick up his own left hand. He will feel across his abdomen, grasp your hand and hold it triumphantly aloft, never realizing the error. It is to such una-

Anosognosia

wareness of neurologic deficits that the term _____ applies.

I. *Testing for tactile inattention (tactile suppression) to simultaneous stimuli.* In visual field testing, Pts sometimes fail to attend to one of two bilateral simultaneous stimuli. Similarly sensory inattention to simultaneous bilateral stimuli occurs with hearing and with touch or pain.
 1. *Testing for tactile inattention to the right or left sides.* Advise the Pt that you may touch more than one site. With the Pt's eyes closed and using light pressure, brush one or simultaneously both cheeks randomly with the tips of your index finger. The Pt reports whatever is felt and should perceive one or both stimuli. Then similarly test the dorsum of the hands and then the feet. If the Pt reports only one stimulus after the Ex has applied simultaneous stimuli, the Ex again states, "I may be touching you in more than one place. Don't let me fool you." Then alternate, randomly touching only one or both sides, until you determine whether the Pt consistently does or does not feel bilateral simultaneous stimuli.
 2. *Testing for unilateral inattention to simultaneous stimuli.* On one side, simultaneously touch the face and hand several times, and then the foot and hand. The Pt normally reports both stimuli. With parietal lesions, the Pt does not attend to the hand stimulus and reports only the face or foot stimulus.
 3. *Interpretation of tactile inattention*
  a. Inattention to simultaneous bilateral stimuli is most prominent after right parietal lobe lesions, in which case the Pt fails to attend to the stim-

ulus on the left (Bender, 1952; Critchley, 1966). The test is valid when the lesion spares the afferent pathways and postcentral gyrus, leaving the sensory thresholds but little altered. With impairment of the sensory pathways on one side, the apparent inattention may represent merely hypesthesia.

b. Just why inattention occurs more commonly with right parietal lesions is unknown. Occasionally, with left parietal lesions, the Pt will not attend to the right side on simultaneous stimulation. After simultaneous stimulation of both sides, the Pt with a right parietal lesion *inattends* to stimuli from the ☐ right/ ☐ left side.

☑ *Left*

J. *Testing for inattention to one entire half of space*
1. Some Pts with lateralized cerebral lesions, usually right parietal, fail to attend to the entire left half of space. The Ex gains evidence for this unilateral neglect by observing that the Pt ignores persons, objects, or any stimuli from the affected side, fails to dress that side of the body, and fails to eat the food from that half of the plate.
2. For formal testing, the Ex asks the Pt to draw a cross or any geometric figure such as a bicycle wheel with spokes or the face of a clock. The Pt will draw one half of the figure accurately but will make mistakes in completing the drawing on the other side (Fig. 11-3) (Critchley, 1966; Stone et al, 1991). For another simple test, ask the Pt to make a pencil mark that exactly bisects a long horizontal line drawn on a sheet of paper. The Pt with a right parietal lobe lesion will make the mark considerably to the right of the true center because of neglect of the left half of space (Tegner and Levander, 1991).
3. Although only right parietal lesions regularly cause contralateral hemi-inattention, lesions of either parietal lobe regularly cause contralateral astereognosia, agraphognosia, astatognosia, and atopagnosia. The sensations of touch, pain, temperature, pressure, and vibration may remain intact. They are relatively more impaired by lesions in the infracortical pathways or PNS.

K. *Testing for prosopagnosia*
1. Prosopagnosia, the inability to recognize faces, either in person or by photos, ranks as one of the most intriguing agnosias. The Ex presents photos of acquaintances or well-known celebrities, such as the President of the United States, for the Pt to identify. The Pt realizes that a photo of a face or a person's actual face is before them and can even describe its parts, but cannot recognize the person by visual cues. If the person speaks the Pt may identify the person instantly by the sound of the voice.
3. The lesion destroys the inferomedial temporooccipital region, a region irrigated by cortical branches of the posterior cerebral artery (Damasio and Damasio, 1989). The lesion is usually bilateral and ischemic or anoxic in origin. Lesions in this region also cause color agnosia (achromatopsia or chromatagnosia).
4. In summary, lesions of *either* parietal lobe may cause contralateral astereognosia, astatognosia, agraphognosia, and atopopognosia, but inattention and anosognosia are commoner with ☐ right/ ☐ left parietal lobe lesions.
5. In contrast, finger agnosia and right-left disorientation are commoner with ☐ right/ ☐ left parietal lobe lesions.

☑ *Right*

☑ *Left*

L. *Summary of somatic sensory testing*
Rehearse section VII, steps A and B of the Summarized Neurologic Examination and section VI, E–K of this chapter.

M. Review of the lobes of the cerebrum.

Celsus around A.D. 25 remarked, ". . . nor can a diseased portion of the body be treated by one who does not know what that part is." This principle remains true today. If you cannot draw the lobes of the brain and define their boundaries, review Chapter 2, section I.D, and Fig. 2-2.

REFERENCES FOR AGNOSIAS

Bender M: *Disorders in Perception, with Particular Reference to the Phenomena of Extinction and Displacement.* Springfield, Charles C Thomas, 1952

Bender M, Stacy C, Cohen J: Agraphesthesia: a disorder of directional cutaneous kinesthesia or a disorientation in cutaneous space. *J Neurol Sci* 1982;53:531–555

Benton A: *Right-Left Discrimination and Finger Localization: Development and Pathology.* New York, Harper & Row, 1959

Caselli RJ: Rediscovering tactile agnosia. *Mayo Clin Proc* 1991a;66:129–142

Cope E, Antony J: Normal values for two-point discrimination test. *Ped Neurol,* 1992;8:251–257

Critchley M: *The Parietal Lobes.* New York, Hafner Publishing, 1966

Damasio H, Damasio AR: *Lesion Analysis in Neuropsychology.* New York, Oxford University Press, 1989

Heimburger R, DeMyer W, Reitan R: Implications of Gerstmann's syndrome. *J Neurol Neurosurg Psychiat* 1964;27:52–57

Levine DN, Calvanio R, Rinn WE: The pathogenesis of anosognosia for hemiplegia. *Neurology* 1991;41:1770–1780

Poeck K. Orgass B: An experimental investigation of finger agnosia. *Neurology* 1969;19:801–807

Reed J: Lateralized finger agnosia and reading achievement at ages 6 and 10. *Child Develop* 1967;38:213–220

Stone SP, Wilson B, Wroot A et al: The assessment of visuo-spatial neglect after acute stroke. *J Neurol Neurosurg Psychiatry* 1991;54:345–350

Tegner R, Levander M: The influence of stimulus properties on visual neglect. *J Neurol Neurosurg Psychiatry* 1991;54:882–887

Weinstein EA, Friedland RP (eds): *Hemi-attention Syndromes and Hemisphere Specialization.* (vol 18: *Advances in Neurology*). New York, Raven, 1977

VII. Steps in the clinical analysis of a sensory complaint

A. Inquire whether the complaint is intermittent or constant.

B. Inquire about any factors or maneuvers which exacerbate or relieve the complaint. Have the Pt demonstrate any postures or maneuvers which may exacerbate the complaint. Ask the Pt's opinion as to the cause for the complaint. Frequently the Pt discloses fears of cancer or some other dread malady. Even if you learn nothing of immediate clinical value, Pts appreciate your interest in their observations and opinions.

C. Ask the Pt to delineate the area of pain or sensory loss. If intelligent, observant, and nonpsychiatric, the Pt will map it out as well or better than the Ex can with pin and cotton, and much more quickly.

D. Before each test, establish communication. State clearly what you expect. Don't equivocate, yet don't suggest responses. Ask for "Yes" or "No" responses, or "Is (stimulus) 1 different from (stimulus) 2?"

E. *Isolate the modality for testing from other sensory modalities.* Do most sensory tests with the Pt's eyes closed.

F. *Monitor the suggestibility and attentiveness of the Pt by sometimes withholding the stimulus and asking whether the Pt perceived it.*

G. *Draw the area of deficit on the Pt or on a diagram.* Delineate the borders only as sharply as the results warrant. Repeat the examination on another day to test the reproducibility of the deficit.

H. *Think through the anatomic pathway for the modality.* Know the location of the secondary sensory neuron and therefore the site of decussation of the pathway.

I. *Make a decision on the probable distribution of the sensory complaint (Fig. 10-13).*

J. *Try to match the Pt's sensory findings against known patterns.* Work through Figs. 10–14 to 10–17.

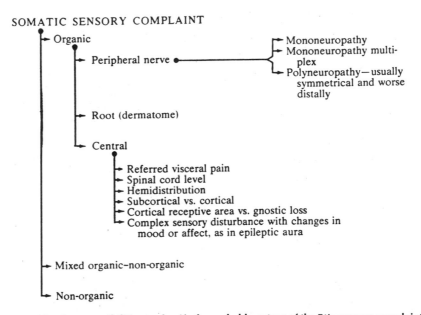

FIG. 10-13. Consider these possibilities to classify the probable nature of the Pt's sensory complaint. See also Fig. 10-14.

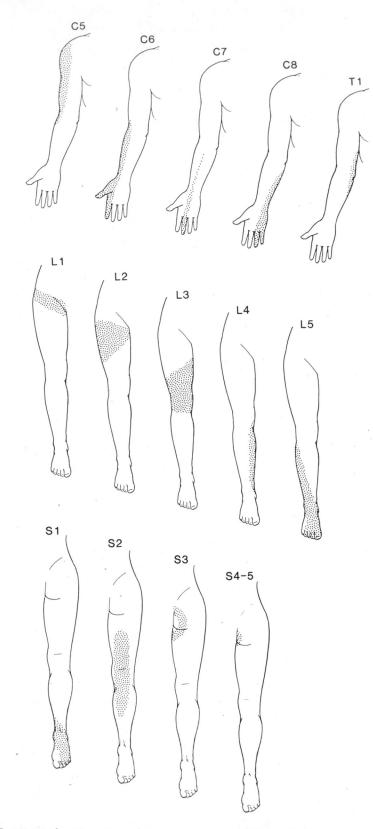

FIG. 10-14. **Dermatomal patterns of sensory deficit caused by interruption of various dorsal roots. C = cervical dermatomes; T = thoracic; L = lumbar; S = sacral; compare also with Fig. 2-10.**

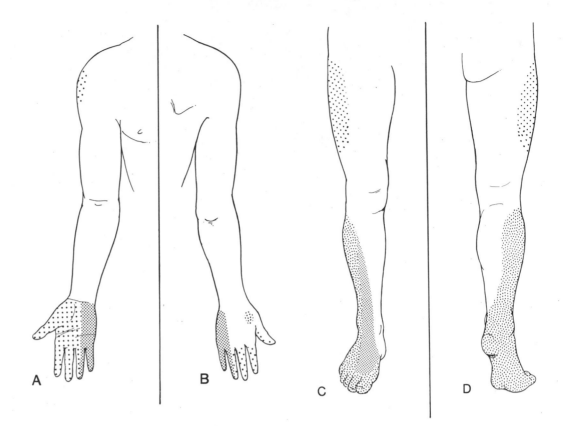

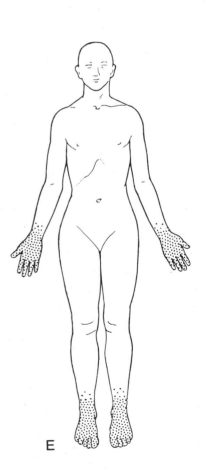

FIG. 10-15. Patterns of sensory deficit caused by lesions of specific peripheral nerves. (*A*) Palmar view of the hand: large dots, median nerve; small dots, ulnar. The dots over the shoulder indicate the sensory loss after interruption of the axillary (circumflex) nerve. (See Fig. 2-11.) (*B*) Dorsal view of the hand: large dots, median nerve; small dots, ulnar; intermediate dots (near base of the thumb), radial. (*C*) Anterior view of the lower extremity: dots on upper thigh indicate the area of sensory loss caused by interruption of the lateral femoral cutaneous nerve. The sparse dots below the knee indicate the sensory deficit caused by interruption of the tibial division of the sciatic nerve. The denser dots represent the peroneal division of the sciatic nerve. (*D*) Posterior view of the lower extremity: the dots on the thigh represent the distribution of the lateral femoral cutaneous nerve. The dots below the knee represent the tibial division of the sciatic nerve. (*E*) Areas of sensory loss caused by a diffuse, symmetrical polyneuropathy. The demarcation between affected and nonaffected areas fades imperceptibly. Hysterical sensory loss tends to cause sharp margins between the affected and nonaffected zones (Chap. 14).

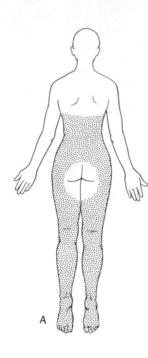

A

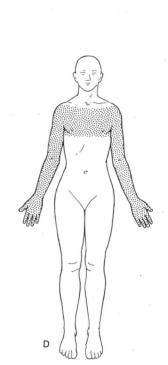

B

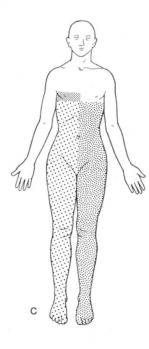

C

D

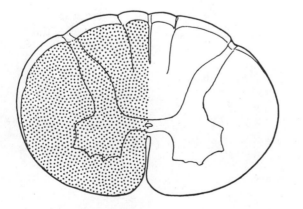

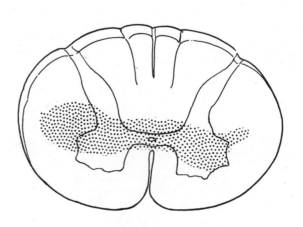

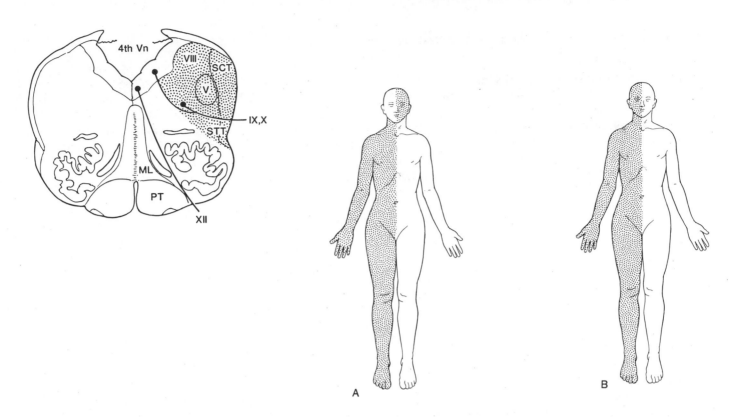

FIG. 10-17. Areas of sensory loss with intracranial lesions. (*A*) Wallenberg's lateral medullary wedge syndrome, usually due to infarction in the distribution of the posterior inferior cerebellar artery. The patient shows ipsilateral loss of facial sensation due to interruption of the descending root of cranial nerve five (V) and contralateral loss of pain and temperature sensation due to interruption of the spinothalamic tract (STT). The patient also has vertigo, nausea, and vomiting due to involvement of vestibular connections and also has a Horner's syndrome because of interruption of autonomic fibers that descend through the reticular formation in the area occupied by the lesion (Fig. 4-31). Interruption of the ninth and tenth nerves (IX and X) causes dysarthria and dysphagia. The patient has ipsilateral ataxia due to interruption of the spinocerebellar tracts (SCT) and the overlying cerebellar hemisphere, irrigated by the posterior inferior cerebellar artery. Notice that the lesion spares the medial lemniscus (ML) and the pyramidal tract (PT) and twelfth nerves (XII). (*B*) Hemisensory loss due to interruption of sensory pathways through the medial lemniscus-thalamo-cortical pathway. (See Fig. 2-27.) Hysteria can also cause hemisensory loss. Chapter 14 discusses the differentiation from organic anesthesia.

< —————————————————————————

FIG. 10-16. Patterns of sensory loss after various lesions of the spinal cord. (*A*) A lesion at the midthoracic level may cause sensory loss caudal to the lesion, commencing at a transverse line at the level of the lesion. Because the ascending fibers from the sacral area occupy the extreme periphery of the cord the lesion may spare these fibers, a phenomenon called sacral sparing. (See Fig. 2-12*B*.) (*B*) Sacral loss of sensation caused by lesion of the distal or sacral part of the spinal cord (the conus medullaris). The conus gives rise to the cauda equinus, consisting of the lumbosacral roots that descend from the conus to exit through the intervertebral foramina. (*C*) Sensory loss in the Brown-Sequard syndrome of hemisection of the spinal cord (see the inset). With the lesion at T4, the patient has a small band of sensory deficit at that level from interruption of the dorsal root, indicated by the dense dots. The patient loses dorsal column modalities ipsilaterally because of interruption of the dorsal column. The patient has leg paralysis because of interruption of the ipsilateral corticospinal tract of the lateral columns (Fig. 2-12*A*). The patient loses pain and temperature sensation on the contralateral side of the body up to the level of the lesion because of interruption of the spinothalamic tract, which has crossed. (*D*) Pattern of sensory loss with syringomyelia (see second inset). When a syrinx or cavitating lesion affects the spinal cord it interrupts the axons that cross to ascend in the spinothalamic tract. With a syrinx extending from C4 to T5, the patient loses pain and temperature sensation in the distribution indicated by the dots in the figure. The lesion does not encroach on the pain and temperature pathways from the trunk and leg, since these pathways run in the periphery of the spinal cord (Fig. 2-12).

Learning Objectives for Chapter 10

I. Introduction to testing general somatic sensations

1. List the special senses and the general senses tested in the screening neurologic examination.
2. Describe differences in sensitivity to stimuli, particularly touch, in different areas of skin.
3. Recite and define the words used to describe deficient or excessive senses of touch, pain, and temperature.
4. Define hyperpathia, neuralgia, and causalgia.
5. Give one common example of paresthesias or dysesthesias experienced by everyone.
6. Give examples of positive or irritative phenomena caused by lesions of the II and VIII cranial nerves.
*7. Discuss some neurophysiological theories to explain the positive or irritative sensations caused by lesions that affect afferent fibers.

II. Examination of somatosensory functions of cranial nerve V

1. Explain how the concept of a 3D "mask of Trigeminus" enables you to recall the posterior border of the innervation field of cranial nerve V on the surface skin and deep structures (teeth, oral cavity, nasal passages, and sinuses).
2. Describe how observing the facial, feeding, and respiratory-related reflexes and certain autonomic reflexes of a newborn infant provides a rational mnemonic for remembering the range of functions mediated by the Vth nerve.
3. Draw a lateral view of the face to show the area of distribution of the three major sensory divisions of the Vth cranial nerve (Fig. 10-2).
4. Draw a dorsal view of the brainstem and show the three subdivisions of the trigeminal sensory nucleus.
5. Diagram the sensory pathway that connects the sensory nuclei of V with the thalamus (Fig. 10-2).
*6. Explain the unique anatomic features of the mesencephalic nucleus of the Vth nerve.
7. Describe and demonstrate how to test touch over the trigeminal area.
8. Explain how to monitor the Pt's attentiveness and suggestibility during testing for pain, touch, and temperature sensation.
9. Explain why, if you suspect a numb area from the Pt's history, you should begin sensory testing with a normal area.
10. Describe and demonstrate how to test the corneal reflex.
11. Name the cranial nerves which mediate the corneal reflex.
*12. Describe the corneomandibular and glabellar blink reflexes.
13. Explain why you should use subtle rather than great differences in testing temperature sensation.
14. Describe and demonstrate how to test for temperature discrimination by the tuning fork versus finger test and the warm and cool tube tests.
15. Explain why you should always test for temperature discrimination before testing for pain, especially with a child.
16. State which nerve root innervates the skin over the angle of the mandible. Explain how knowledge of this fact helps distinguish organic from hysterical loss of facial sensation.
17. Explain, in principle, how the pattern of sensory loss found on the examination distinguishes organic from hysterical loss of sensation, and describe the usual pattern of hysterical loss of sensation in the arm.
18. Describe the clinical characteristics of trigeminal neuralgia.

III. Testing somatosensory functions of the body and extremities

1. State the location of the nerve cell body for the primary, secondary, and tertiary neurons in the pathways for general somatic sensation (Fig. 2-27).
2. Explain why, in testing for a dermatomal loss of sensation, the Ex moves the stimulus *up* and *down* the trunk but *around* the limbs (Fig. 2-10).
3. Describe the pathways by which touch reaches conscious appreciation from the body and extremities.
4. Explain the importance of knowing the location of the secondary neuron in the somatic sensory pathways.
5. Define a lemniscus and name the lemnisci (Table 10-1).
6. Define the spinal lemniscus.
7. On a generalized cross section of the brainstem, locate the lemnisci (Fig. 2-14).
8. Name the one sensation that does not, in fact or theory, have a specific thalamic relay nucleus. (In answering this question, recall how to use your own body to systematically enumerate the senses, as previously taught.)
*9. Given specific cross sections of the medulla, pons, and midbrain (Figs. 2-15 to 2-18), locate the lemniscal sector.
10. Name the thalamic nuclei which relay impulses for somatic sensation, sight, and hearing to the cerebral cortex.
11. Describe the distribution of loss of general somatic sensation after unilateral destruction of the entire nucleus ventralis posterior.
12. Describe the type of pin to use to test pain sensation and how to hold it to ensure a uniform stimulus for the pinpricks.
13. Explain why you make multiple pinpricks at each site rather than single pricks in testing pain sensation.

14. Explain why the Ex always discards a pin after using it to test pain sensation.
15. Explain why the Ex tests temperature and pain sensation on the dorsum of the hands and feet rather than the palms and soles.
16. Describe how to test temperature and pain sensation over the body and extremities.
17. State the evidence suggesting that a neonate or possibly even a fetus might feel pain. Describe how this evidence may be used to accurately and reliably determine the level of a spinal cord transection in a newborn or young infant.
18. Describe the two types of pain in response to a pinprick and relate these to the kind of peripheral nerve fiber that conducts each type of pain.
19. Diagram the pathway for pain and temperature sensation from the trunk and extremities to the cerebral cortex (Fig. 10-6).
20. Explain how the pain and temperature pathway from the face resembles and differs from the pathway for the rest of the body (Figs. 10-2 and 10-6).
21. Describe the order of representation of the entire face and body in the pain and temperature nucleus (substantia gelatinosa of Rolando), and state the location of that nucleus.
22. Describe a neurosurgical operation on the spinal cord that would abolish pain and temperature sensation but would not abolish touch or cause motor disturbances.
*23. Describe how to test for delayed pain and deep pain.
24. Define referred pain and give an example.

IV. Pain in the back, shooting down the leg: the sciatica syndrome

1. Describe the findings on the NE of a Pt with an acute L-5 intervertebral disc herniation.
2. Describe how to do the sciatic nerve stretching tests and the biomechanics involved.
3. Explain why, in the straight-knee leg-raising test, when the Ex stops just short of eliciting pain, and then manually dorsiflexes the Pt's foot, pain is produced.
4. Describe the results and significance when the straight leg-raising test on one side produces radicular pain in the other leg.

V. Proprioception, position and vibration sense: the dorsal column or deep modalities

1. Define proprioceptive sensation.
2. Explain how the etymology of the word *proprioception* applies to its use in neurology.
*3. Summarize the reasoning which led Sherrington to recognize a proprioceptive system.
4. Diagram the skeletomuscular proprioceptive pathway from the foot and hand (Fig. 10-9).
5. Describe the location of the second order neuron in the dorsal column proprioceptive pathway from the

extremities. State where its axon decussates and the name of the pathway it takes to the thalamus.
*6. Diagram the sensory homunculus in the dorsal columns and give the technical terms for the fasciculi of the dorsal columns (Fig. 2-12).
*7. Contrast the nature of the stimuli received by deep and superficial receptors.
*8. Discuss the relationship between the concepts of the mechanoreceptors (dorsal column modalities), and classical Newtonian physics.
9. Describe and demonstrate how to test for position sense in the digits.
10. Demonstrate the proper method for separating the toes to test position sense in toe four (Fig. 10-10).
11. Explain why testing digits three or four provides a greater challenge to the Pt's position sense than digits one, two, or five and why, if you find normal position sense in digits three and four, you do not have to test other digits or proximal joints in the routine screening NE (Fig. 10-11).
12. State what joints you examine next to determine the severity of the loss, if the Pt has no position sense in digits three and four in the hands or feet.
13. State whether a normal person who is attending to the stimulus will make any errors in digit position.
14. State the probability that a Pt who has no position sense will correctly guess the *up* or *down* position of the digit.
15. Describe methods of making position sense testing more challenging than simple *up* or *down* alternatives.
16. In *up* or *down* position sense testing, state the minimum number of trials necessary to make success by chance improbable.
17. Discuss the clinical interpretation when the Pt consistently gives the wrong or exactly opposite answer each time to the *up* or *down* position of the digit.
18. Discuss the reasons why the sensory examination requires such a high degree of skill on the part of the Ex.
19. Recite the instructions the Ex gives the Pt for the swaying (Romberg) test.
20. Describe the result of the swaying test in a normal person, in a hysteric, in Pts with lesions of the cerebellum or dorsal column, and in Pts with vertigo.
21. Give an operational description of the Romberg test.
22. Give an interpretational description of the Romberg test.
23. State the critical sensory pathway for maintaining the upright posture with the eyes closed.
24. Explain why you ask the Pt to stand with the feet together for the Romberg test.
25. Describe how to divert the hysterical patient into performing well in the Romberg test.
26. Describe how to differentiate sensory and cerebellar ataxia (Table 10-2).
27. Describe the effect of closing the eyes on cerebellar and sensory dystaxia.

28. Describe and demonstrate how to test for vibration sense.
29. Describe how to monitor the vibration sense of the Pt by use of your own digits.
30. Explain how to monitor the Pt's attentiveness and reliability in testing vibration sense.
*31. Describe the directional scratch test for dorsal column dysfunction.
32. Review the pathways for conscious perception of touch, temperature and pain, position, and vibration.
33. Compare the relative impairment of the foregoing sensations by lesions of the PNS or central pathways up to the somesthetic cortex, versus cortical lesions themselves.

VI. The multimodal sensations, the gnosias or knowing sensations

1. On a lateral diagram of the cerebral hemisphere shade the posterior parasylvian region.
2. Discuss the presumed special role in sensation of the cortex, which extends from the primary somatosensory, auditory, and visual cortex, and which becomes confluent in the posterior parasylvian area.
3. Describe the location of the primary cortical receptive area for somatic sensation and the location of its association area.
4. Define *gnosia* as used in neurology and give examples of gnosia using the following roots: stato-, stereo-, topo-, grapho-, and noso-.
5. Define *agnosia* and enumerate several agnosias.
6. Describe what the terms *stereoanesthesia* and *asterognosia* imply about the location of the lesion along the sensory pathway.
7. Distinguish between deafness and auditory agnosia, and blindness and visual agnosia, and explain what these terms imply about the location of the lesion along the course of the sensory pathways.

8. Define, give examples of, and describe how to test for astereognosis.
*9. Distinguish between astereognosis and tactile agnosia.
10. Discuss what is meant by the concept of a body scheme or somatognosia.
11. Give some examples of distortion of the body scheme by neuropsychiatric disorders and purely psychiatric disorders.
12. Demonstrate how to test for finger agnosia and right-left disorientation.
13. State whether finger agnosia, right-left disorientation, sensory inattention, and anosognosia are more characteristic of right or left parietal lobe lesions.
14. Describe how to test for agraphognosia (agraphesthesia) and its localizing significance.
15. Define and describe how to test for anosognosia and give its localizing significance.
16. Define and describe how to test for tactile inattention (tactile supression) and its localizing significance.
17. Describe the typical clinical findings in a Pt who does not attend to the left half of space.
*18. Define and demonstrate how to test for prosopognosia, and state its localizing value.
19. Summarize the parietal lobe gnostic tests.
20. Describe and define the lobes of the cerebrum (Fig. 2-2).

VII. Steps in the clinical analysis of a sensory complaint

1. Enumerate the steps in the clinical analysis of a sensory complaint and describe the distributions which implicate an organic sensory abnormality (Fig. 10-13).
2. Rehearse section VII of the Summarized Neurologic Examination and section VI, E–L of this chapter.

Chapter Eleven

The Patient's Mental Status and Higher Cerebral Functions

As not only the disease interested the physician, but he was strongly moved to look into the character and qualities of the patient. . . . He deemed it essential, it would seem, to know the man, before attempting to do him good.
                                                    Nathaniel Hawthorne (1804–1864)

I. The mental status examination: a nonprogrammed interlude

A. *How to derive the mental status information*

  1. The Ex derives most of the information for judging the Pt's mental status as a natural consequence of the questions posed during the standard medical history, which this text does not cover. Although doing the basic NE by a set routine, the Ex probes the Pt's mental status unobtrusively and flexibly. If the Ex blurts out questions obviously designed to test the mental status, such as, "Do you hear voices?" the Pt may respond with annoyance, sullen silence, or outright anger. Yet, just such a question introduced at the proper time encourages the disclosure of distressing thoughts. The Pt then may describe the voice that repeats, "You have the duty to kill your family." The Ex cannot gain access to such thoughts by secretly watching the Pt's behavior through a one-way glass. Because the Ex's characteristics and interview techniques condition what the Pt can and will disclose, the Ex must remain flexible, empathetic, and nonjudgmental. This is the first point: *The interview technique is everything.*

  2. By monitoring the Pt's responses, the Ex determines which questions to use and how far to pursue any particular line of inquiry. As long as the Pt talks productively, continue the inquiry. If the Pt changes the subject or becomes evasive, flustered, or silent, you have pressed too hard. The Pt isn't ready to talk about that. Take another tack. A mentally ill Pt may permit a full NE, yet completely resist inquiries designed to disclose thoughts. Pts will talk about whatever problems and anxieties occupy their thoughts, if they can tolerate the thought and its communication. This is the second point: *Pts will disclose their mental state, if you provide a free opportunity.* Nathaniel Hawthorne marvelously describes the correct interview technique in *The Scarlet Letter:*

  > So [Dr.] Roger Chillingworth—the man of skill, the kind and friendly physician—strove to go deep into his patient's bosom, delving among his principles, prying into his recollections, and probing everything with a cautious touch, like a treasure-seeker in a dark cavern. Few secrets can escape an investigator, who has opportunity and

license to undertake such a quest, and skill to follow it up. A man burdened with a secret should especially avoid the intimacy of his physician. If the latter possess native sagacity, and a nameless something more,—let us call it intuition; if he show no intrusive egotism, nor disagreeably prominent characteristics of his own; if he have the power, which must be born with him, to bring his mind into such affinity with his patient's that this last shall unawares have spoken what he imagines himself only to have thought; if such revelations be received without tumult, and acknowledged not so often by an uttered sympathy as by silence, an inarticulate breath, and here or there a word, to indicate that all is understood; if to these qualifications of a confidant be joined the advantages afforded by his recognized character as a physician,—then, at some inevitable moment will the soul of the sufferer be dissolved, and flow forth in a dark, but transparent stream, bringing all its mysteries into the daylight.

B. Goals of the metal status examination

1. Although avoiding a strict routine of questions, the Ex must keep the goals of the mental status examination in mind to avoid omitting areas of inquiry that may provide critical diagnostic data (Strub and Black, 1977). Learn Table 11-1.
2. Since much of the mental status examination properly belongs to the psychiatric history, the text describes only the *sensorium,* the part of special significance for organic brain disease.

C. The concept of a sensorium

We all intuitively realize that somehow, somewhere, within the body, a mechanism integrates all of the senses, all of the memories, all of the hopes and desires, into a stream of consciousness. The ancient savants long debated the locus of this

---

TABLE 11-1 Outline of mental status examination

I. *General behavior and appearance*	Is the patient normal, hyperactive, agitated, quiet, immobile? Is the patient neat or slovenly? Does the patient dress in accordance with age, peers, sex, and background?
II. *Stream of talk*	Does the patient converse normally? Is the speech rapid, incessant, under great pressure, or is it slow and lacking in spontaneity? Is the patient discursive and unable to reach the conversational goal?
III. *Mood and affective responses*	Is the patient euphoric, agitated, inappropriately gay, giggling, or silent, weeping, and angry? Does the mood swing in a direction appropriate to the subject matter of the conversation? Is the patient emotionally labile?
IV. *Content of thought*	Does the patient have illusions, hallucinations or delusions, and misinterpretations? Is the patient preoccupied with bodily complaints, fears of cancer or heart disease, or other phobias? Does the patient suffer delusions of persecution and surveillance by malicious persons or forces?
V. *Intellectual capacity*	Is the patient bright, average, dull, or obviously demented or mentally retarded?
VI. *Sensorium*	A. Consciousness B. Attention span C. Orientation for time, place, and person D. Memory, recent and remote E. Fund of information F. Insight, judgment, and planning G. Calculation

sensorial mechanism that receives and integrates all of the impressions of the individual senses. Hippocrates (fifth century B.C.) advocated the brain as the site of the sensorium:

> And men should know that from nothing else but from the brain come joys, delights, laughter and jests and sorrows, griefs, despondency, and lamentations. And by this, in especial manner, we acquire wisdom and knowledge, and see and hear and know what are foul and what are sweet and what unsavory.

But Aristotle (384–322 B.C.) located the sensorium in the heart. In his *De Partibus Animalium,* he stated:

> For the heart is the first of all the parts to be formed; and no sooner is it formed than it contains blood. Moreover the motions of pleasure and pain, and generally of all sensations plainly have their source in the heart and find in it their ultimate termination.

Charaka, the Indian savant, asserted around A.D. 100, "The heart is the one seat of consciousness." Even today we reflect the Aristotelian view when we speak of a person in love as having an affair of the heart, or we speak of a person who lacks tender sensibilities as one who has no heart—no organ or place for a sensorium. We can understand Aristotle's confusion on this point when we realize that when the heart stops, consciousness stops. In the Athens of his time, human dissection was forbidden. He probably never dissected a human body nor saw the human brain in situ, nor did he clearly know the difference between nerves and tendons. But even his successor, Theophrastus (371–287 B.C.), cast doubt on the master's locating the sensorium in the heart. Then across the Mediterranean, in Egyptian Alexandria, Herophilus (about 300 B.C.), who was probably only a boy when Aristotle died, located the sensorium in the calamus scriptorius of the fourth ventricle. Another Alexandrian, Erasitratus (310–250 B.C.), opposing on principle the dogmatic views of his senior, Herophilus, shifted the site to the cerebellum, and suggested that the superior intelligence of humankind resulted from the richness of the cerebral cortical convolutions. Nevertheless, Aristotle's views prevailed for 400 years, until the time of Galen (A.D. 130–200?). Galen, apparently during his period of study in Alexandria, supported the doctrines of Herophilus, Erasitratus, and Hippocrates, and established forever the brain as the site of the sensorium. (Paraphrased from Keele K: *Anatomies of Pain.* Springfield, IL, Charles C Thomas, Publisher, 1957.)

In retrospect, it would almost seem as if these early seekers, who suggested that a sensorium knit all of the individual sensory impressions into a stream of consciousness, anticipated modern studies in sensory deprivation. A person kept in a stimulus-free, totally dark, totally soundproof, constant-temperature chamber, completely sequestered from environmental fluctuations and human contact, finds that the sensorium weakens. The person becomes alternately bored, then frightened. The person's thoughts become loose, detached; hallucinations follow. If the person remains isolated long enough, the sensorium will disintegrate completely. The sensorium requires incessant change—the interplay of light and dark, sound and silence, pain and pleasure—to function. The philosophic ideal of pure thought, free from the fetters of the flesh and its environment, is, therefore, exposed as a fraud. The sensorium does not function like a free-floating cloud. It functions in respect to particular environmental stimuli. Thus, in a classroom you behave differently than in a swimming pool, but you survive in both.

D. *Interpretational definition of the sensorium commune:* The sensorium commune is the mechanism for consciously perceiving ongoing events, relating them to the past and to future goals, and responding with behavior appropriate to one's role in life. The sensorium then:

1. Receives the ongoing afferent information and relates it to memory traces of past events and to future possibilities.
2. Invests the stream of thought with emotion, significance, and priority.
3. Programs behavior appropriate to one's role and station.
4. The whole process constitutes perception, integration, and execution. As such, the sensorium has no localized residence but represents the integration of all neural activity within the brain.

E. *The sensorium as communal experience:* If you have ever wondered where the concept and the term *common sense* came from, this section explains it. The ancients recognized that every person who is sound of mind has a common sense of:
1. *Who* they are, and *what* their role and station in life is.
2. *Where* they are.
3. *When* it is: morning, noon, or night; yesterday, today, or tomorrow.
4. *What* is happening: if it's raining, the house is on fire, or a dog is barking.
5. *How* the wise and prudent person should respond. Thus, we have the common sense to come in out of the rain, to get out of a burning house, and to yell at the damned dog to stop yapping, because we all, in common, sense these circumstances as dangers or nuisances. Thus, historically, the term *common sense* derives from the intuition that all normal human beings share a common sense of who, where, and what they are, what is happening in daily affairs, and how to respond appropriately to the exigencies.

F. *Quick operational testing of the sensorium:* A common real circumstance best illustrates the operational testing of the sensorium.
1. *Patient analysis.* A 21-year-old athlete has received a blow to the head causing a two-minute period of unconsciousness. As the Ex reaches the player, who is still lying on the playing field, consciousness appears to have returned. The Ex's quick neurologic appraisal shows normal breathing, pupils, and eye movements, and spontaneous movements of all extremities, precluding an immediate emergency such as spinal-cord compression or a large cerebral lesion. To evaluate the athlete's sensorium immediately, the Ex asks a series of *who, where, when, what* questions, posing them seriatum because of the emergency of the circumstances:

> What is your name?
> Who am I? (Recognition of the Ex's person and role.)
> What has just happened to you? (To determine what the player last remembers—that is to say, what the sensorium has last processed.)
> Who are you playing?
> Where is the game taking place?
> What is the date?
> What is the score of the game?

2. By answering all questions correctly, the athlete demonstrates the first five sensorial functions: consciousness, attention span, orientation for time, person, and place, and recent memory (Table 11-1). The Ex will then ask further questions about neurologic symptoms such as clarity of vision, double vision, numbness, etc. One single question summarizes the goal of testing the Pt's sensorium: Does the Pt know what's going on? Literally, does

the Pt know the score? Or in street language, "Hey man, what's coming down?"

3. Setting aside the practical concerns, we may poetically define the sensorium as the place of knowing, that place where we know what we see, hear, and feel; or paradoxically, in Aristotelian terms, it's where the heart is, where we have our perceptions, feelings, and priorities.

G. *Detailed examination of the sensorium*

1. *Consciousness.* To start with the most elemental consideration, let us ask whether you can respond intelligently to sensory stimuli when you are asleep. Obviously not. Therefore, the sensorium is a property of the waking, conscious state. For the moment, we will define consciousness interpretatively as *awareness of self and environment.* (Chapter 13 discusses operational tests of consciousness.) Is the Pt aware of self and environment?

2. *Attention span.* If the first aspect of a sensorium is consciousness, the second is attentiveness, the attention span of the individual. Can the Pt attend to stimuli long enough to comprehend and respond to them, or attend to a task long enough to complete it? For a simple, effective test, ask the Pt to recite the months backwards or spell *world* backwards.

3. *Orientation.* If conscious and attentive, does the Pt comprehend *who* he or she is, and *where,* and *when* it is? This orientation as to person, place, and time depends on the ongoing sensory impressions. Have you ever awakened from a deep sleep to find that momentarily you did not know the day, the hour, or even where you were? Weren't your mental functions impaired until you became oriented, until all of the pieces of the puzzle suddenly fell into place? Judge the Pt's orientation:

   a. As to *person:* Does the Pt recognize him- or herself and role as a Pt and recognize other people, their roles, and yours as a doctor?

   b. As to *place:* Does the Pt understand the nature and geography of the place? Does the Pt recognize that he or she is in a hospital, its name, and the name of the city and state?

   c. As to *time:* Does the Pt know the time of day, day of week, month, and year?

4. *Memory.* Memory, orientation, and attention span intertwine inextricably. For quick screening purposes, appraise memory this way:

   a. Note how well the Pt recalls and relates the events of the medical history.

   b. Inquire, "Does your memory work all right?" Or more bluntly, "Do you have trouble with your memory?" If you suspect a memory disturbance, say to the Pt, "Suppose we try out your memory?", and provide the Pt with an address, a color, and an object to remember; nonsense items that have no special relationship: 53 Broadway, orange, and table. Have the Pt repeat the items to be sure that they have registered. Then, at the end of the NE, ask the Pt to recite them. Ask the Pt to name the presidents, from the present backwards. Although also requiring a longer attention span, this task requires more memory than reciting the months backwards.

   c. Determine whether the Pt differs in the ability to recall recent or remote events. Can the Pt give his date of birth, but not the present day, month, and year? Can the Pt remember what he or she ate for breakfast? Recent memory suffers most in aging or brain diseases in general. To remember this difference easily, recall that grandfather cannot remember where he just laid his glasses, but he can wax eloquent about events of long ago.

5. *Fund of information.* The oriented, attentive Pt with a good memory knows what is going on in the world. If unable to discuss current events, the Pt has organic brain disease or cultural deprivation, or is so withdrawn as to need psychiatric care.

6. *Insight, judgment, and planning.* Simply ask what the Pt plans to do. Do the proffered goals and plans match the Pt's physical and mental capabilities? The quadriplegic Pt who expects to work as a carpenter or the individual with a borderline IQ who expects to become a chemist lack insight, judgment, and planning. Does the Pt recognize the illness and its implications?

7. *Calculation.* Test calculation by asking whether the Pt can balance a checkbook, make change, do formal paper-and-pencil calculations, and subtract sevens serially from 100.

H. *Summary of the questions used to test the sensorium*

1. Apart from emergencies like the acute head injury described above, the Ex should not machine-gun the Pt with a series of questions with simplistic answers: "Do you know your name? What city are you in? What is the day, date, and week? Who is the President? Can you remember an item, color, and address?" If you ask questions that crudely, Pts, especially if somewhat demented or mentally ill, will quickly realize that you are testing mental status and often reply (not a little piqued), "What's the matter Doc, do you think I'm crazy?" The Ex should ultimately derive answers to the questions posed in Table 11-2 but derive them artfully in the natural course of the interview. The Pt should experience it all as an ordinary discussion, not an inquisition. From the clues provided by the history, NE, and mental status screening questions, the Ex decides whether to ask additional questions or to order formal neuropsychological testing.

I. *Neurologic implications of sensorial defects:* Although sensorial defects usually imply organic disease of the brain, they do not specifically localize lesions. Common sense does not reside snugly in some specifiable series of nuclei and tracts. While memory loss implicates bilateral lesions of the medial temporal lobe and hippocampal-fornix-mammillary body circuit (Fig. 11-12), and dyscalculia suggests a left posterior hemisphere lesion, in general, such sensorial defects also occur with diffuse brain disease. As a rule, neither defects of the sensorium generally, nor of its arbitrary subdivisions in particular, predict the site of the lesion as do sensory and motor defects. This disparity exists because we know enough about the sensory and motor pathways to devise tests that parallel their anatomic and physiologic organization, but we do not know enough about the mind to devise tests that parallel its anatomic and physiologic organization.

J. *Affective responses:* Besides being conscious, attentive, and oriented, and having a good memory, a fund of information, and insight, judgment, and planning, the standard person reacts emotionally to ongoing events. Picture your reaction to a hand grenade thrown onto your table or merely to a cockroach. Your alarm or *aversion* differs in the two cases. Affective response should have the appropriate quality and quantity.

1. Assay affective responses not by direct inquiry, but by comparing the observed with the expected reactions. What affect would you expect as a Pt discusses her paralyzed arm? What affect would you expect if the Pt complains that the "apparatus" plots to kill him? A blunted, bland, or indifferent

TABLE 11-2 Outline of sample questions to screen the patient's sensorium

Questions	Area of sensorium tested
What is your name? How old are you? When is your birthday? What is your address? Are you staying there now? What kind of work do you do? Do you have a family/wife/husband or children? What are their names/occupations/ages/addresses? Where are they now?	Orientation to person, time and place; recent and remote memory; consciousness of self and environment
Do you happen to know the time of day? Have you been waiting long to see me? What is the day/date/month/year? What is the season/weather? What did you do yesterday?	Orientation to time, recent memory
What have you come to see me about?, or, How does it come about that you are seeing me? Do you feel that you need any medical help?	Doctor/patient role recognition, insight as to presence of an illness or need for medical attention, and judgment
What are your plans for the future?, or, How long do you expect you will be off work?	Judgment and planning
What do you think of . . . (mention some item in the news). How has your memory been? Are you worried about it? Suppose we test it. See whether you can remember . . . (give a name, color, and address) Can you name the last several presidents?	Recent memory, fund of information, attention span
Subtract 7 from 100, then take off seven more and continue subtracting 7's. Spell "world" (or other word) backward.	Calculation, attention span

affect occurs most commonly with schizophrenia and with bifrontal lobe lesions.

2. If you have cause to cry or laugh, how much provocation does it take to make you start and how much time does it take you to get over it? If the Pt cries for 15 seconds and then starts to laugh when you ask him to tell you a funny story, the Pt has affective lability, the opposite of affective blunting. Affective lability commonly accompanies bilateral UMN disease, as we have seen in pseudobulbar palsy, or diffuse brain diseases.

K. *Perceptual distortions, illusions, hallucinations, and delusions*
  1. *Illusions.* We have all experienced the illusion of water shimmering on a hot highway on a summer's day. The water is an illusion. *An illusion is a false sensory perception based on natural stimulation of a sensory receptor.* The healthy person realizes that such an experience is an illusion, but the sick person may not.
  2. *Hallucinations.* Observe that sweating, tremulous man cowering on the bed, screaming about dogs and snakes in the corner of his room. Or observe

this calm woman with an expressionless face who tells you in a flat voice that she hears God's voice ordering her to drown her baby. Both Pts display characteristic hallucinations; the man has delirium tremens, the woman schizophrenia. Before an epileptic seizure, many patients experience visual, auditory, or somatic hallucinations. *A hallucination is a false sensory perception not based on natural stimulation of a sensory receptor.* The mentally ill Pt usually does not recognize the hallucination as a false representation of reality, while the epileptic does.

3. *Delusions.* This Pt is eyeing a nurse carrying a tray into the room. He says to you *sotto voce,* "There is one of them now. She's trying to poison me." You err in responding to this remark if you try to reason with him that she has merely come to take his temperature. Somehow, his psychic economy needs to misperceive the nurse as a conspirator, and all the reason in the world will not dispel his belief. *A delusion is a false belief that reason cannot dispel.*

4. Literary geniuses frequently depict illusions, hallucinations, and delusions. Try to identify these perceptual distortions (and get reaccustomed to the programming that follows in the next section):

   a. Here, Macbeth muses alone after murdering Duncan:

   > Is this a dagger which I see before me,
   > The handle toward my hand? Come, let me clutch thee:
   > I have thee not, and yet I see thee still.
   > Art thou not, fatal vision, sensible
   > To feeling as to sight? Or art thou but
   > A dagger of the mind, a false creation,
   > Proceeding from the heat-oppressed brain? . . .
   > Mine eyes are made the fools o'th'other senses.
   > Or else worth all the rest: I see thee still . . .

   This exemplifies ☐ an illusion/ ☐ a hallucination/ ☐ a delusion, which is defined as _____
   _____.

Ans: ☑ *Hallucination. A false sensory perception not based on natural stimulation of a sensory receptor*

   b. Here is a passage from Gérard De Nerval's poem *The Dark Blot:*

   > He who has gazed against the sun sees everywhere he looks thereafter, palpitating on the air before his eyes, a smudge that will not go away.

   This exemplifies ☐ an illusion/ ☐ a hallucination/ ☐ a delusion, which is defined as _____
   _____.

Ans: ☑ *Illusion. A false sensory perception based on natural stimulation of a sensory receptor.*

   c. Here, lawyer Porfiry Petrovitch, in Dostoevsky's *Crime and Punishment,* discusses a client:

   > "Yes, in our legal practice there was a case almost exactly similar, a case of morbid psychology," Porfiry went on quickly. "A man confessed to murder and how he kept it up! It was a regular hallucination; he brought forward facts, he imposed upon every one and why? He had been partly, but only partly, unintentionally the cause of a murder and when he knew that he had given the murderers the opportunity, he sank into dejection, it got on his mind and turned his brain, he began imagining things, and he persuaded himself that he was the murderer. But at last the High Court of Appeals went into it and the poor fellow was acquitted and put under proper care."

☑ *No*
☑ *Delusion*

(1) Was lawyer Petrovitch correct in stating that his client suffered from a regular hallucination"? ☐ Yes/ ☐ No.
(2) Is the client's mental aberration ☐ an illusion/ ☐ a delusion?
(3) Define a delusion: _____

_____.

Ans: A delusion is a false belief that reason cannot dispel.

Editorial Note: Although lawyer Petrovitch stated that his client had hallucinations rather than delusions, his legal instinct was right. Even a harsh, oppressive society like Czarist Russia recognized that a confession does not establish guilt, because delusions may cause people to confess to crimes that they did not commit. Moreover, if the police concentrate too much on obtaining confessions (often by physical and mental duress) they may not concentrate enough on obtaining conclusive, objective evidence of the real perpetrator. This magnificent insight against self-incrimination, reflected in our Fifth Amendment, protects a person against his or her own mental quirks as well as against overzealous prosecution.

5. *Localizing significance of hallucinations.* Although hallucinations may accompany a variety of mental illnesses or diffuse metabolic diseases, repetitively experienced hallucinations may indicate a lesion of the appropriate sensory cortex (Benson and Blumer, 1982). A lesion in the occipital cortex might cause hallucinations of vision; in the uncus, of smell; and in the postcentral gyrus, of somatic sensation. Such hallucinations often constitute part of the aura, or forewarning, of an epileptic seizure produced by a focal lesion in one of these areas.

II. Agnosia, apraxia, and aphasia

I translate into ordinary words the Latin of their corrupt preachers, whereby it is revealed as humbug.   **Bertolt Brecht** (1898–1956)

A. Introduction to agnosia, apraxia, and aphasia

Fate foredooms every neurology text to address the deficits signified by these three mystifying Greek terms. In spite of the fascinating subject matter, the name-plagued literature on agnosia, apraxia, and aphasia discourages even the hardiest student. Aphasiologists, in particular, are a contentious lot. Each one, compulsively, it seems, must disagree with the methods, conceptions, and nomenclature of predecessors (Alexander and Benson, 1991; Brown, 1972; Critchley, 1970; Geschwind, 1971; Gloning, 1970; Goodglass and Kaplan, 1972; Head, 1963; Luria, 1966; Nielsen, 1962; Weisenberg and McBride, 1964). Many authors expend too much effort philosophizing and inventing polysyllabic words, resulting in humbug; hence the quote from Brecht. Salvation arrives if we shun the rhetoric and simply ask: By what operations do we discover the deficits signified?

B. Agnosia

1. *Review of agnosia.* The term *agnosia* means literally *not knowing.* We may, therefore, specify what the Pt does not know. As a review from Chapter 10, list some common types of agnosia tested in the NE: _____

_____.

Ans: Astereognosia, agraphognosia, finger agnosia, astatognosia, atopagnosia, anosognosia, prosopagnosia, etc.

2. *General definition of agnosia.* Since we know the operations to perform to disclose agnosia (e.g., give the Pt certain stimuli to identify), we may

attempt a general definition. *Agnosia is the inability to understand the meaning (import or symbolic significance) of ordinary sensory stimuli even though the sensory pathways and sensorium are relatively intact.*

3. An optimum definition not only states what something is, but also what it is not and the conditions necessary to diagnose it. The necessary conditions to diagnose agnosia are:
   a. The Pt's sensory pathways are sufficiently intact to deliver afferent impulses to the cerebrum.
   b. The Pt's sensorium and mental status are relatively intact.
   c. The Pt previously understood the symbolic significance of the stimulus—in other words, was familiar with it.
   d. The Pt has an organic cerebral lesion as the cause of the deficit.

4. These conditions eliminate Pts with interrupted sensory pathways, mental retardation, and functional mental illnesses such as hysteria and negativism, or advanced dementia, to whom agnosia does not apply (Brown, 1972; Nielsen, 1962). Early in the course of dementia from diffuse brain disease, Pts may show varieties of agnosia, apraxia, and aphasia.

C. *Apraxia*

1. *Definition of apraxia. Apraxia is the inability to perform a willed act even though the motor system and mental status are relatively intact.* The ability to execute a voluntary act is called *praxia* (praxis = action, as in practice). By negating praxia, the ability to act, we describe apraxia, the inability to act.

2. *Tests for apraxia:*
   a. The Ex tests for apraxia almost inadvertently in giving various commands, such as: "Stick out your tongue." "Make a fist." "Walk across the room." These commands disclose tongue, hand, or gait apraxia. More complicated apraxias include ideomotor apraxia, tested by asking the Pt to mime a sequence, such as striking a match and lighting a candle.
   b. Apraxic Pts may do an act automatically that they cannot do on command. For example, apraxic Pts who fail to stick out their tongue on command may lick their lips automatically. The Pt may fail to make a fist when asked to close the fingers but may automatically grasp an object, such as a spoon.

3. *Requisites to distinguish apraxia from other motor defects:*
   a. The Pt's motor system is sufficiently intact to execute the act.
   b. The Pt's sensorium is sufficiently intact to understand the act. The Pt comprehends and attempts to cooperate.
   c. The Pt's previous skills were sufficient to do the act.
   d. The Pt has an organic cerebral lesion as the cause of the deficit.
   e. If reading the definition and conditions for diagnosing apraxia causes the strange feeling of repeating a previous experience (the déjà vu of anterior temporal lobe lesions), we are on the right track. Review Frame B2, which defines agnosia. These requisites exclude Pts with paralysis and with functional mental illnesses, such as hysteria or negativism, profound dementia, and mental retardation, to whom *apraxia* is not meant to apply.

4. *Distinction between apraxia and other motor deficits.* With pyramidal lesions, paralysis precludes the act, violating a necessary condition for the diagnosis of apraxia. The paralyzed Pt may also have apraxia, but the paralysis prevents its recognition. With cerebellar lesions, the Pt retains the abil-

ity to perform an act, but cannot perform it smoothly. With basal motor nuclei lesions, involuntary movements or rigidity impede the act, but the sequence of the act remains possible.

    D. *Pt analysis for identification of constructional and dressing apraxia*
        1. *Medical history.* A 67-year-old right-handed salesman with a college education had noticed dizziness, fatigue, and blurring of vision for three months. Three weeks before hospitalization, he began to have right frontal headaches. For one week, he had noticed weakness and slight numbness of his left extremities. Although he appeared dull and apathetic and did arithmetic poorly, his sensorium was otherwise intact.
        2. *Motor examination.* The Pt could walk, but movements on the entire left side were moderately weak, except for normal frontalis and orbicularis oculi strength. He had no atrophy, tremor, dystaxia, or involuntary movements. The Ex's manipulation of the Pt's left extremities showed an initial catch followed by yielding of the part. Fig. 11-1 shows the reflex pattern.

✓ UMN

          a. His facial weakness was ☐ UMN/ ☐ LMN.

Clasp-knife
* spasticity*

          b. The Pt has the type of hypertonus called _____
_____.

          c. Integrate the total information from the physical examination and Fig. 11-1 to diagnose the motor deficits thus far detected: _____
_____
_____.

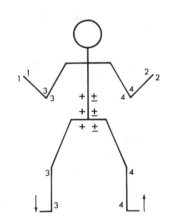

FIG. 11-1. Reflex figurine of the Pt.

Ans: Spastic, hyperreflexic left hemiparesis with extensor toe sign and reduced left-sided abdominal and cremasteric reflexes.

        3. *Sensory examination*
          a. Although the Pt could feel light touch on either side, perhaps less well on the left, he consistently failed to report a left-sided stimulus when the Ex simultaneously touched both of the Pt's hands. He failed to report left-sided stimuli when simultaneous sound stimuli were presented. This type of sensory deficit is called sensory _____.

Inattention or
* suppression*

          b. He recognized coins or a safety pin by vision or when they were placed in the right hand, but not in the left. This deficit is called
_____.

Astereognosis

          c. He had difficulty recognizing numbers traced on the left palm, a defect called _____.

Agraphognosia

Complete left homonymous hemianopsia (Fig. 3-5)

Left eye   Right eye

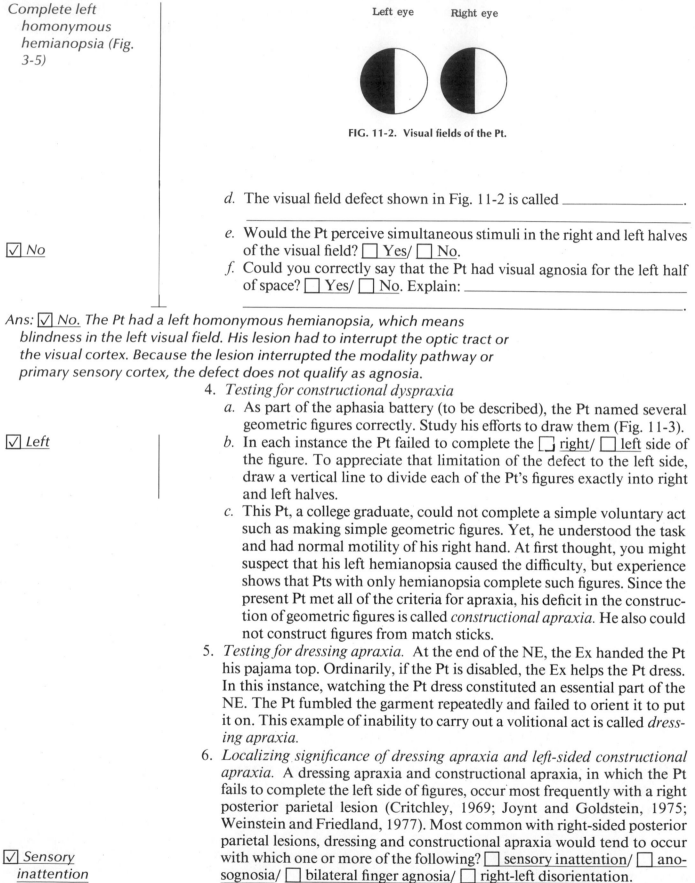

FIG. 11-2. Visual fields of the Pt.

d. The visual field defect shown in Fig. 11-2 is called _____.

☑ *No*

e. Would the Pt perceive simultaneous stimuli in the right and left halves of the visual field? ☐ Yes/ ☐ No.

f. Could you correctly say that the Pt had visual agnosia for the left half of space? ☐ Yes/ ☐ No. Explain: _____.

Ans: ☑ *No. The Pt had a left homonymous hemianopsia, which means blindness in the left visual field. His lesion had to interrupt the optic tract or the visual cortex. Because the lesion interrupted the modality pathway or primary sensory cortex, the defect does not qualify as agnosia.*

4. *Testing for constructional dyspraxia*

   a. As part of the aphasia battery (to be described), the Pt named several geometric figures correctly. Study his efforts to draw them (Fig. 11-3).

☑ *Left*

   b. In each instance the Pt failed to complete the ☐ right/ ☐ left side of the figure. To appreciate that limitation of the defect to the left side, draw a vertical line to divide each of the Pt's figures exactly into right and left halves.

   c. This Pt, a college graduate, could not complete a simple voluntary act such as making simple geometric figures. Yet, he understood the task and had normal motility of his right hand. At first thought, you might suspect that his left hemianopsia caused the difficulty, but experience shows that Pts with only hemianopsia complete such figures. Since the present Pt met all of the criteria for apraxia, his deficit in the construction of geometric figures is called *constructional apraxia*. He also could not construct figures from match sticks.

5. *Testing for dressing apraxia.* At the end of the NE, the Ex handed the Pt his pajama top. Ordinarily, if the Pt is disabled, the Ex helps the Pt dress. In this instance, watching the Pt dress constituted an essential part of the NE. The Pt fumbled the garment repeatedly and failed to orient it to put it on. This example of inability to carry out a volitional act is called *dressing apraxia*.

6. *Localizing significance of dressing apraxia and left-sided constructional apraxia.* A dressing apraxia and constructional apraxia, in which the Pt fails to complete the left side of figures, occur most frequently with a right posterior parietal lesion (Critchley, 1969; Joynt and Goldstein, 1975; Weinstein and Friedland, 1977). Most common with right-sided posterior parietal lesions, dressing and constructional apraxia would tend to occur with which one or more of the following? ☐ sensory inattention/ ☐ anosognosia/ ☐ bilateral finger agnosia/ ☐ right-left disorientation.

☑ *Sensory inattention*
☑ *anosognosia*

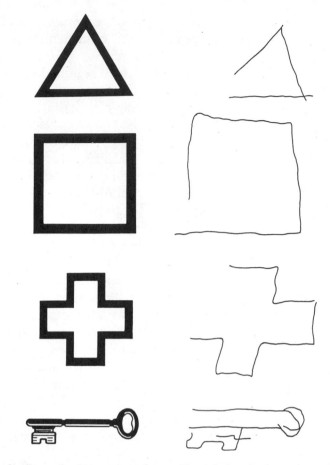

FIG. 11-3. Stimulus figures for Pt to name and copy. The right-hand column shows the attempts of the Pt to copy the figures after he had named them correctly.

7. *Summary of the Pt's clinical deficits:*
   a. *Motor.* Mild spastic, hyperreflexic left hemiparesis with an extensor toe sign. Severe constructional and dressing apraxia.
   b. *Sensory.* Slight left hemihypesthesia and hemihypalgesia, left-sided astereognosis, left-sided tactile and auditory inattention, and complete left homonymous hemianopia.
8. *Localizing significance of the totality of neurologic signs.* How to "think circuitry."

Pyramidal

   a. This Pt's hemiparesis implicates a _____ tract lesion.
   b. To cause hemiparesis, the pyramidal lesion would have to involve the cervical cord, brainstem, or cerebrum. If rostral to the cord, the lesion might involve the brainstem, deep cerebral white matter, or motor cortex. What *motor* finding locates the pyramidal tract lesion at or rostral to the pons? _____
   _____.

Ans: UMN facial palsy from interruption of corticobulbar fibers that activate the lower part of the face.

☑ *Association cortex or its intracerebral connections*

   c. The agnosia and apraxia implicate a lesion at the level of the ☐ brainstem/ ☐ sensorimotor cortex/ ☐ association cortex or its intracerebral connections.

☑ *Right*
☑ *Parietal*

   d. The particular types of agnosia and apraxia implicate a lesion of the ☐ right/ ☐ left/ ☐ both cerebral hemisphere(s), mainly in the frontal/ ☐ parietal/ ☐ occipital/ ☐ temporal region.

9. *The principle of parsimony.* While we might account for the Pt's left hemiparesis and mild hemihypesthesia by a brainstem lesion, we now know that his apraxia-agnosia require a lesion of the dorsolateral cerebral wall in the parietal region. Thus, while we might postulate lesions at two levels, brainstem and cerebral wall, we should now invoke one of the most important principles in diagnosis, the principle of parsimony. This principle, otherwise known as Occam's razor (William of Occam, 1280–1349), requires us to try to pare everything down to the simplest explanation: a single lesion and a single diagnosis. In other words, we seek the simplest, the most *parsimonious,* explanation. Thus, if a single lesion caused the hemiparesis, hemihypesthesia, and agnosia-apraxia, it involves the ☐ spinal cord/ ☐ brainstem/ ☐ dorsolateral cerebral wall.

☑ *Dorsolateral cerebral wall*

    a. The complete hemianopsia indicates a lesion at some level along the optic pathway. Review the optic pathway in Fig. 3-5 and the course of the optic radiation through the lateral cerebral wall in Fig. 3-6. Hemianopia implicates a lesion:

       ☐ (1) In the retina or optic nerve.

       ☐ (2) In the anterior part of the temporal lobe.

☑ *(3)*

       ☐ (3) Between the optic chiasm and the visual cortex of the calcarine fissure.

    b. Applying the principle of parsimony, could the previously postulated lesion of the dorsolateral cerebral wall in the parietal lobe also interrupt the optic pathway? If so, where? See Fig. 3-6A. ☐ Yes/ ☐ No. Explain: _____.

Ans: ☑ *Yes. The geniculocalcarine tract runs through the deep white matter of the parietotemporal region. See Fig. 3-6A.*

    c. In addition to the agnostic-apraxic and visual field deficits, implicating the posterior parietal area, the slight hemihypalgesia and hemihypesthesia implicate the primary somesthetic receptive region of the _____ gyrus of the ☐ right/ ☐ left _____ lobe.

Postcentral; ☑ *right; parietal*

    d. The mild left hemiparesis implicates the motor area located in the right _____ gyrus.

Precentral

    e. The left-sided auditory inattention implicates the auditory association area in the ☐ anterior/ ☐ posterior part of the ☐ right/ ☐ left temporoparietal region.

☑ *Posterior;*
☑ *Right*

    f. Shade Fig. 11-4 to show the presumed extent of the lesion. Use dark shading for the regions which have produced the severest or most complete deficits and lighter shading for the regions responsible for the lesser deficits. Frame D7, above, summarizes the deficits that require a localizing explanation.

10. *Neuropathologic considerations*

    a. By causing edema and compressing vessels, lesions may impair the function of surrounding brain tissue. The severest signs usually reflect the site of maximum tissue damage and, therefore, best predict the lesion site. The Pt's severest defects, the hemianopia and dressing and constructional apraxia, suggest maximum damage to the right posterior parasylvian area, with less involvement of the sensorimotor cortex of the paracentral region.

    b. Radiographic examination showed a mass in the predicted right parieto-occipital region. Craniotomy and biopsy disclosed a large, expanding neoplasm, a glioblastoma multiforme, causing pressure on the surrounding brain. The surgeon removed the right occipital lobe, pro-

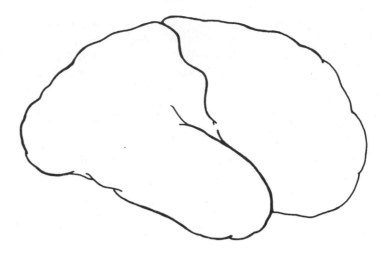

FIG. 11-4. Blank of right cerebral hemisphere. Shade it to show the presumed location of the Pt's lesion.

viding internal decompression. Post-operatively, the left hemiparesis disappeared, suggesting that pressure and edema from the neoplasm had caused it rather than direct extension of the neoplasm to the paracentral area (Fig. 11-5).

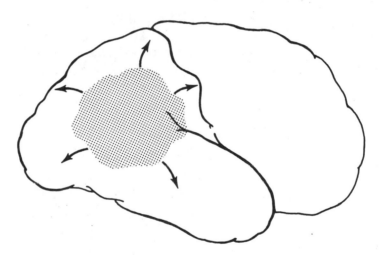

FIG. 11-5. Lateral view of right cerebral hemisphere to show the actual location of the Pt's lesion, as determined at autopsy examination. The arrows indicate the surrounding edema of the hemisphere, which led to additional clinical signs such as hemiparesis, implicating damage to tissue beyond the immediate confines of the neoplasm.

    c. Ordinarily, a Pt with a lesion in the right posterior parasylvian area might also have anosognosia. The Pt failed to show it before operation, but afterwards he failed to recognize that he had a left hemianopia. Anosognosia occurs more commonly with large, acute lesions, such as infarcts, than when lesions evolve relatively slowly, as with neoplasms.

E. *Summary of common apraxias tested in the NE*
  1. *Gait apraxia.* Ask the Pt to walk.
  2. *Tongue apraxia.* Ask the Pt to protrude the tongue and move it up, down, right, and left.
  3. *Everyday activity (ideomotor) apraxia.* Ask the Pt to demonstrate how to use silverware, strike a match and light a candle, and use a key, etc.

4. *Constructional apraxia.* Ask the Pt to copy geometric figures or construct them out of match sticks.
5. *Dressing apraxia.* Watch the Pt try to put on an article of clothing.
6. *Writing and speaking apraxia (aphasia).* Explained in the next section.

III. Aphasia: agnosia and apraxia of language

A. *Definition of aphasia* (literally *a* = lack of, and *phasis* = speech). *Aphasia is the inability to understand or express words as symbols for communication, even though the primary sensorimotor pathways to receive and express language and the mental status are relatively intact.* The definition excludes language disorders caused by functional mental illness, global retardation, or advanced dementia, blindness, deafness, stuttering, or neuromuscular disease.
   1. The purist would use *aphasia* for total loss of language, and *dysphasia* for partial loss, but clinicians use the prefixes *a-* and *dys-* interchangeably.
   2. Strokes and head trauma cause aphasia in about 300,000 Pts per year (Damasio, 1992).

B. *The four avenues of language*
   1. A moment's introspection discloses that we normally employ four major avenues of language. We express language by *speaking* or *writing,* and we receive it by *reading* or *listening* (not to mention Braille, sign language, and Morse code). Thus we *speak/listen* and *write/read.*
   2. Some Pts with brain lesions, while neither deaf nor blind, fail to understand the meaning of spoken or written words. The general term for failure of a Pt with intact sensory pathways to understand the meaning of a stimulus is *Agnosia* _____. Because of the special significance of language for human communication, we call language agnosia *receptive* or *sensory aphasia.*
   3. Some Pts with brain lesions produce the wrong syllables or wrong words when speaking or writing, thus failing in communication. The general term for failure of a nonparalyzed Pt to do such voluntary acts is *Apraxia* _____. We call language apraxia *expressive* or *motor aphasia.*
   4. Recite the four ordinary avenues of receiving and expressing language: *Reading, listening, writing, and speaking* _____ing, _____ing, _____ing, and _____ing.

C. *Volitional, propositional, or representational speech versus exclamatory speech*

Some speech, *exclamatory speech,* serves to communicate the emotional state of the instant, rather than ideas. Exclamations, particularly expletives, erupt spontaneously, unwilled, without deliberation or forethought. On stubbing a toe, we automatically exclaim "Ouch!" Contrarily, we communicate ideas by volitional *propositions* or *representations.* These may consist of a simple declaration, "The fire engine is red," or a distinct proposition. A proposition states something for analysis that was, is, or could be. "Fire engines ought to be red." A proposition is preeminently willful, planned, and often crafty. Aphasics lose propositional speech out of proportion to exclamatory speech. Thus, after struggling but completely failing to produce a propositional statement, the aphasic Pt sighs in anger, exclaiming spontaneously and with perfect clarity, "Oh damn, I can't." Yet when asked to repeat the automatically uttered sentence, the Pt fails again. It has now become propositional or willful speech. In analogy, recall that in pseudobulbar palsy, the Pt loses willful movements but retains or even shows exaggarated automatic laughing or crying. These facts demonstrate that the brain uses different circuits for propositional, as contrasted to emotional, speech. In general, aphasics also retain humming and singing better than spoken language.

   D. *Clinical testing for aphasia*

      1. *Detecting early aphasia during the interview.* Aphasia testing begins as the history begins. You will detect gross defects in language reception or expression immediately. The mildly aphasic Pt produces less than the expected amount of written and spoken language. Although the Pt's conversation remains goal-directed, the Pt fails to hit the nail on the head with crisp, logical narratives. The speech may degenerate to circumlocutions, platitudes, and clichés, dredged more from memory than composed of willful, novel, or artful word combinations. Less commonly, the aphasic Pt becomes wordy, as if by preempting the conversation, the Pt can prevent the other person from saying something that the Pt cannot understand, and may show a gratuitous redundancy in searching for *le mot juste* (just the right word).

      2. *Formal aphasia screening tests.* The Ex uses a formal protocol (Table 11-3) to test the Pt's ability to read, write, name things, repeat words and sentences and copy them to dictation, and to follow written and verbal commands. Do not memorize the protocol, because the summarized NE includes it. Place the Pt's worksheet in the medical chart. Damasio (1992) lists several longer aphasia tests, but they merely extend the principles of the Halstead-Reitan-Wepman protocol given here.

TABLE 11-3 Instructions for use with the stimuli of Fig. 11-6 to test for cerebral dysfunction

Patient's task	Examiner's instructions to the patient
1. Copy SQUARE (A).	FIRST, DRAW THIS ON YOUR PAPER (Point to square, item A). I WANT YOU TO DO IT WITHOUT LIFTING YOUR PENCIL FROM THE PAPER. MAKE IT ABOUT THIS SAME SIZE (Point to square.) Elaborate on the requirement for a continuous line if necessary. If the patient is concerned about making a heavy or double line, point out that only a reproduction of the shape is required. If the patient has obvious difficulty in drawing any of the figures, encourage him to proceed until it is clear that he can make no further progress. If he does not accomplish the task reasonably well on his first try, ask him to try again, and instruct him to be particularly careful to do it as well as he can.
2. Name SQUARE	WHAT IS THAT SHAPE CALLED?
3. Spell SQUARE	WOULD YOU SPELL THAT WORD FOR ME?
4. Copy CROSS (B)	DRAW THIS ON YOUR PAPER. (Point to cross). GO AROUND THE OUTSIDE LIKE THIS UNTIL YOU GET BACK TO WHERE YOU STARTED. (Examiner draws a finger-line around the edge of the stimulus figure.) MAKE IT ABOUT THIS SAME SIZE. (Point to cross.) Additional instructions, if necessary, should be similar to those used with the square.
5. Name CROSS	WHAT IS THAT SHAPE CALLED?
6. Spell CROSS	WOULD YOU SPELL THAT WORD FOR ME?
7. Copy TRIANGLE (C)	Similar to 1 and 4 above.

TABLE 11-3 Instructions for use with the stimuli of Fig. 11-6 to test for cerebral dysfunction

Patient's task	Examiner's instructions to the patient
8. Name TRIANGLE	WHAT IS THAT SHAPE CALLED?
9. Spell TRIANGLE	WOULD YOU SPELL THAT WORD FOR ME?
10. Name BABY (D)	WHAT IS THIS? (Show baby, item D.)
11. Write CLOCK (E)	NOW I AM GOING TO SHOW YOU ANOTHER PICTURE BUT DO *NOT* TELL ME THE NAME OF IT. I DON'T WANT YOU TO SAY ANYTHING OUT LOUD. JUST WRITE THE NAME OF THE PICTURE ON YOUR PAPER. (Show clock, item E.)
12. Name FORK (F)	WHAT IS THIS? (Show fork, item F.)
13. Read 7 SIX 2 (G)	I WANT YOU TO READ THIS (Show item G). If the subject has difficulty, attempt to determine whether he can read any part of the stimulus figure.
14. Read M G W (H)	READ THIS. (Show item H.)
15. Reading I (I)	NOW I WANT YOU TO READ THIS. (Show item I.)
16. Reading II (J)	CAN YOU READ THIS? (Show item J.)
17. Repeat TRIANGLE	NOW I AM GOING TO SAY SOME WORDS. I WANT YOU TO LISTEN CAREFULLY AND SAY THEM AFTER ME AS CAREFULLY AS YOU CAN. SAY THIS WORD: TRIANGLE.
18. Repeat MASSACHUSETTS	THE NEXT ONE IS A LITTLE HARDER BUT DO YOUR BEST. SAY THIS WORD: MASSACHUSETTS.
19. Repeat METHODIST EPISCOPAL	NOW REPEAT THIS ONE: METHODIST EPISCOPAL.
20. Write SQUARE (K)	DON'T SAY THIS WORD OUT LOUD. (Point to stimulus word "square," item K.) JUST WRITE IT ON YOUR PAPER. If the patient prints the word, ask him to write it.
21. Read SEVEN (L)	CAN YOU READ THIS WORD OUT LOUD? (Show item L.)
22. Repeat SEVEN	NOW, I WANT YOU TO SAY THIS AFTER ME: SEVEN.
23. Repeat-explain. HE SHOUTED THE WARNING	I AM GOING TO SAY SOMETHING THAT I WANT YOU TO SAY AFTER ME, SO LISTEN CAREFULLY: HE SHOUTED THE WARNING. NOW YOU SAY IT. WOULD YOU EXPLAIN WHAT THAT MEANS? Sometimes it is necessary to amplify by asking the kind of situation to which the sentence would refer. The patient's understanding is adequately demonstrated when he brings the concept of impending danger into his explanation.
24. Write: HE SHOUTED THE WARNING	NOW I WANT YOU TO WRITE THAT SENTENCE ON THE PAPER. Sometimes it is necessary to repeat the sentence so that the patient understands clearly what he is to write.
25. Compute 85 − 27 = (M)	HERE IS AN ARITHMETIC PROBLEM. COPY IT DOWN ON YOUR PAPER ANY WAY YOU LIKE AND TRY TO WORK IT OUT. (Show item M.)
26. Compute 17 × 3 =	NOW DO THIS ONE IN YOUR HEAD: 17 × 3
27. Name KEY (N)	WHAT IS THIS? (Show item N.)
28. Demonstrate use of KEY (N)	IF YOU HAD ONE OF THESE IN YOUR HAND, SHOW ME HOW YOU WOULD USE IT. (Show item N.)
29. Draw KEY (N)	NOW I WANT YOU TO DRAW A PICTURE THAT LOOKS JUST LIKE THIS. TRY TO MAKE YOUR KEY LOOK ENOUGH LIKE THIS ONE SO THAT I WOULD KNOW IT WAS THE SAME KEY FROM YOUR DRAWING. (Point to key, item N.)

TABLE 11-3 Instructions for use with the stimuli of Fig. 11-6 to test for cerebral dysfunction	
Patient's task	Examiner's instructions to the patient
30. Read (O)	WOULD YOU READ THIS? (Show item O.)
31. Place LEFT HAND TO RIGHT EAR	NOW, WOULD YOU DO WHAT IT SAID?
32. Place LEFT HAND TO LEFT ELBOW	NOW I WANT YOU TO PUT YOUR LEFT HAND TO YOUR LEFT ELBOW. The patient should quickly realize that it is impossible.

E. *Technique for administering the Halstead-Reitan-Wepman test for cerebral dysfunction (including aphasia)*

1. First, instruct the Pt, "I have several things for you to do. Please do them carefully, and be sure to do your best. First write your name, address, and the date on the page." The latter command also subtly tests temporal orientation without a direct question and gives immediate insight into the Pt's ability to comprehend and write.

2. Repeat or amplify instructions as necessary to elicit the Pt's best performance, but avoid actual help with any item (Reitan, 1984). As with the mental status questions, Pts may become upset or distressed if they perform poorly. Continue to offer sympathetic encouragement. If necessary, defer the test for a second session if the Pt seems tired or discouraged.

3. Now, get a colleague and practice administering the test. Relate the instructions in Table 11-3 to Fig. 11-6.

F. *Interpretation of the results of the Halstead-Reitan-Wepman cerebral dysfunction battery*

1. The normal person with a (legitimate) high-school degree makes no errors on this test. Even normal 10- to 12-year-old Pts generally make no errors. Illiterate Pts will make some spelling errors. Any errors raise the question of a cerebral lesion. Expect 100 percent correct answers from a 100 percent intact brain.

2. When the screening test indicates a deficit, explore it with further examples. If the Pt has trouble recognizing or naming objects, give the Pt several alternatives, including the correct one to select from; e.g., if the Pt cannot say "baby," say alternatives, such as "dog, man, woman, or baby," for the Pt to select from.

G. *Analysis of a Pt for aphasia:* This 44-year-old male store clerk had an epileptic seizure and over the past several weeks gradually became somewhat lethargic. His speech became slow, somewhat hesitant, and marked by circumlocutions. For example, instead of saying "the President," he said "That brun (one) at the top. Uh, that top one." He had no sensory deficits or clinically evident hemiparesis but had slight flattening of his right nasolabial fold, and the tapping speed with his right hand, his dominant hand, was slightly slower than the left. Work carefully through Table 11-4 and Fig. 11-7 that record the results of the aphasia screening battery. Refer to Fig. 11-6 and the instructions in Fig. 11-3 as needed.

1. In addition to aphasia, this Pt showed a type of constructional apraxia different from that shown in Fig. 11-3. In Fig. 11-3, the Pt failed to complete the left side of the drawings. Notice in Fig. 11-7 that the present Pt's deficits in drawing the shape of objects affect the whole figure, not just one side.

2. The performance on the arithmetic part of the test shows severe dyscalculia.

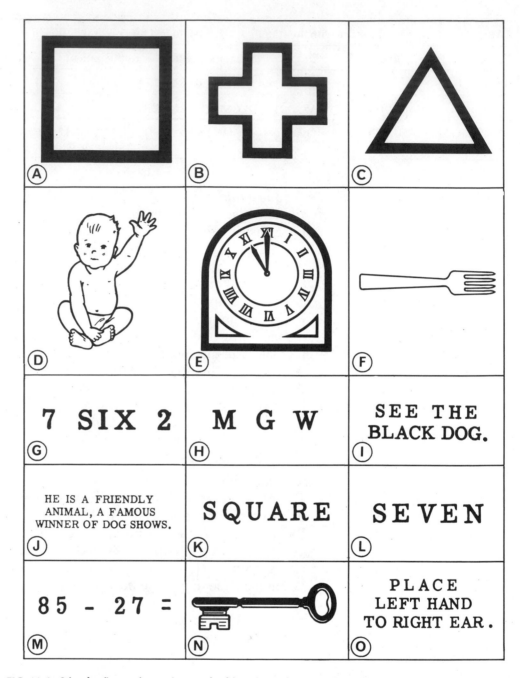

FIG. 11-6. Stimulus figures for testing cerebral functions. This test is the Halstead-Reitan-Wepman screening test as modified by Dr. Ralph Reitan (1984) and currently used in the Neuropsychology Laboratory at Indiana University and many other testing centers.

TABLE 11-4 Test results on patient with severe aphasia (*An asterisk means to look at Fig. 11-7 to see what the patient did in response to the test item.)	
Patient's task	Patient's response
1. Copy SQUARE*	The patient started to draw on the test booklet. See Fig. 11-7, 1.
2. Name SQUARE	OK.
3. Spell SQUARE	OK.
4. Copy CROSS*	See Fig. 11-7, 4-1 to 4-3.

TABLE 11-4 Test results on patient with severe aphasia (*An asterisk means to look at Fig. 11-7 to see what the patient did in response to the test item.)

Patient's task	Patient's response
5. Name CROSS	"Square"—did not respond to examiner's further questioning.
6. Spell CROSS	"un hu"; "c-r-o-w-s-s-"
7. Copy TRIANGLE*	See Fig. 11-7, 7-1 to 7-5.
8. Name TRIANGLE	Patient made no response after repeated questioning.
9. Spell TRIANGLE	Patient was asked three times to spell triangle; then asked how the word started: "TR," patient could go no further.
10. Name BABY	OK.
11. Write CLOCK*	Patient took test booklet from examiner and put it sideways. He finally drew Fig. 11-7, 11.
12. Name FORK	OK.
13. Read 7 SIX 2	"Six." (Examiner pointed to the letter.) "7, six and 7 -a four."
14. Read M G W	"Meg - m-i-g"
15. Reading I	Patient had a long pause and then read quickly, "See that dog."
16. Reading II	"He is a" (long pause) "friend of family - oh - woman of a dog." (Read very quickly after pause.)
17. Repeat TRIANGLE	Mushy articulation.
18. Repeat MASSACHUSETTS	Massachuses
19. Repeat METHODIST EPISCOPAL	"Methodiss epis fi tul."
20. Write SQUARE*	See Fig. 11-7, 21.
21. Read SEVEN*	"S s s - sev - s-e-v-e-n." Patient said the word and wrote it although not requested to write. See Fig. 11-7, 22.
22. Repeat SEVEN	"Sevun"
23. Repeat-explain HE SHOUTED THE WARNING.	Repeated the phrase but could not explain its meaning.
24. Write HE SHOUTED THE WARNING*	See Fig. 11-7, 24.
25. Compute 85 − 27 = *	Patient confused—did not know what (−) meant. See Fig. 11-7, 25, 1 to 4. The examiner wrote the problem in 25-5 and the patient answered 9.
26. Compute 17 × 3 = *	Patient could not compute; See Fig. 11-7, 26-1. Examiner gave 2 × 3; See Fig. 11-7, 26-2, Patient just scribbled.
27. Name KEY	OK with much prompting.
28. Demonstrate use of KEY	Patient could not: "You could show a fellow how."
29. Draw KEY*	Patient turned book upside down to draw. See Fig. 11-7, 29.
30. Read PLACE LEFT HAND TO RIGHT EAR	"Please the left-left hand behind me."
31. PLACE LEFT HAND TO RIGHT EAR	Patient placed right hand to right ear.
32. PLACE LEFT HAND TO LEFT ELBOW	Patient placed right hand to left elbow.

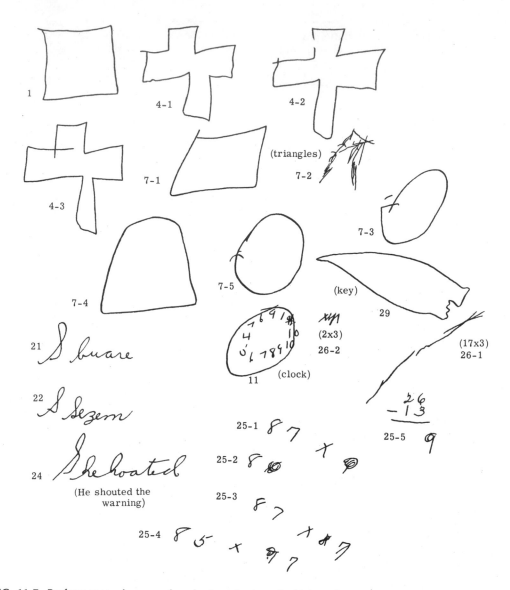

FIG. 11-7. Performance of a severely aphasic patient on the Halstead-Reitan-Wepman screening test for cerebral dysfunction. The number beside each figure refers to the number of the test item in Table 11-1. A number such as 4-2, refers to the fourth test item, the second attempt of the Pt to do the task.

The Pt could not even multiply 2 × 3. The Ex adds such additional tests when the Pt fails one of the items on the screening battery.

3. After radiographic examination disclosed a mass in the left hemisphere, a biopsy disclosed a malignant neoplasm. The Pt died 28 days after the operation, about a month after the test results obtained in Table 11-2 and Fig. 11-7. Autopsy disclosed a large multicentric glioblastoma in the left hemisphere, with one mass of neoplastic tissue in the posterior inferior frontal region and the other in the posterior parasylvian region.

4. Fig. 11-8 illustrates aphasic errors from other Pts when they were asked to write, "He shouted the warning."

H. *General classification of aphasia*

1. *Expressive/receptive aphasia.* Traditionally, neurologists have classified aphasia as *receptive, expressive,* or *mixed expressive-receptive* aphasia. Most Pts have mixed expressive and receptive language deficits, with impairment of all four avenues of language. In judging relative loss of

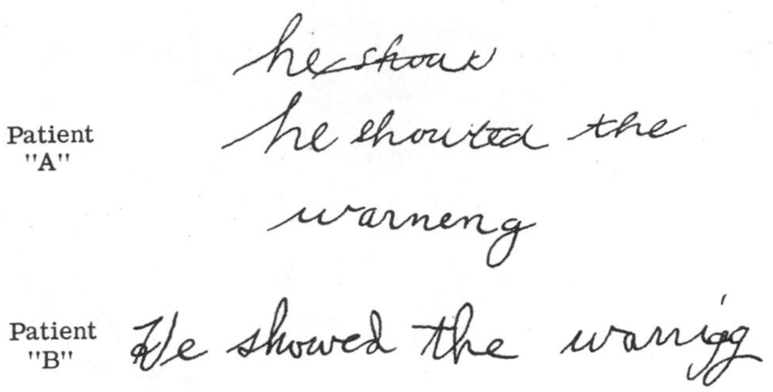

Patient "A"

he shoue

he shouted the

warneng

Patient "B"   *He showed the warigg*

FIG. 11-8. Some typical performances of aphasic Pts with left hemisphere lesions when attempting to write, "He shouted the warning." The disturbance in letter formation is called *dysgraphia*.

receptive and expressive language, recall that the active expression of language requires more effort than receiving it. Therefore, aphasics typically comprehend language better than they express it.

2. *Fluent and nonfluent aphasia.* Many authors prefer to classify aphasia as *fluent* or *nonfluent,* depending on the amount of retained language, rather than following the traditional expressive-receptive scheme (Geschwind, 1971).

I. *General localization of lesions causing aphasia*
  1. *Localization to the dominant hemisphere*
    a. The lesion that causes aphasia is in the left cerebral hemisphere in almost all right-handed and most left-handed Pts (Hecaen and Ajuriaguerra, 1964). Therefore, we say that the left hemisphere is usually dominant for language. Operationally, in designating a hemisphere as dominant for language, we mean that a lesion of that hemisphere will result in aphasia and that physiological tests, such as cortical stimulation (Penfield and Roberts, 1952), electrocorticography (Ojemann et al, 1989), and radioactive scans show activation of one or more zones of the left hemisphere during language tasks.
    b. Normally the hemispheres are asymmetric, with the left hemisphere larger than the right, particularly the planum temporale (area between the transverse temporal gyri and posterior end of the sylvian fissure) (Galaburda et al, 1978).
  2. *Localization within the dominant hemisphere.* The lesion usually involves the parasylvian region of the left hemisphere, subjacent deep white matter, caudate-putamen, or the thalamus, interrupting the corticocortical circuits of the parasylvian cortex or its connections with the deep nuclear masses (Bruyn, 1989; Damasio, 1992; Damasio and Damasio, 1989; Naeser et al, 1982; Geschwind, 1971; Russell and Espir, 1961). Uncommonly, mostly in left-handers, the lesion occupies the homologous regions of the right hemisphere. The type of aphasia fairly well predicts the site of the lesion within the aphasiogenic zone depicted in Fig. 11-9.

J. *Nonfluent (Broca's) motor aphasia (expressive aphasia)*
  1. *Clinical features:*
    a. The nonfluent aphasic Pt speaks telegraphically and sparsely (Mohr et al, 1978). The Pt uses some nouns and verbs, but omits the small connecting words, conjunctions such as *but, or,* and *and,* and articles such as *a, an,* or *the.* The Pt says, "I go house," instead of, "I go to the house." In fact, as an excellent test sentence, ask the Pt to repeat "No *if's, and's, but's,*

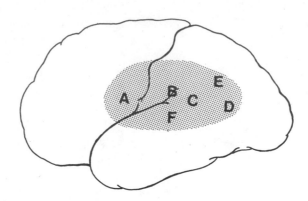

FIG. 11-9. Lateral view of the left cerebral hemisphere to show the expected lesion sites in aphasic Pts.

for's, or *or's.*" The nonfluent aphasic loses the normal rhythms and inflections of speech, and thus has one form of *dysprosody.* The Pt shows a poverty of associations, such as naming all of the makes of automobiles or all objects that are red.

  b. The Pt with Broca's aphasia also has difficulty writing, suggesting that the posterior inferior part of the frontal lobe contains the executive center for language expression, consisting of the funnel through which language plays on the motor cortex to express speech by speaking or writing.

  c. Importantly, the Pt retains the ability to audit language and to read.

 2. *Lesion site.* Relatively pure expressive or nonfluent aphasia indicates a lesion of the anterior part of the aphasic zone, in the posterior inferior part of the frontal lobe (Broca's area, A in Fig. 11-9). This region conveniently abuts on the classical motor area and correlates with the predominantly motor function of this region of the cerebrum. Because of the inverted representation of the body in the motor strip, the face area abuts on the aphasic zone. Thus, an upper motor neuron palsy of at least the right side of the face, if not a frank right hemiplegia, frequently accompanies expressive aphasia.

 K. *Fluent (Wernicke's) receptive aphasia*

  1. *Clinical features.* In direct contrast to Broca's nonfluent aphasia, the fluent aphasic produces plentiful or even an excessive number of words, but the words are often wrong or assembled of the wrong sounds (phonemes). The substitution of erroneous phrases, words, or parts of words is called *paraphasia.* The Pt crams in numerous word substitutions, circumlocutions, and neologisms, perhaps best described as a "word salad" or "word potpourri," which rob the speech of meaning. Yet, the jargon may retain normal prosody, normal rhythm, and inflection, thus sounding like speech but deficient in communicative content. Thus, the term *fluent,* implying fluent communication, is misleading. Pts with fluent aphasia lose the ability to audit their own words and the words of others. They cannot use their auditory feedback to correct their own errors in word production, resulting in their barrage of word errors. Children may also have fluent aphasia (Klelin et al, 1992).

  2. *Lesion site.* The lesion causing fluent aphasia occupies the region around the posterior end of the sylvian fissure at the parieto-occipito-temporal confluence (sites B, C, and F of Fig. 11-9). Thus, the lesion affects the aphasic zone more posteriorly and temporally than in nonfluent aphasia. It disconnects the auditory cortex in the superior temporal gyrus from the rest of the posterior parasylvian area, the word association area.

L. *Dyslexia, or visual word agnosia*

1. *Clinical features.* Dyslexia consists of a relatively pure agnosia for the meaning of written words, in spite of adequate intelligence and exposure to conventional methods of instruction. Frequently, dyslexics cannot name colors. If the history or aphasia screening test suggests dyslexia, give the Pt additional statements or a paragraph to read and ask the Pt to explain the material. Many learning disabled children have dyslexia. Contrarily, some children—normal, learning disabled, or retarded—have hyperlexia. They read prematurely at very young ages but may lack the ability to interpret what they read (Mehagan, 1972).

2. *Lesion site.* In dyslexia, the lesion usually occupies the posterior end of the aphasic zone (site D in Fig. 11-9). It damages the word association cortex of the occipital lobe or disconnects it from afferents that arrive via the corpus callosum, or from the lingual and fusiform gyri (Greenblatt, 1977). Benson (1977) describes a type of dyslexia after lesions of the dominant frontal lobe that may be associated with Broca's aphasia. Congenital, hereditary, or developmental dyslexia, as seen in children, constitutes a common problem (Critchley, 1964; Drew, 1957; Flynn and Deering, 1989). It may reflect disorders of hemispheric symmetry or migrational disorders of the neurons of the visual association cortex, which can be visualized by MRI scan (Cohen et al, 1989; Humphreys et al, 1990). Dyscalculia often accompanies dyslexia in children (Gordon, 1992; O'Hare et al, 1991).

M. *Auditory agnosia*   The Pt with relatively pure auditory aphasia fails to understand spoken words but can write and speak. The lesion occupies the posterior part of the superior temporal gyrus (site F of Fig. 11-9) next to the primary auditory receptive area in the transverse gyri, in the floor of the sylvian fissure.

N. *Global aphasia*

1. *Clinical features.* The Pt has severe expressive and receptive dysphasia, virtually eliminating all receptive and expressive communication by words. Any speech retained is mainly exclamatory or severely telegraphic.

2. *Lesion site.* In global aphasia the lesion destroys virtually all of the left parasylvian cortex (sites A–F, entire shaded area of Fig. 11-9) or its connections with the caudate-putamen, or thalamus. Since the middle cerebral artery exclusively irrigates the entire parasylvian cortex and most of the caudate-putamen, global aphasia and all other types of aphasia commonly result from infarction. Shade this zone in Fig. 11-10.

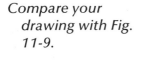

Compare your drawing with Fig. 11-9.

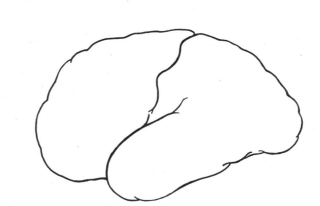

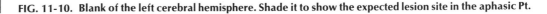

FIG. 11-10. Blank of the left cerebral hemisphere. Shade it to show the expected lesion site in the aphasic Pt.

O. *Review of the neurologic findings associated with the types of aphasia*

1. The neurologic deficits associated with aphasia will vary depending on the location of the lesion within the aphasic zone, but they follow a definite logic, if you understand the location of the motor area and the primary receptive cortex for vision and hearing (Fig. 2-2C). A lesion in the anterior part of the parasylvian zone abuts on the motor area, while a more posterior lesion may interrupt the optic radiation (geniculocalcarine tract). Review Fig. 3-6, if necessary.

2. The Pt with nonfluent aphasia would more likely have ☐ hemiparesis/ ☐ hemianopsia/ ☐ right-left confusion, because the lesion is located ____

Ans: ☑ *Hemiparesis; anteriorly in the aphasic zone next to the motor area.*

3. The fluent aphasic would more likely have ☐ hemiparesis/ ☐ hemianopsia/ ☐ anosognosia, because the lesion is located _____

Ans: ☑ *Hemianopsia; posteriorly in the aphasic zone, overlying the geniculocalcarine tract.*

4. The fluent aphasic would most likely have a severe receptive aphasia, because the lesion is located _____

Ans: *posteriorly in the aphasic zone in the auditory and visual word association region.*

P. *Role of the right hemisphere in language*

1. The right hemisphere can interpret words as symbols for verbal communication only to a limited extent, after the brain reaches developmental maturity (Ledoux et al, 1977; McClone and Young, 1991). The right hemisphere has to deliver the language stimuli it receives to the left hemisphere via the corpus callosum for interpretation and motor expression (Greenblatt, 1977). The parasylvian zone of the right hemisphere interprets and modulates the prosody of emotional expression, the rhythm, melody, and inflections that add emotion to speech. Pts with lesions in the right parasylvian zone or its subcortical connections cannot invest their own speech with its emotional coloring nor interpret the emotional connotation or gestures of others. In analogy to aphasia, the Pt whose speech lacks emotional inflection has expressive aprosody. The Pt who cannot differentiate the emotional inflections of language spoken by others has receptive aprosody, or the Pt may have global aprosody (Ross, 1981).

2. *Testing for right hemisphere aprosody*

   a. To detect *expressive aprosody,* the Ex listens for flat emotionless speech during the medical history and asks the Pt to say a test phrase while investing it with different emotional inflections. Say, "Would you come here," out loud, investing it with as much seduction as possible and then as much anger as possible. Play with this phrase as a thespian might, to discover how many different emotions it can convey.

   b. To detect *receptive aprosody,* the Ex says a test phrase in different emotional inflections, and asks the Pt to interpret the emotion conveyed. Tape recordings can provide standardized phrases.

3. *Differential diagnosis.* A flat expressionless speech can also occur with various other neuropsychiatric disorders: depression, dementia, Broca's aphasia, and diseases of the thalamus or basal motor nuclei, such as parkinsonism.

□ *Apraxia*
□ *Agnosia*

4. Expressive aprosody would qualify as a form of □ apraxia/ □ agnosia, while receptive aprosody would qualify as □ apraxia/ □ agnosia.

Q. *The levels and types of speech disturbance*

1. Communicative speech derives from words arranged according to rules of grammar and syntax, and invested with prosody. A variety of factors—thought disorders like schizophrenia, neuroses, structural lesions of the brain, and cultural exposure—can alter the communicative content and emotional connotation of speech.

2. We have now distinguished four levels of disturbance in speech production: *dysphonia, dysarthria, dysprosody,* and *dysphasia.* At the lowest level, *dysphonia* consists of a disturbance in, or a lack of, the production of sounds in the larynx. *Dysarthria* is a disorder in articulating speech sounds. Then, the *dysprosodies:* consist of scanning speech (cerebellar), plateau speech (basal motor nuclei/parkinsonian), and stuttering, cluttering, and absence of emotional inflections (cerebral). At the highest level, *dysphasia* consists of a disturbance in the understanding or expression of words as symbols for communication. Review (or if you wish, write out) the definitions of these terms and check your definitions against the ones given in Section III of the Summarized Neurologic Examination.

3. One end of the neuropsychiatric spectrum of speech disorders consists of little or no speech, called mutism or aphonia: deaf mutism, elective mutism, hysterical mutism, akinetic mutism, autism and other retardation syndromes, catatonia, depression, postictal confusion, and the mutism or bradylalia after bilateral lesions of the thalamus or basal motor nuclei. Delayed or no speech in a child always raises the question of a form of mutism, mental retardation, or deafness.

3. The other end of the speech spectrum consists of too much speech, an increase in the amount and rate of speech, of logorrhea, fluent aphasia, cluttering, echolalia, and pressure of speech (and that ineffable bore, the compulsive talker, or conversational narcissist).

R. *Gerstmann's syndrome*

1. *Clinical features.* The core components of Gerstmann's syndrome consist of dysgraphia, dyscalculia, finger agnosia, and right-left disorientation, but most Pts have other features of aphasia. The Pt often has agraphia for spontaneous writing, but can copy. Children normally go through a stage that is called a developmental Gerstmann's syndrome (Gordon, 1992; O'Hare et al, 1991).

2. *Lesion site.* Although a lesion of the left angular gyrus, at the parietooccipitotemporal junction (site E in Fig. 11-9), may cause the four core components of Gerstmann's syndrome, one or all of the components can occur with lesions of more distant sites (Heimberger et al, 1964). Even though the lesion is unilateral, the finger agnosia and right-left disorientation affect both sides of the body, thus representing bilateral asomatognosias.

S. *A review of the definitions of agnosia, apraxia, and aphasia*

Now that you know the operational methods to test for these disorders, give a general interpretational definition of:

1. Agnosia: _____

_____.

Ans: See Frame IIB2, p 387.

2. Apraxia: _____

_____.

Ans: See Frame IIC1, p 388.

3. Aphasia: _____

_____

_____.

Ans: See Frame IIIA, p 394.

4. The requisites to distinguish any type of agnosia from other disturbances of sensation, comprehension, or perception are: _____

_____

_____.

Ans: See Frame IIB3, p 388.

5. The requisites necessary to distinguish any type of apraxia from other disorders of execution are: _____

_____

_____.

Ans: See Frame IIC3, p 388.

IV. A resume of cerebral localization

A. *The concept of cerebral localization:* The philosopher seeks to localize functions in the brain and to find the seat of mind and emotion. The practicing physician seeks to localize lesions in the brain. Sometimes, the philosopher-physician confuses the process. Just because an Ex can localize a lesion from the deficit of function does not localize the function; localizing the function in this circumstance indulges in the sin of circular reasoning:

Sequence 1:
    Child: "Daddy, why do things fall to the ground?"
    Daddy: "Why, that's simple, because there is gravity."

Sequence 2:
    Child: "Daddy, why do you say there is gravity?"
    Daddy: "Why, that's simple, because things fall to the ground."

B. *Clinicopathologic correlation:* Relation of functional deficit to lesion site.
   1. Fig. 11-11 does not require that functions localize in the regions labeled. It means that a given clinical deficit, determined according to a specific test procedure, implies a lesion in a particular site. We do not worry ourselves with localizing functions if we recall the operational steps: Give a test, executing it and judging the results according to standard procedure. Match the results against the site of brain lesions in a number of Pt's and note the correlation between particular deficits and particular lesion sites (Adams and Victor, 1989; Brazis et al, 1990; Joynt and Goldstein, 1975; McClone and Young, 1991; Pincus and Tucker, 1985). That method, the method of clinicopathologic correlation, leads to the construction of Fig. 11-11. Current studies by electrocorticography, radioactive (PET) scanning that discloses regional variations in blood flow and metabolism, and the Wada test (unilateral carotid injections of amytal) confirm and extend the localizing conclusions reached by clinicopathologic correlation.

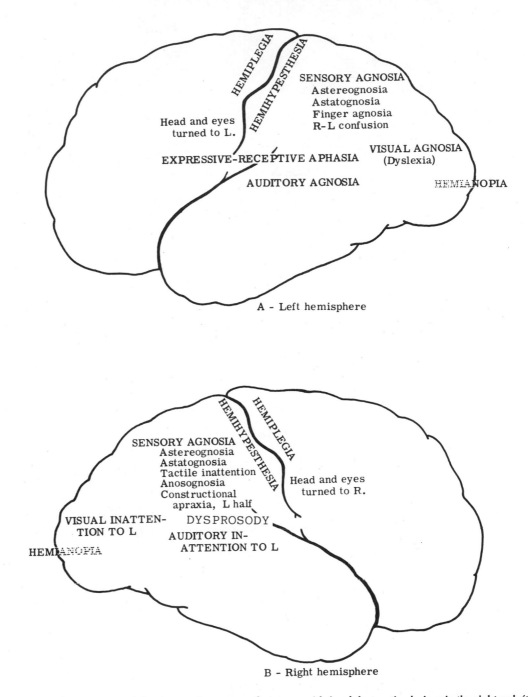

FIG. 11-11. Summary of the signs and symptoms that occur with focal destructive lesions in the right or left cerebral hemispheres. (*A*) Lateral view of left cerebral hemisphere. (*B*) Lateral view of the right cerebral hemisphere. Note that some signs, such as hemiplegia, appear after lesions of either hemisphere, but that other signs depend on which hemisphere contains the lesion.

2. *Localization of memory.* Although diffuse disease of the cerebrum impairs memory, bilateral lesions restricted to the medial temporal lobe or diencephalon cause relatively selective memory loss, the *pure amnestic syndrome,* in which Pts retain their previous IQ and have no other frank neurologic signs (Adams and Victor, 1989) (Fig. 11-12).

3. We cannot now answer and cannot ever answer the questions of the Book of Job: But where shall wisdom be found? And where is the place of understanding?

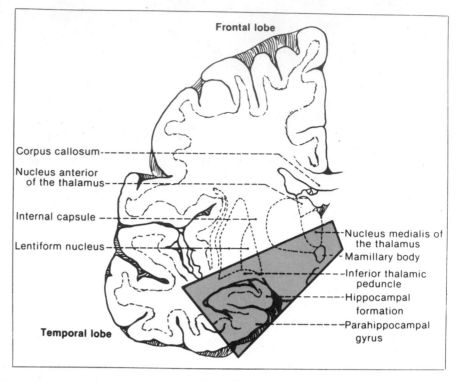

FIG. 11-12. Coronal section of a cerebral hemisphere showing the region which when damaged bilaterally causes loss of recent memory.

C. *Diagnostic value of agnosia, apraxia, and deficits of the sensorium in the functional-organic dichotomy*

1. After completing the history and NE, the Ex has to reach a tentative diagnosis for guidance in whether to select ancillary diagnostic tests. If required, these tests then confirm or reject the tentative diagnosis.
2. Diagnosis requires the Ex to proceed through a labyrinth, or dendrogram (Fig. 11-13).

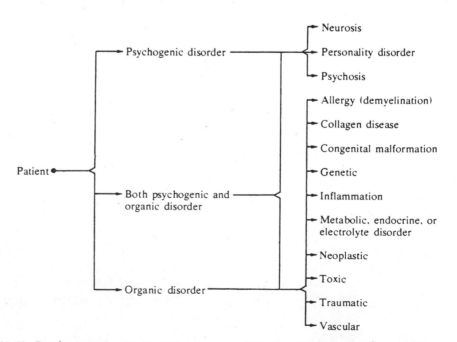

FIG. 11-13. Dendrogram showing the initial diagnostic dichotomy into functional versus organic disease.

3. Each turn you take in the dendrogram depends on the evidence accumulated from the history, physical examination, and laboratory tests. The first diagnostic dichotomy requires a decision as to whether the Pt most likely has an organic or a so-called functional disorder. If you realize that a large percentage of Pts seeking medical help have functional or emotional disorders—perhaps as many as half of the adults who will come to your office—you will realize the importance of making the first dichotomy in diagnosis correctly.

4. In essence the Ex must recite this catechism:

    a. Does the Pt have a lesion (biochemical or anatomical)?

    b. Where is the lesion?

    c. What is the lesion?

    d. What critical diagnostic procedures are required?

5. If the Pt has frank neurologic signs, such as hemiplegia or hemianopsia, agnosia, or apraxia, the first diagnostic dichotomy is easy; the Pt has ☐ organic/ ☐ functional disease.

    ☑ *Organic*

6. Most functional diseases spare most of the sensorium. Therefore, the average neurotic or mildly psychotic Pt has no sensorial defect. Brain lesions may impair memory, orientation, and consciousness—sensorial functions—without causing more obvious neurologic signs. Therefore, sensorial defects themselves may indicate organic disease.

    a. Disorderered memory, orientation, or consciousness in a mentally disturbed Pt most likely indicates ☐ organic/ ☐ functional disease.

    ☑ *Organic*

    b. Preservation of memory, orientation, or consciousness in a mentally disturbed Pt, most likely indicates ☐ organic/ ☐ functional disease.

    ☑ *Functional*

7. *Warning:* Read this. Although useful, the organic/functional dichotomy is artificial. The absence of sensorial defects and frank neurologic signs, although reducing the likelihood of organic brain lesions, never guarantees their absence. The lesion may not have exceeded the safety factor of the tissue to cause frank neurologic signs, even though it has produced changes recognized by the Pt or associates. Contrarily, severely psychotic Pts with schizophrenia or depression may display sensorial defects and perform poorly on the Halstead-Reitan-Wepman cerebral dysfunction test. Many so-called functional disorders—schizophrenia, depression, hyperactivity, anorexia nervosa, bulimia, obesity, sleep disorders, and headaches—have a biological basis, but no identifiable lesions in the classical sense; or, as in schizophrenia, they require subtle measurement to demonstrate (DeMyer et al, 1992). We often walk the fine edge between triumph and disaster in trying to identify or exclude organic cerebral dysfunction.

V. Special features of the mental status and neurologic examination in dementia and aging

A. Symptoms and signs disclosed by history, mental status, and NE in dementia and aging. Certain findings help establish diffuse organic disease, but do not signify single, focal lesions (Allison, 1962; Chui, 1989; Cummings and Benson, 1992; DePaulo and Folstein, 1978; Huff et al, 1987; Jenkyn and Reeves, 1981).

    1. *Alterations in intellectual function caused by diffuse brain disease.*

        a. Poor planning, judgment, and decision making, with poverty of thought and action, negativism, childishness, and loss of flexibility. Family members often express these changes as, "The Pt just does not act like himself or herself any more."

      b. Loss of interest in current events with circumscription of activities, hypochondriasis, and self-preoccupation.

      c. Forgetfulness, with recent memory worse than remote memory—"living in the past."

  2. *Alterations in affect*

      a. Depression with mixture of apathy and irritability and often complaints of undue fatigability. Less frequently, aggression or mania.

      b. Anxious worrying over trivial matters.

      c. Lability of emotions (pseudobulbar affect).

  3. *Alterations in vegetative function and personal hygiene*

      a. Sudden or premature aging in facial appearance and posture. (The Pt who looks 80 years old usually is not that old, or, if you look 80 at 70, you aren't going to make it to 80.)

      b. Slovenly personal appearance, often with bladder and bowel incontinence.

      c. Alterations in appetite, usually with weight loss.

      d. Disordered sleep cycle, often with nocturnal disorientation.

      e. Decrease in sexual activity and interest or, less commonly, hypersexuality or inappropriate sexuality.

C. *Neurologic findings in aging and dementia*

  1. *Alterations in speech*

      a. Dysarthria

      b. Poverty of speech and associations, circumlocutions, aphasia-like word searching and anomia

      c. Monotonous or plateau speech, lacking in prosody

      d. Perseveration and echolalia

  2. *Alterations in gait* (Joseph and Young, 1992 and see the gait essay, page 301).

      a. Unsteadiness, falling, broad base

      b. Marche à petits pas

      c. Gait apraxia

      d. Loss of verticality with retropulsion or anteropulsion and festination

  3. *Alterations in overall motor function*

      a. Poverty and slowness of all volitional movements.

      b. Increasing flexion posture. See Section D, next.

      c. Hypertonicity, either lead-pipe rigidity or paratonic rigidity (Gegenhalten). Facial immobility.

      d. Deterioration of handwriting (dysgraphia and micrographia). Inspect samples of the Pt's signature over several years (using old checks, etc.).

      e. Involuntary movements: orolingual hyperkinesias and mild resting or action tremors.

      f. Disinhibition of primitive reflexes (explained in the next section).

      g. *Disordered motor functions in subcortical dementia:* Alzheimer's disease causes predominantly cortical degeneration. The so-called subcortical dementias affect basal motor nuclei and rostral brainstem as much or more than the cortex. Such Pts with Huntington's chorea, thalamic degeneration, parkinsonism, or Wilson's hepatolenticular degeneration present with early or conspicuous motor signs along with their dementia (Chui, 1989; Cummings and Benson, 1992). Whether the Ex can clearly separate on clinical grounds the dementia per se of cortical and subcortical dementia remains controversial (Adams and Victor, 1989).

4. *Alterations in MSRs.* All MSRs brisk (including jaw jerk) except for reduced or absent triceps surae (due to mild distal senile peripheral neuropathy).

5. *Alterations in visual function*
   a. Apparent reduction in vision.
   b. The pupils become miotic and, in the very elderly, may fail to react to light and in accommodation (Jenkyn and Reeves, 1981).
   c. Poor fixation and smooth pursuit, with limited upward gaze.

6. *Alterations in sensation*
   a. Anosmia common
   b. Reduced deep modalities, such as vibratory sensation in feet
   c. Presbyacusis

D. *Primitive reflexes in aging and dementia*

> *Sometimes the convolutions [gyri] are simply reduced in volume, at other times they are puckered; in other cases there is induration. The patient lives a life of mere excito-motory and nutritive kind. The cerebral functions are obliterated. The true spinal and ganglionic functions remain alone. There is much for the physiologist to investigate in this singular return to a sort of infantile existence.*
>
> **Marshall Hall** (1790–1857)

1. *The theory of primitive reflexes.* At term the infant's pre-programmed primitive reflexes, such as breathing and sucking, determine its behavior (O'Doherty, 1986). As the infant's cortex matures, it comes to dominate or inhibit the primitive inborn behaviors. Then, with aging or dementia, the cortex loses neurons, disinhibiting the primitive reflexes, allowing the Ex to elicit them in the brain-impaired adult (Huff et al, 1987; Jenkyn et al, 1977; Paulson and Gottlieb, 1968).

2. *The flexion attitude or posture*
   a. The newborn infant emerges at term in an attitude of universal flexion, the so-called fetal posture, with the head flexed on the chest, the chest flexed on the pelvis, and the arms and legs flexed upon the body. Paul Yakovlev (1947) interpreted this posture as a "grasp reflex of the body upon the body." The flexion attitude dominates in the normal newborn to the point that the infant cannot completely extend its knees and elbows, nor can the Ex by passive manipulation.
   b. During the first year, as the cerebral cortex matures, the normal infant unfolds from this attitude, unfolding from itself and unfolding in defiance of gravity, to reach an erect posture and to extend and free the limbs for action.
   c. In advanced senility or advanced dementia, as the cerebral cortex degenerates, the flexed fetal posture re-emerges, and the Pt again folds up on himself and again succumbs to gravity. Shakespeare spoke of this life cycle of flexion–vertical posture–flexion as once an adult, twice an infant (Fig. 11-14).

E. *Table of primitive reflexes and other signs of organic dementia in adults:* The primitive reflexes and related findings, while nonlocalizing as to lesion site, reflect diffuse organic dysfunction of the cerebrum. Hence, they provide a valuable adjunct to the standard NE (Huff et al, 1987; Jenkyn et al, 1977; Katzman and Rowe, 1992; Koller et al, 1982). See Table 11-5.

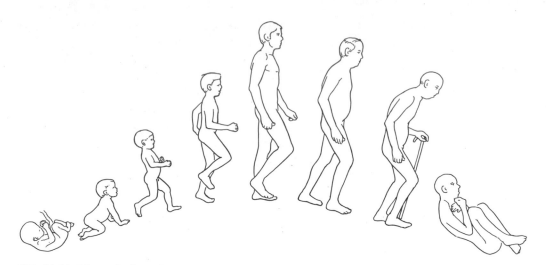

FIG. 11-14. The cycle from flexion-to-verticality-to-flexion during the lifespan of the individual: once an adult, and twice an infant (after Yakovlev, 1947).

TABLE 11-5 Nonlocalizing neurologic signs in diffuse organic brain dysfunction

1. *Range of eye movement and smooth pursuit.* Instruct Pt to hold head still and follow Ex's finger through extremes of horizontal gaze and vertical gaze. Hold a transparent ruler in front of cornea to measure range of deviation.
   Normal: Eyes move smoothly, without nystagmus, 7 mm upwards and 10 mm in other directions.
   Abnormal: Irregular, hesitant, or saccadic smooth pursuit. Upward gaze usually most limited. Upgaze and lateral gaze should equal at least 5 and 7 mm respectively.
2. *Lateral gaze impersistence.* Pt holds head still and deviates the eyes as far as possible to the left to maintain persistent fixation on a point on the wall for a timed 30-second period. Instruct the Pt to blink, if necessary, but not to allow the eyes to deviate back to the middle.
   Normal: Pt persists in maintaining fixation for 30 seconds.
   Abnormal: Pt unable to persist for 30 seconds.
3. *Tongue impersistence.* Instruct Pt to protrude the tongue in the midline as far as possible for a timed 30-second period.
   Normal: Pt persists for 30 seconds.
   Abnormal: Pts with involuntary movement syndromes, such as chorea, invariably fail, as often do demented Pts or Pts with a short attention span.
4. *Glabellar blink.* Pt looks at a point across room. Ex stands at sides, and brings index finger down from above the forehead and taps the glabella rapidly ten times.
   Normal: Reflex closure of eyelids inhibited after several taps; lids remain open.
   Abnormal: Continuous reflex blinking of upper or lower lid or both, with or without lid closure (disinhibition). Some normal individuals may continue to blink.
5. *Snout reflex.* The Pt closes the eyes. The Ex taps the philtrum several times at a medium rate, or the Ex may press the tip of a test tube firmly (not so as to cause pain) against the philtrum, compressing the upper lip against the gum.
   Normal: No response
   Abnormal: Puckering or pursing of the lips
6. *Suck reflex.* The Pt closes the eyes. Using the rounded tip of a test tube, stroke the Pt's lips from the center of the crevice to the sides.
   Normal: Sucking response in young infant. Thereafter, no response.
   Abnormal: Any pursing or sucking motion of lips (disinhibited) in Pt older than early infancy. Failure of young infant to suck.
7. *Nuchocephalic reflex.* Pt stands relaxed, eyes lightly closed. Ex tells Pt to relax and let the body and arms be loose and floppy. The Ex briskly turns the Pt's shoulders ⅛- to ¼-turn to the right and to the left several times, stopping randomly with shoulders turned in one direction or another.

TABLE 11-5 Nonlocalizing neurologic signs in diffuse organic brain dysfunction

---

Normal: Head reflexly turns in direction of shoulder movement after about ½-second lag to realign straight ahead with the new shoulder position. (Exclude cervical spondylosis.)

Abnormal: Head holds original position and does not turn to align with the new position of the shoulders. (The reflex is "disinhibited.")

8. *Grasp reflex.* Ex uses index and middle finger to stroke the Pt's palm from the hypothenar eminence toward the junction of the Pt's thumb and index finger.

   Normal: Present in early infancy but not thereafter.

   Abnormal: The Pt grasps the Ex's fingers. Forced groping may ensue, in which the Pt maintains the grasp and moves the hand wherever the Ex moves the hand, or the Pt may involuntarily grope for an object presented to vision.

9. *Palmomental reflex.* The Ex instructs the Pt to relax. Pt sits or reclines. Break a wooden tongue blade transversely, and use the serrated margin to stroke proximodistally along the Pt's thenar eminence on the right and left hands.

   Normal: No contraction of mentalis muscle, but the reflex occurs in most Pts if the stimulus is very strong (Koller et al, 1982).

   Abnormal: Readily elicited ipsilateral and sometimes bilateral mentalis contraction.

10. *Arm dropping test.* Ex instructs Pt, "Relax your arms completely. Let me do all of the work." Ex grasps Pt's arm by wrist, elevates it, and lets it drop. The Ex catches the Pt's arm with the other hand to avoid injury. This test is most successful when done after the nuchocephalic test, which gives the Pt experience in what a totally floppy arm feels like.

    Normal: Free fall of the arm.

    Abnormal: Failure to let the arm drop freely. Occasionally, a normal subject cannot relax to allow free fall of the arm.

11. *Leg dropping test.* Repeat as for arm dropping. The Pt sits with the legs dangling over a table edge. The Ex grasps the ankle, extends the leg, and allows it to drop.

12. *Paratonia* (Gegenhalten). Ex grasps Pt's wrist and passively moves Pt's arms in various directions.

    Normal: Free, non-oppositional response.

    Abnormal: More or less continuous opposition to movement in any direction, which may give in and then resume. Must differentiate from parkinsonian rigidity (Yakovlev, 1947).

F. *Additional methods of assessing the demented Pt:* Applegate et al (1990) list several additional tests to evaluate the physical, cognitive, and emotional status of Pts suspected of dementia. Generally the Ex should order an MRI of the brain (Caplan et al, 1990).

VI. Review of tests for cerebral dysfunctions

A. *Rehearsal time again:* Define the sensorium, state the seven areas of the sensorium, and give an example of a question designed to test each of the areas.

B. *Distinguish between an illusion, a hallucination, and a delusion.*

C. *Define agnosia, aphasia, and apraxia, and describe tests for each.*

D. *With a partner, work through the Halstead-Reitan-Wepman screening test for cerebral dysfunction, using section VIII, steps A and B, of the Summarized Neurologic Examination.* Know the procedures, but, to avoid memorization, use the instruction sheet to administer the test.

E. *With a partner, practice how to elicit the nonlocalizing signs of cerebral dysfunction (Table 11-5).*

BIBLIOGRAPHY FOR AGNOSIA, APRAXIA, AND APHASIA

Adams RD, Victor M: *Principles of Neurology* (4th ed). New York, McGraw-Hill, 1989

Alexander MP, Benson DF: The aphasias and related disturbances, in Joynt RJ (ed): *Clinical Neurology* (vol 1). Philadelphia, Lippincott, 1991

Allison R: *The Senile Brain: A Clinical Study.* London, Edward Arnold, 1962

Applegate JP, Blass JP, Williams TP: Instruments for the functional assessment of older patients. *N Engl J Med* 1990;322:1207–1214

Benson D, Blumer D: Psychiatric aspects of neurologic disease, in Greenblatt M: *Seminars in Psychiatry* (2d ed). New York, Grune & Stratton, 1982

Benson D: The third alexia. *Arch Neurol* 1977;34:327–331

Brazis PW, Masdeau JC, Biller J: *Localization in Clinical Neurology* (2d ed). Boston, Little, Brown, 1990

Brown J: *Aphasia, Apraxia, and Agnosia: Clinical and Theoretical Aspects.* Springfield, IL, Charles C Thomas, 1972

Bruyn RPM: Thalamic aphasia: a conceptual critique. *J Neurol* 1989;236:21–25

Caplan L, Shuren J, De Witt L: Abnormal mental states: Decision strategies for imaging referral. *MRI Decisions* 1990;4:14–25

Chui HC: A review emphasizing clinicopathologic correlation and brain–behavior relationships. *Arch Neurol* 1989;46:806–814

Cohen M, Campbell R, Yaghmai F: Neuropathological abnormalities in developmental dysphasia. *Ann Neurol* 1989;25:567–570

Critchley M: *Aphasiology and Other Aspects of Language.* London, Edward Arnold, 1970

Critchley M: *The Parietal Lobes.* New York, Hafner Publishing, 1969

Critchley M: *Developmental Dyslexia.* London, William Heinemann Medical Books, 1964

Cummings JL, Benson DF: *Dementia: A Clinical Approach.* Stoneham, MA, Butterworth-Heinemann, 1992

Damasio H, Damasio AR: *Lesion Analysis in Neuropsychology.* New York, Oxford University Press, 1989

Damasio AR: Aphasia. *N Engl J Med* 1992;326:531–539

DeMyer M, Gilmore RL, Hendrie HC, et al: Magnetic resonance brain images in schizophrenic and normal subjects: Influence of diagnosis and education. *Schizophren Bull* 1988;14:21–37

DePaulo JR, Folstein MF: Psychiatric disturbances in neurological patients: Detection, recognition, and hospital course. *Ann Neurol* 1978;4:225–228

Drew A: A neurological appraisal of familial congenital word-blindness. *Brain* 1956;79:440–460

Flynn JM, Deering WM: Subtypes of dyslexia: Investigation of Boder's system using quantitative neurophysiology. *Dev Med Child Neurol* 1989;31:215–223

Galaburda AM, LeMay M, Kemper TL, et al: Right-left asymmetries in the brain. *Science* 1978;199:852–856

Geschwind N: Aphasia. *N Engl J Med* 1971;284:654–656

Gloning I: Eine Klassifizierung der Aphasie aufgrund einer quantitativ-experimentellen Untersuchung. *Fortschr Neurol Psychiatr* 1970;38:246–264

Gordon N: Children with developmental dyscalculia. *Dev Med Child Neurol* 1992;34:459–463

Goodglass A, Kaplan E: *Assessment of Aphasia and Related Disorders.* Philadelphia, Lea & Febiger, 1972

Greenblatt SH: Neurosurgery and the anatomy of reading. A practical review. *Neurosurg* 1977;1:6–15

Head H: *Aphasia and Kindred Disorders of Speech.* New York, Stechert-Hafner, 1963

Heimberger R, De Myer W, Reitan R: Implications of Gerstmann's syndrome. *J Neurol Neurosurg Psychiatr,* 1964;27:52–57

Hecaen H, Ajuriaguerra J: *Left-Handedness, Manual Superiority and Cerebral Dominance.* New York, Grune & Stratton, 1964

Huff FJ, Boller F, Lucchelli F, et al: The neurologic examination in patients with probable Alzheimer's disease. *Arch Neurol* 1987;44:929–933

Humphreys P, Kaufmann WE, Galaburda AM: Developmental dyslexia in women: Neuropathological findings in three patients. *Ann Neurol* 1990;28:727–738

Jenkyn LR, Reeves AG: Neurologic signs in uncomplicated aging (senescence). *Seminars Neurol* 1981;1:21–30

Jenkyn LR, Walsh DB, Culber CM, et al: Clinical signs in diffuse cerebral dysfunction. *J Neurol Neurosurg Psychiatr* 1977;40:956–966

Joseph AB, Young RR: *Movement Disorders in Neurology and Neuropsychiatry.* Cambridge, Blackwell, 1992

Joynt RJ, Goldstein MN: Minor cerebral hemisphere, in Friedlander WJ (ed): *Advances in Neurology* (vol 7). New York, Raven, 1975, pp 147–183

Katzman R, Rowe J: *Principles of Geriatric Neurology.* Philadelphia, FA Davis, 1992

Klelin SK, Masur D, Farveer K, et al: Fluent aphasia in children: Definition and natural history. *J Child Neurol* 1992;7:50–59

Koller WC, Glatt S, Wilson RS, et al: Primitive reflexes and cognitive function in the elderly. *Ann Neurol* 1982;12:302–304

LeDoux JE, Wilson DH, Gazzaniga MD: A divided mind. Observations on the conscious properties of the separated hemispheres. *Ann Neurol* 1978;2:417–421

Luria AR: *Higher Cortical Functions in Man.* New York, Basic Books, 1966

McGlone J, Young B: Cerebral localization, in Joynt RJ (ed): *Clinical Neurology* (vol 1). Philadelphia, Lippincott, 1991

Mehegan H, Dreifuss F: Hyperlexia. *Neurology* 1972;22:1105–1111

Mohr JP, Pessin MS, Finkelstein S, et al: Broca aphasia: Pathologic and clinical. *Neurology* 1978;28:311–324

Naeser MA, Alexander MP, Help-Estabrooks N, et al: Aphasia with predominantly subcortical lesion sites. *Arch Neurol* 1982;39:2–14

Nielsen JM: *Agnosia, Apraxia, Aphasia: Their Value in Cerebral Localization.* New York, Stechert-Hafner, 1962

O'Doherty N: *Neurologic Examination of the Newborn.* Lancaster, MTP Press, 1986

O'Hare AE, Brown JK, Aitken K: Dyscalculia in children. *Dev Med Child Neurol* 1991;33:356–361

Ojemann FI, Lettich E: Electrocorticographic (ECoG) correlates of language. I. Desynchronization in temporal language cortex during object naming. *Electroencephalog Neurophysiol* 1989;73:453–463

Paulson GW, Gottlieb G: Developmental reflexes: The re-appearance of fetal and neonatal reflexes in aged patients. *Brain* 1968;91:37–52

Penfield W, Roberts L: *Speech and Brain Mechanisms.* Princeton, Princeton University Press, 1959

Pincus JH, Tucker GJ: *Behavioral Neurology* (3d ed). New York, Oxford University Press, 1985

Reitan RM: *Aphasia and Sensory-Perceptual Deficits in Adults.* Tucson, Reitan Neuropsychology Laboratories, 1984

Ross ED: The aprosodias. *Arch Neurol* 1981;38:561–569

Russell W, Espir M: *Traumatic Aphasia.* London, Oxford University Press, 1961

Strub RL, Black FW: *The Mental Status Examination in Neurology.* Philadelphia, FA Davis, 1977

Weinstein EA, Friedland RP (eds): Hemi-inattention syndromes and hemisphere specialization, *Advances in Neurology* (vol 10). New York, Raven, 1977

Weisenburg T, McBride KE: *Aphasia: A Clinical and Psychological Study.* New York, Stechert-Hafner, 1964

Wells CE (ed): Dementia, in Plum F, McDowell FH (eds): *Contemporary Neurology Series* (no. 15). Philadelphia, FA Davis, 1977

Yakovlev P: Paraplegia in flexion of cerebral origin. *J Neuropath Exp Neurol* 1954;13:267–296

Learning Objectives for Chapter Eleven

I. The mental status examination

1. Describe how the Ex monitors the appropriateness of any particular line of inquiry in the mental status examination and describe some of the adverse responses Pts make when the Ex makes a mistake in the technique of the mental status examination.

2. Explain the need for flexibility in collecting the data for the mental status examination; yet, the need for a specific outline to arrange it.

3. Outline the goals or areas of inquiry of the mental status examination (Table 11-1).

**4. Describe in historical perspective the concept of a common sensorium (sensorium commune) and its localization in the brain.

5. Give an interpretational definition of the sensorium commune.

6. Describe how the *who, where, when, what,* and *how* questions illustrate the concept of the sensorium.

7. Recite the actual questions that the Ex would use to test whether a person who had just received a head injury had regained full sensorial function.

8. Explain why the Ex should not, except in emergencies, ask the questions that screen the sensorium in serial order.

9. Describe how to test orientation to time, person, and place.

10. Describe how to test a Pt's memory.

11. List the seven areas of the sensorium (Table 11-1, item VI) and give examples of questions designed to test each area (Table 11-2).

12. Discuss the localizing significance of sensorial defects.

13. Explain what is meant by a *blunted* or a *labile* affect.

14. Define *illusion, delusion,* and *hallucination.*

II. Agnosia, apraxia, and aphasia

1. Describe the operational tests for several common types of agnosias and give a general interpretational definition of agnosia.

2. Recite the qualifications that separate agnosia from other disturbances of sensory reception.

3. Give a general interpretational definition of apraxia.

4. Recite the qualifications that separate apraxia from other disturbances of execution.

5. Explain how the principle of parsimony (Occam's razor) applies to localizing a neurologic lesion.

6. Explain how a mass lesion, like a neoplasm, may produce signs or symptoms of impairment of neural tissue beyond the actual border of the lesion.

7. Describe the operational tests for several common types of apraxia tested in the neurologic examination.

III. Aphasia: agnosia and apraxia of language

1. Name the two avenues by which the normal person receives language, and the two for expressing it. Describe how to test these four avenues of language.

2. Explain the difference between emotional, or expletive, speech and volitional, or propositional, speech.

3. Demonstrate how to use an instruction sheet and page of stimulus-figures to screen a Pt for cerebral dysfunction (Fig. 11-6 and Table 11-3).

4. Describe the difference in the constructional apraxia shown by Pts with left parasylvian as contrasted to right parasylvian area lesions.

5. Explain how to determine the dominant hemisphere for language operationally. State which hemisphere is dominant in most persons, whether right- or left-handed.

6. Describe the usual location within the dominant hemisphere of the lesion that causes aphasia.

7. Describe the differences in speech output of a nonfluent and a fluent aphasic patient.

8. Distinguish between expressive dysphasia, receptive dysphasia, dyslexia, auditory agnosia, mixed aphasia, and global aphasia.

9. Draw a lateral outline of the proper cerebral hemisphere and shade the zone within which lesions cause aphasia. Give the general name for this region (Fig. 11-9).

10. Describe where, within the aphasic zone, a lesion would most likely produce: relatively pure expressive or nonfluent aphasia; auditory aphasia; dyslexia; combination of fluent aphasia, auditory aphasia, dysgraphia, and dyslexia; global aphasia (Fig. 11-9).

11. Describe which type of aphasia would most likely occur with hemiparesis, and which type with hemianopia.

**12. Describe the role of the right hemisphere in language and how to test its function.

**13. Recite the components of Gerstmann's syndrome and state the expected site of the lesion.

14. Distinguish between dysphonia, dysarthria, dysprosody, and dysphasia.

15. Give general (interpretational) definitions of aphasia, agnosia, and apraxia, and state the requisites or qualifications that distinguish each of them from other defects of reception and execution.

IV. A resume of cerebral vocalization

1. Contrast in principle the effect of a lesion of the posterior parasylvian region of the left cerebral hemisphere with a similar lesion on the right (Fig. 11-11).

2. On a lateral outline drawing of the two cerebral hemispheres, write down the neurologic findings resulting from acute destructive lesions in various locations (Fig. 11-11).

3. Describe the location of the lesion which would selectively impair recent memory, giving a pure amnestic syndrome (Fig. 11-12).

3. Recite the four questions of the catechism that the Ex must address in analyzing the presence or absence of a lesion.

4. Explain how to use testing of the sensorium and the nonlocalizing signs of diffuse cerebral dysfunction (Table 11-5) to differentiate functional and organic mental illness in Pts who do not have frank localizing signs on the standard NE.

5. Discuss the pitfalls in trying to dichotomize disease into functional and organic types.

**V. Special features of the mental status and neurologic examination in dementia and aging

1. Describe typical alterations in intellectual, affective, and vegetative functions in dementia and aging.

2. Describe typical alterations in speech in dementia and aging.

3. Describe typical alterations in gait and overall motor function in dementia and aging.

4. Name the signs of motor dysfunction suggesting dementia with subcortical lesions.

5. Name a MSR typically reduced in aged individuals, and explain.

6. Describe the changes disclosed by the NE in smell, hearing, vision, and pupillary responses in aging and dementia.

7. Explain the concept of primitive reflexes as related to dementia and aging and the phrase, "once an adult, twice an infant" (Fig. 11-14).

8. State which direction of eye movements is usually most impaired in diffuse cortical disease.

9. Describe the technique and normal result of testing for motor impersistence, glabellar blink, snouting and sucking reflexes, nuchocephalic reflex, grasp reflex, palmomental reflex, arm- and leg-dropping tests, and paratonia (Table 11-5).

Chapter Twelve

Examination of the Patient Who Has a Disorder of Consciousness

I may speak alike to you and my own conscious heart.
Percy Bysshe Shelley (1792–1822)

I. Evaluation of consciousness

A. *Interpretational definition:* From the endless philosophic definitions of consciousness, let us choose one: *Consciousness is the awareness of self and environment.* We might add that consciousness implies the awareness of thought.

B. *Operations that establish consciousness:* Physicians employ *inspection, conversation,* or, if necessary, *pain* to determine the Pt's awareness of self and environment. To prove conscious awareness, the Pt must have sufficiently intact receptors to receive stimuli and a sufficiently intact effector to produce a behavior, verbal or nonverbal, that depends on consciousness.
   1. *Inspection.* Does the Pt respond appropriately to the ongoing visual, auditory, and tactile stimuli of the ordinary environment?
   2. *Conversation.* Does the Pt respond appropriately to conversational voice or arouse to loud commands and questions?
   3. *Pain.* Does the Pt respond appropriately to pain?

C. *Pathologic alterations in the level of consciousness:* Disease may alter consciousness in one of two directions, elevation or depression. What we classify as elevations of consciousness may precede depression of consciousness, as part of the same cycle of events—e.g., during the evolution of hepatic coma (Table 12-1).
   1. *Nomenclature note.* The terms used to describe altered consciousness vary (Adams and Victor, 1989; Plum and Posner, 1982). Table 12-2 gives serviceable, if not universal, definitions.
   2. *Delirium (acute confusional state) and mania.* The Pt displays a transient, global impairment of the sensorium, with abnormally decreased or increased psychomotor activity and a disturbed sleep–wake cycle (DSM-III-R; Lipowski, 1989). The Pts then return to their previous mental state. Although demented Pts may also suffer periods of delirium, the term *delirium* means only a temporary state of sensorial impairment, whereas *dementia* means permanent impairment. The causes of delirium extend from sleep deprivation to various drugs and toxic-metabolic states. In aged persons, delirium occurs most commonly at night. Withdrawal from alco-

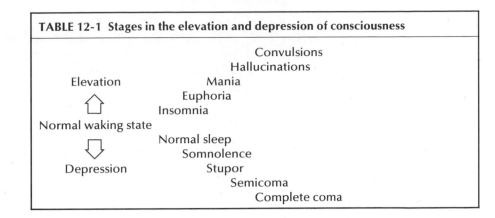

TABLE 12-1 Stages in the elevation and depression of consciousness

	Convulsions
	Hallucinations
Elevation	Mania
⇧	Euphoria
	Insomnia
Normal waking state	
⇩	Normal sleep
	Somnolence
Depression	Stupor
	Semicoma
	Complete coma

TABLE 12-2 Definition of terms used to describe depression of consciousness

1. *Normal waking state:* Sensorium fully intact. The person sleeps at appropriate times, arouses fully, and appropriately maintains the waking state.
2. *Somnolence:* The Pt arouses spontaneously at times or after normal stimuli but drifts off inappropriately. The sensorium functions adequately when aroused.
3. *Stupor:* Appears asleep but arouses to vigorous verbal stimuli. May awaken spontaneously for brief periods, but sensorium clouded. Shows some spontaneous movements and follows some brief commands.
4. *Semicoma (light coma):* No response to verbal stimuli. Moves mainly in response to painful stimuli. Reflexes (corneal, pupillary, etc.) intact. Breathes adequately.
5. *Coma (deep or complete coma):* No spontaneous movements or arousal. Reflexes absent. Breathing impaired or absent.

---

hol or other depressant drugs causes delirium tremens, the classical example of delirium with excitement (Chap. 11). Any such state of excessive cerebral excitation may cause tremors and convulsions. Mania, characterized by pressure of speech, grandiosity, flight of ideas, hyperactivity, and insomnia, may also develop in the course of disorders that cause unconsciousness (Starkstein et al, 1990).

3. Put So (somnolence), St (stupor), SC (semicoma), or C (coma) before the appropriate statements in Table 12-3.

✓	*C*
✓	*So*
✓	*St*
✓	*SC*

TABLE 12-3 Characteristics of depressed consciousness

_____	Pt is unarousable to any stimuli and is areflexic.
_____	Pt can be aroused to normal consciousness but drifts back to sleep.
_____	Pt can be partially awakened to follow some commands but lapses quickly.
_____	Pt cannot be aroused to voice, moves mainly in response to painful stimuli and reflexes and breathing are present.

D. *The Glascow Coma Scale for grading the level of consciousness*
  1. A grading scale forces the Ex to observe systemically and accurately. I guarantee that the necessity to grade a response, as in eliciting MSRs, makes you observe better than if you do not face such a reckoning.

> *Depend on it, sir, when a man knows he is to be hanged in a fortnight, it concentrates his mind wonderfully.*
>
> **Samuel Johnson** (1709–1874)

2. For the Glascow Coma Scale, the Ex periodically grades eye opening 0–5, the best verbal response 0–5, and the best motor response to pain 0–6 (Teasdale et al, 1978). The trend lines derived from these simple tests readily disclose any deterioration or improvement. In Fig. 12-1, the trend lines document a declining level of consciousness in a Pt with cerebral edema. After the Pt received IV mannitol, a hyperosmolar agent that reduces edema, the trend lines document the abrupt improvement.

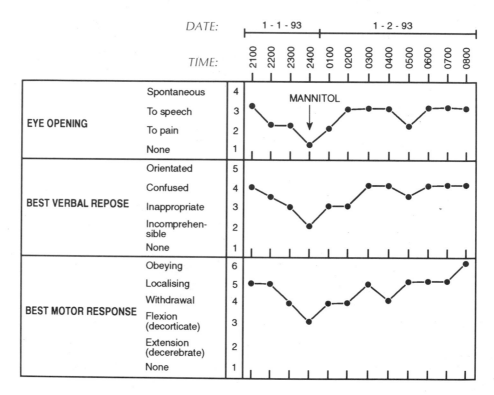

FIG. 12-1. The Glascow coma scale. Notice the declining level of consciousness until after treatment with mannitol, which reduces brain edema.

3. Like the Apgar score, the total score for the three categories provides a prognosis (Bates et al, 1991; Evans et al, 1976; Teasdale et al, 1978). A Glascow Coma Scale score of 3–8 implies a poor prognosis (Levin et al, 1992).

II. Anatomical basis of consciousness

A. *Parts of the neuraxis unnecessary for consciousness*

To identify the parts of the CNS necessary for consciousness, we will cut away and discard the parts unnecessary for consciousness. To insure your familiarity with the gross subdivisions of the CNS that we will have to cut off, review and actually draw them, as shown in Fig. 2-1. Then use scissors to cut away the parts of your drawing as described in the text.

In search of the parts unnecessary for consciousness, excise the entire spinal cord. Next excise the cerebellum. Then excise the medulla and caudal half of the pons. Surgical transection of the neuraxis at any level from the sacral cord to the midpons spares consciousness (if we artificially maintain respiration and blood pressure). (Actually go ahead and scissor these parts off of your drawing. This seeming busy work will lead to permanent retention.) The pile of parts discarded as unnecessary for consciousness now contains the entire spinal cord, medulla, caudal half of the pons, and the cerebellum. But now, complete transection of the brainstem between the midpons and the rostral end of the midbrain will abolish consciousness.

Next, instead of completely transecting the pons and midbrain, let us make partial transections to determine what must remain to support consciousness. To appreciate the partial cuts, review brainstem anatomy by drawing the generalized cross section of the brainstem (Fig. 2-14, page 55). Again, actually cut the parts off of your drawing as called for.

We find that complete transection or even removal of the entire basis of the midbrain or pons bilaterally does not abolish consciousness. If we start with a completely intact nervous system, bilateral destruction of the basis of the pons or midbrain spares vertical eye movements but causes complete paralysis of all other volitional movements. The Pt retains full sensation and full consciousness but can communicate that consciousness by the only available effector mechanism, the vertical eye movements. (See the *locked-in syndrome,* Section VII). Thus, snip off the brainstem basis bilaterally, and place it on the discard heap.

After transecting the basis, we can insert the knife blade a little deeper to transect the medial and lateral lemnisci. The Pt loses the sensations mediated by these pathways, but consciousness remains. We can then start cutting dorsally on the brainstem and transect or remove the tectum. Consciousness remains. Next, core out the cranial nerve motor nuclei. Consciousness remains. Thus, from your cross-sectional drawing of the brainstem, cut away the tectum, lemnisci, and cranial nerve nuclei and add them to the discard heap. Now, transection of the tegmentum bilaterally between midpons and rostral midbrain abruptly abolishes consciousness. For consciousness, the midbrain and rostral pontine tegmentum must remain intact (Reznick, 1983) and in continuity with the cerebrum at the diencephalon; but except for the rostral half of the pontomesencephalic tegmentum, we have discarded all other parts of the neuraxis caudal to the diencephalon.

From your original drawing, you now have left in your hand a cerebrum in continuity with its diencephalon and pontomesencephalic tegmentum. Now, we will determine the role of the remaining parts of the CNS in consciousness by transecting the diencephalon and basal ganglia at successively more rostral levels. We must insert the knife from the bottom of the cerebrum to transect these gray masses bilaterally without damaging the surrounding white matter or cortex. Bilateral transection of the diencephalon permanently and irreversibly abolishes consciousness. As we extend more rostrally into the basal ganglia, the evidence becomes a little less secure because of the lack of pure lesions in human disease. Tentatively, we can state that acute bilateral destruction of the globus pallidus and caudate nuclei also abolishes consciousness—at least, if the lesion extends a little into the neighboring diencephalon or septal region, as it usually does, or into the neighboring medial hemispheric wall (Freemon, 1971). Thus, we find that bilateral lesions at any level, from the pontomesencephalic tegmentum up through diencephalon and basal ganglia to the medial hemispheric wall, abolish consciousness (Figs. 12-2 and 12-3).

Notice in Figs. 12-2 and 12-3 that as the lesions involve structures rostral to the midbrain, particularly basal ganglia and medial hemispheric wall, they must become increasingly larger than those required in the pontomesencephalic tegmentum and diencephalon.

The next anatomical region consists of the deep white matter surrounding the diencephalon and basal ganglia, which conveys axonal circuits between those neuronal masses and the cortical neurons. If we destroy the deep white

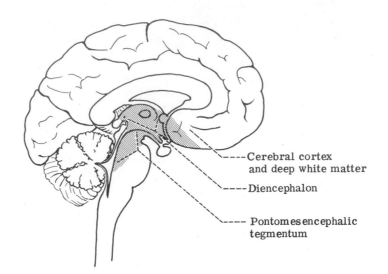

FIG. 12-2. Sagittal section of the brain. The stippled area includes the part of the pontomesencephalic tegmentum and the diencephalon in which bilateral lesions abolish consciousness.

matter of one hemisphere, or scrape off all of its cerebral cortex, or remove both white matter and cortex by a hemispherectomy, the Pt can retain consciousness (see, however, Albert et al, 1976). Actually trace a hemisphere from Fig. 12-2, cut it out, and add it to the discard heap. The discard heap of the gross parts unnecessary for consciousness thus includes _____ _____ _____ .

Ans: The spinal cord, medulla, caudal pons, cerebellum, entire basis and tectum of pons and midbrain, the lemnisci and cranial nerve nuclei, and either one of the two cerebral hemispheres.

Although we can dispense with either one of the two cerebral hemispheres, we cannot dispense with both. We can discard any pair of the frontal, parietal, occipital, and temporal lobes. We profoundly alter personality and sensorimotor functions, but consciousness per se remains. But if we remove too much of the cerebrum bilaterally, or if we scrape the cerebral cortex off of *both* hemispheres, or destroy the cortex by hypoxia or hypoglycemia, the Pt permanently loses consciousness. If we suck out the deep white matter from both hemispheres, disconnecting the cortical shell from the brainstem and diencephalon, the Pt permanently loses consciousness. Such severe, bilaterally destructive decorticating or demyelinating lesions stand in direct contrast to the tiny, confined bilateral pontomesencephalic tegmental lesions that exquisitely and selectively abolish consciousness with little effect on functions mediated through other pathways. Review Fig. 12-3 which shows the smallest, most discrete lesion that will permanently abolish consciousness.

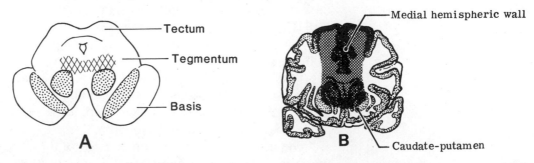

FIG. 12-3. Coronal section of the midbrain (*A*) and of the cerebrum (*B*) at the level of the caudate nuclei. The shaded area shows the sites and comparative sizes of lesions that abolish consciousness.

B. *Summary of the parts of the neuraxis necessary and unnecessary for consciousness*

1. The foregoing observations disclose that full consciousness requires the pontomesencephalic tegmentum of at least one half of the brainstem and the ipsilateral diencephalon, and most of the ipsilateral cerebral hemisphere. This may, just may, constitute the minimal amount of brain required to function as a person. Although a necessary condition for consciousness, an intact pontomesencephalic tegmentum alone is not a sufficient condition, or at least not sufficient to provide operational evidence of consciousness. That requires, in addition, a cerebral hemisphere, or most of a hemisphere with access to some effector to produce behavioral responses that signify consciousness. What is not expendable bilaterally is:

    a. Medial hemispheric wall
    b. Caudate-putamen (striatum)
    c. Diencephalon
    d. Midbrain tegmentum: Bilateral tegmental lesions of modest size completely and permanently abolish consciousness.
    e. Rostral pontine tegmentum

2. To justify your having learned the structure unnecessary for consciousness, note this supreme fact: If your Pt has a lesion confined to one of these structures and is or becomes unconscious, something else has caused the unconsciousness. The usual explanation is that the lesion has herniated or shifted the brain to compress the structures indispensable for consciousness. Without medical or surgical intervention, the Pt will die. Section III discusses these brain herniations and their clinical recognition.

C. *To prove your mastery of the neuroanatomical basis of consciousness, do these things:*

1. Enumerate the parts of the neuraxis that we can discard without abolishing consciousness. _____

Ans: *Spinal cord, medulla, and caudal half of pons (but we must support breathing and blood pressure); cerebellum; tectum; basis; lemnisci; cranial nerve nuclei of the brainstem; any pair of the four cerebral lobes, or one cerebral hemisphere (and maybe a little of the other hemisphere).*

2. Enumerate the various sites of lesions within the neuraxis that will abolish consciousness. Assume artificial support of breathing and blood pressure, insuring that the neural lesion causes loss of consciousness, not hypoxia or ischemia. _____

Ans: *Make the lesions bilaterally at any level from the rostral pontine midbrain tegmentum, diencephalon, basal ganglia, or medial hemispheric wall, including the septal region. Or destroy bilaterally the cerebral cortex or the deep white matter.*

3. State where to put the smallest lesion that will most selectively abolish consciousness. _____

Ans: *Place the lesion bilaterally in the midbrain tegmentum (Fig. 12-3A).*

4. Microscopically, the critical region for consciousness is the reticular formation of the pontomesencephalic tegmentum, as explained in Section VI of Chap. 2.

D. Operational demonstration of the pathways for consciousness

1. Insert a *stimulating* electrode into the midbrain reticular formation of an animal.
2. Apply *recording* electrodes over the scalp. The record obtained from the scalp electrodes is called an *electroencephalogram* (EEG).
3. After the animal goes to sleep, stimulate the reticular formation and observe:
   a. That the animal opens its eyes and looks around. This is the fundamental observation.
   b. That the EEG shows a distinct change in the electrical activity of the brain. This is the correlative observation (Fig. 12-4).

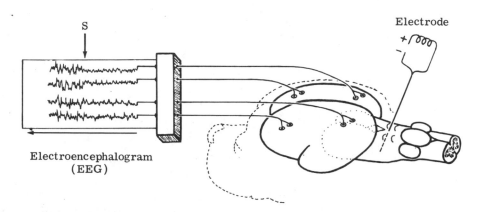

FIG. 12-4. **Notice the alerting response recorded in the EEG after stimulation of an electrode which has been inserted into the rostral reticular formation. The animal initially is asleep. S marks the point of stimulation during the EEG recording. Notice the abrupt change from the high amplitude slow waves of sleep to the low amplitude, fast activity of the waking state.**

4. After having awakened the animal with a stimulus to the reticular formation, the experimenter can greatly increase the current to make an electrolytic lesion around the tip of the electrode. The animal will lapse into unconsciousness.
5. Similarly, stimulation of the midline and intralaminar nuclei of the thalamus will produce an alerting response.
6. *Interpretation of the experiment:* Demonstration of a nonspecific ascending pathway
   a. The initial stimulation through the electrode was like throwing on a master switch: The whole brain lit up. Since the whole cortex responded, we say that a *diffuse* or *nonspecific* ascending pathway has been stimulated. Since these impulses run through the thalamus, we conclude that the experiment demonstrates an ascending reticulo-thalamo-cortical pathway. We call this entire pathway the *ascending reticular activating system* (ARAS). Although the physiologic evidence strongly points to a thalamocortical projection of the ARAS, the actual axons have yet to be demonstrated.
   b. Notice that the operational definition of the ARAS depends on two lines of evidence: Stimulation of the system ☐ heightens/ ☐ decreases consciousness, whereas destruction ☐ heightens/ ☐ decreases consciousness.

☑ *Heightens*
☑ *Decreases*

7. Give an operational definition of the ARAS based on the effects of stimulation or destruction. _____

_____

_____

Ans: The ARAS consists of the neuronal groups in the pontomesencephalic tegmentum and diencephalon which increase consciousness when stimulated and decrease it when destroyed.

E. *Demonstration of specific thalamocortical pathways*

1. The thalamocortical pathways of the sensory nuclei have a very specific, point-to-point relation to the cerebral cortex, in contrast to the ARAS, which projects diffusely or nonspecifically. To demonstrate this contrasting, specific system, do this:

    a. Insert a *stimulating* electrode into one of the sensory relay nuclei of the thalamus.

    b. Apply *recording* electrodes over the cortical receptive area of the nucleus. In Fig. 12-3, the stimulating electrode is inserted into the nucleus ventralis posterior and the recording electrodes are placed over the somesthetic receptive area in the postcentral gyrus. Study Fig. 12-5.

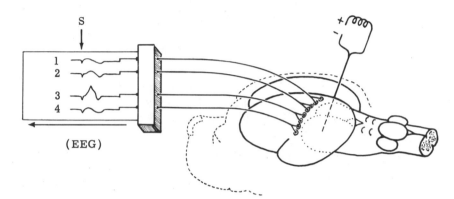

FIG. 12-5. Notice in the EEG the specific point of cortical excitation (third lead) after stimulating a thalamic sensory relay nucleus. Computer averaging is necessary with scalp recording to separate the signal from the background activity.

2. Although neuroanatomists have not identified the axons that project the diffuse, nonspecific pathway of the ARAS to the cortex, they have identified the axons of the specific thalamic relay nuclei. The specific systems are so specific that stimulation of minute retinal areas, stimulation of the cochlea by discrete sound frequencies, or stimulation of the skin of the individual digits evokes a response in a tiny, specific cortical sensory area. Review the specific thalamic sensory relay nuclei and their cortical projection areas in Table 12-4.

TABLE 12-4 Specific sensory relay nuclei of the thalamus		
Modality	Thalamic nucleus	Cortical receptive area
Vision		Calcarine cortex in _____ lobe
Hearing		Superior temporal gyrus in _____ lobe
Somatic sensation		Postcentral gyrus in _____ lobe

1. Lateral geniculate body, occipital
2. Medial geniculate body, temporal

3. N. ventralis posterior, parietal

3. The ☐ specific/ ☐ nonspecific pathways of the ARAS mediate the general state of consciousness, whereas the ☐ specific/ ☐ nonspecific thalamocortical pathways mediate consciousness of particular sensory events.

☑ *Nonspecific*
☑ *Specific*

BIBLIOGRAPHY FOR CONSCIOUSNESS

Adams R, Victor M: *Principles of Neurology* (4th ed). New York, McGraw-Hill, 1989.

Albert ML, Silverberg R, Reches A, et al: Cerebral dominance for consciousness. *Arch Neurol* 1978;33:453.

Bates D: Defining prognosis in medical coma. *J Neurol Neurosurg Psychiatr* 1991;54:569–571.

Evans BM: Patterns of arousal in comatose patients. *J Neurol Neurosurg Psychiatr* 1976;39:392–402.

Freemon FR: Akinetic mutism and bilateral anterior cerebral artery occlusion. *J Neurol Neurosurg Psychiatr* 1971;34:693–698.

Levin HS, Williams DH, Eisenberg HM: Serial MRI and neurobehavioural findings after mild to moderate closed head injury. *J Neurol Neurosurg Neuropath* 1992;55:255–262.

Lipowski ZJ: Delirium in the elderly patient. *N Engl J Med* 1989;52:578–582.

Plum F, Posner J: *The Diagnosis of Stupor and Coma* (2d ed). Philadelphia, F.A. Davis, 1972.

Reznick M: Neuropathology of seven cases of locked-in syndrome. *J Med Sci* 1983;60:67–68.

Starkstein SE, Mayberg HS, Berthier ML, et al: Mania after brain injury: Neuroradiological and metabolic findings. *Ann Neurol* 1990;27:652–659.

Teasdale G, Knill-Jones R, van der Sande J: Observer variability in assessing impaired consciousness and coma. *J Neurol Neurosurg Psychiatr* 1978;41:603–610.

III. Internal herniations of the brain

A. *Lethal consequences of space-occupying intracranial lesions:* Cerebral contusions, hematomas, abscesses, and neoplasms, either by their size or by inciting edema, increase the volume of the intracranial contents. Lesions that increase intracranial pressure cause internal shifts or herniations of the brain that compress the diencephalon and brainstem (Davis and Robertson, 1991; Plum and Posner, 1982). This compression impairs consciousness and the life-sustaining functions of breathing, blood pressure control, and temperature regulation.

B. *Anatomy of the intracranial partitions and compartments:* To understand how space-occupying lesions kill Pts, study Figs. 12-6 to 12-8, and complete the subsequent exercises.

Falx; tentorium

1. The cranial cavity is divided by tough, dural partitions called the _____ cerebri and the _____ cerebelli.

Falx cerebri

2. The dural partition that divides the supratentorial space into right and left halves is the _____.

3. The tentorium cerebelli forms a tent over the cerebellar hemispheres by inserting itself between the cerebellar hemispheres below and the

Occipital

_____ lobes above.

4. The free, medial edges of the tentorial halves form the tentorial

Notch (opening)

_____.

5. The part of the cerebellum that protrudes through the tentorial notch is the

Vermis

superior tip of the _____.

6. The tentorial notch surrounds the ☐ pons/ ☐ mesencephalon/

☑ *Mesencephalon*

☐ diencephalon.

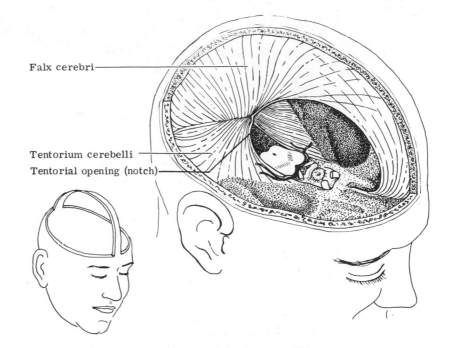

FIG. 12-6. Basket-handle dissection of the skull and removal of the cerebral hemispheres. Notice how the falx cerebri and tentorium cerebelli, folds of the dura mater, partition the intracranial space. Notice that the mesencephalon was transected from the cerebral hemispheres and left *in situ*. Locate the IIId nerve issuing from the mesencephalon, going under the posterior cerebral artery, and piercing the dura. Notice the posterior cerebral artery then passing over the free edge of the tentorium to reach the overlying temporo-occipital portions of the cerebrum.

7. In Figs. 12-6 and 12-7 notice that:
   a. The transected brainstem remains *in situ* after removal of the cerebral hemispheres, and notice that the posterior cerebral artery passes over the free edge of the tentorial notch to reach the temporo-occipital portions of the cerebrum.
   b. The IIId nerve issues from the mesencephalon and passes under the posterior cerebral artery.

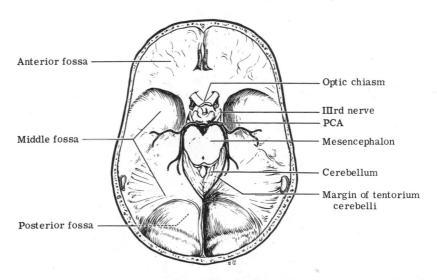

FIG. 12-7. Base of the skull after removal of the basket handle and its attached falx cerebri. The mesencephalon remains *in situ,* as in Fig. 12-6. Notice that the cerebellar vermis occupies the apex of the tentorial opening. Notice that the posterior fossa is under the tentorium. Notice the IIId nerve traveling under the posterior cerebral artery (PCA). *(Redrawn from F. Plum and J. Posner: The Diagnosis of Stupor and Coma. Philadelphia, F.A. Davis, 1966)*

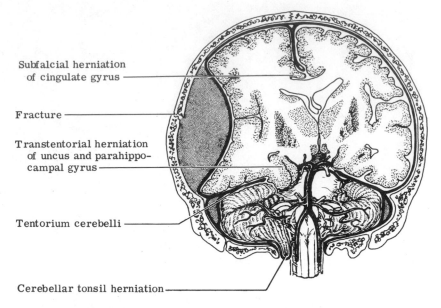

Subfalcial herniation of cingulate gyrus

Fracture

Transtentorial herniation of uncus and parahippo-campal gyrus

Tentorium cerebelli

Cerebellar tonsil herniation

FIG. 12-8. Coronal section of the head with ventral view of the brainstem and cerebrum. A large epidural hematoma has shifted the brain from right to left. Notice that the uncus has herniated over the tentorial edge on the right. Follow along the vertebral and basilar arteries to their terminal branches, the posterior cerebral arteries. Notice how the posterior cerebral artery on the right impinges on the IIId nerve. *(Redrawn from F. Netter: Ciba Symposia, (vol 18, plate XI), 1966)*

C. Responses of the fluid pools of the intracranial space to increased pressure

1. *Intracranial fluid pools.* Water comprises 80 to 90 percent of the brain. Brain water is physically incompressible and biologically relatively immobile, since it is confined within the tissue, but it increases greatly in cerebral edema. This relatively immobile brain water contrasts with the two rapidly mobile liquid pools of the intracranial space, the *intravascular blood* and the *cerebrospinal fluid* (CSF). If brain tissue swells, what will happen to the lumen of the veins and capillaries? _____.

2. From studying Figs. 12-8 and 12-9, describe what pressure does to the ventricles, sulci, and subarachnoid space of a swollen hemisphere. _____ _____.

3. Thus, the first compensation for increased pressure depends on the two rapidly mobile intracranial fluid pools, the _____.

Collapse

Collapses or displaces them

CSF and intravascular blood

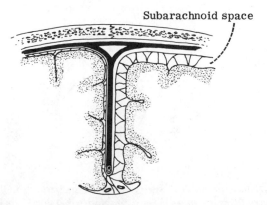

Subarachnoid space

FIG. 12-9. Coronal section through falx and adjacent portions of the cerebrum along the interhemispheric fissure. Notice that the swollen hemisphere (reader's left) has collapsed the subarachnoid space and that the cingulate gyrus has begun to herniate under the free, inferior edge of the falx.

4. The infant has additional ways to compensate for increased intracranial pressure, manifested by the following physical signs: _____
_____ .

Ans: Bulging fontanels, split sutures, and increased OFC.

Puberty (10 to 12 yr)

5. As the skull matures, it no longer yields to increased intracranial pressure. If you find split sutures on a skull radiograph of an 18-year-old Pt, the increased pressure must have started before the age of _____ .
6. If the hemispheric swelling exceeds the compensatory mechanisms in infant or adult, the affected hemisphere can only respond by herniating out of the hemicranium. Study Fig. 12-8 and state the only *two* places the shifting hemisphere can go.
   a. _____ .
   b. _____ .

Ans: Medially under the falx, or downward over the edge of the tentorial notch.

D. *Anatomy of transtentorial herniation of the cerebrum*
1. With a space-occupying lesion in one hemicranium, the bony wall of the calvarium prevents herniation or decompression outward. The cerebral hemisphere can only herniate *medially* or *downward* (Fig. 12-8).
   a. The dural membrane that opposes *medial* shift of the cerebrum is the

Falx cerebri

   _____ _____ .
   b. The dural membrane that opposes *downward* shift of the cerebrum is the

Tentorium cerebelli

   _____ _____ .
2. *Trans* means *over* or *across;* hence *trans*continental. Since part of the swollen hemisphere has shifted *across* the free edge of the tentorium cerebelli,

Transtentorial

   this lesion is called _____ *tentorial* herniation.
3. Since part of the swollen hemisphere has shifted *under* the falx cerebri, this

subfalcial (the x becomes c)

   shift is called *sub*_____ herniation.

4. Hence, the two internal herniations of a swollen hemisphere are

Transtentorial; subfalcial

   _____ herniation and _____ herniation.

5. The part of the cerebrum that undergoes subfalcial herniation is the

Cingulate

   _____ gyrus
6. The parts that undergo transtentorial herniation are the medial parts of the temporal lobe, namely the _____ and _____ gyrus.

Ans: Uncus; parahippocampal (see Fig. 12-8 if you missed).

7. Fig. 12-10 shows the brain of a Pt, as freshly removed at autopsy. Fill in the labels, and in the blanks below, describe what is wrong. _____
_____ .

Ans: The left uncus and parahippocampal gyrus have herniated across the tentorial notch, compressing the IIId nerve and midbrain.

E. *Effect of transtentorial and subfalcial herniation on consciousness.* Since subfalcial and transtentorial herniation compress the medial hemispheric wall, diencephalon, and mesencephalon, they interfere with the ARAS and alter the Pt's level of consciousness. Medial shift of the brain may correlate better with changes of consciousness than downward displacement (Ropper, 1989). Initially, the change may consist of excitement, but usually the Pt descends

Somnolence, stupor, semicoma, and coma

through the levels of decreased consciousness, namely, _____
_____ .

A. *IIId nerve*
B. *Uncus*
C. *Parahippocampal gyrus*
D. *Mesencephalon*
E. *Tentorial notch*

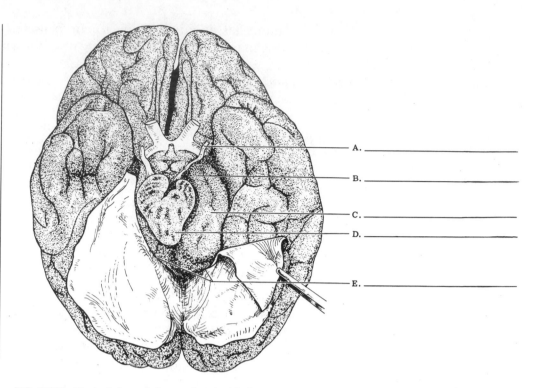

FIG. 12-10. Ventral view of the cerebrum with the tentorium cerebelli reflected on the left side. Complete the labels on the right side. *(Redrawn from T. Peele: The Neuroanatomic Basis for Clinical Neurology (2d ed). New York, McGraw-Hill Book Company, 1961)*

F. Effect of transtentorial herniation on the IIId nerve

1. As transtentorial herniation increases, the uncus displaces the posterior cerebral artery and the IIId nerve. The IIId nerve contains parasympathetic fibers which, when stimulated, cause the pupil to _____.

Constrict

2. After interruption of the IIId nerve, what happens to the pupillary size? _____. Explain. _____.

Ans: *Increases; the unopposed action of the pupillodilator muscle (sympathetic) enlarges the pupil.*

3. Since the pupilloconstrictor fibers occupy the superomedial part of the IIId nerve, the caudally displaced posterior cerebral artery impinges on them first when the temporal lobe herniates (Fig. 12-11).

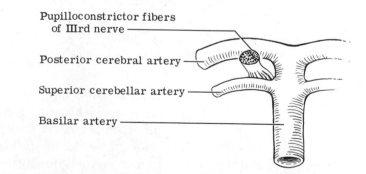

Pupilloconstrictor fibers of IIIrd nerve

Posterior cerebral artery

Superior cerebellar artery

Basilar artery

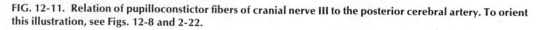

FIG. 12-11. Relation of pupilloconstictor fibers of cranial nerve III to the posterior cerebral artery. To orient this illustration, see Figs. 12-8 and 2-22.

4. In a Pt suspected of a space-occupying intracranial lesion, what would an increasing pupillary size and a decreasing level of consciousness imply?

_____

_____.

Ans: Transtentorial herniation, brainstem compression, and death

5. As transtentorial herniation advances, both of the IIId nerves may cease to function. Both pupils become *dilated* and *fixed,* no longer responding to light. Prior to dilating, the opposite pupil may go through a phase of mild constriction (Ropper, 1990). Whereas a unilateral dilated and fixed pupil announces danger requiring prompt or even heroic intervention, bilateral dilated and fixed pupils from brainstem compression are almost synonymous with death (Hasler, 1967; Walker, 1963).

G. *Effect of transtentorial herniation on motor function*
   1. Consider now a Pt with a large acute right hemisphere lesion. It would cause a ☐ left/ ☐ right-sided hemiplegia.

☑ *Left*

   2. As the herniating right hemisphere compresses the mesencephalon, the left basis gets pushed across against the opposite free edge of the tentorium on the left side, indenting the basis (Kernohan-Woltman notch). Notice in Fig. 12-7 the close relation of the basis mesencephali to the tentorial edges, affording virtually no safety factor.

   3. After compression of the left basis, the UMN fibers cannot transmit impulses. The Pt now shows a _____-sided hemiplegia in addition to the original left-sided hemiplegia. The new hemiplegia is ☐ ipsilateral/ ☐ contralateral to the right hemisphere lesion.

Right
☑ *Ipsilateral*

   4. Such an ipsilateral hemiplegia is called a *paradoxical* hemiplegia because it is on the ☐ same/ ☐ opposite side as the hemispheric lesion. Sometimes the paradoxical hemiplegia appears first, constituting a false localizing sign of the side of brain herniation.

☑ *Same*

   5. Hence, if a Pt started out with a large right hemispheric lesion and left hemiplegia, and then had a right hemiplegia, the Pt has double hemiplegia. If the double hemiplegia evolves very rapidly, the Pt might display cerebral shock. What would happen to the MSRs and tone? _____.

Decreased or absent

   6. Thus, depending on the rapidity of evolution of the lesion, the MSRs and tone may vary time to time and from side to side.
   7. Recite now the neurologic findings in cerebral herniation in respect to the IIId nerve, the ARAS, and the pyramidal tracts in the basis mesencephali. Check the preceding frames to insure that you have recited the effects correctly.

H. *Bilateral transtentorial herniation*
   1. Many pathologic conditions cause *bilateral* transtentorial herniation. The lesion may consist of cerebral edema from trauma, encephalitis, or metabolic disorders, such as uremia and hepatic coma. Of the structural lesions, head injuries, subdural hematomas, hydrocephalus, multiple metastatic neoplasms or abscesses, and intracranial hemorrhage lead the list. If both hemispheres swell, the unci and parahippocampal gyri of both sides try to squeeze down through the tentorial notch. The ring of swollen tissue acts exactly like a ligature around the midbrain, tied in a slip knot, and pulled at both ends.

2. The *coup de grace* to the Pt with transtentorial herniation, bilateral or unilateral, is mesencephalic and pontine hemorrhage (Friede and Roessmann, 1966). As the brainstem vessels become stretched and compressed by the advancing herniation, the blood flow to the stem is interrupted. The vessel walls rupture. The consequent brainstem hemorrhage is usually the terminal event that causes the Pt to die (Fig. 12-12).

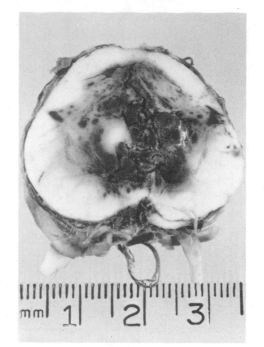

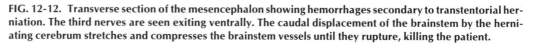

FIG. 12-12. Transverse section of the mesencephalon showing hemorrhages secondary to transtentorial herniation. The third nerves are seen exiting ventrally. The caudal displacement of the brainstem by the herniating cerebrum stretches and compresses the brainstem vessels until they rupture, killing the patient.

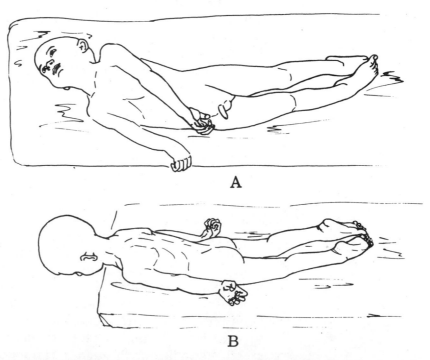

FIG. 12-13. Decerebrate posture. (*A*) Pt placed on his side. (*B*) Pt placed with his head over the edge of the table to show the rigid extension of his neck. (*Redrawn from W. Penfield and H. Jasper: Epilepsy and the Functional Anatomy of the Human Brain. Boston, Little, Brown and Company, 1954*)

I. *Decerebrate rigidity, a postural syndrome of rostral brainstem lesions*

1. *Description of the decerebrate posture.* Extensive midbrain lesions, either intrinsic or from unilateral or bilateral transtentorial herniation, disconnect the cerebrum from the rest of the brainstem, i.e., decerebrate the individual. The decerebration can, in fact, be toxic-metabolic decerebration rather than anatomic. Along with IIId nerve signs, double hemiplegia, and loss of consciousness, the Pt shows a diagnostic postural syndrome called *decerebrate rigidity.* Study Fig. 12-10 and assume the decerebrate posture yourself. Can you maintain it easily? After carefully inspecting the limb and trunk postures of the Pt, cover Fig. 12-13, and test your powers of observation by completing Table 12-5.

Closed

Extended

Extended
Extended, internally rotated
Flexed

Flexed
Extended, internally rotated
Plantar flexed, inverted (equinovarus)
Plantar flexed

TABLE 12-5 · Posture in decerebrate rigidity
The mouth is ☐ open/ ☐ closed.
The head is ☐ extended/ ☐ flexed.
The trunk is ☐ extended/ ☐ flexed.
The arms are _____.
The wrists are _____.
The fingers are _____.
The legs are _____.
The feet are _____.
The toes are ☐ plantar flexed/ ☐ dorsiflexed.

2. *Muscle tone in decerebrate rigidity.* Testing of the muscle tone of the Pt in Fig. 12-10 would disclose rigid extension of the extremities and spine, but if you once bend the part, it will yield like a clasp knife. Hence the tonic disturbance seems to combine features of spasticity and rigidity.

3. *Descriptive definition of decerebrate rigidity.* The Pt displays an involuntary posture with the
    a. Proximal joints (spine, shoulders, hips, elbows and knees) rigidly ☐ extended/ ☐ flexed.
    b. Distal joints (wrists/ankles, fingers/toes) rigidly ☐ extended/ ☐ flexed.
    c. Forearms and legs ☐ internally/ ☐ externally rotated.

☑ *Extended*
☑ *Flexed*
☑ *Internally*

4. *Pathophysiologic explanation of the decerebrate posture.* As a prelude to interpreting the decerebrate posture, review the strength of the muscle actions listed in Table 12-6. Actually test a normal subject to complete the table.

Ans: If you tested carefully, you should have checked the <u>stronger than</u> column every time.

    a. We conclude that the direction of pull of the strongest muscles determines the posture of the spine and extremities assumed by the decerebrate Pt.
    b. Fig. 12-14 shows the posture of a quadruped with decerebrate rigidity. A quadruped with decerebrate rigidity will stand, if set on its feet. Review also Fig. 7-2.

TABLE 12-6 Comparative strength of postural deviations in decerebrate rigidity

Action	Stronger than/	Weaker than/	Action
1. Jaw closure is	☐	☐	jaw opening
2. Head extension is	☐	☐	head flexion
3. Trunk extension is	☐	☐	trunk flexion
4. Arm extension is	☐	☐	arm flexion
5. Forearm pronation when the arm is extended is	☐	☐	supination
6. Wrist flexion is	☐	☐	wrist extension
7. Finger flexion is	☐	☐	finger extension
8. Leg extension is	☐	☐	leg flexion
9. Inversion of the foot is	☐	☐	eversion
10. Ankle flexion is	☐	☐	ankle extension
11. Toe flexion is	☐	☐	toe extension

☑ *Quadruped*
(Review Table 12-5 and Fig. 7-2, if you missed.)

c. The extended head, tail, and extremities, and the closed jaw of the quadruped indicate that all muscles acting to cause the decerebrate posture support the animal's posture against collapse due to the pull of gravity. These same muscles cause it to leap and locomote in defiance of gravity. Hence, we interpret decerebrate rigidity as that posture maintained by excessive contraction of the antigravity muscles of the quadruped. In general, the strongest muscles of humans are the true antigravity muscles of a ☐ quadruped/ ☐ biped.

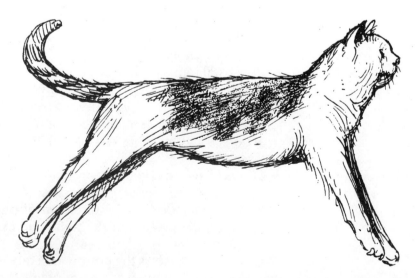

FIG. 12-14. Decerebrate posture in cat. (From L. Pollock and L. Davis: The reflex activities of a decerebrate animal. Comp Neurol 50:377–411, 1930)

d. What anatomic operation would you do to the animal to produce the posture of Fig. 12-14? _____

_____ .

5. *Role of the vestibular system in decerebrate rigidity.* After decerebration by midbrain transection interrupts the impulses descending from the cerebrum, the vestibular system becomes overactive, causing it to overstimulate or drive the powerful antigravity muscles.

a. Explain whether you should classify the decerebrate posture as a deficit or release phenomenon. _____

_____ .

Ans: Decerebrate rigidity is a new behavior, released by interruption of descending pathways.

b. Describe a surgical experiment or series of experiments to prove that the drive for the decerebrate posture comes from the vestibular system. Think carefully! _____

See next frame

_____

_____ .

c. Like any release phenomenon, decerebrate rigidity not only requires a lesion to release it, but an intact neural mechanism to produce, drive, and perpetuate it. Sherrington showed that destruction of the vestibular nerves, nuclei, or of the vestibulospinal tracts abolished the decerebrate posture. This means that activity via these tracts drives the decerebrate posture. Dorsal or ventral root transection also abolish it.

d. In order for decerebrate rigidity to appear, the critical neural structure transected or compressed is the _____; the critical neural structures which must remain intact are the _____

Midbrain

*Vestibular system,
vestibulospinal
tract, and dorsal
and ventral roots*

_____ .

6. Give a succinct clinical description of the decerebrate posture. Be sure to separate observation from interpretation. _____

_____

_____ .

Ans: The decerebrate posture consists of the rigid extension of the neck, trunk, arms, and legs with wrist pronation and wrist and finger flexion, and ankle and toe flexion with internal rotation of the feet.

7. Give the pathophysiologic interpretation of decerebrate rigidity. _____

_____

_____ .

Ans: It is a release of the antigravity posture of the quadruped, maintained by the vestibulospinal system and dorsal root afferents, after mesencephalic lesions or toxic-metabolic states that functionally decerebrate the Pt.

8. Some unconscious Pts show decerebrate posturing only in response to pain. To elicit the posture, press the ball of your thumb or a knuckle hard for several seconds against the Pt's sternum.

J. *Decorticate versus decerebrate posture*

1. It is instructive to compare the posture of decerebrate rigidity with chronic hemiplegia after the stage of cerebral shock or diaschisis in acute hemiplegia has passed (Fig. 12-15).

2. Describe the major difference in the posture of the arm in decerebrate rigidity versus hemiplegic spasticity? _____

_____ .

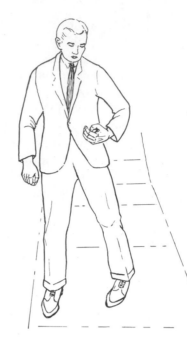

FIG. 12-15. Posture in chronic adult hemiplegia. Compare the arm position with Fig. 12-12.

Ans: The hemiplegic arm is held flexed at the elbow, rather than extended.
Otherwise, the wrist and finger postures are similar (as is the leg posture).

    K. *Respiratory and autonomic effects of brainstem lesions and transtentorial herniation*
        1. The unconscious Pt may display strong inspiratory stridor because of collapse of the oropharyngeal muscles. Simply place your fingers behind the ramus of the mandible and pull the mandible forward. The Pt will immediately breathe freer. An oropharyngeal airway then solves the problem.
        2. Lesions at various levels from the diencephalon to the medullocervical junction cause characteristic alterations in the pattern of breathing. Learn Fig. 12-16.
        3. Transtentorial herniation, by external compression, caudal displacement, and kinking of the brainstem, causes a "wave of failure" to pass caudally from diencephalon to medulla. The Pt passes in succession through the various respiratory dysrhythmias in Fig. 12-16 that reflect the effects of lesions at various rostrocaudal levels. The one type of dysrhythmia seen with intrinsic brainstem lesions but not with transtentorial herniation is apneustic breathing, C of Fig. 12-16 (Plum and Posner, 1982).
        4. The effect of transtentorial herniation or other brainstem lesions on blood pressure and pulse varies. While either hypertension or hypotension and either tachycardia or bradycardia may occur, typically increased intracranial pressure causes a slowing of the pulse rate and an increasing blood pressure (Cushing's phenomenon). Many factors, such as the ventilatory efficiency, may alter this formula. Thus, the Ex must expect changes in these vital signs and monitor them carefully.

    L. *Transforaminal herniation*
        1. *Anatomy of transforaminal herniation.* The diffusely swollen brain or the hydrocephalic brain may impose the death penalty by another mechanism. As increased pressure pushes the intracranial contents caudally, the cere-

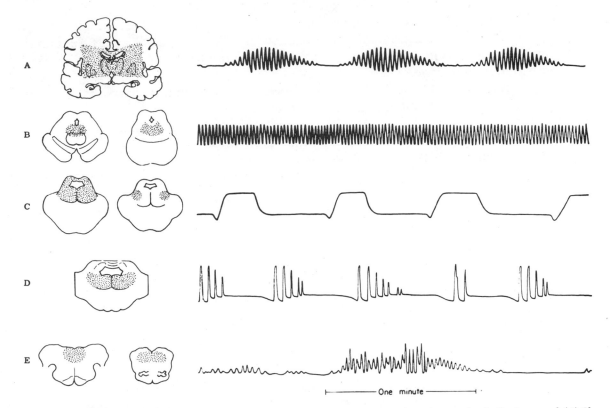

FIG. 12-16. Correlation of intra-axial brainstem lesions at successive levels, with the type of respiratory dysrhythmia caused. (*A*) Cheyne-Stokes respiration. (*B*) Central neurogenic hyperventilation. (*C*) Apneustic breathing. (*D*) Cluster breathing. (*E*) Ataxic breathing. (*Redrawn from F. Plum and J. Posner: The Diagnosis of Stupor and Coma. Philadelphia, F.A. Davis Company, 1966*)

bellum and medulla herniate into the foramen magnum. This aperture is designed to accommodate only the cervicomedullary junction.

    a. Since the caudalmost part of the cerebellum, the cerebellar *tonsil,* is the part of the cerebellum to herniate, this type of brain herniation is called *tonsilar herniation,* or *transforaminal herniation.* See the herniated right cerebellar tonsil in Fig. 12-8.

    b. Transforaminal herniation may result from expanding *supra*tentorial lesions, as of the cerebrum, or from expanding *infra*tentorial lesions, such as a cerebellar neoplasm.

  2. *The clinical syndrome of transforaminal herniation.* The clinical syndrome mimics transection of the neuraxis at the level of the medullocervical junction. The Pt becomes quadriplegic, anesthetic, and totally apneic. The Pt has complete respiratory arrest because of compression of the reticulospinal tracts that transmit the respiratory drive to the LMNs that innervate the diaphragm and intercostal muscles. Review Fig. 6-13.

 M. *Summary of the internal herniations of the brain*

  1. Name the common internal herniations of the brain. _____

    _____.

Subfalcial,
  transtentorial, and
  transforaminal

  2. Name the parts of the brain which herniate in each case. _____

    _____.

Cingulate gyrus;
  parahippocampal
  gyrus and uncus;
  cerebellar tonsil

3. State, in principle, how brain herniations kill the Pt. _____

Ans: By impairing vital functions like breathing, P rate, and BP, and ultimately by causing brainstem hemorrhage.

4. Could you test for cerebellar function in a comatose Pt? ☐ Yes/ ☐ No. Explain. _____

Ans: ☑ No. The cerebellum plays no known role in consciousness or mentation. Since the comatose Pt makes no voluntary movements, cerebellar function cannot be tested.

5. If a comatose Pt removed from a wrecked car shows distinct decerebrate rigidity only in the upper extremities with the lower extremities totally flaccid, what would be the best clinical conclusion? Think circuitry to figure out and explain the answer. _____

Ans: The Pt had suffered spinal cord transection as well as a brain injury, a not uncommon association. In this case, a single lesion does not explain the clinical picture but a single cause, trauma, does.

O. *Brain herniations: A clinical summation*

1. When any modern gladiator, a boxer, a football player, or a race driver, dies after a head injury, in sacrifice to our appetite for brutality, you can surmise that the mechanism of death was brain edema and herniation (Jordan, 1992). If we do not, as a people, value above all else the preciousness and fragility of life, one might suppose that we would, at least, value and protect the organ of advantage. (For the brain is not, as you might have misbelieved, an organ of intelligence; it functions, as Szent-Györgyi said, as an advantage-seeking organ.) The television hero or athlete stunned by a head injury who immediately resumes normal activity represents not only a cultural travesty, but also an egregious error in medical management. *Any person stunned or unconscious from a blow to the head requires careful medical observation.* The physician must recognize that any Pt with any head injury or any suspicion of a space-occupying intracranial lesion is the most imperative type of medical emergency; as imperative as cardiac arrest, respiratory arrest, or hemorrhage, which may then ensue. Almost anyone can recognize when the Pt is in coma. The physician must read the clinical warnings to anticipate when coma may evolve. That is to say, we must deal with prediction, the most difficult of all the arts. To predict the predictable and prevent the preventable, you must know how brain lesions kill and how to anticipate the circumstances and read the evolving signs that can lead to death.

2. The Ex must carefully monitor every Pt who has a potential brain herniation. Record *all* physical signs: vital signs, such as blood pressure and pulse, and physical signs such as the pupillary diameters in millimeters. Given a Pt with a head injury and left hemiparesis who is initially conscious, outline the sequence of events in an order that will predict transtentorial herniation, and list the sequence of events to death:

Answer given in next frame.

a. Consciousness: _____

b. Condition of extremities: _____

c. Pupillary changes: _____

    d. Respiration: _____

_____.

    e. Pulse and blood pressure: _____

_____.

    f. Final pathologic change in brainstem _____

_____.

3. Answers to frame 2:
   a. May have some excitement, then pathologic sleep, stupor, semicoma, and coma.
   b. Left hemiparesis may worsen, right hemiparesis appears, then quadriplegia, often followed by decerebrate rigidity and then complete flaccidity just preceding death.
   c. The right pupil becomes dilated and fixed, then the left. Both eyes become immobile.
   d. Cheyne-Stokes, central neurogenic hyperventilation, cluster breathing, and ataxic, or Biot's, respiration, and finally total apnea.
   e. Pulse and blood pressure may fluctuate, but tendency to increasing blood pressure with decreasing pulse rate.
   f. Hemorrhage into the brainstem, secondary to stretching of the brainstem vessels.
4. The time to help has essentially passed when the Pt has reached the stage of deep coma, bilateral pupillodilation, and decerebrate rigidity. At that point, many Pts are irretrievable. The Ex must have recognized the Pt's increased pressure and potential for herniation and called for neurological help. If the physicians can relieve the pressure early, the Pt recovers; if not, the Pt dies. That is why you have to understand the mechanisms we have studied and the clinical signs they produce.

REFERENCES FOR BRAIN HERNIATIONS

Davis RL, Robertson DM: *Textbook of Neuropathology* (2nd ed). Baltimore, Williams and Wilkins, 1991.

Friede R, Roessmann U: The pathogenesis of secondary midbrain hemorrhages. *Neurology* 1966;16:1210–1216.

Hasler O: Arterial pattern of human brainstem: Normal appearance and deformation in expanding supratentorial conditions. *Neurology* 1967;17:368–375.

Jordan B: *Medical Aspects of Boxing.* Boca Raton, CRC Press, Inc., 1992.

Plum F, Posner J: *The Diagnosis of Stupor and Coma* (2d ed). Philadelphia, F.A. Davis, 1982.

Ropper AH: A preliminary MRI study of the geometry of brain displacement and level of consciousness with acute intracranial masses. *Neurology* 1989;39:622–627.

Ropper AH: The opposite pupil in herniation. *Neurology* 1990;40:1707–1709.

Walker A: The syndromes of the tentorial notch. *J Nerv Ment Dis* 1963;136:118–129.

REFERENCES FOR DECEREBRATE RIGIDITY AND OTHER BRAINSTEM SIGNS OF COMA

Brendler SJ, Selverstone B: Recovery from decerebration. *Brain* 1970;93:381–392.

Halsey J, Downie A: Decerebrate rigidity with preservation of consciousness. *J Neurol Neurosurg Psychiatr* 1966;29:350–355.

Pollock L, David L: The reflex activities of a decerebrate animal. *J Comp Neurol* 1930;50:377–411.

Sherrington C: *The Integrative Action of the Nervous System.* New Haven, Yale University Press, 1947.

Zeman W, Youngue E: Decortication as a result of widespread circulatory and anoxic damage. *J Neuropath Exp Neurol* 1957;16:492–506.

IV. Neurologic examination of the unconscious Pt

A. *Introduction*

1. For the most difficult diagnostic challenge of all, I would ask you to evaluate a Pt brought in comatose off of the street, with no history available. Review the *Neurologic Examination of the Unconscious Patient* on page xxi, at the front of the text. Recite the ABCDEEs, 5H mnemonics, and review the differential diagnostic dendrogram. See also Fisher (1966) and Plum and Posner (1982) for additional descriptions of the NE in the unconscious Pt.

2. The seemingly unresponsive Pt may have a toxic-metabolic state, an anatomic lesion, trauma, or a mental illness. The Ex has to determine immediately whether either an anatomic lesion or a metabolic-toxic disorder threaten the Pt's life. Asymmetric neurologic signs, such as a hemiparesis or a cranial nerve palsy, provide the best evidence of anatomic coma. The mental disorders get sorted out in the course of the evaluation for life-threatening disorders. Mental illnesses include hysteria, malingering, and psychosis with catatonia [catatonia consists of catalepsy (waxy flexibility), negativism, mutism, posturing, and rigidity].

B. *Inspection of the comatose Pt*

1. If the Pt can breathe adequately, so can the Ex. The Ex has at least a little time for contemplation. Proceed to look for what is good and favorable and what is bad and evil. Anything that works normally, i.e., breathing, pupillary light reflexes, is good. What does not work at all signifies evil. Therefore, we extract a cosmic law about the NE of the unconscious Pt. *Whatever behavior the Pt shows, a pupil constricting or a limb moving, establishes the integrity of some neuroanatomic circuit and the function of some intact neurophysiologic mechanism.* When the Pt shows no behavior, the Ex has to decide whether this results from interruption of neuroanatomic circuits, the depth of the coma, or total effector paralysis, as in severe Guillain-Barré syndrome, or the Pt curarized for management on a respirator.

C. *"Good" behaviors disclosed by the four-glance, instant screening NE of the acutely unconscious Pt.* Given that the Pt is not comatose with no reflexes or behavior at all, the Ex can complete quite an adequate survey of the Pt's neuroanatomic circuits in four glances.

1. *Blinking or tonic closure of the eyelids.* Cranial nerves V and VII work, hence the pontine tegmentum is intact.

2. *Random slow conjugate drifts of the eyes to the sides.* Cranial nerves III, IV, and VI and the frontopontine pathway that drives eye movements work (Fig. 2-31) (Rodriguez-Barrios, 1966).

3. *Normal breathing and oropharyngeal reflexes.* Coughing, swallowing, hiccuping, and yawning: cranial nerves IX, X, and XII and the pontomedullary reticular formation and cervical and thoracic levels of the spinal cord work. (Fig. 6-13).

4. *Random spontaneous, particularly semipurposive symmetrical movements of all four extremities.* Both pyramidal tracts, from motor cortex to the sacral level of the spinal cord, work (Fig. 2-28). At this point, the Ex knows that the whole length of the neuraxis more or less works. If after the four glances, the Ex then finds intact pupillary, corneal, vestibular, and audito-palpebral reflexes, further documenting the functional integrity of the midbrain, pons, medulla, and their cranial nerves, the Ex has completed a cerebral-cortex-to-sacral-cord screening NE that virtually excludes a large anatomic lesion as the cause for the unconscious episode.

5. In addition to random or semipurposive movements, the unconscious Pt may show myokymia, and a variety of mutterings, shivers, shudders, twitches, and myoclonias difficult to classify, as well as more patterned movements of choreiform, athetoid, or dystonic type; or aimless picking at the bedclothes, a sign called *carphologia*. These actions are of uncertain localizing or prognostic import.

D. *"Bad" behaviors disclosed by inspection of the unconscious Pt*
   1. Worst of all is no behavior whatsoever: flaccid eyelids and no pupillary responses, no eye drifts (in deep coma and brain death, the eyes return to and remain fixed in the neutral position), no breathing, and no spontaneous movements; a totally flaccid, dumped-in-a-heap posture, and no response to any stimulus. But the Ex does not know whether the absence of behavior results from neurologic destruction with neural shock, widespread LMN paralysis, or merely the depth of the coma—e.g., as in a massive overdose of barbiturates.
   2. Next worst is a sustained or driven posture: sustained deviation of the head and eyes, or decerebrate rigidity.
      a. Focal seizures may cause deviation of the head and eyes. In the absence of convulsions, you would expect a destructive lesion in the conjugate gaze center in the ☐ ipsilateral/ ☐ contralateral posterior frontal region, or in the ☐ ipsilateral/ ☐ contralateral half of the pons.

☑ *Ipsilateral*
   ☑ *Contralateral*
Review Figs. 2-31 and 5-2

VI and VII (Fig. 2-31)

      b. List which cranial nerve(s) would most likely be paralyzed by a lesion affecting the region of the pontine conjugate lateral gaze center.

      _____.

   3. *Prognostically evil findings.* Of Pts who fail to recover corneal and pupillary light reflexes within 24 h, virtually all die, but no prognostic formula can, in fact, unerringly predict death. Prognostic scales have an error rate of 5 to 20 percent when applied to nontraumatic coma and cannot be used as an excuse to terminate life-support systems prematurely (Bates, 1991).

E. *Detecting hemiplegia in the unconscious Pt.* The Ex looks for asymmetry of movement, posture, and muscle tone. Unless deeply comatose, the unconscious Pt with intact pyramidal tracts moves all four extremities spontaneously or in response to pain. The acute, severe anatomic lesions that cause unconsciousness, or the hemiplegia that follows focal seizures (Todd's paralysis), usually cause flaccid hemiplegia (cerebral shock). The face and extremities on the intact side continue to show some muscle tone. A tip-off posture of flaccid hemiplegia is that the leg rests in external rotation, with the foot turned out. Hemiplegia and a broken hip are the two commonest reasons for this posture. Flaccidity on one side and absence of spontaneous or pain-induced movements identify hemiplegia.

1. *Flaccidity of the cheek.* When the unconscious hemiplegic Pt inhales, the cheek on one side sucks in; when the Pt exhales, that cheek puffs out. It will be on the ☐ hemiplegic/ ☐ nonhemiplegic side. Explain. _____

_____ .

Ans: ☑ *Hemiplegic. The buccinator and other facial muscles on the hemiplegic side have a flaccid paralysis from cerebral shock. Therefore, the cheek on the hemiplegic side sucks in and puffs out. Facial muscles on the other side have tone.*

2. *The eyelid-release test*
   a. Review of facial motor innervation
      (1) Make a drawing to show the UMN and LMN innervation of the right side of the face in Fig. 12-17. Check against Fig. 6–3*B*.

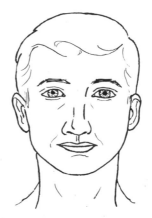

FIG. 12-17. **Blank to draw in the UMN innervation of the VIIth nerve nucleus and the LMN innervation of the facial muscles.**

      (2) Recall that the LMNs for the orbicularis oculi muscle may receive innervation by many crossed as well as uncrossed UMNs. Hence, in acute hemiplegia, after sudden interruption of UMNs, the eyelid shows ☐ flaccid/ ☐ spastic weakness. The eyelid-release test demonstrates this, because even in the unconscious (but not completely comatose) Pt, the eyelids close because of tonic innervation; i.e., by a positive drive.

☑ *Flaccid*

   b. *Procedure for eyelid-release test.* Gently pull both eyelids up with your two thumbs and then release them simultaneously (Fig. 12-18).
   c. *Results.* The eyelid of the hemiplegic side glides down slowly while the opposite lid closes rapidly—in fact, almost snaps shut, unless the Pt is deeply comatose. Why does the eyelid on the nonhemiplegic side close faster? _____

_____ .

Ans: The orbicularis oculi muscle of the normal side is not paralyzed and retains muscle tone.

3. *The limb-dropping tests.* The limb-dropping tests demonstrate flaccid paralysis of the extremities.
   a. *The wrist-dropping test.* Grasp both of the Pt's forearms just proximal to the wrist. Hold the forearms vertical, as in Fig. 12-19. The hemiplegic wrist drops at right angles, while the nonhemiplegic wrist, having some tone, remains to some degree vertical.

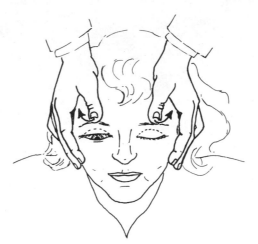

FIG. 12-18. Eyelid-release test in a comatose Pt with right hemiplegia. Standing at the head of the Pt's bed, the Ex elevates both lids and releases them simultaneously. The lid of the hemiplegic side closes slowly because of flaccidity of its orbicularis oculi muscle, while the lid of the normal side closes briskly because of tonus in its orbicularis oculi muscle.

b. *The arm-dropping test.* Grasp both forearms, as in the wrist-dropping test, and release them simultaneously. The hemiplegic arm drops limply, while the normal arm glides or floats down (see Fig. 12-20). Lift the arm only a few inches and cushion its drop. Beware of ulnar nerve injury.

c. *The leg-dropping test.* Crook the Pt's knees on your arm. Extend one leg first and drop it; then the other (Fig. 12-21). The Ex can both see and hear the difference as the hemiplegic leg drops more rapidly to strike the bed.

d. The dropping tests depend on the principle of asymmetry of muscle tone. For correct interpretation, the nonhemiplegic side must have some muscle tone. Hence, deep coma or LMN paralysis invalidates the tests.

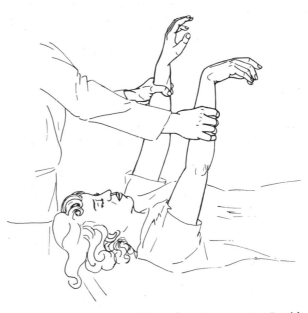

FIG. 12-19. The wrist-dropping test for flaccid hemiplegia in a comatose Pt with right hemiplegia.

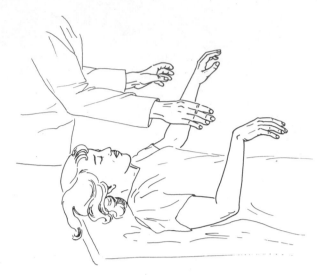

FIG. 12-20. The arm-dropping test for flaccid hemiplegia in a comatose Pt with right hemiplegia.

4. Summarize the methods of detecting acute flaccid hemiplegia in an unconscious Pt. _____

_____

_____.

Ans: Inspect for asymmetry of movement and puffing out of one cheek. Test for asymmetry of muscle tone by manipulation of the extremities and by the eyelid- and extremity-dropping tests.

F. *Resistance to movement: Paratonia*
1. The Pt with paratonia resists movement of any part of the body in any direction. It commonly occurs in unconscious Pts. It is as if the Pt divines every movement you impose and automatically counteracts it.
2. Paratonia, like any resistance dependent on muscular contraction, does not occur on the side of acute flaccid hemiplegia, or in the deeply comatose Pt, when all tone is lost. The novice often misidentifies the nonhemiplegic side as hemiplegic because of mistaking paratonia for the increased tone of a UMN lesion.

G. *Resistance to movement: Nuchal rigidity and meningeal irritation signs*
1. *Definition of nuchal rigidity.* The term *nucha* refers to the back of the neck. Nuchal rigidity means that neither the Pt nor the Ex can flex the Pt's head

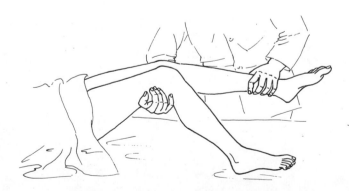

FIG. 12-21. The leg-dropping test for flaccid hemiplegia in a comatose Pt with right hemiplegia.

because of reflex spasm of the nuchal (extensor) muscles. Irritation of the subarachnoid space, most commonly by inflammation (encephalitis or meningitis), or subarachnoid blood, causes nuchal rigidity.

2. *Suspension or tethering of the spinal cord.* The spinal cord is buoyed by the surrounding CSF and suspended, or tethered, in position by its attachment to the medulla, by the nerve roots, and by special suspensory ligaments, the denticulate ligaments (Emery, 1967) (Fig. 12-22).

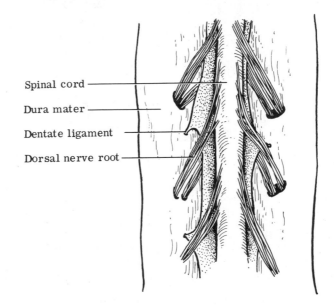

Spinal cord
Dura mater
Dentate ligament
Dorsal nerve root

FIG. 12-22. Dorsal view of the spinal cord, with the dura split open. Notice the dentate (denticulate) ligaments that suspend the spinal cord.

3. *Biomechanics of neck flexion and extension.* By understanding the mechanics involved in eliciting nuchal muscle spasm, you get a bonus: You learn how to position a Pt who has suffered a vertebral fracture and how to interpret Lhermitte's sign. Study Figs. 12-23 and 12-24.

   a. The line A–A′ in Fig. 12-23 impales the neuraxis. It simulates a lever with the fulcrum at the top of the vertebral column. Thus, flexion of the head causes ☐ relaxation/ ☐ stretching of the spinal cord.

☑ *Stretching*

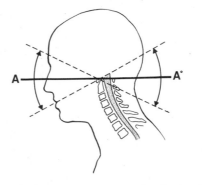

A ――――――――――――――― A°

Fig. 12-23. Sagittal section of the head to show the effect of head extension and flexion in stretching and relaxing the spinal cord. Imagine a steel rod driven through the head (A-A′). It acts as a lever with the fulcrum over the body of the first cervical vertebra.

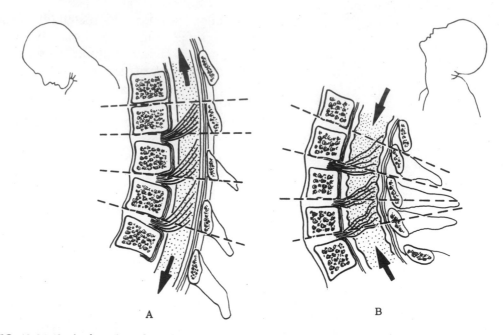

FIG. 12-24. Sagittal sections through the cervical spinal cord and vertebrae. (*A*) Head flexion. (*B*) Head extension. Notice that the spinal cord and nerve roots are stretched and lengthened in *A*, and relaxed and pleated in *B*.

    b. During neck flexion and extension, movement occurs not only between the skull and first cervical vertebra, but also between all other cervical vertebrae. The neck does not flex as though hinged at one point: When bent, it curves like a sapling. The interrupted lines in Fig. 12-24*A* and *B* show the actual changes in vertebral angulation with flexion-extension and the accompanying changes in tension on the nerve roots and spinal cord (Breig, 1978; Goel, 1989).

  4. *The mechanism of spasm of the nuchal (extensor) muscles: The pain-spasm-pain cycle.*

    a. During ordinary movement, the cord changes from a relaxed accordion-like wrinkling to simple straightening (Fig. 12-24), with little or no actual traction on the spinal cord or roots (Breig, 1978). When, however, roots, meninges, and cord are inflamed and swollen, the ordinarily innocuous act of flexing the head puts tension on the inflamed structures. It's like pressing on a boil. As long as the part with the boil remains still, it does not hurt. Movement of the part, however, placing tension on the swollen tissues, causes intense pain. Any pain of this type elicits immediate muscle spasm, which acts to prohibit the painful movement (O'Connell, 1946; Wartenberg, 1950). If you have ever tried to take a deep breath when you had a "stitch" in your side from a pleuritic rub, you will know how effectively pain inhibits the muscular contraction which causes it. Other examples of pain-avoiding muscle spasm are the abdominal wall rigidity of peritonitis, and back rigidity from lumbar sprains, a "crick in the back."

    b. With inflamed meninges, the movement which causes pain from tension on the cord and nerve roots would be neck ☐ extension/ ☐ flexion.

☑ *Flexion*

  H. *Technique of testing for nuchal rigidity*

    1. With the Pt supine and relaxed, place your hand under the Pt's occiput and gently attempt to flex the neck. Normally, it bends freely. If the Pt has nuchal rigidity, the neck resists flexion and the Pt winces with pain. If

nuchal rigidity is severe, the Ex can lift up the Pt's head and trunk as if the spine were a rigid rod or as if the Pt were a statue (Fig. 12-25*A*).

2. Because true nuchal rigidity indicates meningeal irritation, the Ex must distinguish it from other forms of cervical rigidity. With true nuchal rigidity, the neck resists only flexion. The neck moves freely through rotation and extension, because they do not put tension on the spinal cord. To demonstrate that rigidity affects only the nuchal muscles, place your hand on the Pt's forehead. Passively roll the Pt's head from side to side to demonstrate free head rotation, in spite of the resistance to flexion (Fig. 12-25*B*). Then, lift the Pt's shoulders to let the head fall backwards, testing for freedom of extension (Fig. 12-25*C*).

3. *Cervical* rigidity means any resistance to neck movement, in any direction. In contrast, *nuchal* rigidity specifically means resistance to neck flexion, that is, rigidity of the ☐ back/ ☐ front of the neck due to meningeal irritation. Fig. 12-26 lists some of the numerous causes of cervical rigidity.

☑ *Back (nape)*

I. *Neck manipulation and spinal cord injury*

   2. *Contraindications to neck manipulation.* Study Fig. 12-27. It shows a fracture dislocation of the cervical vertebrae but can represent any mass lesion, such as a tumor or herniation of an intervertebral that compromises the cervical cord.

     a. Head flexion would place tension on the swollen spinal cord. The cord will impinge on any intruding mass. For this reason, do not test for nuchal rigidity in a Pt suspected of a cervical cord lesion. Also suspect any Pt unconscious from trauma to have a cervical fracture and obtain cervical spine films (Trunkey, 1991; Gisbert et al, 1989). Be cautious about any neck manipulation in any unconscious Pt, particularly a neonate. The pain-protective reflexes may be abolished.

     b. In addition to cervical cord injury, neck manipulation may compress the vertebral artery (Fig. 12-32) and cause vertebrobasilar stroke (Garg and Walshe, 1993), or cause vascular insufficiency of the cord (Linssen et al, 1990). This complication also follows chiropractic manipulation, as explained in section X, G, 3.

   2. *Positioning of a Pt with known or suspected cervical cord injury.* Your natural tendencies urge you to place an injured Pt supine with the head flexed on a pillow; exactly the wrong position. In a suspected cervical cord injury, splint and transport the Pt with the neck in a position to reduce tension on the cord—in other words, in a neutral or slightly _____ position.

Extended

   3. *Lhermitte's sign after neck flexion.* Neck flexion in the alert Pt may cause a shocklike sensation extending from the neck to the feet. Coughing, sneezing, or straining may elicit the same sensation. The explanation is mechanical stretch of the cord in the presence of a cervical cord lesion, causing irritation of the sensory pathways. It is common in multiple sclerosis (Gutrecht, 1989).

J. *Review of nuchal rigidity*

   1. In nuchal rigidity, the neck moves freely in all directions except for _____.

Flexion

   2. State the maneuvers to show that a Pt with resistance to neck flexion has nuchal, and only nuchal, rigidity. _____

_____

_____

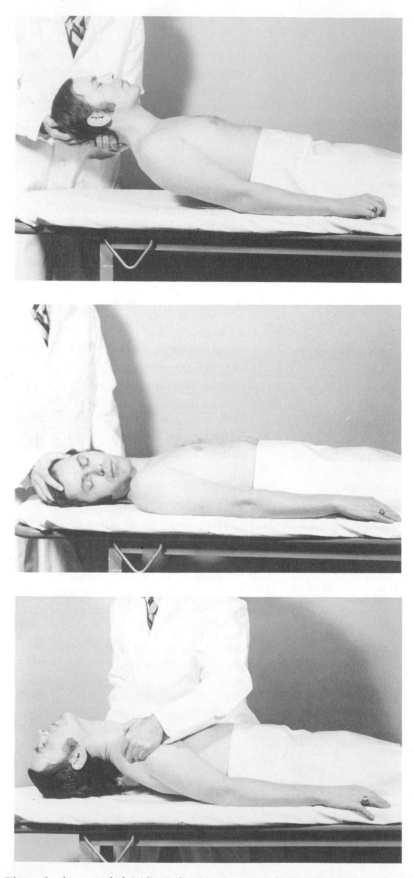

FIG. 12-25. Diagnosis of pure nuchal rigidity, indicative of meningeal irritation. (*A*) The neck strongly resists flexion, often to the degree that the Ex can actually pick up the Pt's head and spine like a statue. (*B*) The neck rotates freely in spite of extreme nuchal rigidity that resists flexion. (*C*) The head falls back freely when the Ex lifts the Pt's shoulders.

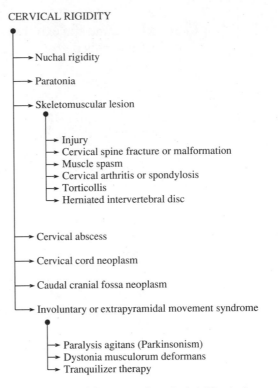

CERVICAL RIGIDITY

→ Nuchal rigidity

→ Paratonia

→ Skeletomuscular lesion

→ Injury
→ Cervical spine fracture or malformation
→ Muscle spasm
→ Cervical arthritis or spondylosis
→ Torticollis
→ Herniated intervertebral disc

→ Cervical abscess

→ Cervical cord neoplasm

→ Caudal cranial fossa neoplasm

→ Involuntary or extrapyramidal movement syndrome

→ Paralysis agitans (Parkinsonism)
→ Dystonia musculorum deformans
→ Tranquilizer therapy

FIG. 12-26. Differential diagnosis of cervical rigidity (reference only).

Ans: With the Pt supine, roll the Pt's head from side to side and lift the shoulders to allow the head to drop back, thus showing free movement in all directions except flexion.

Subarachnoid Meningitis and subarachnoid hemorrhage

3. Then, and only then, is it a reliable sign of an irritative process in the _____ space, the most common causes of which are _____.

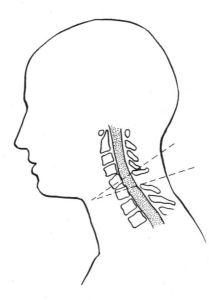

FIG. 12-27. Fracture-dislocation of C₅ on C₆. The displaced vertebrae have impinged on the contused and swollen cord.

Paratonia

4. If the head of the Pt with decreased consciousness resists movement in all directions, and the extremities do likewise, then the Pt has the generalized hypertonia called _____.

K. *Confirmatory signs of meningeal irritation: Brudzinski's and Kernig's signs*
1. *Brudzinski's sign.* When testing for nuchal rigidity, watch for adduction and flexion of the legs (Brudzinski's sign) as you attempt to flex the head (Wartenberg, 1950). Why would the Pt's knees flex? _____
_____.

Ans: Flexion of the neck places tension on the entire cord and roots (review nerve root stretching tests, Fig. 10-7 if you missed). Flexion of the legs reduces stretch on nerve roots.

2. *Leg raising tests.* With the Pt supine, do the bent-knee and straight-knee leg raising tests of Kernig and Laseague (Fig. 10-7). Meningeal irritation causes the Pt to resist leg movement in both cases.

L. *Absence of meningeal irritation signs in the presence of meningeal irritation.* The usual meningeal irritation signs may fail to occur in three circumstances: infancy, senility, and coma. In these Pts, the Ex has to tap the subarachnoid space with a needle to diagnose inflammation or subarachnoid hemorrhage. Chapter 13 discusses indications and contraindications for a lumbar tap.

M. *Opisthotonos, a driven posture*
1. First of all, learn to pronounce the word correctly: ah-piss-*THAH*-tonos, not oh-*PISS*-tho-tonos.
2. *Definition.* Opisthotonos consists of a bowed-backward, or hyperextended, position, resembling a "wrestler's bridge" (Fig. 12-28).

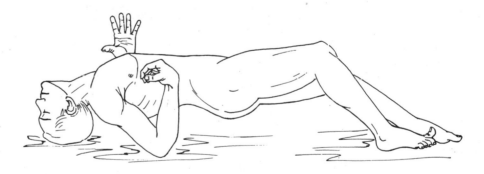

FIG. 12-28. Severe opisthotonus. (Redrawn from Dorland's Illustrated Medical Dictionary. Philadelphia, W.B. Saunders Co., 1965)

3. *Causes.* Opisthotonos results from overcontraction of the immensely powerful extensor muscles of the spine. It occurs with meningeal irritation, decerebrate rigidity, tetanus, and strychnine intoxication; thus, from at least three different pathophysiologic mechanisms. Opisthotonos also occurs in hysteria and catatonic schizophrenia, conditions without a demonstrable lesion (Fig. 12-29).
a. In meningeal irritation, opisthotonus results from spasm of the powerful extensor muscles, splinting the neck and back against flexion, which causes pain. We can regard it as a pain-protective reflex posture in these cases.

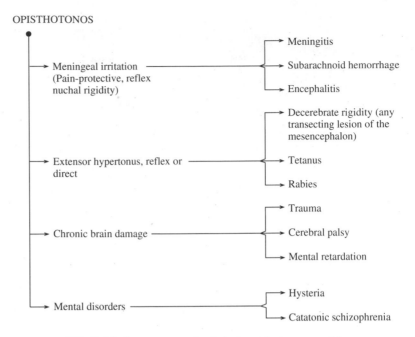

FIG. 12-29. Some causes of opisthotonus (reference only).

b. In decerebrate rigidity, the opisthotonic posture results from the hypertonus of the quadrupedal antigravity muscles, driven by the vestibular system after an anatomic midbrain lesion or metabolic lesion has inactivated or disconnected the cerebrum from the brainstem.

c. In tetanus and strychnine intoxication, muscle stretch reflexes and LMN excitability increase tremendously. All skeletal muscles become extremely hypertonic. Tetanus toxin, in addition to its central excitatory effects, also has a contractile action on muscles, causing them to remain cramped even after transection of their nerves (Dastur et al, 1977). When all muscles contract maximally, the strongest muscles dictate the posture by overpowering their weaker antagonists. However, in tetanus, in particular, local factors based on variability in the excitability of the LMN pools and the direct cramping action of the toxin may cause violations of the strongest-muscle law. Thus, as shown in Fig. 12-25, the arm flexors may overcome their stronger antagonists, the extensors. If you want to know what the opisthotonic Pt suffers, lie down supine, extend your neck and legs into the wrestler's bridge position, clench your teeth (lockjaw), and contract every muscle in your body as hard as you can for one minute.

4. In summary, opisthotonos results from at least three different pathogenic mechanisms.

a. In decerebrate rigidity: _____

_____.

b. In meningeal irritation: _____

_____.

c. In strychnine or tetanus intoxication: _____

_____.

a. Hypertonus of antigravity muscles.
b. Reflex pain-protective extensor spasm
c. Increased reflex and muscular irritability

REFERENCES FOR NEUROLOGIC EXAMINATION OF THE UNCONSCIOUS PATIENT

Fisher CM: The neurological examination of the comatose patient. *Acta Neurol Scand* 1969;45(suppl 36):1–56.

Rodrigues-Barrios R: The study of ocular motility in the comatose patient. *J Neurol Sci* 1966;3:183.

Plum F, Posner J: *The Diagnosis of Stupor and Coma.* (2d ed). Philadelphia, F.A. Davis, 1982.

REFERENCES FOR MENINGEAL IRRITATION SIGNS: NUCHAL RIGIDITY AND OPISTHOTONOS

Breig A: *Adverse Mechanical Tension in the Central Nervous System: An Analysis of Cause and Effect.* New York, Wiley, 1978

Dastur FD, Shahani WT, Dastoor DH, et al: Cephalic tetanus: Demonstration of a dual lesion. *J Neurol Neurosurg Psychiatr* 1977;40:782–786.

Emery J: Kinking of the medulla in children with acute cerebral oedema and hydrocephalus and its relationship to the dentate ligaments. *J Neurol Neurosurg Psychiatr* 1967;30:267–275.

Garg B, Walsh L: Submitted to *Neurology,* 1993.

Gisbert VL, Hollerman JJ, New AL, et al: Incidence and diagnosis of C7-T1 fractures and subluxations in multiple trauma patients: evaluation of the advanced trauma life support guidelines. *Surgery* 1989;106:702–708.

Goel VK, Weinstein JN: *Biomechanics of the Spine: Clinical and Surgical Perspective.* Boca Raton, CRC Press, 1989

Gutrecht JA: Lehrmitte's sign: from observation to eponym. *Arch Neurol* 1989;46:557–558.

Linssen WHJP, Praamstra P, Fons JM, et al: Vascular insufficiency of the cervical cord due to hyperextension of the spine. *Ped Neurol* 1990;6:123–125.

O'Connell J: The clinical signs of meningeal irritation. *Brain* 1946;69:9–21.

Thorner J: Modification of meningeal signs by concomitant hemiparesis. *Arch Neurol* 1948;59:485–495.

Trunkey D: Initial treatment of patients with extensive trauma. *N Engl J Med* 1991;324:1259–1263.

Wartenberg R: The signs of Brudzinski and Kernig. *J Pediatr* 1950;37:679–684.

V. Sensory examination of the unconscious Pt

A. *First principles*

1. *Necessity for effector integrity.* Bedside testing of sensation in the unconscious Pt requires observing some motor response. Three conditions may reduce or block a response: LMN paralysis, UMN paralysis with cerebral shock, or simply the depth of coma. If no response occurs, then the Ex does not know whether the afferent or efferent limb of the arc has failed. To bypass the necessity for intact effectors, the Ex can assess the integrity of sensory pathways by electronically recording evoked responses to somatosensory (SSER), visual (VER), and auditory stimuli (BAER) (Chap. 13).

2. *Follow a rostrocaudal routine.* As with an alert Pt, the Ex adopts a rostrocaudal routine to test the sensory systems of the unconscious Pt. Start with the rostralmost cranial nerves and proceed caudally over the body. Skip cranial nerve I.

B. *Cranial nerve II and the pupillary light reflex*

    1. The Ex tests cranial nerve II indirectly by the pupillary light reflex. Thus, in the unconscious Pt, the Ex tests cranial nerves II and III simultaneously.

    2. In Fig. 12-30, draw the pupilloconstrictor reflex pathway. Start, as usual, at the receptor and trace through the pathway.

Compare your drawing with Fig. 4-30.

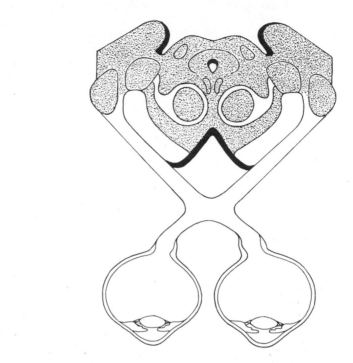

FIG. 12-30. Blank for drawing the pathway of the pupilloconstrictor reflex. Start with a retinal neuron.

    3. *Abnormal pupillary responses in the unconscious Pt.* Measure and record the size of the pupils in millimeters. Before concluding they do not react, darken the room completely, then suddenly turn on the overhead lights and flash a flashlight in the eyes while watching with a magnifying glass. Many factors may alter pupillary size (Table 12-7).

C. *Cranial nerve V.* Test the afferents of V by the corneal reflex, by painful compression in the supraorbital notch, and by trying to elicit a jaw jerk (Fig. 7-6). To test the afferent arc of the Vth nerve by pain requires VIIth nerve function to express a trigeminofacial reflex.

    1. *Corneal reflex.* Test with a wisp of cotton, as in the conscious Pt.

    2. *Supraorbital compression test for V–VII reflex*

        a. Press your thumbnail strongly into the Pt's eyebrow over the superciliary notch, the exit site of the ophthalmic division of V. Locate your own notch by pressing the ball of your thumb from medial to lateral along your eyebrow. Then press your fingernail in until you feel pain.

        b. The expected response in an unconscious Pt is an *ipsilateral* facial grimace. Hence, the Ex can test each half of the face separately. In the comatose Pt with acute hemiplegia, the grimace would be absent or weaker on the ☐ hemiplegic/ ☐ nonhemiplegic side. Explain. _____

Ans: ☑ Hemiplegic. *After acute UMN lesions, the excitability of reflexes is temporarily reduced during the phase known as cerebral shock.*

TABLE 12-7 Pupillary findings in the unconscious Pt		
Size and reactions	Toxic-metabolic agents	Anatomic lesions
Widely dilated, nonreactive	Strong cholinergic blocker or sympathomimetic drugs	Midbrain failure or bilateral IIIrd nerve lesions
Widely dilated but reactive	Mild anticholinergics found in some OTC sleeping & cold medications; adrenergic vasopressors	May mean early midbrain failure
Midposition or mildly dilated (4–6 mm) and sluggish or nonreactive	Glutethimide (Doriden®)	May mean both sympathetic and parasympathetic paralysis; Adie's syndrome
Pupilloconstriction	Normal sleep, anoxia, and uremia; glaucoma drugs or other parasympatho-mimetics	Interruption of sympathetic pathways
Pinpoint but reactive if bright light used	Opiates	Massive pontine lesion, frequently hemorrhage, that disrupts descending sympathetic pathways

    c. If the Ex suddenly and unexpectedly flicks the closed eyelashes of the Pt in feigned coma, the Pt often shows an exaggerated response with grimacing and head retraction. This is practically never seen in organic coma (Wiggs, 1973).

D. *Auditory division of VIII (auditopalpebral reflex.* Test by a sudden loud sound, such as a clap or clanging pans, and observe the Pt for a startle response.

E. *Vestibular division of VIII.* Two tests, caloric irrigation and the counter-rolling test, elicit a vestibulo-ocular reflex that causes conjugate deviation of the eyes. The receptors for the tests are essentially the cupulae of the semicircular canals, but the cristae and neck proprioceptors may add somewhat to the response (Beuttner and Zee, 1989). The vestibular nuclei relay the vestibular impulses through the MLF to activate the VIth and IIId nerve nuclei.

    1. *The counter-rolling test for the vestibulo-ocular reflex (doll's eye test, or oculocephalic reflex).*

        a. Principle of the test. If you have an old-fashioned doll, hold it up in front of you. If you turn the doll's head *down,* the eyes will turn *up* to remain looking at you in the eye. If you turn the doll's head *up,* the eyes will rotate *down* to remain looking at you in the eye. Counterweights behind the eyes cause this counter-rolling action, which essentially keeps the eyes on the visual target when the head moves.

        b. Technique for the counter-rolling test. Hold the Pt's head in a neutral position with your hands and briskly rotate it to the *right* and *left* and *up* and *down,* and stop it in each rotated position. For example, rotate the head to the right and stop it in that position. During the initial rotation to the right, the eyes counter-roll *against* the direction of head turning, to the left relative to the head, but actually they simply maintain their original position. As the Ex holds the head in the rotated position, the eyes quickly turn and align straight ahead from the new head position. Failure of the eyes to counter-roll indicates failure of the vestibulo-ocular reflex.

2. *Review of caloric irrigation*

a. *Indication.* Do caloric irrigation when the counter-rolling test fails. Caloric irrigation provides a more powerful stimulus than head turning, but the counter-rolling action added to caloric irrigation is more effective than either alone (Fisher, 1969).

b. *Precaution.* What precaution must you take before injecting water into the external auditory meatus? _____
_____.

Ans: *Inspect it, and remove wax and inspect for otitis or a perforated eardrum. The Pt's coma might have come from extension of a middle-ear infection into the brain.*

c. *Technique.* Review the technique for caloric irrigation from Chap. 7. Give details of position and materials to be used. _____
_____.

Ans: *Flex the supine Pt's head 30 degrees. Irrigate the auditory canals with 100 ml of water at 30°C over a period of 40 sec or with 5 ml of ice water.*

d. *Normal response to cold caloric irrigation.* The Pt shows nystagmus featured by slow deviation of the eye ipsilaterally, and quick, saccadic jerks that restore the eyes to the primary position. As the coma deepens, the saccade disappears, while the vestibular deviation remains. In yet deeper coma, the deviation lessens until no response is obtained at all, even though the pathways remain anatomically intact.

e. Describe how to analyze the absence of any response to caloric irrigation of either ear. _____
_____
_____.

See next frame.

f. Think through the reflex arc and consider the various possible reasons for absence of a response: The stimulus may have been inadequate. Try colder water and irrigate longer. The Pt's labyrinths are inexcitable, or the VIIIth nerves are interrupted. The vestibular nuclei, or MLF, are interrupted by an extensive tegmental lesion. The peripheral nerves to the ocular muscles are interrupted, or neuromuscular transmission has failed. The Pt may be in a stage of profound coma, or brain dead. Obviously, any response provides more useful information than no response.

g. *Significance.* Normal pupillary reactions to light and full normal conjugate counter-rolling of the eyes in response to the vestibulo-ocular stimuli virtually exclude an anatomic lesion of the pontomesencephalic tegmentum as the cause for the unconsciousness. The Pt has a supratentorial lesion, or metabolic-toxic coma. Fixed eyeballs, thus no vestibulo-ocular reflex, with normally reactive pupils, suggests depressant drugs—generally, barbiturates.

3. Name the two methods of testing the comatose Pt for the integrity of the MLF in its course through the tegmental core of the brainstem. _____
_____.

Caloric irrigation and the counter-rolling test.

4. Which method should you choose to test the MLF in a Pt unconscious from head trauma? ☐ caloric irrigation/ ☐ counter-rolling test. Explain. _____
_____.

Ans: ☑ *Caloric irrigation. Do not manipulate the neck in a Pt suspected of head trauma, because of the possibility of a cervical fracture.*

5. An alternative to caloric irrigation is galvanic stimulation of the labyrinth (Toglia et al, 1981).

F. *Cranial nerves IX and X.* Spontaneous swallowing or groaning constitutes a sufficient test. Actually eliciting the gag reflex may induce vomiting and aspiration of stomach contents into the lungs.

G. *General somatic sensation*

1. To test the somatic pathways in unconscious Pts, the Ex applies stimuli that would be perceived as painful by the conscious Pt. Make a fist and press your knuckles strongly against the Pt's sternum. Observe for an arousal response with eye opening or decerebrate posturing.

2. Test for localized pain responses by stimulating each extremity separately. Pinch the Pt's fingernails or toenails hard, or press them with the rubber tip of a pencil. To insure a painful stimulus, the Ex must apply the pinch correctly. Grasp your left thumbnail between the tip of your right thumbnail and index finger and pinch it hard. You may or may not feel much pain. Next grasp the left thumbnail by placing the center of the tip of the right thumb over the margin of the left thumbnail where it attaches to the flesh, and this time squeeze and torque, or twist, the left nail, as though trying to screw on a bottle cap. Try the technique with other fingers. With practice, you can learn to torque only the fingernail, not the whole digit, which might injure the Pt's finger joints.

3. As an alternative pain stimulus, try pinching the Pt's skin between your thumb tip and index finger. Avoid pinpricks (because of AIDS) or the use of your fingernails, which may leave wounds. Try the various ways of testing facial and body pain on yourself to learn the proper strength of stimulus to use.

4. Do not overdo pain testing in the Pt suspected of feigned coma. The Pt may have a steely resolve not to respond. Sudden, unexpected stimuli, such as flicking a closed eyelid, are more likely to elicit a response than extremely strong ones (Wiggs, 1973).

REFERENCES FOR SENSORY TESTING OF THE UNCONSCIOUS PATIENT

Buettner UW, Zee DS: Vestibular testing in comatose patients. *Arch Neurol* 1989;46:561–563.

Fisher CM: The neurological examination of the comatose patient. *Acta Neurol Scand* 1969;(suppl 36)45:1–56.

Toglia JU, Adam RU, Stewart G: Galvanic vestibular tests in the assessment of coma and brain death. *Ann Neurol* 1981;9:294–295.

Wiggs JW: Detection of feigned coma. *N Engl J Med* 1973;289:379.

VI. Factors that compound and complicate the neurologic examination of the unconscious Pt

A. *The MSRs and toe signs.* You may wonder why I have waited so long to discuss the MSRs and toe signs, that prove so valuable in the alert Pt. Because of cerebral shock, the unconscious Pt may have decreased, equal, or increased MSRs after UMN interruption, or no MSRs depending on the depth of coma. Even when the MSRs are unequal, the Ex does not know whether one side is pathologically depressed or the other pathologically hyperactive. Depression of consciousness for any reason, even deep sleep in some individuals, may cause bilateral extensor toe signs. This is not to say that the Ex neglects the MSRs and toe signs as valueless and unworthy of testing. They may well disclose a diagnostic pattern which supports conclusions from inspection and other sources. This does say that in coma, neither the presence nor the absence of the typical UMN signs have the significance that they do in the alert Pt.

B. *Pre-existing neurologic signs.* Some relatively common pre-existing conditions may confuse the diagnosis. The apparent unconsciousness may be the result of petit mal, or psychomotor seizure status epilepticus; the failure to react to sound may represent pre-existing deafness; the immobile eye with the nonreactive pupil may be a glass eye; the Pt may have congenital ptosis or anisocoria; the pupils may react sluggishly, and the MSRs may be absent because of Adie's syndrome; and the hemiplegia may be a postictal paralysis after a focal seizure (Todd's paralysis); or the Pt may have had a pre-existing hemiplegia or other neurologic signs before the coma. Is the coma just another complication or a new illness entirely? Mild disuse atrophy, brisk MSRs, and spasticity, particularly of the fingers, will identify a pre-existing hemiplegia.

C. *How to address the unconscious Pt: The law of respect.* Because of the difficulties in judging the level of consciousness, the Ex must never, *never* make flippant or pejorative remarks at the bedside of a presumably unconscious or anesthetized Pt. Pts often hear and remember more than expected (Baier and Schomaker, 1990; Cheek, 1960). *Always assume that the Pt hears and understands everything said at the bedside.* Some authors recommend that the physician, ward personnel, and family always address the Pt by name and talk to the Pt as if he were conscious (La Puma et al, 1988). Although such stimulation may not speed recovery (Pierce et al, 1990) at least it does not violate the first principle of medical practice: primum nonnocere. Addressing unconscious Pts by name and avoiding thoughtless comments at least causes no harm and does affirm the Pt as a human being rather than as a carcass.

REFERENCES FOR HOW TO ADDRESS THE UNCONSCIOUS PATIENT

Baier S, Schomaker MZ: *Bed Number Ten: A Patient's View of Long Term Care.* Boca Raton, CRC Press, 1990.

Cheek DB: What does the surgically anesthetized patient hear? *Rocky Mtn Med J* 1960; 57:49–53.

La Puma J, Schiedermayer DL, Gulyas AE, et al: Talking to comatose patients. *Arch Neurol* 1988;45:20–22.

Pierce JP, Lyle DM, Quine S, et al: The effectiveness of coma arousal intervention. *Brain Injury* 1990;4:191–197.

VIII. The locked-in syndrome (deafferentated state, ventral pontine syndrome)

A. *Clinical features*

1. Bilateral extensive lesions—infarction, trauma, abscess, hemorrhage, demyelination, or neoplasm—may destroy both pyramidal tracts in the basis pontis or midbrain (Chia, 1991; Feldman, 1971; Resnick, 1983; Turazzi and Bricolo, 1977). The Pt suffers complete bilateral hemiplegia, anarthria, aphagia, and incontinence. The only volitional movements possible

are vertical eye movements. Automatic breathing continues. The Pt retains full consciousness and sensation because the lesion spares the tegmentum and its contained lemnisci. Volitional vertical eye movements remain since the pathways enter the pretectum and tectum rostral to the lesion, but the lesion interrupts the conjugate lateral gaze pathways to the pons (Fig. 2-31). In those rare instances where the lesion destroys the pyramidal tracts at midbrain level, the Pt may also retain volitional blinking and horizontal eye movements (Chia, 1991).

2. The Pt communicates consciousness by vertical eye movements, the only volitional effector mechanism remaining, using upward movements for "Yes" and downward for "No." Otherwise, the Pt's consciousness, devoid of any efferent pathways to other effectors, remains "locked-in."

3. If unrecognized by the Ex, the locked-in state condemns the Pt to the cruelest of existences. Perfectly conscious and in possession of all senses and faculties, the Pt cannot avoid even the trifling annoyances. The Pt cannot adjust a heel to relieve pressure, nor scratch an itch, nor flick a fly from the face, nor voluntarily swallow to relieve a flooded pharynx. Although thought and emotion remain as powerful as ever, the Pt cannot utter the faintest whisper nor write a single letter. Even the total helplessness is not the worst of it, if others make unintended but dehumanizing remarks at the bedside, as if the Pt were a non-person. Moreover, since a Pt may pass through the locked-in state during recovery from coma (Turazzi and Bicolo, 1977), the Ex must always anticipate the return of sentiency and monitor for it daily by meticulous NEs.

REFERENCES FOR THE LOCKED-IN SYNDROME

Chia LG: Locked-in syndrome with bilateral ventral midbrain infarcts. *Neurology* 1991;41:445–446.

Feldman M: Physiological observations in a chronic case of "locked-in syndrome." *Neurology* 1971;21:459–478.

Reznick M: Neuropathology in seven cases of locked-in syndrome. *J Neurol Sci* 1983;60:67–78.

VIII. The persistent vegetative state (PVS)

A. *Definition.* Jennet and Plum (1972) defined the *PVS* as a persistent state following coma, characterized by eye opening and ". . . a return of wakefulness accompanied by an apparent total lack of cognitive function" with no evidence of "a working mind." In essence, the Pt, while appearing awake, remains unconscious, thus implying the separation of these two functions.

1. *Persistent* emphasizes that the PVS has already lasted for some weeks, and implies that the Pt may remain that way for an extended period.

2. *Vegetative* emphasizes the assumption that the Pt, devoid of awareness or mind, exists only physically, retaining only autonomic, vegetative, or reflex functions, such as BP control, breathing, digestion, and automatic elimination (Munsat et al, 1989).

3. Some states, the *akinetic mutism* of Hugh Cairns (1941; 1952), the decorticate or *apallial state* of Kretschsmer (Dalle et al, 1977), and the coma vigile of the French, resemble, or are synonymous with, the PVS, but Adams and Victor (1989) identify coma vigile with the locked-in syndrome.

B. *Pathogenesis of the PVS.* A catastrophe, e.g., severe hypoxia, head trauma, or massive infarction, has caused coma and permanent bilateral diffuse damage, usually at multiple levels from the rostral brainstem through diencephalon, basal ganglia, deep white matter, and cerebral cortex. After such a catastrophe, the stage of eyes-closed unconsciousness usually lasts no more than a month. Then the Pt will enter the stage of eyes-open unconsciousness, the so-called PVS. Pts with progressive cerebral degenerative diseases may also end in a vegetative state.

C. *Clinical features of the PVS*
   1. PVS Pts exhibit apparent sleep-wake cycles, but even though their eyes open, the Pts remain mute and completely devoid of any verbal or nonverbal communication, or of any purposeful or adaptive behavior that offers operational proof of consciousness.
   2. PVS Pts may blink, move their eyes spontaneously, and may fixate and pursue to some degree. They do not actively fixate and selectively move the eyes from target to target, which would imply consciousness. Vestibulo-ocular reflexes generally remain.
   3. PVS Pts will awaken or, at least, open their eyes to putatively painful stimuli. They extend or flex their limbs in response to pain but show no purposive or adaptive avoidance. They fail to orient actively to light, sound, or touch, but may startle in response to these stimuli.
   4. PVS Pts are akinetic or hypokinetic. Although the Pt may display more or less severe paralysis, spasticity, rigidity, or paratonia and sometimes hypotonia, the akinesia is out of proportion to and not directly caused by the UMN syndrome. They cannot do any self-help tasks such as dressing or feeding.
   5. PVS Pts retain many autonomic and somatic reflexes. They are incontinent of urine and feces but generally support their own BP and respiration.
   6. PVS Pts show many of the primitive reflexes reviewed in Table 11-5: grasping, sucking, automatic yawning, and chewing, but not purposeful chewing and swallowing. Feeding is by tube or gastrostomy. Some Pts display the spontaneous crying or laughing of pseudobulbar palsy (Higashi et al, 1977).

D. *Prognosis for survival and recovery from the PVS.* Operational proof of consciousness has returned to Pts who have been in the PVS for as long as 18 to 36 months (Arts et al, 1985; Higashi et al, 1981; Rosenberg, 1977). Seen in this light, the PVS may represent a phase, after coma, preceding the return of consciousness. For these reasons, the Ex must periodically repeat the NE in all Pts with altered consciousness and must never hastily dismiss the Pt as a "vegetable" or too quickly render a DNR, or disconnect judgment. The burden does not rest on the Pt to prove consciousness and personhood, but on the neurologic evaluation of the Ex to refute it. If all of this makes you feel uncertain and humble about our ability—yours and mine—to judge consciousness, I won't worry about you: You have the right attitude for a physician.

REFERENCES FOR THE PERSISTENT VEGETATIVE STATE

Adams R, Victor M: *Principles of Neurology* (4th ed). New York, McGraw-Hill, 1989.

Arts W, van Dongen H, van Hof-van Duin J, et al: Unexpected improvement after prolonged post-traumatic vegetative state. *J Neurol Neurosurg Psychiatr* 1985;48:1300–1303.

Cairns H, Oldfield R, Pennybacker JB, et al: Akinetic mutism with an epidermoid cyst of the third ventricle. *Brain* 1941;64:273–290.

Cairns H: Disturbances of consciousness with lesions of the brain stem and diencephalon. *Brain* 1952;75:109–146.

Dalle Ore G, Gerstenbrand F, Lucking CH, et al (eds): *The Apallic Syndrome.* New York, Springer-Verlag, 1977.

Higashi K, Hatano M, Abiko S, et al: Five-year follow-up study of patients with persistent vegetative state. *J Neurol Neurosurg Psychiatr* 1981;44:552–554.

Jennett B, Plum F: The persistent vegetative state: A syndrome in search of a name. *Lancet* 1972;1:734–737.

Munsat TL, Stuart WH, Cranford RE: Guidelines on the vegetative state: Commentary on the American Academy of Neurology statement. *Neurology* 1989;39:123–124.

Rosenberg GA, Johnson SF, Brenner RP: Recovery of cognition after prolonged vegetative state. *Ann Neurol* 1977;2:167–168.

IX.   The neurologic examination in the diagnosis of brain death

A. *Traditional definition of death.* The traditional definition of death reflected the Aristotelian idea that placed consciousness and, therefore, personhood in the heart. Until about 1960, physicians generally pronounced a person dead after the heartbeat and breathing had irreversibly stopped—that is to say, when these functions did not recommence spontaneously.

B. *Changes in the definition of death necessitated by advances in scientific knowledge and technology*
   1. The advance in scientific knowledge consisted of finally acknowledging the brain as the site of consciousness and of personhood.
   2. The two advances in technology consisted of:
      a. Techniques to maintain or restart breathing and the heartbeat when, formerly, they would have irreversibly stopped.
      b. Techniques of organ transplantation (first kidney transplant in 1954; first heart transplant in 1967). Harvesting of organs requires prompt, absolute determination of brain death. These developments made the traditional definition of death obsolete.
      c. The United States now accepts death as the irreversible cessation of all brain function, including the brainstem (Walker, 1985). The United Kingdom and some other countries define death as irreversible cessation of all brainstem function.

C. *The brain-death protocol (BDP) and ethical considerations in brain death*
   1. The BDP (Table 12-8) outlines a sequence of operations that enable physicians to recognize and certify—in a word, *diagnose*—that the death of the brain and, therefore, of the person has taken place. The physician has no ethical responsibility or purpose in maintaining a brain-dead body, and may end all therapy and support systems, and harvest organs for transplantation.
   2. The BDP utilizes exactly the same principles and procedures that are required to diagnose any other condition, e.g., gangrene of the leg or hepatitis. *The process of diagnosing brain death and terminating support for a brain-dead body is entirely separate from and has nothing to do with euthanasia.* Euthanasia means killing a person who has a living brain. After brain death, no person remains to be killed.

TABLE 8 Criteria for the brain death protocol

A. *Primary clinical criteria*
   1. The Pt has suffered a clinical disaster that could cause brain death and is completely comatose with no respiration or other movements that could arise in the brain.
   2. The Pt is receiving artificial respiration and is adequately oxygenated.
   3. The Pt has a minimum core body temperature of 36.1° for a child or 32.2° for a mature individual.
   4. The Pt is normotensive (but may require dopamine, etc., for support), and is in as good a metabolic balance as the circumstances allow.
   5. The Pt has no significant level of depressant or neuroparalytic (synaptic-blocking) medications. Determine by history, chart review, and toxicology screen.
   6. The Pt shows no brainstem functions whatsoever.
      a. Absolute coma
      b. Midposition or dilated pupils, nonreactive to light, not paralyzed by neuroactive drugs
      c. Absolutely no spontaneous or induced eye movements
      d. Absolutely no response to Vth nerve stimulation: no glabellar blink, corneal reflex, supraorbital pain response, jaw jerk, faciociliary (pupillodilation) reflex, or oculocardiac reflex
      f. Absolutely no spontaneous or reflex facial movements
      e. Absolutely no oropharyngeal responses: no gag reflex, tongue thrusting, sucking, chewing, snouting, or rooting; no tongue movements
      f. Absolutely no auditopalpebral or vestibulo-ocular reflexes
      g. Complete apnea on adequate testing by temporary stoppage of the respirator
   8. A second complete NE done 12 to 24 h after the first demonstrates absolutely no responses.
B. *Ancillary diagnostic tests for brain death*
   1. Isoelectric EEG
   2. Absence of cerebral blood flow by radionuclide or Doppler studies or direct angiography

---

D. *The assumptions underlying the BDP are*
   1. Since personhood and consciousness reside in the brain, the death of the brain is the death of the person, irrespective of the state of the other organs.
   2. Competent physicians can reliably—essentially, infallibly—distinguish a live brain from a dead brain. The living brain, if at the right temperature and not simply depressed by toxic-metabolic states, displays:
      a. Clinically demonstrable functions.
      b. Recordable electrical activity.
      c. Blood flow.
   3. Conversely, a dead brain displays:
      a. No clinically demonstrable function.
      b. No recordable electrical activity.
      c. No blood flow.

E. *Causes for brain death and initiation of the BDP.* The medical catastrophes which commonly lead to life-support systems and may cause brain death are hypoxia, irreversible brain edema, head injuries, and necrotizing meningitis or encephalitis. The Pt is always intubated for mechanical ventilation, is catheterized, and has an intravenous or intra-arterial line to monitor and control the BP and metabolism. The attending physician who suspects brain death requests a consultation by a specialist in neurology or neurosurgery. The physician does not generally request a BDP until at least 12 to 24 h after the medical catastrophe that jeopardized the brain, to allow some time to assess any potential for recovery of the brain.

F. *Role of the neurologic specialist in the BDP*

1. The neurologist completes a printed BDP that lists the criteria for brain death (Table 12-8). Steps 2–5 of Table 12-8 insure that the brain is not too cold nor too depressed by metabolic imbalance or drugs, nor too poorly oxygenated to display functions if it remains alive. The Ex must exclude neuromuscular-blocking drugs that would prevent the motor responses relied on to demonstrate brain function.

2. The Ex does the most searching cranial nerve examination possible (Table 12-8, steps 6a–g). Since the endotracheal tube obstructs visibility in the mouth, the Ex inserts a gloved finger along the side of the tongue and palpates it for any movements and then stimulates the palatal arch for a gag reflex. The Ex decides whether to order an EEG or blood flow study (Plum and Posner, 1982; Walker, 1985).

G. *Apnea testing in the BDP*

1. Finally, if the NE, EEG, or flow study fail to demonstrate any brain function, the Ex tests for permanent apnea. *Any* brain function shown by the NE or the laboratory tests terminates the BDP at that point, obviating the apnea test. The Ex tests for apnea last because it is the only test of the BDP that can cause harm. Hypoxia during apnea testing can cause ventricular fibrillation and cardiac arrest and may add further anoxic insult to any surviving brain tissue.

2. For apnea testing, the Ex turns off the ventilator for 3 to 10 min in order to achieve a CO_2 level of 60 mmHg or more that provides a maximum stimulus to the pontomedullary respiratory centers (Gutmann and Marino, 1991; Marks and Zisfein, 1990). The Ex checks for any respiratory efforts by placing one hand flat, spanning the lower ribcage and abdomen, and the other on the mouth, jaw, and neck muscles. Palpation provides a more sensitive and certain way to detect slight movement than sight. The Ex cannot maintain absolute vigilance by sight for many minutes, but can do so by employing touch.

3. The neurologic specialist repeats the NE and the apnea test in no less than 6 h, preferably 12 to 24 h later, depending on circumstances.

H. *What constitute the minimum criteria to diagnose brain death?*

1. If the NE discloses no evidence of function after two NEs separated by 12 to 24 h, some physicians will then diagnose brain death. They consider the NE as the necessary and sufficient condition.

2. Other physicians, with whom I agree, regard the NE as a necessary condition to diagnose brain death, but prefer one of two further safeguards (see, for example, the Pt of Ringel et al, 1988):

   a. An isoelectric EEG, which shows no cerebral electrical activity.

   b. Absence of cerebral blood flow as proven by radionuclide, or direct, angiography, or Doppler flow studies.

3. These ancillary procedures prove useful if something prevents a full, adequate NE, such as severe burns of the face and head, or traumatic destruction of facial parts.

4. Radionucleide scan or EEG may be added to conclude the BDP after only one NE in order to facilitate organ transplantation rather than waiting for a prolonged period for a second clinical examination (Ashwal and Schneider, 1989).

I. Rationale for involving more than one physician in the BDP
Involvement of at least three separate physicians—the attending physician, the neurologist, and radiologist or electroencephalographer—to diagnose brain death increases the probability that at least one of them will be honest, competent, and unpurchasable. Then, if a pathologist does an autopsy, a fourth physician insures the validity of the diagnosis. The pathologist, by gross and microscopic examination, can determine whether the brain had died many hours before removal, as distinguished from one subjected to prompt fixation shortly after death (Walker, 1985). The involved physicians do *not* meet as a committee and do not "vote" on whether the Pt's brain is dead. They all ascertain independently of each other that brain death criteria have been met, according to the techniques which each knows and understands best. With these safeguards, the diagnosis of brain death then becomes as infallible as possible.

J. Brain death protocol in infants. Because of presumably greater resistance to hypoxia, the BDP for infants, particularly prematures, is somewhat more conservative than for older Pts (Ashwal and Schneider, 1989; Ashwal, Schneider, and Thompson, 1989; Kohrman and Spivack, 1990).

K. Pitfalls and precautions in the diagnosis of brain death
   1. The two greatest pitfalls in the diagnosis of brain death are hypothermia or an overdose of depressant drugs. In both circumstances, the NE may show no brain function, and the EEG may be isoelectric, *yet the Pt may recover completely.* Nuclide scans or direct angiography will still demonstrate cerebral blood flow in these Pts who show no clinical or electrical evidence of brain function, but whose brains remain alive. And consider this scenario: A murderer who wanted to make a Pt appear brain dead could administer atropine to block pupillary and cardioinhibitory responses and curarize the Pt to block skeletomuscular responses. Such a Pt would have no effector responses and meet brain death criteria on the purely clinical examination, but the EEG would demonstrate electrical activity, and the radionuclide study would demonstrate cerebral blood flow.
   2. The physician insures a rational response to the BDP by informing the family on a day-to-day basis of the Pt's condition and prognosis. The family must understand that the purpose of the BDP is to verify beyond doubt that the person has already died and that continued support of the remaining organs is futile. Otherwise the family may misperceive termination of support as an effort to save money for an insurance company or the hospital, to provide organs for transplantation, or to commit euthanasia or genocide.

REFERENCES FOR BRAIN DEATH

Ashwal S, Schneider S: Brain death in the newborn. *Pediatrics* 1989;84:429–437.

Ashwal S, Schneider S, Thompson J: Xenon computed tomography measuring cerebral blood flow in the determination of brain death in children. *Ann Neurol* 1989;25:539–546.

Gutmann DH, Marino PL: An alternative apnea test for the evaluation of brain death. *Ann Neurol* 1991;30:852–853.

Kohrman MH, Spivack BS: Brain death in infants: Sensitivity and specificity of current criteria. *Pediatr Neurol* 1990;6:47–50.

Marks SG, Zisfein J: Apneic oxygenation in apnea tests for brain death: A controlled trial. *Arch Neurol* 1990;47:1066–1068.

Plum F, Posner J: *Diagnosis of Stupor and Coma* (2d ed). Philadelphia, F.A. Davis, 1982.

Ringel RA, Riggs JE, Brick JF: Reversible coma with prolonged absence of pupillary and brainstem reflexes: An unusual response to a hypoxic-ischemic event in MS. *Neurology* 1988;38:1275–1277.

Walker AE: *Cerebral Death* (3d ed). Baltimore, Urban and Schwarzenberger, 1985

X. The neurologic examination in intermittent disturbances of consciousness: syncope, fainting, or blackout spells

A. Definition. Syncope is a sudden, temporary loss and return of consciousness, not caused by epilepsy.

B. Proximate pathophysiologic mechanisms of syncope. Syncope, whether psychogenic or organic, usually results from cerebral ischemia induced by:

   a. Vagal inhibition of the heart, causing bradycardia-asystole
   b. Loss of vasoconstrictor tone by sympathetic inhibition or insufficiency
   c. Mechanical decreases in cerebral blood flow because of pooling of blood in the large venous tributaries with inadequate cardiac output or inadequate arterial flow (as in transient ischemic attacks)
   d. Cardiac dysrhythmias

C. Inciting factors for syncope (Fig. 12-31)

   1. *Psychogenic syncope* results from an identifiable emotional stimulus. Look for anxiety, fright, or secondary gain.
   2. *Neurogenic syncope.* An identifiable physical event serves as a stimulus. Look for the inciting stimulus, such as cough syncope, carotid sinus hypersensitivity, etc. This type of syncope and psychogenic syncope act through

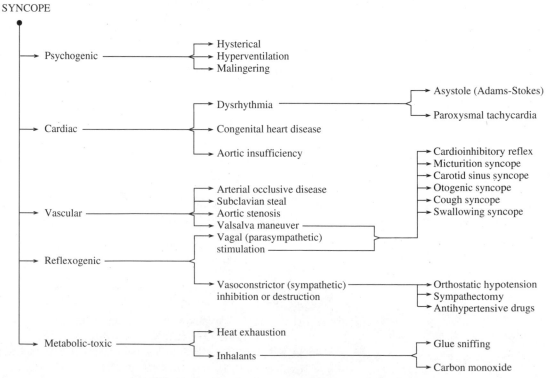

FIG. 12-31. Common types of syncope (reference only).

vasovagal mechanisms (Arnold et al, 1991). The syncope evolves usually over minutes with premonitory feelings of fear, anxiety, impending doom, dizziness, and nausea. Cholinergic stimulation predominates, producing sweating, increased peristalsis, salivation, and bradycardia. The definition of vasovagal syncope differs from author to author (Eagle and Black, 1983).

3. *Hypovolemic syncope* results from inadequate circulation of blood. Look for severe anemia, or the mechanical insufficiency in the heart and vessels, or in the return of blood to the heart. This category includes orthostatic hypotension, parade-ground syncope, and micturition syncope.

4. *Cardiac dysrhythmia syncope* results from a disturbance in impulse generation or transmission in the heart (Fujimura et al, 1989). Look for the heart disease underlying it. Of special importance, look for Adams-Stokes AV block and for the prolonged QT interval-syncope syndrome, since treatment of it prevents death. Syncope frequently requires a cardiac workup (Fujimura et al, 1989; Kulbertus and Frank, 1988; Natelson, 1985).

D. *Historical factors in syncope*
1. *Critical historical data.* Since syncope has so many causes, the Ex must rely on the history to delimit the proper steps in the physical examination. Most important of all, learn the mode of onset. *The clue to the cause comes from how the attack starts, not how it ends.* The critical questions are:
   a. What symptoms, posture, activities, and social circumstances prevail when the attacks come on? Is the Pt standing, sitting, moving, changing position, coughing, urinating, or hyperventilating?
   b. Is the Pt alone or with people, and, if with people, which ones?
   c. Does each attack follow the same pattern?
   d. What happens during the attack: falling, convulsive movements, sweating, cyanosis, etc.?
   e. What are the events of the recovery stage?
   f. Insure that you have obtained a detailed step-by-step beginning-to-end description from the Pt and observers.
2. *Reproducing the circumstances of the attack.* Try to reproduce as closely as possible the circumstances of the attack. If the Pt reports that a posture, such as head turning, elicits an attack, have the Pt turn the head. If hyperventilation or coughing precedes the attack, have the Pt hyperventilate or cough. If the Pt faints in the presence of his mother, observe him in the presence of his _____.

Mother

E. *Observation of the Pt during an attack.* If the Ex has the fortune to witness an attack, have the Pt describe the symptoms—dizziness, weakness, nausea, flashing lights, etc. Protect the Pt during the unconscious phase.
1. Place the Pt on a soft surface.
2. Insure that the Pt has an open airway. Turn the Pt's head to the side to prevent aspiration in case of vomiting.
3. Check vital signs, blood pressure, pulse, respiratory rate, pupillary size, muscle tone, and reflexes.
4. Until you establish a diagnosis, draw a blood sample for hypoglycemia or hypocalcemia whenever you observe any attack that alters consciousness, and consider giving IV glucose.

F. *Psychogenic syncope and hyperventilation syncope*
1. Some emotion-provoking event—the sight of blood, a needle prick, or bad news—triggers psychogenic syncope. For repeated, inappropriate psycho-

genic syncope, investigate the Pt's emotional status. Emotional illness never manifests solely by syncope. It is only one shadow in the pattern of emotional turmoil (Leis et al, 1992).

b. Hysterical attacks usually occur in the presence of people emotionally entangled with the Pt. At the end of the NE, call in the family to see how the family and Pt interact. The Pt may faint on the spot, thus clinching the diagnosis. Organic syncope is not "socially dependent."

c. Preceding psychogenic attacks, Pts commonly hyperventilate. When they fall, they usually do not hurt themselves nor become incontinent. Often, as in the swaying (Romberg) test, the Pt conveniently falls into the observer's arms. In organic attacks, the fall often injures the Pt, but this distinction is by no means absolute.

d. Always ask about changes in breathing and any associated symptoms (Hoefnagels et al, 1991), and consider doing the hyperventilation test (Chap. 9).

F. *Mechanical or hydraulic hypovolemic syncope.* In these types of syncope, pooling of blood in the veins results in inadequate cardiac output.

1. *Micturition syncope.* During urination, particularly with a very full bladder, the Pt faints (Lyle, 1961). Release of a large volume of fluid from the bladder and sudden relaxation of the abdominal wall drops abdominal pressure. The sudden drop in abdominal pressure allows blood to stagnate in the tributaries of the inferior vena cava, curtailing venous return to the heart. Also, cardioinhibitory reflexes may arise from the bladder itself (Lukash et al, 1964). The same drop in abdominal pressure causes syncope after rapid removal of ascitic fluid from the abdomen.

2. *Parade-ground syncope.* If a person stands still for a period of time, as a soldier on a parade ground, blood pools in the inferior vena cava and its tributaries in the lower extremities. After the person faints and becomes horizontal, blood returns to the circulation, and the person recovers promptly.

3. *Orthostatic syncope (orthostatic hypotension)*

   a. Upon suddenly arising from a sitting or reclining position, the Pt feels giddy or may faint. The BP has dropped rather than automatically adjusting to the erect position. Everyone experiences this phenomenon to some degree.

   b. Take the BP and P with the Pt reclining and upright. Normal young persons display an acceleration of the P by 5 to 25 beats and a drop in systolic BP of as much as 25 mmHg and an increase of up to 10 mmHg in the diastolic (Arnold et al, 1991). In association with symptoms, a consistent drop of 30 mmHg systolic and 15 diastolic (the 30/15 rule) or a drop below 90 mmHg systolic pressure, establishes orthostatic hypotension. The elderly show a lower BP on standing than young persons. A tilt table test refines the analysis of orthostatic hypotension, and the Valsalva maneuver provides further evidence of autonomic insufficiency (Almquist et al, 1989; Chen et al, 1989; Thomas et al, 1989).

4. *Stretch syncope.* The Pt faints when extending the head while stretching. The syncope may result from a combination of Valsalva maneuver and vertebral artery occlusion (Pelekanos et al, 1990).

5. How much cardiac inhibition or vasodilation from loss of sympathetic vasoconstrictor tone contributes to the mechanical effects in these types of syncope is unknown (Scherrer et al, 1990). At any rate, the final reason the

⊥ Pt faints, whether from cardioinhibitory reflexes, inhibition of vasoconstrictor tone, or Valsalva effect, is _____.

Ans: Cerebral ischemia from hypotension or inadequate cardiac output.

F. *Reflexogenic vasovagal syncope from coughing, swallowing, and ear disease*
   1. *Swallowing or glossopharyngeal syncope.* The Pt faints when swallowing or
      in association with spontaneous pain in the ear and throat (glossopharyn-
      geal neuralgia analogous to trigeminal neuralgia).
   2. *Cough (ptussive) syncope.* The Pt, usually one with lung disease, has syn-
      cope after prolonged coughing. The syncope may result from a vagal reflex
      or from the Valsalva effect, that reduces the return of blood via the vena
      cava. In some cases, coughing or sneezing may precipitate syncope in Pts
      with the Chiari malformation (Corbett et al, 1976; Weig et al, 1991), or
      other posterior fossa lesions or with neck masses.
   3. *Otogenic syncope.* The Pt faints after stimulation of the external auditory
      canal, as during the insertion of an otoscope, or as a result of ear disease.
      Because the auditory canal and drum originate from the branchial arches,
      they receive sensory twigs from the branchial arch nerves, including IX and
      X. Thus, stimulation of the external auditory canal or drum may directly
      stimulate IXth or Xth nerve cardioinhibitory afferents.

G. *Reflexogenic syncope from carotid sinus hypersensitivity*
   1. *Pathophysiology.* Increased BP stimulates baroreceptors in the carotid
      sinus that compensate by causing vasodilation or cardiac inhibition.
      Hypersensitivity of the reflex causes syncope.

IXth

Xth .

   a. The carotid sinus is innervated by the _____ cranial
      nerve.
   b. Cardiac inhibition is a parasympathetic reflex with the efferent arc
      through the _____ cranial nerve.
   c. If carotid sinus hypersensitivity causes syncope by bradycardia-asystole,
      it is *cardioinhibitory syncope.*
   d. If carotid sinus hypersensitivity causes syncope from inhibition of sym-
      pathetic vasoconstrictor tone, the syncope is *vasodepressor carotid sinus
      syncope.*
   e. A third, controversial type of carotid sinus syncope is the *cerebral type*
      in which neither the pulse nor the blood pressure changes radically
      (Reese et al, 1962; Engle, 1962).
   f. Paradoxical reflex inhibition of the sympathetic nervous outflow rather
      than the expected vasoconstriction and tachycardia may exacerbate
      hypotension from hemorrhagic shock and during isoproterenol infusion
      (Almquist et al, 1989; Sherrer et al, 1990).
   2. Complete Table 12-9.

Decreased
  sympathetic
  vasoconstrictor
  tone
Reflex asystole or
  bradycardia
Unknown

TABLE 12-9 Mechanisms of carotid sinus syncope	
Type of carotid sinus syncope	Mechanism of syncope
Vasodepressor	
Cardioinhibitory	
Cerebral	

3. *Role of head turning and neck manipulation in syncope*
    a. A Pt with a hypersensitive carotid sinus or with swollen lymph nodes may faint upon turning the head because of inadvertent mechanical stimulation of the carotid sinus.
    b. Head turning may also cause fainting by temporarily occluding a carotid or vertebral artery. In a normal young person, occlusion of a major cerebral artery may cause no symptoms or signs. In elderly, hypertensive, or arteriosclerotic Pts with occlusive arterial disease, the other arteries may fail to supply the brain adequately after one is occluded (Kubular and Millikan, 1964; Sheehan et al, 1960) (Fig. 12-32).

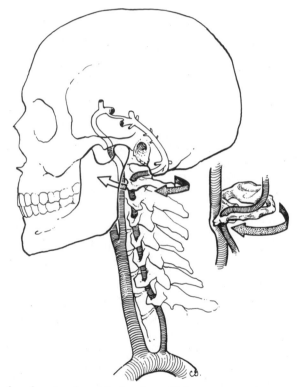

FIG. 12-32. Diagram to show how turning of the head may kink or compress the carotid or vertebral arteries, interfering with blood flow to the brain.

    c. Chiropractic neck manipulation, which lacks any scientific justification in the first place, may cause death or severe neurologic disability from vertebrobasilar infarction (Frumkim and Baloh, 1990; Mas et al, 1989).
4. *Contraindications to the carotid sinus massage test for carotid sinus sensitivity.* Consider carotid sinus massage only after completing the entire neurovascular examination to exclude these contraindications:
    a. Hypertensive, elderly, or arteriosclerotic Pts. Cardiac asystole or hypotension may cause death or a brain infarct (Beal et al, 1981).
    b. Known or suspected heart disease.
    c. Loud carotid bruits (Chap. 1).
5. *Indications for the carotid sinus massage test*
    a. A Pt with lapses of consciousness for which the history and physical examination disclose no cause.
    b. A Pt with syncope precipitated by head turning or who has enlarged cervical lymph nodes.

6. *Procedure for carotid sinus massage test*

    a. Complete the general physical and NE, including palpating the neck for nodes and listening over the head and neck for bruits. Monitor the Pt by EKG and preferably also EEG.

    b. Place the Pt upright in a chair. A standing Pt may fall during the test or, if reclining, may not have sufficient hypotension to faint even though the Pt has a hypersensitive carotid sinus.

    c. Have the Pt repeat whatever head maneuver or position results in syncope.

    d. The Ex must utilize a control test for suggestibility to exclude psychogenic syncope. State that you will rub the Pt's neck, but do not suggest the outcome. Select any point on the neck away from the carotid sinuses, and massage gently for 5 to 15 seconds. Fainting establishes psychogenic syncope.

    e. Locate the carotid sinus by gently palpating the carotid bifurcation. Press your fingers gently backward, just below the angle of the mandible and anterior to the sternocleidomastoid muscle. Record the BP and P. Massage the carotid bulb with very gentle pressure for 5 to 15 seconds and again record the BP and P. After 5 minutes, massage the other carotid bulb.

    f. In normal subjects, the pulse slows by about 15 percent (Arnold et al, 1991). Carotid sinus hypersensitivity is established by asystole lasting more than 3 seconds, or a drop of more than 50 mmHg in the systolic BP (Fujimura et al, 1989).

    g. While it is merely bad to miss an untreatable disorder, it is criminal to miss a treatable disorder. Carotid sinus hypersensitivity can be treated by surgical denervation of the sinus or by parasympathetic-blocking agents. Therefore, do not overlook this treatable cause of syncope.

7. Name two mechanisms by which head turning can cause loss of consciousness. _____ .

Ans: Stimulation of a hypersensitive carotid sinus or occlusion of a major cerebral artery.

8. Name the contraindications to the carotid sinus massage test. _____ _____ .

Ans: Old person, arteriosclerosis, heart disease, occlusion of one carotid artery.

9. What is the position of the Pt for the carotid sinus massage test? ☐ sitting/ ☐ standing/ ☐ reclining. Explain. _____ .

Ans: ☑ Sitting. If standing, the Pt may fall. If reclining, the Pt may not faint even with a hypersensitive carotid sinus.

    H. Subclavian steal syndrome. The Pt has stenosis, or occlusion, of the left subclavian artery prior to the origin of the left vertebral artery. The Pt has a bruit over the supraclavicular fossa and sometimes a thrill. The BP in the left arm is reduced. Exercise of the left arm "steals" blood from the vertebral system, resulting in dizziness, syncope, and other brainstem signs.

    I. Breathholding spells. The most common syncope in children six months to four years of age has a stereotyped tetrad of provocation by anger or frustration;

expiratory apnea and cyanosis; unconsciousness and opisthotonic rigidity; and stupor. The child may have literally dozens of these attacks. The history is all-important. The NE shows nothing abnormal.

J. *Epilepsy versus syncope*
  1. The most common differential diagnosis in syncope is epilepsy. Careful history and an epileptiform EEG generally separate epilepsy.
  2. Since cerebral ischemia disrupts brain metabolism, the Pt not only may faint, but may also have a convulsion—an epileptic seizure—as part of an attack of syncope or breathholding.

K. *Subsequent workup of syncope when the initial evaluation fails to establish a diagnosis.* Proceed with EKG and EEG if the history and physical exam fail to establish the cause for syncope, but insure first that you have tried all of the bedside tests. Occasionally, MRI examination will disclose an unsuspected lesion, particularly of the posterior fossa, that causes the syncope (Weig et al, 1991). In spite of a full workup, a significant number of Pts with blackout spells will remain undiagnosed after the initial evaluation (Eagle and Black, 1983; Kapoor et al, 1983). Above all, follow the Pt. The number of Pts with no diagnosis will drop as the follow-up visits continue.

REFERENCES FOR SYNCOPE

Almquist A, Goldenberg IF, Milstein S, et al: Provocation of bradycardia and hypotension by isoproterenol and upright posture in patients with unexplained syncope. *N Engl J Med* 1989;320:346–351.

Arnold RW, Dyer JA, Gould AB, et al: Sensitivity to vasovagal maneuvers in normal children and adults. *Mayo Clin Proc* 1991;66:797–804.

Beal MF, Park TS, Fisher CM: Cerebral atheromatous embolism following carotid sinus pressure. *Arch Neurol* 1981;38:310–311.

Chen MY, Goldenberg IF, Milstein S, et al: Cardiac electrophysiologic and hemodynamic correlates of neurally mediated syncope. *Am J Cardiol* 1989;63:66–72.

Corbett JJ, Butler AB, Kaufman B: "Sneeze syncope" basilar invagination and Arnold-Chiari type I malformation. *J Neurol Neurosurg Psychiatr* 1976;39:381–384.

Duvoisin R: Convulsive syncope induced by the Weber maneuver. *Arch Neurol* 1962;7:219–226.

Eagle KA, Black HR: Evaluation of patients with syncope. *N Engl J Med* 1983;309:1650.

Engel G: *Fainting* (2nd ed). Springfield, IL, Charles C Thomas, Publisher, 1962

Engle GL: *Fainting: Physiological and psychological considerations.* (2d ed). Rochester, University of Rochester, 1962.

Frumkin LR, Baloh RW: Wallenberg's syndrome following neck manipulation. *Neurology* 1990;40:611–615.

Fujimura O, Yee R, Klein GJ, et al: The diagnostic sensitivity of electrophysiologic testing in patients with syncope caused by transient bradycardia. *N Engl J Med* 1989;321:1703–1706.

Hoefnagels WAJ, Padberg GW, Overweg J, et al: Syncope or seizure? The diagnostic value of the EEG and hyperventilation test in transient loss of consciousness. *J Neurol Neurosurg Psychiatr* 1991;54:953–954.

Kapoor WN, Karpf M, Wieand S, et al: A prospective evaluation and follow-up of patients with syncope. *N Engl J Med* 1983;309:197–204.

Kubala M, Millikan C: Diagnosis, pathogenesis, and treatment of "Drop Attacks." *Arch Neurol* 1964;11:107.

Kulbertus HE, Franck G (eds): *Neurocardiology.* Mount Kisco, NY, Futura Publishing, 1988.

Leis AA, Ross MA, Summers AK: Psychogenic seizures: ictal characteristics and diagnostic pitfalls. *Neurology* 1992;42:94–99.

Lukash WM, Sawyer GT, David JE: Micturition syncope produced by orthostasis and bladder distention. *N Engl J Med* 1964;270:341–344.

Lyle C et al: Micturition syncope. Report of 24 cases. *N Engl J Med* 1961;265:982.

Mas JL, Henin D, Bousser MG, et al: Dissecting aneurysm of the vertebral artery and cervical manipulation: A case report with autopsy. *Neurology* 1989;39:512–515.

Natelson BH; Neurocardiology: An interdisciplinary area for the 80s. *Arch Neurol* 1985;42:178–184.

Pelekanos JT, Dooley JM, Camfield PR, et al: Stretch syncope in adolescence. *Neurology* 1990;40:705–708.

Reese C, Green J, Elliott F: The cerebral form of carotid sinus hypersensitivity. *Neurology* 1962;12:492.

Scherrer U, Vissing S, Morgan BJ, et al: Vasovagal syncope after infusion of a vasodilator in a heart transplant recipient. *N Engl J Med* 1990;322:602–604.

Sheehan S, Bauer R, Meyer J: Vertebral artery compression in cervical spondylosis. *Neurology* 1960;10:968.

Thomas JE, Schirger A, Fealey RD, et al: Orthostatic hypotension. *Mayo Clin Proc* 1981;56:117–125.

Weig SG, Buckthal PE, Choi SK, et al: Recurrent syncope as the presenting symptom of Arnold-Chiari malformation. *Neurology* 1991;41:1673–1674.

Learning Objectives for Chapter Twelve

I. Evaluation of consciousness

1. Give a succinct, general (interpretational) definition of consciousness.
2. Describe the standard bedside operations to test for consciousness.
3. Recite and define the terms for elevation and depression of consciousness (Tables 12-1 and 12-2).
4. Describe the degree of arousability that characterizes somnolence, stupor, semicoma, and true coma or deep coma (Table 12-2).
5. State what happens to the reflexes in deep or strictly defined coma.
6. Define delirium and mania.
7. Describe the advantages of a quantitative scale for numerical grading of consciousness (Fig. 12-1).
8. Recite the three responses graded for the Glasgow Coma Scale.

II. Anatomical basis of consciousness

1. Enumerate which parts of the CNS can be excised without abolishing consciousness (assuming artificial support of breathing and blood pressure).
2. Enumerate the parts of the CNS required for consciousness.
3. Enumerate all sites of lesions that abolish consciousness and state where to place the most restricted lesions that will most selectively abolish consciousness.
4. Name the neuronal system that mediates alerting and consciousness, and describe as precisely as possible its location and components.
5. Give an operational definition of the ascending reticular activating system (ARAS) based on the effects of its stimulation or destruction (Figs. 12-4 and 12-5).
6. Describe the difference in the EEG response to stimulation of the ARAS and a specific thalamic sensory relay nucleus.

III. Internal herniations of the brain

1. Give some examples of space-occupying intracranial lesions.
2. Name the large, tough dural membranes which separate the intracranial space into compartments (Figs. 12-6 to 12-8).
3. Make a drawing of the skull base (calvarium removed) to show the tentorium and the transected mesencephalon, posterior cerebral artery, and IIId nerves in situ, after removal of the cerebral hemispheres (Fig. 12-7).

4. Draw the outline of the tentorial opening (incisura tentorii cerebelli), and state which part(s) of the brain occupy the the tentorial notch.
5. Name the parts of the brain which the tentorium cerebelli separates (Fig. 12-8).
6. Explain in terms of its consistency and water content why the brain readily herniates out of its normal position.
7. State the two fluids which respond or readjust most readily to shifts or compression of the brain.
8. State the only two places a herniating cerebral hemisphere can go, and give the names of these two types of internal brain herniation.
9. Name the major artery and nerve encountered by the herniating medial edge (uncus and parahippocampal gyrus) of the temporal lobe (transtentorial herniation) (Figs. 12-8 and 12-10).
10. Describe the clinical effects of transtentorial herniation on consciousness.
11. Describe the effect of transtentorial herniation on pupillary size.
12. Make a drawing which shows the location of the pupilloconstrictor fibers in the IIId nerve and the relation of the IIId nerve to its adjacent arteries (Fig. 12-9).
13. Describe the clinical significance of an alteration of consciousness and increasing pupillary size in a Pt who may have an intracranial space-occupying lesion.
14. Describe the pupillary changes as transtentorial herniation advances.
15. State the clinical implications of dilated, fixed pupils in an unconscious patient (who has no pharmacological reason for dilated pupils).
16. Explain how transtentorial herniation can give rise to an ipsilateral or paradoxical hemiplegia.
17. Describe and explain the altering UMN signs that may evolve during transtentorial herniation.
18. Describe the terminal pathologic event in the brainstem of Pts with transtentorial herniation (Fig. 12-12).
19. Assume the decerebrate posture, and describe how it affects the position of the jaws, neck, trunk, arms, wrists, hands, legs, and feet (Fig. 12-13 and Table 12-5).
20. Describe the body's posture when it assumes the position dictated by the pull of its strongest muscles.
21. State the site of the anatomic lesion that causes decerebrate rigidity.
22. Discuss the neurophysiologic explanation for the decerebrate posture. State which neural systems must remain intact for the posture to appear.
23. Describe the disturbance in muscle tone seen in the decerebrate state.
24. Classify the decerebrate state as a release or a deficit phenomenon, and explain.
25. Contrast the posture of the arm in the decerebrate and decorticate (hemiplegic) postures (Fig. 12-15).
26. Describe how to elicit decerebrate posturing in an unconscious Pt.

27. Describe the characteristic respiratory dysrhythmias that result from brainstem lesions, and state the location of the responsible lesion (Fig. 12-13).
28. Describe the typical effect of increased intracranial pressure on P and BP (Cushing's phenomenon).
29. Define and describe transforaminal herniation of the brain, and explain how it may kill the patient.
30. Give an orderly description of the signs of transtentorial herniation as related to:
    a. Consciousness
    b. Motor signs in the extremities
    c. Pupillary and IIId nerve signs
    d. Respiration
    e. Pulse and blood pressure
31. Name the common internal herniations of the brain. Name the parts of the brain which herniate in each instance. Describe, in principle, how brain herniations kill the Pt.

IV. **Neurologic examination of the unconscious Pt**
1. Recite the ABCDEE mnemonic that reminds the Ex of the priorities in first approaching an unconscious Pt.
2. Enumerate some causes for coma that the Ex can discover by smelling the Pt's breath.
3. Describe the type of findings on the NE that best help to differentiate anatomic from toxic-metabolic causes of coma.
4. Describe the positive, favorable motor findings apparent immediately on inspection that suggest an anatomically intact nervous system in an unconscious but not completely comatose Pt (the "four-glance" NE).
5. Describe the immediate findings that suggest a poor prognosis for the unconscious Pt.
6. Describe the series of observations and maneuvers that detect acute hemiplegia in the unconscious Pt (Figs. 12-18 to 12-21).
7. Explain the significance of paratonia on the opposite side from a flaccid hemiplegia in an acutely unconscious Pt.
8. Define the term *nucha*, and state the clinical significance of *nuchal rigidity.*
9. Name and describe the ligaments which tether the spinal cord to the dura (Fig. 12-22).
10. Describe how extension and flexion of the head affect the tension on the spinal cord and nerve roots (Figs. 12-23 and 12-24).
11. Explain the pathophysiology of nuchal rigidity in response to meningeal irritation.
12. Describe the maneuvers to separate pure nuchal rigidity from other forms of a stiff neck (Fig. 12-25*A–C*).
13. Describe how to position the head of a Pt who may have suffered a neck injury before moving or transporting the Pt. State which position to avoid and why.
14. State a catastrophic result of excessive or forceful neck

manipulation in a Pt with a mass lesion in the cervical vertebral canal.

**15. Describe Lhermitte's sign of a cervical cord lesion.

16. Describe and name the leg signs of meningeal irritation.

17. List three circumstances in which a Pt with meningeal irritation may fail to show the classical signs.

18. Pronounce *opisthotonos* correctly, and describe the opisthotonic posture (Fig. 12-28).

19. Enumerate several conditions which cause the opisthotonic posture (Fig. 12-29).

20. Describe at least two different basic pathophysiologic mechanisms that cause opisthotonos.

V. Sensory examination of the unconscious Pt

1. State the only bedside method for determining the integrity of the IId cranial nerve in an unconscious Pt.

2. Describe two different methods of testing the integrity of the afferent arc of the Vth cranial nerve in the unconscious Pt.

3. Describe how the facial muscles of an unconscious Pt with an acute, completely flaccid hemiplegia respond to an ipsilateral and contralateral corneal stimulus, or supraorbital compression.

4. Describe how to test the integrity of the VIIIth cranial nerve in an unconscious Pt.

5. Describe and demonstrate how to do the doll's eye, or counter-rolling, test in an unconscious Pt.

6. Explain the significance of intact vestibulo-ocular reflexes in the unconscious Pt.

**7. State which phase of caloric-induced nystagmus disappears first in the unconscious Pt.

8. Describe a possible danger in eliciting the gag reflex in an unconscious Pt.

9. Describe how to test for somatic pain responses in an unconscious Pt, and explain why the Ex should not use a pin.

10. Describe the responses of a partially unconscious, acutely hemiplegic Pt to fingernail compression (painful stimulus) on the hemiplegic and intact sides.

VI. Factors that compound and complicate the neurologic examination of the unconscious Pt

1. Describe how the MSRs in unconscious Pts may differ from normal and explain why their interpretation is more difficult than in the alert Pt.

2. Describe the effect of decreased levels of consciousness on the plantar responses.

3. State whether the Ex can elicit MSRs or a plantar reflex in a deeply comatose Pt.

4. Describe several pre-existing neurologic findings that confound the NE of the comatose Pt.

5. Discuss the question of addressing the Pt assumed to be unconscious.

Note: Learning objectives are not listed for sections VII–IX, because they apply the NE to special states rather than imparting knowledge required for the everyday practice of medicine.

**VII. The neurologic examination in the locked-in syndrome (differentiated state)

**VIII. The neurologic examination in the persistent vegetative state

**IX. The neurologic examination in the diagnosis of brain death

X. Intermittent disturbances of consciousness: Syncope.

1. Define *syncope*.

2. Enumerate several pathophysiologic mechanisms that may result in syncope.

3. State the most important historical information you need to diagnose the cause of syncope.

4. Enumerate the cholinergic signs that occur during vasovagal syncope.

5. State two types of cardiac dysrhythmia that may lead to syncope.

6. State the most important observations the Ex should make in witnessing an attack of syncope and describe how to protect the Pt.

7. State what blood test should always be considered when the Ex witnesses any unexplained episode of altered consciousness.

8. Describe the most common change in breathing that precedes psychogenic syncope and describe how to test for it.

9. Describe several types of mechanical or hydraulic hypovolemic syncope.

10. State the normal limits for changes in BP and P in testing for orthostatic syncope (orthostatic hypotension).

11. Describe the pathogenic mechanism(s) involved in swallowing, cough, and otogenic syncope.

12. Describe three types of carotid sinus syncope.

13. Explain how turning of the head may cause syncope, and how chiropractic neck manipulation may cause death or severe neurologic impairment.

**14. Describe and demonstrate how to test for a hyperactive carotid sinus, and enumerate the contraindications to the test.

15. Describe the diagnostic physical findings in a Pt with the subclavian steal syndrome.

16. Describe the clinical features of the most common nontraumatic, nonepileptic cause of loss of consciousness in young children between six months and four years of age, and the findings, if any, on the NE.

17. State the ancillary neurodiagnostic procedures that the Ex should consider when the initial history and NE fail to disclose the cause for syncope.

Ancillary Neurodiagnostic Procedures

We have instruments of precision in increasing numbers with which we and our hospital assistants at untold expense make tests and take observations, the vast majority of which are but supplementary to, and as nothing compared with, the careful study of the patient by a keen observer using his eyes and ears and fingers and a few simple aids.

Harvey Cushing (1869–1939)

I. Array of neurodiagnostic procedures

After completing the history and neurologic examination (NE) and proposing a tentative diagnosis, the Ex has to decide whether further studies are required. If so, the Ex should review the array of diagnostic tests (Table 13-1) to choose the one or two safest, least invasive, and most economical procedures that will _best_ confirm or refute the tentative diagnosis. Do not order every conceivable test to cover every diagnostic possibility. Go for the jugular. If those fail to establish the diagnosis, then select successive tests in a logical "decision tree" order.

II. The cerebrospinal fluid (CSF) examination

A. _Location, origin, and circulation of the CSF_
  1. _Location._ The CSF, totaling about 150 cc, occupies the ventricles and subarachnoid space of the craniovertebral cavity.
  2. _Origin and circulation_
     a. The CSF derives from the choroid plexuses of the lateral, third, and fourth ventricles, from water produced by oxidative metabolism, and as an ultrafiltrate from the blood-brain barrier of the cerebral capillaries (Fishman, 1992; May et al, 1990). The production rate is 0.3 to 0.4 ml/min.
     b. The CSF escapes from the ventricles by flowing out of foramina in the fourth ventricle, the _L_ateral foramina of _L_uschka and the _M_edian foramen of _M_agendie. The ependymal and leptomeningeal surfaces and root sleeves also provide routes of absorption (Rando and Fishman, 1992). Learn Fig. 13-1.
     c. After exiting from the foramina of the fourth ventricle, the CSF enters the subarachnoid space, between the arachnoid and pia mater. It may then percolate _down_ around the spinal cord or _up_ over the cerebral hem-

TABLE 13-1 Ancillary neurodiagnostic procedures

A. *Neuroradiologic imaging*
   1. *Plain films*
      a. Skull
      b. Vertebrae
   2. *MRI scan* (enhanced and unenhanced)
      a. Brain
      b. Spinal cord
   3. *CT Scan* (enhanced and unenhanced)
      a. Brain
      b. Spinal cord
   4. *Angiography*
      a. Arteriography
      b. Venography
   5. *Doppler imaging*
      a. Blood flow
      b. Ventricular and cerebral contours in premature and young infants
   6. *Radionuclide scanning*
      a. Scan for blood flow
      b. PET and SPECT scans for regional blood flow and metabolism
      c. Cisternography for CSF flow
B. *Electroneurodiagnosis*
   1. EEG (electroencephalography)
   2. EMG (electromyography)
   3. NCV (motor or sensory nerve conduction)
   4. Evoked responses
      a. SSER (somatosensory evoked responses)
      b. BAER (brainstem auditory evoked responses)
      c. VER (visual evoked responses)
      d. ERG (electroretinogram)
   5. ENG (electronystagmogram)
   6. Audiogram
C. *Punctures*
   1. Subarachnoid (LP or cisternal) for CSF
   2. Subdural for blood, pus, or fluid
   3. Ventricular for blood or CSF
   4. Stereotaxic for lesion biopsy
D. *Blood biochemistry*
   1. Chem 17
   2. Toxicology screening
   3. Quantitative amino acid and organic acid screening

   4. Serum enzymes
   5. Long chain fatty acids
   6. Serum ceruloplasmin
   7. B_{12} and folic acid
   8. Serum ceruloplasmin
   9. Long chain fatty acids
   10. Lysosomal enzymes
E. *Neuro-ophthalmology*
   1. Visual acuity
   2. Visual fields
   3. Ophthalmoscopy direct and indirect, and slit-lamp inspection of media and fundus
   4. Color vision
   5. Fluorescence angiography for papilledema
F. *Urinalysis*
   1. Routine including specific gravity
   2. Amino and organic acid screen
   3. Toxicology screening
   4. Catecholamines
G. *Neuropsychologic tests*
   1. Developmental
   2. IQ
   3. Achievement
   4. Neuropsychological battery
   5. Personality profile
H. *Biopsy*
   1. Muscle
   2. Nerve (sensory)
   3. Skin
   4. Brain
   5. Leukocyte/fibrocyte culture for respiratory and lysosomal enzymes, karyotyping, genotyping, and immunologic analysis of T cells
I. *Microbiologic tests*
   1. Serologic
   2. Culture of microorganisms
   3. Immunologic
J. *Genetic*
   1. Karyotype
   2. Genotype

ispheres to the superior sagittal sinus. There, Pacchionian granulations extend from the subarachnoid space into the lumen of the sinus, permitting absorption of the CSF into the venous blood (Fig. 13-2).

d. Trace a drop of CSF from the temporal horn of the lateral ventricle to its absorption into the blood: _____

_____.

Ans: Temporal horn, trigone (atrium) anterior horn, interventricular foramen, IIId ventricle, IVth ventricle, subarachnoid space, and Pacchionian granulation

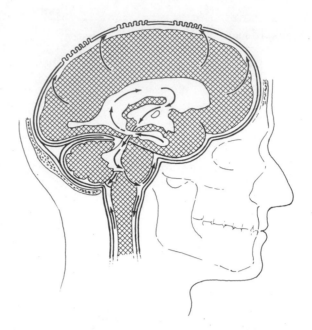

FIG. 13-1. Lateral view of the ventricular system and cerebrospinal fluid (CSF) circulation. Beginning in the temporal horn, trace a drop of CSF through the ventricular system, into the subarachnoid space, and up over the convexity of the hemisphere to the Pacchionian granulations along the superior sagittal sinus.

B. *Functions of the CSF*
    1. The CSF in the subarachnoid space provides a flotation layer around the brain and spinal cord that cushions them from trauma. All entering and exiting vessels and craniospinal nerves must cross the subarachnoid space.
    2. The CSF permits circulation of neurohumors, peptide hormones, antibodies, and leukocytes.
    3. The CSF aids in regulating the pH and electrolyte balance of the CNS.

C. *Composition of the CSF:* The CSF is a sparkling-clear salt solution containing a few white blood cells (WBCs), proteins, sugar, and traces of enzymes, neurohumors, and neurotransmitters (Fishman, 1992; Herndon and Brumback, 1989). See Table 13-2.

D. *Normal pressure of the CSF:* The normal pressure of the CSF varies with the age of the Pt (Table 13-2): 10–100 mm water for young infants, 80–180 for

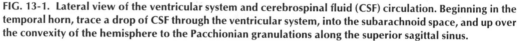

Superior sagittal sinus

Skull

Dura mater

Subarachnoid space

Pacchionian granulation

Cerebrum

Falx

FIG. 13-2. Coronal section through the cerebral falx to show the Pacchionian granulations projecting directly into the superior sagittal sinus. CSF passes through the granulations into the venous blood of the sinus.

TABLE 13-2 Typical CSF profiles in normal individuals and those with various diseases

| | Color | Pressure | Cytology | | | Chemistry | | Immuno-electro-phoresis |
			Cell count/ mm^3	Cell type	Stained smear or culture	Glucose: % of blood sugar	Total protein	
Normal young infant	Sparkling clear	10–100 mm H$_2$O	<10	Mononuclear	No bacteria	≈66% of blood	20–170 mg %	Normal
Normal adult	Sparkling clear	80–180 mm H$_2$O	<5	Mononuclear	No bacteria	≈66% of blood	10–40 mg %	Normal
Meningitis Acute bacterial	Cloudy	↑	500 to 1000s	Polymorphonuclear	Bacteria present	<50% of blood	↑	†CIE shows bacterial antigens
Tuberculous	Cloudy, xanthochromic	*N or ↑	10–500	Mostly mononuclear	Bacteria present	<50% of blood	↑	Not diagnostic
Fungal	Cloudy, xanthochromic	N or ↑	<500	Mostly mononuclear	Fungi present	<50% of blood	↑	Not diagnostic
Encephalitis	Clear to faintly cloudy	N or ↑	<500	Mononuclear after first hours	Stain negative	N	N to moderate ↑	Use serologic testing, DNA analysis
Subarachnoid hemorrhage	Erythrochromic or xanthochromic	N or ↑	100s to 1000s to 10,000s	RBCs	Negative	N	Varies with amount of bleeding	Not helpful
Demyelinating diseases	Sparkling clear	N	N or slight ↑	Mononuclear, plasma cells	Negative	N	N to slight ↑	Increased γ-globulin
Neoplasm	Sparkling clear or xanthochromic if protein ↑	N or ↑	N or slight ↑	Neoplastic cells sometimes present	Negative	N	N to slight ↑	Normal or nondiagnostic

*N = Normal
†CIE = Counter-immunoelectrophoresis

TABLE 13-3 Common causes for cessation of CSF flow and their remedies

Cause	Remedy
Blood clot in the needle lumen	Replace stilet to ream out the needle.
Nerve root has fallen over the bevel of the needle	Rotate the shaft of the needle.
Displacement of the tip of the needle from the subarachnoid space or incomplete penetration	If you think the needle tip is too deep, withdraw it slightly; or, if too shallow, insert it further.

normal mature individuals, and up to 250 mm water for grossly obese individuals, because of increased intra-abdominal pressure. Disease may cause increased or decreased intracranial pressure, with increased intracranial pressure by far the most common problem.

E. *Increased intracranial pressure*
  1. *Symptoms and signs of increased intracranial pressure*
      a. Increased pressure in infants causes a bulging fontanel, split sutures, and an increasing OFC (Chap. 1).
      b. *Symptoms* consist of headaches, nausea and vomiting, dizziness, transient blurring of vision (amaurosis), and mild obtundation.
      c. *Signs* consist of papilledema, and often VIth nerve palsy as a consequence of compression of the nerve during its long intracranial course.
  2. *Causes of increased intracranial pressure*
      a. *Expanding lesions* within the craniovertebral space, such as hematomas, neoplasms, abscesses, and brain edema. Rarely, increased production of CSF may cause increased pressure.
      b. *Prolonged status epilepticus or hypoxia,* which causes edema
      c. *Metabolic encephalopathies:* hepatic, uremic, Reye's syndrome, pseudotumor cerebri, and endocrinopathies
      d. *CNS infections:* Meningitis and encephalitis may incite extreme edema and increased pressure.
      e. *Occlusive lesions* which impede the flow of CSF from the ventricles to the subarachnoid space and through the Pacchionian granulations. The most common sites of blockage are:
          (1) The interventricular foramen of Monro, usually by a neoplasm
          (2) The cerebral aqueduct, usually by congenital atresia or stenosis, inflammatory adhesions, or neoplastic compression
          (3) The fourth ventricle and its outlets, usually by posterior fossa neoplasms or inflammatory adhesions
          (4) Subarachnoid space, usually by adhesions after meningitis or subarachnoid hemorrhage
          (5) Pacchionian granulations, usually by adhesions, high CSF protein, or thrombosis of dural sinuses
  3. *Increased intracranial pressure and Pascal's law*
      a. Physically, the CSF is essentially water and the CNS is about 80 percent water. Students who have only handled the stiff, formalin-fixed brain of the cadaver do not appreciate the supple softness of the living brain. Its compliancy resembles a balloon (the pia-arachnoid) filled with molasses. Therefore, a physicist, in studying intracranial hydrodynamics, might represent the CNS and the CSF as a single homogeneous fluid. To duplicate biologic conditions, the CNS–CSF model includes the vascular space within the craniovertebral space, as shown in Fig. 13-3A.
      b. The CNS–CSF in the craniovertebral space is incompressible. According to Pascal's law, pressure exerted on a fluid in a closed container is transmitted equally in all directions. The pressure transmission is independent of the size or shape of the container. Therefore, pressure in the lumbar CSF reflects the intracranial pressure. As intracranial pressure increases, it displaces CSF and the intravascular blood. As these compensations fail, any further increase in pressure causes the brain to herniate down through the foramen magnum (Chap. 12).

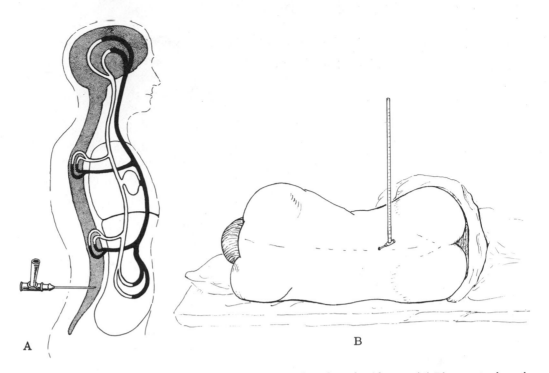

FIG. 13-3. Manometer attached to a needle inserted into the subarachnoid space. (*A*) Diagram to show the continuity of vessels inside and outside of the craniovertebral cavity. A needle inserted into the lumbar sub-arachnoid space has a vertical manometer attached. For this and subsequent illustrations, regard the Pt as lying on the left side with the manometer vertical (see *B*). (*B*) Pt in left lateral position with legs and back flexed.

F. *Low CSF pressure syndrome*

1. *Symptoms and signs.* The Pt experiences headache, vertigo, tinnitus, nausea, and vomiting, especially when arising from a reclining to a vertical position, and may faint. The symptoms could occur because of loss of flotation, allowing the cerebrum to sag onto the brainstem. The headache may result from traction on meninges, or vasodilation and increased intracranial blood volume in compensation for the loss of CSF (Grant et al, 1991).

2. *Causes of low CSF pressure*

   a. Procedures that pierce the meninges and establish a CSF leak include lumbar puncture and neurosurgical operations.

   b. Basal skull fractures create fistulae in the nose or middle ear causing CSF rhinorrhea or otorrhea.

   c. Severe dehydation

   d. Leakage along nerve roots (Rando and Fishman, 1992)

   e. Idiopathic aliquorrhea (Bell, Joynt, and Sahs, 1960; Rando and Fishman, 1992)

3. *Treatment of low CSF pressure.* Recumbency, hydration, repair of fistulae, and an epidural blood patch (Seebacher et al, 1989). Some authors advocate bed rest in the prone position for 3 to 12 h after a lumbar puncture (Petito and Plum, 1974), but others doubt its efficacy (Fischman, 1992, Kuntz et al, 1992). Intracranial subdural hematomas may result from low CSF pressure (Rando and Fishman, 1992).

G. *Indications for lumbar puncture (LP, spinal puncture, rachiocentesis)*

1. To identify bacterial, viral, spirochetal, fungal, or viral infections of the CSF. Repeated LPs serve to monitor the effect of treatment.

2. To identify subarachnoid bleeding
3. To identify neoplastic invasion or seeding of the subarachnoid space by gliomas, carcinomas, or leukemias and lymphomas
4. To introduce contrast agents into the CSF for myelography or radionuclides for study of CSF flow dynamics, and to locate leaks (Herndon and Brumback, 1989)
5. To measure and fractionate CSF proteins in suspected immunologic diseases, especially multiple sclerosis, and for the differential diagnosis of some neuropathies, such as Landry-Guillain-Barré-Strohl polyradiculitis
6. To measure pH, enzymes, neurotransmitters, and trace constituents

H. *Contraindications to an LP*
   1. *Infection of the lumbar skin* through which the needle must pass
   2. *Coagulopathies.* Diseases such as hemophilia and thrombocytopenia, or anticoagulant therapy, represent relative rather than absolute contraindications. Lumbar hematomas may follow an LP in these Pts (Masdeu, Breuer, and Schoene, 1979; Plum, 1974).
   3. *Cervical cord lesions.* Removal of CSF from the lumbar region may cause the cord to shift against the lesion, resulting in quadriplegia, apnea, and death.
   4. *Increased intracranial pressure, or a suspected or known intracranial mass*
      a. If the history, NE, or ophthalmoscopic examination suggests a mass lesion, or increased pressure, avoid an LP. The most common mass lesions which cause brain herniation include neoplasms, hematomas, abscesses, cerebral edema, and massive cerebral hemispheric infarction. Of 22 Pts with brain abscess, 5 showed evidence of herniation within 2 h of an LP (Samson and Clark, 1973). Posterior fossa lesions which may cause transformational herniation also pose a great threat. *If the clinical findings raise the question of a mass lesion that may cause brain herniation, always order a CT or MRI scan before doing an LP.* The radiographic examination may clinch the diagnosis and render the LP useless as well as potentially harmful.
      b. Sometimes the Ex will elect to do an LP even in the presence of increased pressure in order to identify or exclude a specifically treatable disorder. Conditions with possible increased pressure that may require an LP include suspected meningitis or encephalitis and pseudotumor cerebri. Then the Ex has to weigh the indications against the contraindications, a type of guesswork known as "clinical judgment" (Clarke, 1985; Fishman, 1992; Lorber and Sutherland, 1980).

I. *Complications of an LP*
   1. *Headache and post-LP low CSF pressure syndrome.* See Section F, above
   2. *Iatrogenic infection.* Extremely rare
   3. *Bleeding.* Epidural, subdural, or subarachnoid; a so-called bloody tap (Masdeu, Breuer, and Schoene, 1979)
   4. *Back pain at the puncture site*
   5. Name two circumstances in which the Ex generally should order a CT or MRI scan prior to an LP: _____

_____.

Ans: Suspicion of increased intracranial pressure, or high cervical lesion that impinges on the spinal cord.

J. Technique for lumbar puncture (LP)

  1. *Psychological preparation of the Pt for an LP.* Everyone dreads needles, particularly a stab in the back. Every layman, it seems, knows of someone who had one of "those taps" and afterward had a permanent backache or never walked again. Of course the layman has reversed cause and effect: the Pt's disease caused the disability, not the LP, but today's litigious Pts always blame the doctor, not the disease. The Ex must insure that the indications are valid and that the Pt understands the necessity for the procedure.

  2. *Positioning of the Pt for an LP*

   a. Position an acutely ill Pt on the side with the legs drawn up and the spine flexed (Fig. 13-3B). In this position, the distance between the dorsal processes and lamina of adjacent vertebrae is ☐ increased/ ☐ decreased.

Ans: ☑ Increased. Spinal flexion thus increases the target area for the needle. Review Fig. 12-24 if you erred.

   b. If the Pt is not acutely ill, some Exs prefer to place the Pt in the sitting position, but again with the spine flexed.

  3. *Needle insertion and manometry*

   a. Scrub the skin with antiseptic and, under sterile technique, insert a 20-gauge needle, its stilet in place, in the interspace between the dorsal processes of vertebrae L_{4-5} or L_5–S_1. Angle the needle slightly cephalad and insert it with the bevel of the needle turned parallel to the long axis of the spine. The bevel then cleanly separates the longitudinal fibers of the dura rather than transecting them; this reduces post-LP leakage of CSF.

   b. If the history or ophthalmoscopic examination raises a question of increased pressure, such as pseudotumor cerebri, proceed this way: Insert a needle through the skin but stop it just before it reaches the subarachnoid space. Remove the stilet and attach a manometer. With the manometer in place and with a fingertip blocking the open bore at the top of the manometer, advance the needle into the subarachnoid space and allow the fluid to fill the manometer gradually. Otherwise, the Ex may insert the needle with its regular stilet in place and quickly attach a three-way stopcock and manometer after withdrawing the stilet. Record the opening pressure. At the end of the procedure, record the closing pressure.

   c. For premature and young infants, use a standard butterfly needle (Greensher et al, 1971). The Ex should limit the depth of any needle puncture to 2.5 cm in infants.

  4. *Fluctuations in the meniscus in the manometer*

   a. The meniscus of CSF in the manometer will show spontaneous fluctuations around some mean value, for example, 120 mm water (Fig. 13-4).

   b. Let us see why the fluctuations occur. As shown in Fig. 13-3A, the intracranial and intraspinal veins communicate directly with the extracranial and extravertebral veins. Since these communicating channels lack valves, the extracranial veins transmit any change in their pressure directly into the craniovertebral space, particularly the changes in intrathoracic pressure. When a person inhales air, the CNS–CSF pressure ☐ increases/ ☐ decreases/ ☐ does not change.

Ans: ☑ Decreases. The intrathoracic pressure decreases with inspiration. Blood is sucked from the CNS veins and the CNS–CSF pressure drops during

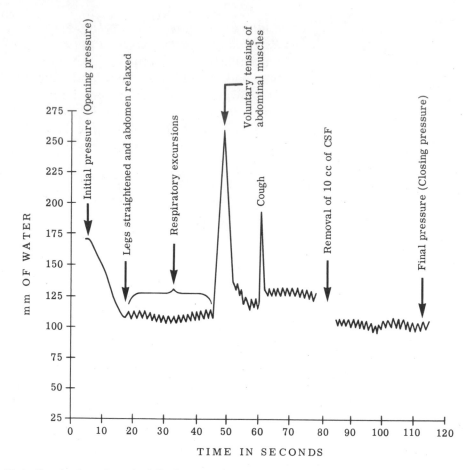

FIG. 13-4. Graph of cerebrospinal fluid pressure, as measured by manometry. Starting at the left, read through the legends just above the arrows.

inspiration. Breathing causes rhythmic excursions of the manometer meniscus at the rate of 16/min, as shown in Fig. 13-4.

    c. Contraction of the abdominal muscles would ☐ increase/ ☐ decrease the intracranial pressure. Explain: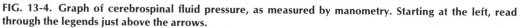

Ans: ☑ *Increase. The intervertebral veins reflect the increased intra-abdominal pressure backwards into the craniovertebral space, reducing the outflow of blood from the CNS. Since the arterial input continues, the CNS–CSF pressure increases.*

    d. The pulse causes smaller excursions at the rate of 72/min, not shown in Fig. 13-4 because of their small amplitude.

    e. Since the arterial walls absorb much of the arterial pressure, the CNS–CSF pressure most closely depends on the capillary and venous pressure.

    K. *Clinical evaluation of increased pressure as registered by CSF manometry*

      1. Assume that the opening pressure in the manometer is 240 mm water, which is ☐ normal/ ☐ low/ ☐ high.

☑ *High*

      2. Two explanations exist:

        a. The intrinsic CNS–CSF pressure is too high.

        b. The pressure reflects factors extrinsic to the craniovertebral space.

      3. An LP always makes the Pt anxious, which causes increased tension in the

skeletal muscles. What, then, is a simple extrinsic cause for increased CNS–CSF pressure? _____

Abdominal muscle tension

4. The Pt's anxiety and flexed posture causes abdominal muscle tension. Encourage the Pt to relax the flexed position and to take a few deep breaths. In the Pt with the opening pressure of 240 mm water, these maneuvers dropped the pressure to 210 mm water. This value is ☐ normal/ ☐ low/ ☐ high.

☑ *High*

5. The flexed posture has caused the Pt to flex the head on the chest, and it may have bent somewhat to the side as it rests on the pillow. Since flexion or turning of the head may compress the jugular veins, the Ex straightens the Pt's head and readjusts it on the pillow. These maneuvers failed to drop the pressure below 200 mm water, indicating that the Pt had slightly increased intrinsic intracranial pressure.
6. If an expanding intracranial lesion raises the CNS–CSF pressure, let us visualize what might happen after removal of CSF from the lumbar region (Fig. 13-5).

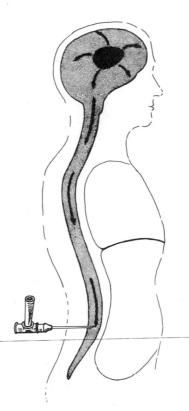

FIG. 13-5. Depiction of an expanding intracranial lesion (oval black mass) causing increased intracranial pressure. The pressure exerts itself equally in all directions. Escape of CSF through a lumbar needle allows the intracranial contents to flow (herniate) toward the region of lowered pressure.

7. The Pt may have early or impending internal herniation of the brain from increased intracranial pressure. The system may be delicately balanced, with the uncus and parahippocampal gyrus poised ready to plunge over the edge of the tentorium, or the cerebellar tonsils ready to herniate through the foramen magnum. These two potentially fatal herniations are called _____ and _____ herniation.

Transtentorial and transforaminal

Die

8. Withdrawal of fluid from the lumbar region will allow the brain to flow down toward the point of low pressure, according to Pascal's law. The potential herniation is converted to actual herniation. The Pt will _____.
9. If, after careful measurement, the Ex concludes that the Pt truly has intrinsic increased intracranial pressure, what is the next step? ☐ Withdraw <u>fluid rapidly</u>./ ☐ <u>Withdraw fluid cautiously</u>./ ☐ <u>Withdraw the needle immediately</u>.

Ans: ☑ *Withdraw the needle immediately! The small amount of fluid in the manometer suffices for a cell count, which is usually the most important information needed.*

10. Describe the maneuvers required to exclude extrinsic factors as the cause for high spinal fluid pressure: _____
_____.

Ans: Have the Pt straighten the legs and take several deep breaths. Extend the Pt's head and reposition it on the pillow.

    L. *Cessation of CSF flow*

1. Frequently, even though the opening CSF pressure was normal, the flow of fluid stops. Very rarely, transforaminal herniation, like a plug in a drain, blocks the transmission of intracranial pressure after a small amount of CSF has drained out. In this case, the Pt shows dramatic signs of apnea and quadriplegia. Most commonly, the cause is far more benign: Something has blocked the needle (Table 13-3).
2. After trying the maneuvers in Table 13-3, the Ex reattaches the manometer to measure the pressure again. If the system from the subarachnoid space through the needle to the manometer is open, the manometer meniscus should show excursions at the rate of 16/min, caused by _____.

Breathing

3. In the absence of respiratory excursions, the Ex can test for the patency of the CSF-needle-manometer system by using a safe method of extrinsic pressure to see whether it will raise the meniscus in the manometer. How could the Ex safely raise the extrinsic venous pressure to test for a rise in the manometer, indicating patency of the system, without increasing the risk of brain herniation? _____
_____.

Ans: Press on the Pt's abdomen (Fig. 13-6). The Ex must avoid the Valsalva maneuver or direct jugular compression because these maneuvers would increase intracranial pressure, risking brain herniation. Therefore, abdominal pressure is the only safe test.

4. The CSF may also stop flowing through the needle if a lesion occludes the vertebral canal, as in Fig. 13-6.
5. Whatever the reason for cessation of CSF flow, the Ex tests the patency of the system by the methods just described. Summarize these methods in proper order:
    (1) _____
    (2) _____
    (3) _____
    (4) _____

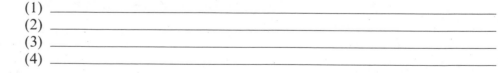

Ans:
(1) Replace and withdraw the stilet to clear a blood clot.
(2) Rotate the shaft of the needle.
(3) Advance or withdraw the needle tip slightly.
(4) Replace manometer and watch for respiratory excursions, or press on the abdomen.

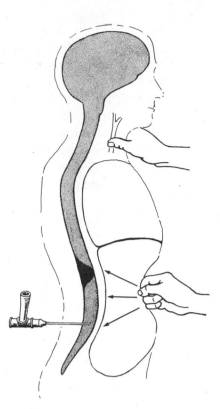

FIG. 13-6. A lesion (black mass) occluding the vertebral canal. (*A*) Compression of the jugular vein. (*B*) Compression of the abdomen. Which will cause a rise of fluid in the manometer or cause a few drops of CSF to flow from the needle? ☐ jugular compression only/ ☐ abdominal compression only/ ☐ **both jugular and abdominal compression.**

Ans: ☑ *Both jugular and abdominal compression*

6. Only one of the tests in the preceding frame will prove that the CSF-needle-manometer system is patent if a lesion occludes the vertebral canal as in Fig. 13-6. That test is ⎽⎽ .

Ans: Watching for a rise of the fluid in the manometer after abdominal compression

7. *What not to do if CSF stops flowing through the needle.* Exasperation may tempt the Ex to try to suck CSF out by a syringe. If at this point you do not understand why you should not forcefully suck out CSF, the text has totally failed.

M. *The jugular compression (Queckenstedt) test:* This test involved detecting a block in the spinal canal by seeing whether digital compression of the jugular veins increased the height of the fluid in the manometer. CT and MRI scan have made this test virtually obsolete.

N. *Collection and appearance of the CSF:* After measuring the opening pressure, the Ex collects 10–15 cc of CSF by allowing several ml to drip into each of three tubes. The normal fluid appears sparkling clear in all three tubes. Inspect all three tubes for *cloudiness, redness (erythrochromia),* and *yellowness (xanthochromia).* The attending physician bears the responsibility for proper inspection of CSF after collection, not the laboratory technician.

O. *Cloudiness of the CSF:* Cloudiness usually means an increased number of WBCs in the CSF. Rarely, numerous bacteria cause cloudiness. Normally, the CSF contains five or fewer WBCs per mm^3. More than 300 per mm^3 of polymorphonuclear WBCs, or more than 400–500 per mm³ of lymphocytes or monocytes, will cause detectable cloudiness, if the Ex inspects the CSF properly. Obvious cloudiness occurs with counts of 600–800 WBCs per mm³. To detect minimal cloudiness with counts in the range of several hundred WBCs per mm³, do the following:

1. Obtain an exact duplicate of the tube used to collect the CSF and add the same amount of water as is in the CSF tube. The duplicate tube must have the same translucency, color, and refractive index as the CSF tube.
2. Hold the duplicate and CSF tubes side-by-side against a white sheet of paper, then against a dark background, and then against a light source. Use daylight, if at all possible. Compare the CSF with the water by looking through the sides of the tubes, as in using a colorimeter. The direct, side-by-side comparison enables the Ex to detect very subtle cloudiness or color changes. Even mild CSF pleocytosis with WBCs and red blood cells (RBCs) may cause the Tyndall effect, a snowy iridescence in bright sunlight.
3. Students often grumble and regard this as all unnecessary because the CSF goes to the lab for the "official" examination and cell count anyway, so why bother? Well, good physicians inspect the CSF personally and do the cell count on the spot, before the cells have undergone the autolysis that commences in an hour, and to gain the information quickly and reliably. In the second place, personal inspection checks the accuracy of the laboratory, a check that is unfortunately necessary (Kaufman and Venderlinde, 1967). If the laboratory reports 20 WBCs per mm³ after the Ex has seen a cloudy fluid, the laboratory must be wrong. If the Pt has meningitis, you simply cannot tolerate an error on this critical point.

P. *Erythrochromia and xanthochromia:* Erythrochromia means a red or pink CSF. An RBC count of 100 to 300/mm³ causes erythrochromia. Normally the RBC count in the CSF is _____.

zero

1. RBCs get into the CSF at one of two times in relation to the tap:
   a. From *preexisting* bleeding caused by a ruptured blood vessel, injury, or other CNS lesion.
   b. From *inadvertent* bleeding caused by the needle puncture, a "traumatic" or "bloody tap".
2. *Differentiation of preexisting bleeding from a bloody tap.* A traumatic tap is inconsequential, while preexisting bleeding may foretell a life-threatening lesion. To distinguish the two sources of RBCs, proceed by the three-tube test, centrifugation, or cytologic demonstration of erythrophagocytosis by monocytes.
   a. *The three-tube test.* Compare the amount of discoloration in the three tubes of CSF. Preexisting blood mixes freely with the CSF, and all three tubes display the same color. A traumatic tap tends to clear by the third tube.
   b. *Centrifugation.* If the three tubes are uniformly bloody, centrifuge one to deposit any intact RBCs in the bottom. Compare the supernatant fluid with a control tube of water, as described above. If the supernatant CSF is sparkling clear, the RBCs entered the CSF recently, either coming from preexisting bleeding that occurred less than 2 to 4 h before the tap, or from the tap itself. Discoloration of the supernatant fluid of a bloody CSF specimen means that the RBCs had entered the CSF more than 2 to 4 h before, and have undergone disintegration. The free hemoglobin in solution colors the supernatant fluid. If the bleeding occurred several

days before the tap, the color is partially from bilirubin, a degradation product of hemoglobin.

    c. *Correction of the CSF WBC count for contamination by blood.* If the CSF is bloody, the Ex can still estimate the CSF white count by subtracting from the total WBC count 1 WBC/mm^3 for every 700 RBCs/mm^3 in the CSF. The remainder, after this correction, is the true CSF WBC count.

    d. *Erythrophagocytosis.* Microscopic proof of preexisting blood comes from the demonstration of RBCs within macrophages. Crenation of RBCs as demonstrated by microscopy once was thought to prove preexisting bleeding, but the greater osmolarity of CSF over serum always tends to crenate cells, making this criterion false.

Q. *Xanthochromia of the CSF:* Xanthochromia means a yellowish discoloration of the CSF, detected by controlled comparison of the CSF sample with water. The most common causes are free hemoglobin, bilirubin, and high protein (Van der Meulen, 1966). Distinguish the possibilities this way:

    1. Xanthochromia from high protein will usually clot quickly when the CSF stands in the tube (Froin's syndrome).

    2. Dip a Hemastix tape (Ames Laboratories) into the CSF to identify hemoglobin. An Ictotest reagent tablet identifies bilirubin. Neither reagent reacts if only protein is present.

R. *Laboratory examination of the CSF:* The routine tests include sugar, total protein, and serologic tests for syphilis. If the cell count excedes 5 WBCs per mm^3, the cells should be smeared on a slide, stained, and examined for organisms, and cultured. Chloride determination has little value on the routine specimen. The success of further examination of the CSF depends on careful planning. The vast array of tests places even more value on the clinical findings to focus on and select the crucial tests for the particular Pt. Fig. 13-7 lists the array of tests done on the CSF.

    1. *Cytological analysis and staining*

        a. *Normal cell content of the CSF.* The normal total CSF WBC is 10 or fewer WBCs/mm^3 for preterm or term infants to one year, and five or fewer for children or adults. Normally lymphocytes make up 75% of the total and monocytes 25%. Normally the CSF contains no RBCs, polymorphonuclear leukocytes, eosinophiles or plasma cells, and no neurons, but it may contain ependymal cells. The most common causes of CSF pleoctyosis are meningitis and encephalitis. Convulsions alone can cause a mild pleocytosis, which may then cause confusion with encephalitis (Clark, 1985; Edwards, Schmidley, and Simon, 1983).

        b. *Staining.* The cells in the CSF are concentrated by centrifugation or by sedimentation methods. Depending on the diseases suspected clinically, the cell stains include the Papanicolaou, Romanowsky, Wright-Giemsa, or the Diff-quik methods, or India ink for fungi (Bigner, 1992).

        c. *Identification of neoplastic cells in the CSF.* In acute encephalitis, the activated lympocytes may resemble neoplastic cells and require differentiation from the various types of neoplastic cells that invade the subarachnoid space. Invasion of the subarachnoid space commonly occurs in lymphomas and in acute leukemia but not commonly in chronic leukemias. Immunophenotyping helps distinguish lymphomas, which are usually monoclonal B-cells. The most common carcinomatoses of the meninges are breast, lung, and melanoma. Various gliomas, mostly medulloblastoma, pineoblastoma, retinoblastoma, and neuroblastoma,

EXAMINATION OF THE CSF

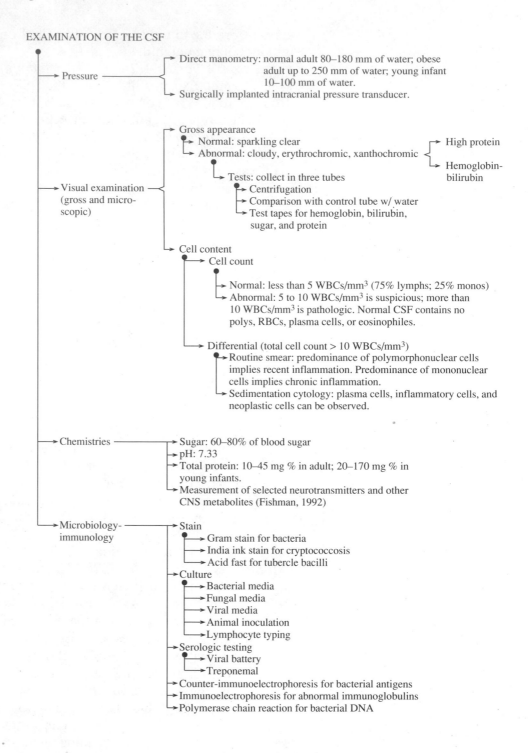

Pressure
- Direct manometry: normal adult 80–180 mm of water; obese adult up to 250 mm of water; young infant 10–100 mm of water.
- Surgically implanted intracranial pressure transducer.

Visual examination (gross and microscopic)
- Gross appearance
  - Normal: sparkling clear
  - Abnormal: cloudy, erythrochromic, xanthochromic
    - High protein
    - Hemoglobin-bilirubin
    - Tests: collect in three tubes
      - Centrifugation
      - Comparison with control tube w/ water
      - Test tapes for hemoglobin, bilirubin, sugar, and protein
- Cell content
  - Cell count
    - Normal: less than 5 WBCs/mm³ (75% lymphs; 25% monos)
    - Abnormal: 5 to 10 WBCs/mm³ is suspicious; more than 10 WBCs/mm³ is pathologic. Normal CSF contains no polys, RBCs, plasma cells, or eosinophiles.
  - Differential (total cell count > 10 WBCs/mm³)
    - Routine smear: predominance of polymorphonuclear cells implies recent inflammation. Predominance of mononuclear cells implies chronic inflammation.
    - Sedimentation cytology: plasma cells, inflammatory cells, and neoplastic cells can be observed.

Chemistries
- Sugar: 60–80% of blood sugar
- pH: 7.33
- Total protein: 10–45 mg % in adult; 20–170 mg % in young infants.
- Measurement of selected neurotransmitters and other CNS metabolites (Fishman, 1992)

Microbiology-immunology
- Stain
  - Gram stain for bacteria
  - India ink stain for cryptococcosis
  - Acid fast for tubercle bacilli
- Culture
  - Bacterial media
  - Fungal media
  - Viral media
  - Animal inoculation
  - Lymphocyte typing
- Serologic testing
  - Viral battery
  - Treponemal
- Counter-immunoelectrophoresis for bacterial antigens
- Immunoelectrophoresis for abnormal immunoglobulins
- Polymerase chain reaction for bacterial DNA

may seed the subarachnoid space. The glial cells stain with antibodies to glial fibrillary acid protein. A full antibody panel aids in differentiating various types of neoplastic cells (Bigner, 1992; Herndon and Brumback, 1989).

2. *Identification of infectious agents in the CSF*

   a. Direct staining, culture, and various antigen-antibody reactions identify viruses, bacteria, and fungi in the CSF. The fields of immunology and molecular biology, particularly the polymerase chain reaction, advance so rapidly that the Ex almost has to consult with a specialist or specialty text to select the best tests to apply to each CSF sample (Fischman, 1992; Herndon and Brumback, 1989; Scheld, Whitley, and Dirack, 1991).

Antibody panels are available for the most common bacteria and viruses that invade the CNS. Many of these tests depend on matching serum and CSF reactions and estimating the rate of production of antibodies and their passage through the blood-brain barrier. Counterimmune electrophoresis (CIE) identifies *H. influenzae, N. meningitidis, S. pneumoniae,* and other streptococci, and the polymerase chain reaction identifies a wide variety of organisms.

b. Herpes simplex is identified by immunoassays of serum and CSF. The detection of this virus, with its predilection for the temporal lobe, is extremely important because of the potential for treatment with acyclovir.

c. Syphilis is identified by a positive FTA-ABS (fluorescent antibody absorption) test.

d. Cryptococcus, the most frequent fungal infection of the CSF, is detected by staining, culture, and latex agglutination tests.

e. Borrelia burgdorferi (Lyme disease) is detected by the Western Blot test.

f. Tuberculous meningitis is detected by staining, culture, and the polymerase chain reaction (Kaneko et al, 1990).

g. HIV can be recovered from the CSF in all stages of the infection, even before any clinical signs of AIDS and in the absence of recovery of the virus from the blood. The neurologic complications span the gamut: dementia, aseptic meningitis, myelopathy, polyneuropathy, secondary opportunistic meningitides, and vasculitis (Sharer, 1992).

3. *Glucose content of CSF.* Typically the CSF glucose is about two-thirds of the blood glucose. The CSF glucose concentration lags some hours behind changes in the blood glucose. Generally the Ex should draw a blood glucose at the time of the LP for comparison. Ideally the LP should be done in the morning to allow for overnight equilibration of blood and CSF values. High CSF glucose virtually always reflects high blood values. Low CSF glucose typically occurs in acute bacterial meningitis. Low CSF glucose may also occur with subarachnoid hemorrhage, with pleocytosis from lymphocytic or neoplastic invasion of the CSF, and idiopathically (aglycorrachia) (Fraser, 1991).

4. *Identification of abnormal proteins in the CSF*
   a. The total protein is measured, and the immunoglobulins are fractionated. Even with blood in the CSF, the Ex can estimate the total CSF protein by subtracting 1 mg/100 ml of protein for each 1000 RBCs present. Abnormal immunoglobulins can be detected even in the absence of elevation of the total protein (Herndon and Brumback, 1989). The normal amount of protein varies with the Pt's age (Table 13-4).

TABLE 13-4 Values for total CSF protein in the first year		
	CSF protein (mg/dl)*	
	Range	Mean
Birth preterm	65–150	115
Full term	20–170	90
One month	20–150	62
Three months	20–100	46
Six months	15–50	37
Nine months	15–30	24

*Normal adult <45 mg/dl

b. CSF findings in multiple sclerosis and other immunopathies. The CSF may display a mild pleocytosis and contain plasma cells and immunologically altered lymphocytes. It shows increased gammaglobulin, mainly IgG, and an increased CSF IgG index. Agarose electrophoresis demonstrates oligoclonal gammopathy as discrete bands, whereas normal CSF immunoglobulins migrate as a diffuse band. Isoelectric focusing shows heavy and light chains of immunoglobulins. Myelin basic protein is frequently increased. The clinical findings, CSF profile, and MRI examination together provide the basis for the diagnosis of multiple sclerosis.

S. Summary of CSF Examination
1. Review Table 13-2 for the CSF changes in various disorders, but do not memorize.
2. State in principle the differences in the pressure, cell count, and protein values during maturation from preterm infants to adults: _____

_____

_____.

Ans: Normal young infants have a lower pressure, higher WBC count, up to 10 cells/mm³, and higher protein than adults. The protein concentration falls during childhood and gradually increases again during the adult years when it has an upper limit of 45 mg/dl.(Table 13-4).

REFERENCES FOR CSF EXAMINATION

Bell W, Joynt R, Sahs A: Low spinal fluid pressure syndromes. *Neurology* 1960;10:512–521

Bigner SH: Cerebrospinal fluid (CSF) cytology: Current status and diagnostic applications. *J Neuropath Exp Neurol* 1992;51:235–245

Clark MA: Convulsions and lumbar puncture. *Dev Med Child Neurol* 1985;27:538–542

Edwards R, Schmidley JW, Simon RP: How often does a CSF pleocytosis follow generalized convulsions? *Ann Neurol* 1983;13:460–461

Fishman RA: *Cerebrospinal Fluid in Diseases of the Nervous System* (2d ed). Philadelphia, Saunders, 1992

Fraser JL: Persistent lumbar aglycorrachia of unknown cause. *Neurology* 1991;41:1323–1324

Grant R, Condon B, Hart I, et al: Changes in intracranial CSF volume after lumbar puncture and their relationship to post-LP headache. *J Neurol Neurosurg Psychiatr* 991;54:440–442

Greensher J, Mofenson HC, Borofsky LG, et al: Lumbar puncture in the neonate: A simplified technique. *J Pediatr* 1971;78:1034–1035

Herndon RM, Brumback RA (eds): *The Cerebrospinal Fluid.* Boston, Kluwer Academic Publishers, 1989

Kaneko K, Onodera O, Miyatake T, et al: Rapid diagnosis of tuberculous meningitis by polymerase chain reaction (PCR). *Neurology* 1990;40:1617–1618

Kaufman W, Vanderlinde R: Medical-laboratory evaluation. *N Engl J Med* 1967;277:1024–1025

Kuntz K, Kokmen E, Miller P, Offord K, Ho M: Post lumbar puncture headache: Experience in 501 consecutive procedures. *Neurology,* 1992;42:1884–1887.

Masdeu JC, Breuer AC, Schoene WC: Spinal subarachnoid hematomas: Clue to a source of bleeding in traumatic lumbar puncture. *Neurology* 1979;29:872–876

May C, Kaye JR, Atack JR, et al. Cerebrospinal fluid production is reduced in healthy aging. *Neurology* 1990;40:500–502

Petito F, Plum F: The lumbar puncture. *N Engl J Med* 1974;290:225–226

Rando TA, Fishman RA: Spontaneous intracranial hypotension: Report of two cases and review of the literature. *Neurology* 1992;42:481–487

Samsom DS, Clark K: A current review of brain abscess. *Am J Med* 1973;54:201–210

Scheld WM, Whitley RJ, Durack DT: *Infections of the Central Nervous System.* New York, Raven, 1991

Seebacher J, Ribeiro V, LeGuillou JL: Epidural blood patch in the treatment of post dural puncture headache: A double blind study. *Headache* 1989;29:630–632

Sharer LR: Pathology of HIV-1 infection of the central nervous system. *J Neuropath Exp Neurol* 1992;51:3–11

Swaiman KF: Spinal fluid examination, in Swaiman KF (ed): *Pediatric Neurology.* St. Louis, CV Mosby, 1989: 105–111

Van Der Meulen J: Cerebrospinal fluid xanthochromia: An objective index. *Neurology* 1966;16:170–178

III. Neuroradiology

A. *Plain skull and spine radiographs*
1. *Information provided.* Plain skull radiographs show bone and some calcified intracranial lesions, but do not show normal brain, ventricles, or subarachnoid spaces.
2. *Indications for plain skull or vertebral radiographs*
   a. Plain radiographs of the skull and vertebrae display their contours, thickness, density, and vascular markings, and any hyperostoses, erosions, or fractures. Plain radiographs of the skull display the air-filled cavities, foramina, and the state of closure of the sutures.
   b. Plain skull radiographs quickly and inexpensively screen for infection in the sinuses and mastoids by showing mucosal thickening, cloudiness, and fluid levels. Order frontal, lateral, Waters, and Towne views to visualize all of the sinuses and the mastoid air cells. Plain films serve little purpose if MRI or CT is required, because these procedures also show sinus disease.
   c. Vertebral radiographs aid in screening unconscious Pts with acute head injuries for cervical fracture-dislocations.
   d. Surveys of the skull, ribs, and long bones by plain radiographs identify previous fractures in battered infants.
   e. In most other instances, the Ex will bypass plain films for CT or MRI scans, which provide far more information.
3. *Risk of plain radiographs.* Minimal radiation.

B. *MRI scan of the head or vertebral column*
1. *The superiority of MRI over CT scan.* Because MRI shows normal CNS anatomy (Fig. 13-8) and almost all CNS lesions (Fig. 13-9) better than CT, MRI scan is the procedure of choice. I am tempted to suggest that the CT scan belongs in the Smithsonian Institution as a relic of a bygone era. CT remains more widely available, requires less time, and costs somewhat less, but these minor advantages do not outweigh its inferiority to MRI.
2. *Typical indications for an MRI scan*
   a. Suspected cerebrovascular disease: infarction (Fig. 13-9*A*), hemorrhage (Fig. 13-9*F*), aneurysms, and arteriovenous malformations. MRI angiography demonstrates the intracranial and neck vessels, in lieu of invasive angiography.
   b. Suspected demyelinating disease (Fig. 13-9*B*)
   c. Neoplasia: primary or metastatic (Fig. 13-9*C*)

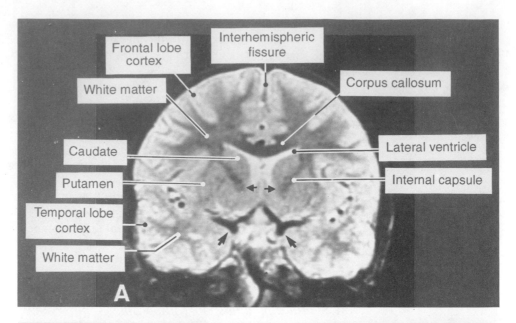

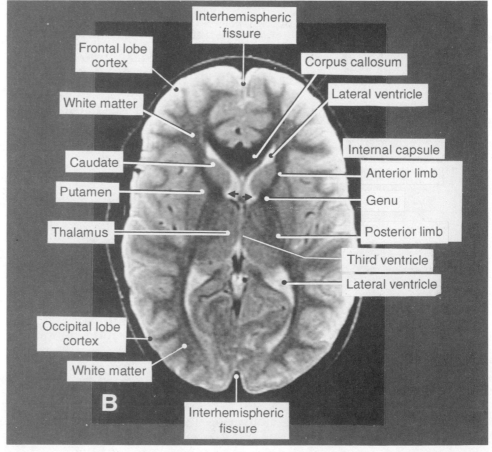

FIG. 13-8. (*A*) Coronal section, T2 weighted image, at the level of the genu of the internal capsule. The upper arrow points to the genu of the internal capsule at the foramen of Monro. Lower arrows show the internal carotid artery as it bifurcates into the middle and anterior cerebral arteries. (*B*) Horizontal section, T2 weighted image, at the level of the genu of the internal capsule. The arrows point to the genu of the internal capsule at the foramen of Monro.

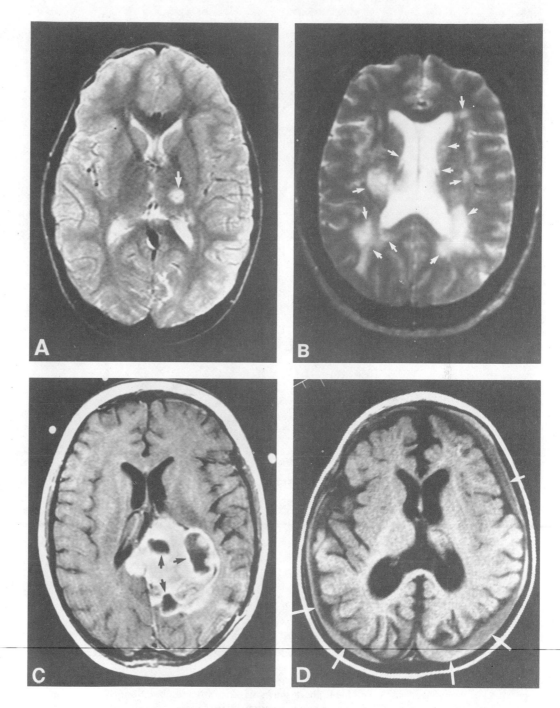

FIG. 13-9. Montage of lesions demonstrated by MRI and CT scan. The left side of the Pt's brain is to the reader's right. All horizontal scans are mounted with the frontal lobes up. (*A*) MRI, horizontal T$_2$ section of the brain, showing a subacute infarct (arrow) in the left thalamus. (*B*) MRI, horizontal T$_2$ section of the cerebrum, showing multiple areas of periventricular demyelinization (arrows) in multiple sclerosis. (*C*) MRI, horizontal T$_1$ section of brain, gadolinium enhanced, showing an astrocytoma with cystic cavities (arrows). The tumor is bright, and the fluid-filled cysts and CSF are black in T$_1$-weighted images, in contrast to bright in T$_2$-weighted images. (*D*) MRI, horizontal T$_1$ section of the brain, showing bilateral hematomas (arrows) and atrophic cerebrum with enlarged ventricles and subarachnoid spaces. The Pt, a battered child, had received

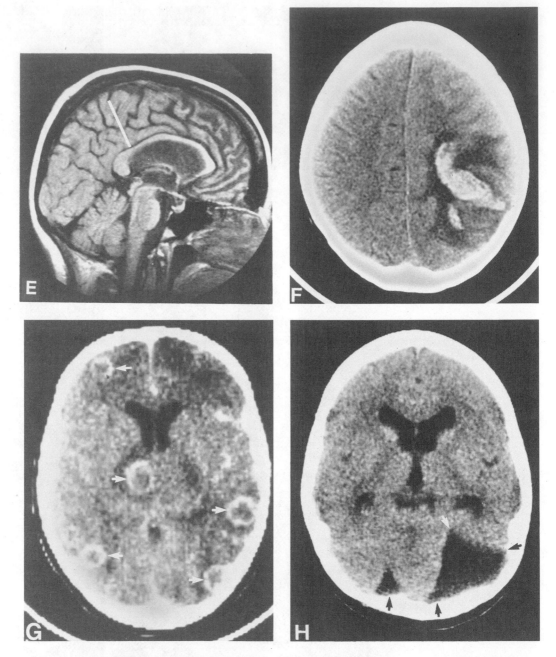

FIG. 13-9. (*Continued*) multiple head injuries. (*E*) MRI, sagittal T₁ section of the brain. The medial wall of the hemisphere shows selective frontal lobe atrophy with extreme widening of the subarachnoid spaces (arrows). Notice the normal size of the sulci in the parts of the cerebrum posterior to the white marker. The Pt has a form of pre-senile dementia called Pick's disease. (*F*) CT scan, horizontal section at a high level of the cerebrum, above the ventricles, showing a recent hemorrhage in the left parieto-occipital region. Edema causes the dark zone around the hemorrhage. (*G*) CT scan, horizontal section of the cerebrum, showing a contrast-enhanced white ring of vascularity around multiple abscess cavities. (*H*) CT scan, horizontal section of the brain, showing congential arachnoid cyst of the posterior fossa (three arrows). It has displaced the cerebellum and caused slight ventricular enlargement from obstructive hydrocephalus. The single arrow (to the reader's left) points to the displaced cisterna magna cerebelli.

    d. Craniospinal trauma (Fig. 13-9*D*)

    e. Dementia (Fig. 13-9*E*)

    f. Acute infections: meningitis, encephalitis, and abscess (Fig. 13-9*G*)

    g. Developmental retardation, microcephaly, macrocephaly, hydroceph-aly, cerebral palsy, and suspected malformation (Fig. 13-9*H*)

   h. Investigation of the cause of seizures
   i. Acute or new onset headaches
   j. Anoxic encephalopathy
3. *Enhancement with gadolinium.* The IV injection of gadolinium increases the value of an MRI scan by showing the blood vessels and sites of increased blood-brain barrier permeability, as in infarcts, neoplasms (Fig. 13-9*C*), or contusions.
4. *Risks of MRI scan.* MRI per se causes no known adverse biological effects, but the strong magnetic field precludes MRI for Pts with implants of magnetic metals and certain electronic devices. Some Pts get claustrophobia when inserted into the MRI tube. Uncooperative Pts and infants require sedation or anesthesia to prevent movement during an MRI scan.

C. *Indications for a CT scan*
1. The one advantage of CT over MRI is the ability to show bone and calcified parenchymal lesions of the CNS. As such, CT serves for any of the previously listed indications for plain radiographs. CT visualizes lesions of the posterior fossa or base of the skull poorly, because the bone and soft-tissue interfaces degrade the image.
2. For demonstration of frank intracranial hemorrhage and the ventricular contours, CT substitutes for MRI when time is critical, as in the diagnosis of acute intracranial bleeding from a head injury, when the Ex has to identify or exclude a lesion requiring surgical intervention quickly. Its wider availability and shorter scanning time then substitute for an MRI.
3. CT also suffices to follow the changes in ventricular size after shunt operations for hydrocephalus.
4. CT provides three-dimensional reconstruction of the skull for plastic surgery to correct craniofacial malformations and some facial injuries.
5. For all other circumstances requiring an imaging procedure, order an MRI scan.
6. *Contrast enhancement of the CT.* As with MRI, contrast material injected into a vein will enhance many lesions and increase the value of the CT scan (Fig. 13-9*E*).
7. *Risk of CT.* Virtually negligible radiation. Some uncooperative Pts and infants require sedation. Pts may have allergic reactions to injected contrast material.

SUGGESTED READINGS FOR MRI AND CT SCAN

Atlas SW: *Magnetic Resonance Imaging of the Brain and Spine.* New York, Raven, 1991

Barkovich JA: *Pediatric Neuroimaging.* New York, Raven, 1989

Berquist TH: *MRI of the Musculoskeletal System* (2d ed). New York, Raven, 1990

Daniels DL, Haughton VM, Naidich TP: *Cranial and Spinal Magnetic Resonance Imaging. An Atlas and Guide.* New York, Raven, 1987

Hayman LA, Hinck VC: *Clinical Brain Imaging. Normal Structure and Functional Anatomy.* St. Louis, Mosby Year Book, 1992

Kucharczyk W: *MRI: Central Nervous System.* Philadelphia, Lippincott, 1990

Latchaw RE: *MR and CT Imaging of the Head, Neck and Spine* (2d ed). St. Louis, Mosby Year Book, 1991

Newton TH, Fillon WP, Hasso AN: *Computed Tomography of the Head and Neck.* New York, Raven, 1988

Pomeranz SJ: *Craniospinal Magnetic Resonance Imaging.* Philadelphia, Saunders, 1989

Peterson H, Kieffer S: Neuroradiology, in Baker A, Baker L (eds): *Clinical Neurology*. New York, Harper & Row, 1977

Ramsey RG: *Neuroradiology* (2d ed). Philadelphia, Saunders, 1987

Salamon G, Raynaud C, Regis J, et al: *Magnetic Resonance Imaging of the Pediatric Brain: An Anatomical Atlas*. New York, Raven, 1990

Schnitzlein HN, Murtaugh FR: *Imaging Anatomy of the Head and Spine* (2d ed). Baltimore, Urgan & Schwarzenberg, 1990

Wolpert SM, Barnes PD: *MRI in Pediatric Neuroradiology*. St. Louis, Mosby Year Book, 1992

Yock DH: *Imaging of CNS Disease. A CT and MRI Teaching File*. St. Louis, Mosby Year Book, 1991

D. *Angiography of the CNS:* arteriography and venography
  1. *Methods*
     a. Direct injection of iodinated contrast material into an intraarterial catheter demonstrates the arteries and veins on radiographs (Fig. 13-8).
     b. By various technical and computer manipulations, CT and MRI scans themselves or in combination with intravenous contrast material show larger CNS vessels. Improvements in MRI angiography have reduced the need for, and may eliminate, invasive angiography by femoral catheterization.
     c. Doppler ultrasound studies demonstrate blood flow in the neck and some intracranial vessels.
  2. *Indications for invasive angiography (as a supplement to MRI angiography)*
     a. Demonstration of narrowed or occluded vessels in the neck and intracranial arteries.
     b. Investigation of subarachnoid hemorrhage and demonstration of aneurysms and arteriovenous malformations.
     c. Preoperative planning of surgical procedures for lesions which may involve or displace vessels.
  3. *Risk of invasive angiography:* arterial thrombosis and allergic reactions to the contrast media. Since the kidneys excrete the contrast material, renal failure may preclude angiography.

SUGGESTED READINGS FOR ANGIOGRAPHY

Berguer R, Caplan LR: *Vertebrobasilar Arterial Disease*. St. Louis, Quality Medical Publishers, 1992

Djindjian R: *Angiography of the Spinal Cord*. Baltimore, University Park Press, 1970

Hyman LA, Hinck VC: *Clinical Brain Imaging. Normal Structure and Functional Anatomy*. St. Louis, CV Mosby, 1992

Huber P: *Cerebral Angiography* (2d ed). Stuttgart, Georg Thieme Verlag, 1982

Newell DW, Asalid R (eds): *Transcranial Doppler*. New York, Raven, 1992

Newton TH, Potts DG (eds): *Radiology of the Skull and Brain*, vol 1, Books 1 and 2, *The Skull;* vol 2, Book 1, *Technical Aspects;* Book 2, *Arteries;* Book 3, *Veins;* Book 4, *Specific Disease Processes,* vol 3, *Anatomy and Pathology*. St. Louis, CV Mosby, 1974

Osborne A: *Introduction to Cerebral Angiography*. Hagerstown, Harper & Row, 1980

Petty GW: Transcranial Doppler ultrasonography. *Neurol Chron* 1991;1:1–7

E. *Head ultrasound.* Head ultrasound demonstrates gross cerebral lesions in fetuses, newborn, and young infants, until the fontanel closure. Although less sensitive than CT or MRI, it has the advantage that it can be done repeatedly prenatally or at the bedside of a sick infant and does not require transportation of the Pt to the radiology suite. Ultrasound has no known risk.

SUGGESTED READINGS FOR ULTRASONOGRAPHY

Fischer AQ (ed): Pediatric Neurosonology (vol 4). *J Child Neurol* (suppl) 1989

Graziana LJ, Pasto M, Stanley C, et al: Neonatal neurosonographic correlates of cerebral palsy in preterm infants. *Pediatrics* 1986;78:88–95

Levene MI, Williams JL, Fawer CL: *Ultrasound of the Infant Brain.* Philadelphia, Lippincott, 1985

G. *Invasive contrast myelography:* Visualization of spinal cord and vertebral lesions by CT or MRI scan has reduced the need for direct injection of contrast material into the subarachnoid space via an LP.

H. *Radionuclide brain scans*
   1. *Information provided.* Radionuclide scans show areas where radioactive substances have accumulated because of disruption of the blood-brain barrier or increased CNS metabolism.
   2. *Indications.* For the diagnosis of intracranial lesions, MRI scan has relegated radioactive brain scanning to special circumstances:
      a. Localizing an active epileptogenic focus prior to surgical removal.
      b. Studying the dynamics of CSF flow.
      c. Determining the absence of cerebral blood flow in the diagnosis of brain death (Chap. 12).
      d. Studying brain activity during various mental and physical tasks by PET (positron emission tomography). Although of great research value, PET scanning is not a routine clinical procedure.

SUGGESTED READING FOR RADIONUCLIDE SCANNING

Brooks D: PET: Its clinical role in neurology. *J Neurol Neurosurg Psychiatr,* 1991;54:1–5

Diksic M, Rega RC: *Radiopharmaceuticals and Brain Pathophysiology Studied with PET and SPECT.* Boca Raton, CRC Press, 1991

IV. Electroencephalography (EEG) and evoked potentials

A. *Principle:* Electrodes attached to the scalp record the changes in electrical potentials in the underlying cerebrum. The voltage differences between pairs of electrodes are amplified and recorded as wavy lines on paper, using an X-Y display system, as in the EKG. The waves may be too high or too low in amplitude, or too fast or too slow. The frequency of the waves in cycles per second and their amplitude vary with the region of the cerebrum, the age of the Pt, and the level of alertness. Sleep has its own distinctive EEG patterns. Brain lesions may alter the frequency of the waves, their amplitude, and their contour or configuration. Diffuse brain disease, such as metabolic encephalopathies or dementia, cause diffuse slowing of the brain waves, while focal destructive cerebral lesions, such as infarcts, abscesses, and neoplasms, cause focal slowing. In epilepsy, the EEG typically shows focal or generalized spikes, or spikes and slow waves (Fig. 13-10).

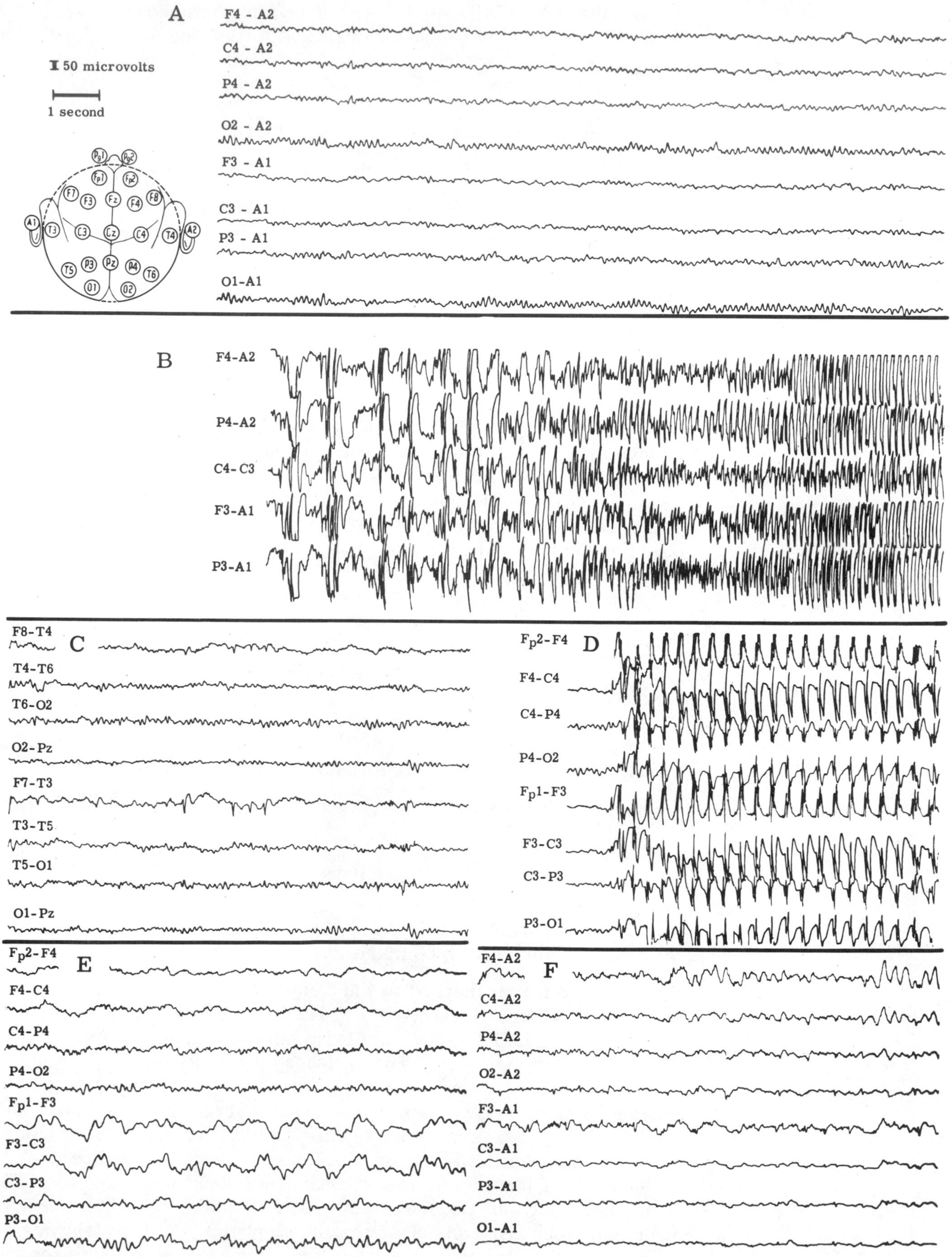
A
50 microvolts
1 second
F4 - A2
C4 - A2
P4 - A2
O2 - A2
F3 - A1
C3 - A1
P3 - A1
O1-A1
B
F4-A2
P4-A2
C4-C3
F3-A1
P3-A1
C
F8-T4
T4-T6
T6-O2
O2-Pz
F7-T3
T3-T5
T5-O1
O1-Pz
D
Fp2-F4
F4-C4
C4-P4
P4-O2
Fp1-F3
F3-C3
C3-P3
P3-O1
E
Fp2-F4
F4-C4
C4-P4
P4-O2
Fp1-F3
F3-C3
C3-P3
P3-O1
F
F4-A2
C4-A2
P4-A2
O2-A2
F3-A1
C3-A1
P3-A1
O1-A1

B. *Use of the EEG in the diagnosis of seizures and pseudoseizures*
   1. The EEG's greatest value lies in differentiating epilepsy from other periodic cerebral dysfunctions and in differentiating true seizures from pseudoseizures. *A seizure is any change in the mental, sensory, or motor state caused by an abnormal, hypersynchronous discharge of neurons. Epilepsy is defined as recurrent seizures.*
   2. Virtually all epileptics have abnormal EEGs during a seizure. Most epileptic Pts have abnormal EEGs in the interval between seizures, but if the hypersynchronous discharge appears only intermittently, any given EEG in the interictal period may be normal. Combined video monitoring and EEG aids in correlating subtle seizures with epileptiform discharges, or in disclosing that a given seizure-like event is a pseudoseizure because no epileptiform activity occurred. Long-term ambulatory monitoring by a portable EEG pack may also disclose epileptiform discharges, when the base-line EEG proves inconclusive in the face of a clinical history suggesting seizures. Clinicians commonly err in expecting an EEG to "rule out epilepsy." The pitfalls are that Pts with epilepsy may have a normal interictal EEG, and occasionally a Pt with hypersynchronous, epileptiform discharges, i.e., spikes, or spikes and waves, will not have clinically detectable seizures. The diagnosis of epilepsy depends on correlating the abnormal discharges with some regular change in the Pt's mental, motor, or sensory state. The diagnosis of epilepsy thus rests on this correlative proof, not simply an EEG pattern.

C. *Activation of hypersynchronous, epileptiform activity during an EEG*
   1. Several procedures may activate spikes, or spikes and waves, in the EEG. These activating procedures increase the likelihood that any given interictal EEG will show an epileptiform abnormality, and, in fact, may precipitate an actual seizure.
   2. The routine activating procedures consist of hyperventilation for 3 to 5 min, photic stimulation, and sleep. Hyperventilation drives off CO_2, reducing the blood pH. This change increases the likelihood of a spike, or spike-wave discharge, particularly in Pts with petit mal seizures. Photic stimulation with different flash frequencies activates the occipital cortex and may bring out epileptiform discharges or a frank clinical seizure. Sleep may also activate a spike focus not seen during the waking record.

D. *EEG in coma and other acute changes in mental state*
   1. Sometimes, an EEG aids in diagnosing the cause of coma or otherwise unexplained changes in mental state. Nonconvulsive status epilepticus, with no convulsive motor activity, may cause acute changes in mental state

FIG. 13-10. Electroencephalograms. The inset at the upper left shows the calibration signals and the position of the electrodes on the head. The electroencephalograph acts as an X-Y recorder. Each line on the EEG represents the difference in electrical potential between a pair of electrodes. Excepting record *B*, the first four lines in each record (even numbers) are from the right side of the head, the second four (odd numbers) are homologous leads from the left side. To read the records (except *B*), mentally "pick up" the top four lines and superimpose them on the bottom four lines. (*A*) Normal record with symmetrical 10 cps (alpha) rhythm in the occipital leads. (*B*) High amplitude, symmetrical hypersynchronous discharge during a grand mal, generalized tonic-clonic seizure. The first portion of the record shows a few myoclonic jerks, the mid-portion shows the tonic phase, and the last portion of the record shows the individual, whole-body jerks of the clonic phase. Succinylcholine has blocked the skeletal muscular action, eliminating artifact from muscle action potentials. (*C*) Spike focus in the left frontotemporal region. This type of focal abnormality usually indicates a chronic, epileptogenic lesion. (*D*) Generalized, 3 cps hypersynchronous burst, usually associated with transient loss of consciousness, without tonic-clonic motor activity. (*E*) Random slow (delta) waves of 1 to 3 cps in the left anterior and central regions. This wave form usually indicates an acute destructive lesion such as an infarct, neoplasm, abscess, or contusion. (*F*) Amplitude asymmetry with flattening of the waves over the left hemisphere, and some generalized slow activity. The Pt has a subdural hematoma with a large amount of blood over the left hemisphere.

with disorientation, delirium, or coma. The EEG may be the only way to document the epileptic cause. Brain death, hypothermia, and intoxication with depressant drugs may result in complete absence of recordable electrical activity in the EEG (Chap. 12).

2. EEG recording aids in monitoring the treatment of status epilepticus with IV anticonvulsant medications.

E. *Space-occupying lesions* such as infarcts, neoplasms, abscesses, and contusions cause focal slow waves over the lesion site. The MRI has supplanted the EEG in the diagnosis of focal destructive lesions.

F. *EEG in apnea and sleep disorders.* Daytime EEGs in narcolepsy and overnight polysomnographic recordings including EEG are often necessary to resolve the cause of nocturnal episodes, apnea, and the parasomnias.

G. *Summary of EEG changes.* Sharp, waves, spikes, or intermixed spikes and slow waves imply an epileptogenic lesion, usually of static type, such as a brain scar, or a slowly advancing lesion. Slow waves alone, if focal, imply a focal destructive lesion or transient metabolic depression. Generalized slow waves imply reduction of consciousness or a generalized brain disease. Flattening of the waves, if not postictal, suggests a fluid, either blood or CSF, between the brain and skull, or absence of, or complete destruction and death of, the part of the cerebrum that underlies the electrodes. Table 13-5 summarizes the indications for an EEG. Order a video-monitored or ambulatory EEG if the routine EEG fails to record one of the Pt's customary episodes, and the diagnosis remains in question.

H. *Risk of EEG:* None.

I. *Editorial note:* EEG has attracted more than its fair share of entrepreneurs, some of whom read EEGs by long-distance telephone. The electroencephalographer must personally attend the laboratory every day to consult with the referring physicians and technicians about the proper recording of each Pt and to insure high quality, artifact-free records. As a general rule, the EEG is worse than useless unless read by a physician:

1. Who is trained in neurology and who personally oversees the EEG laboratory daily.
2. Who personally diagnoses and treats a wide variety of neurologic Pts and thus fully appreciates the clinical meaning of the EEG findings.
3. Who continually checks his EEG interpretations against the clinical course and ultimate diagnosis of the Pts referred to the EEG laboratory and against the opinions of knowledgeable colleagues.
4. Who knows the structure of the brain, understands how lesions affect it, and regularly attends neuroradiological and autopsy sessions to make rueful note of diagnostic errors.

TABLE 13-5 Summary of clinical indications for an electroencephalogram (EEG)

1. Intermittent episodes of brain dysfunction that could be epilepsy.
2. Acute undiagnosed changes in mental state, including coma, seizures, or pseudoseizures
3. Sleep disorders, including sleep apnea
4. Monitoring of the anticonvulsant treatment of status epilepticus
5. Ancillary procedure for the diagnosis of brain death

5. In fact, as you see, these criteria, with slight change in wording, characterize any good physician who runs any laboratory.

J. *Magnetoencephalography:* Recording of the magnetic fields associated with the electrical activity of the brain provides information that supplements standard EEG and evoked potentials (Sato, 1990).

SUGGESTED READINGS FOR EEG AND MAGNETOENCEPHALOGRAPHY

Bennett DR, Hughes JR, Korein J, et al: *Atlas of Electroencephalography in Coma and Cerebral Death: EEG at the Bedside or in the Intensive Care Unit.* New York, Raven, 1976

Daly DD, Pedley TA: *Current Practice of Clinical Electroencephalography* (2d ed). New York, Raven, 1990

Lowenstein DH, Aminoff MJ: Clinical and EEG features of status epilepticus in comatose patients. *Neurology* 1992;42:100–103

Markand ON: Slow spike-wave activity in EEG and associated clinical features: often called "Lennox" or "Lennox-Gastaut" syndrome. *Neurology* 1977;27:746–757

Sato S: Magnetoencephalography, in *Advances in Neurology* (vol 54). New York, Raven, 1990

Stockard-Pope JE, Werner SS, Bickford RG, et al: *Atlas of Neonatal Electroencephalography* (2d ed). New York, Raven, 1992

Thorpy MN (chairman): Diagnostic Classification Steering Committee: *International Classification of Sleep Disorders (ICSD): Diagnostic and Coding Manual.* Rochester, MN, American Sleep Disorders Association, 1990

K. *Evoked responses in the CNS*
1. *Principle.* Electrodes placed at various sites on the skin over the brain or spinal cord record the transmission of the nerve impulses through the sensory pathways to the sensory areas of the cortex. The studies consist of visual-evoked responses (VER), auditory-evoked responses, or brainstem-auditory-evoked responses (BAER), and somatic-sensory-nerve-evoked responses (SSER). The BAER consists of seven different waves, representing the passage of the nerve impulses through the seven levels of the auditory pathway (Fig. 9-7): acoustic nerve, cochlear nuclei, superior olivary complex, lateral lemniscus, inferior colliculus, medial geniculate body, and thalamocortical radiations to the temporal lobe.
2. *Indications for evoked responses*
   a. Objective assessment of the integrity of visual, auditory, and somatosensory pathways in unconscious, uncooperative, and psychiatrically ill Pts or infants
   b. Monitoring of depth of anesthesia and coma
   c. Intra-operative monitoring of the integrity of spinal and cerebral pathways during surgical procedures

SUGGESTED READINGS FOR EVOKED POTENTIALS

Chiappa KH: *Evoked Potentials in Clinical Medicine* (2d ed). New York, Raven, 1990

Cusick JF, Wyklebust JB, Larson SJ, et al: Spinal cord evaluation by cortical evoked responses. *Arch Neurol* 1979;36:140

Liveson JA, Ma DM: *Laboratory Reference for Clinical Neurophysiology.* Philadelphia, FA Davis, 1992

Markand OM, Farlow MR, Stevens JC, et al: Brain-stem auditory evoked potential abnormalities with unilateral brain-stem lesions demonstrated by magnetic resonance imaging. *Arch Neurol* 1989;446:295–299

Singh N, Sachdev KK, Brisman R: Trigeminal nerve stimulation: Short latency somatosensory evoked potentials. *Neurology* 1982;32:97–101

V. Electronystagmography (ENG)

A. *Principle:* ENG provides a quantitative method for recording nystagmus, either spontaneous or that evoked by caloric stimulation, positional change, rotation, or by an optokinetic drum. Recording of eye movements takes advantage of the fact that the eye is polarized (with the cornea positive) in reference to the fundus. Skin electrodes placed on either side of the eye record the electrical changes as the polarized eyeballs move. An X-Y recorder, as with EEG or EKG, then records the movements as waves on a strip of moving paper.

B. *Indications for an ENG:* ENG aids in the analysis of Pts with dizziness or who have symptoms or signs of VIIIth nerve or brainstem disease.

SUGGESTED READING FOR ELECTRONYSTAGMOGRAPHY

Rubin W, Brookler KH: *Dizziness. Etiologic Approach to Management.* New York, Thieme Medical Publishers, 1991

VI. Magnetic stimulation

A. *Principle:* Stimulation of the motor cortex by magnetic energy permits measurement of conduction through the pyramidal tract, allowing objective evaluation of lesions. The technique can also be applied to peripheral nerves. The technique and instrumentation are still in their infancy.

B. *Risk:* Painless and, insofar as is known, harmless unless the Pt has metal implants of some type.

SUGGESTED READINGS FOR MAGNETIC STIMULATION

Chiappa KH: Transcranial magnetic stimulation of the human motor cortex for evaluation of central motor pathways. *Neurol Chron* 1991;1:1–5

Chokroverty S: *Magnetic Stimulation in Clinical Neurophysiology.* Stoneham, MA, Butterworths, 1990

Thompson PD, Day BL, Crockard HA, et al: Intra-operative recording of motor tract potentials at the cervico-medullary junction following scalp electrical and magnetic stimulation of the motor cortex. *J Neurol Neurosurg Psychiatr* 1991;54:618–623

Wassermann EM, Fuhr P, Cohen LG, et al: Effects of transcranial magnetic stimulation on ipsilateral muscles. *Neurology* 1991;41:1795–1799

VII. Electromyography (EMG) and nerve conduction velocity

A. *Principle of EMG:* A needle electrode inserted into a muscle records the electrical potential produced when the muscle fibers depolarize and contract. An X-Y system (an oscilloscope or paper strip as in EKG or EEG) displays the potentials (Fig. 7-22).

B. *Indications for EMG*
   1. *Differentiating neurogenic and myopathic weakness:* The EMG has its greatest value in determining whether weakness is due to neuropathy, defective neuromuscular transmission, or myopathy.
      a. In *neurogenic* atrophy the EMG discloses fibrillations, fasciculations, and giant polyphasic motor units (Fig. 7-22).
      b. In *myasthenia gravis,* the EMG discloses a decremental response in the amplitude of the electrical potentials as the muscle weakens during repetitive stimulation (Jolly test).
      c. In *myopathies,* the EMG discloses a decreased amplitude of the muscle potentials or myotonic potentials.
   2. *Differentiation of root versus peripheral nerve weaknesses.* By detecting exactly which muscles show the effects of denervation, the EMG can aid in differentiating root (myotomal) from peripheral nerve lesions. For example, a nerve root lesion affects different muscles than a peripheral nerve lesion (Table 2-1).

C. *Risk:* The insertion of the needle causes minor pain but virtually never leads to significant complications.

D. *Nerve conduction velocity and nerve trunk stimulation*
   1. *Measuring the conduction velocity of motor nerves.* A stimulating electrode is applied over a large motor nerve trunk, and the response is recorded by EMG from one of its muscles. From the distance and the time elapsed between stimulus and response, the velocity of impulse conduction in the nerve can be calculated directly. Stimuli can be applied at two points along the nerve, and the time for the shorter distance subtracted from the longer to cancel out the delay for neuromuscular transmission.
   2. *Measuring the conduction velocity of sensory nerves.* The time between the electrical stimulus at a distal site and a more proximal site is recorded and the distance measured directly along the course of the nerve. The velocity can also be computed during the recording of SERs.
   3. *Indications for measuring the conduction velocity of nerves.* Conduction velocity determinations aid in diagnosing peripheral neuropathies and in locating the sites of peripheral nerve compression in compression neuropathies. Normal velocities range between 40 to 60 m/sec for adults.
      a. In *peripheral neuropathies,* the nerve conduction velocity is less than 75 percent of normal. The test only establishes that the nerve is diseased. It gives little differential information as to whether the disease is toxic, metabolic, or heredofamilial in origin, but it can help to differentiate demyelinating neuropathies from primary axonopathies.
      b. In *nerve compression syndromes,* stimulation of nerve trunks can localize the lesion site. For example, it is sometimes difficult to decide whether a Pt who has tingling in the thumb and index finger has compression of the C_6 nerve root, or compression of the median nerve in the carpal tunnel at the wrist. Delayed conduction across the wrist estab-

lishes the carpal tunnel syndrome, rather than a nerve root compression syndrome.

4. *Risk of NCV.* Moderately uncomfortable.

SUGGESTED READINGS FOR ELECTROMYOGRAPHY

Aminoff MJ: *Electrodiagnosis in Clinical Neurology.* Edinburgh, Churchill-Livingstone, 1988

Basmajian JV, DeLuca E: *Muscles Alive. Their Functions Revealed by Electromyography.* Baltimore, Williams & Wilkins, 1985

Dorfman LJ, Bosley TM: Age-related changes in peripheral and central nerve conduction in man. *Neurology* 1979;29:38

Goodgold J, Eberstein A: *Electrodiagnosis of Neuromuscular Diseases* (3d ed). Baltimore, Williams & Wilkins, 1983

Kimura J: *Electrodiagnosis in Diseases of Nerve and Muscle: Principles and Practice* (2d ed). Philadelphia, FA Davis, 1989

Liveson JA, Ma DM: *Laboratory Reference for Clinical Neurophysiology.* Philadelphia, FA Davis, 1992

VIII. Muscle, nerve, and brain biopsy

A. *Muscle biopsy:* A moderately affected muscle is biopsied. The operator avoids end-stage muscle consisting mainly of scar tissue. Part of the muscle is fixed in formalin for histologic stains, in glutaraldehyde for electron microscopy, and unfixed tissue is frozen for enzyme histochemistry, biochemistry, and immunoelectrophoresis.

1. *Clinical use.* The biopsy aids in distinguishing muscular weakness of *neuropathic, myopathic,* or *inflammatory* origin.

   a. In *neuropathic* or *LMN* disease, the muscle biopsy shows atrophy of the fibers of individual fascicles that constitute a motor unit, while the neighboring fascicles of muscle fibers which have intact axons remain healthy.

   b. In *myopathic* disease, the muscle biopsy shows uniform involvement of all muscle fibers.

   c. In *inflammatory* disease, the muscle biopsy shows an inflammatory reaction of the tissue, mainly perivascular lymphocytes, granulomas, or parasitic cysts. In polymyositis, the muscle fibers on the periphery of the fascicles display selective damage.

2. *Risk.* Wound infection, bleeding, and anesthetic complications.

SUGGESTED READINGS FOR MUSCLE BIOPSY

Adachi M, Sher JH: *Neuromuscular Diseases (Current Trends in Neurosciences).* New York, Igaku-Shoin Medical Publishers, 1990

Brooke MH: *A Clinician's View of Neuromuscular Diseases* (2d ed). Baltimore, Williams & Wilkins, 1986

Dubowitz V: *Muscle Biopsy. A Practical Approach* (2d ed). Philadelphia, Saunders, 1985

Engle AG, Banker BQ (eds): *Myology.* New York, McGraw-Hill, 1986

Walton J (ed): *Disorders of Voluntary Muscle* (5th ed). Boston, Churchill-Livingstone, 1988

B. *Nerve biopsy*

    1. *Principle.* A few diseases cause pathognomic or highly suggestive lesions in peripheral nerves, demonstrable by the appropriate histologic techniques. Sensory nerves are biopsied.

    2. *Clinical use.* Biopsy of a purely sensory nerve, usually the sural nerve, aids in diagnosing many types of neuropathies, particularly of metabolic or heredofamilial type. It provides the most information in connection with muscle biopsy, EMG, and nerve conduction velocity studies.

    3. *Risk.* Wound infection and anesthesia or paresthesias in the nerve distribution.

SUGGESTED READINGS FOR NERVE BIOPSY

Dyck P, Karnes J, Lais A, et al: Pathologic alterations of the peripheral nervous system of man, in Dyck P, Thomas J, Lambert E, et al (eds): *Peripheral Neuropathy.* Philadelphia, Saunders, 1984

Schochet SS: *Diagnostic Pathology of Skeletal Muscle and Nerve.* Norwalk, CT, Appleton-Century-Crofts, 1986

C. *Brain biopsy:* Brain biopsy is indicated to recover some viruses or to diagnose neoplasms and some degenerative diseases. The risks are infection and hemorrhage.

IX. A perspective on the use of laboratory procedures (from Robert Wartenberg)

Careful history taking and interpreting, minute and repeated clinical examination are time consuming. It is particularly the busy physician who is inclined to delegate the diagnosis to the laboratory in the vain hope of saving time. Too many irrelevant technical procedures often confuse the issue, cloud the essential point, and broaden the margin for error. Time invested in clinical examination might have paid greater dividends. The main point is this: laboratory procedures often seem necessary because the clinical examination has not been adequate. They are all too often superfluous, and a thorough clinical examination would have provided grounds for correct management of the patient. The more clinical neurology we know, the less need there is for laboratory procedures and the more valuable these procedures become when they are necessary. . . .

Before any technical procedure is used, the following points should be considered carefully. (1) Some methods are time consuming. Valuable and irretrievable time may be lost through their use. (2) Some methods are expensive and to some patients may be an incommensurate economic burden. (3) Some methods are not always harmless, are often painful and sometimes fraught with danger. (4) The objective findings depend on the integrity of delicate mechanical apparatus. (5) The interpretation may be equivocal. (6) Even if by laboratory procedures the presence of a definite pathological process has been established, it does not mean that the finding is clinically significant or that it can account for the patient's present condition. (7) The information obtained, however interesting, may not influence the clinical diagnosis and may be completely irrelevant to the actual management of the patient. (8) The correct evaluation of the most informative and illuminating laboratory findings is possible only when correlated with the findings of a complete clinical examination, for which there is no substitute. The laboratory cannot tell the whole story; it can give only a brief passage. (9) The more thorough and exact the neurological examination, the more informative and helpful are the results of the necessary laboratory procedures. (10) If the laboratory findings contradict the clinical findings, it is, in the last analysis, best to base the diagnostic decision on the clinical findings.

—Robert Wartenberg (*Diagnostic Tests in Neurology. A Selection for Office Use. Chicago, Year Book Medical Publishers, 1953. Used by permission.*)

Learning Objectives for Chapter Thirteen _____

I. Array of neurodiagnostic procedures

State the principles that govern the selection of laboratory tests.

II. The cerebrospinal fluid (CSF) examination

1. State the location of the CSF.
2. Trace a drop of CSF from its origin to its absorption.
3. Draw a lateral projection of the ventricular system (Fig. 13-1).
4. List the functions of the CSF.
5. Describe the composition of normal CSF.
6. Enumerate the normal pressure of the CSF at various ages.
7. Describe the signs and symptoms of increased intracranial pressure in infants and older Pts.
8. Describe, in principle, the causes for increased CSF pressure.
9. Recite the kinds of lesions which typically obstruct the flow of CSF at the various critical sites along its flow pathway.
10. State Pascal's law of distribution of pressure in an enclosed container (Fig. 13-3).
11. Describe the signs and symptoms and some causes of low CSF pressure.
12. List several common indications for a lumbar puncture (LP).
13. List and explain the most important contraindications for an LP.
14. Describe the complications of an LP.
15. Discuss the apprehensions of the Pt about an LP.
16. Describe how to position a Pt for an LP and why that position is chosen (Fig. 13-3*B*).
17. Describe how to insert a needle for an LP.
18. Describe how to measure the CSF pressure, and state the normal range.
19. State the precautions the Ex takes in measuring the CSF pressure when the history or clinical examination raise the possibility of increased pressure.
20. State what causes the normal fluctuations in the level of the CSF meniscus in the manometer.
21. State, in principle, the relationship between the CSF pressure and the pressure in the extracranial veins.
22. Describe the changes in CSF pressure with inspiration and expiration and explain why these changes occur.
23. State whether the intracranial-CSF pressure is most closely related to the arterial or capillary/venous pressure.
24. State the mechanism by which an anxious Pt's abdominal muscle tension may increase the opening CSF pressure.
25. Describe how to induce the anxious Pt to relax the abdominal muscles.
26. Explain how neck flexion may increase the CSF pressure.
27. Summarize the actions or instructions the Ex uses to exclude extrinsic causes for a high opening CSF pressure.
28. State how an LP can cause the death of a Pt with intrinsically increased CSF pressure.
29. Explain, according to Pascal's law, why increased intracranial pressure will cause the brain to herniate after an LP (Fig. 13-5).
30. State what actions the Ex should take if the opening CSF pressure remains increased after having completed the usual maneuvers to exclude extrinsic causes for increased pressure.
31. Enumerate the causes and describe what to do if the flow of CSF stops or the manometer excursions cease (Table 13-3).
32. Describe, in principle, the clinical signs of transforaminal herniation.
33. Describe how to determine whether the CSF-manometer system is patent.
34. Explain why the Ex would use abdominal rather than jugular compression to determine whether the CSF-manometer system is patent if the flow of CSF stops.
35. Explain why the Ex should not aspirate CSF with a syringe if the flow suddenly stops.
36. Explain why the Ex collects the CSF in three different tubes.
37. Describe the gross appearance of normal CSF.
38. Enumerate the usual pathologic alterations in the gross appearance of the CSF.
39. Describe the proper way to inspect a sample of CSF for changes in gross appearance.
40. State how many red or white cells must be present to alter the gross appearance of the CSF.
41. State the usual cause for cloudiness of the CSF.
42. Explain how to interpret the situation when the Ex has seen a gross alteration in the CSF, and the laboratory returns a report of a normal gross appearance.
43. Explain how to interpret the situation if the Ex has seen a cloudy CSF, and the laboratory reports a count of less than 50 WBCs/mm^3.
44. Explain why the Ex cannot delegate the immediate gross and microscopic inspection of the CSF to the laboratory.
45. Distinguish between erythrochromia of the CSF and xanthochromia.
46. Define what is meant by a traumatic or bloody tap.
47. Describe the methods for distinguishing a traumatic tap from pre-existing blood in the CSF.
48. Explain the importance of centrifuging red or yellow CSF.
49. State the length of time required for xanthochromia to appear after hemorrhage into the CSF.
50. Describe how to correct the WBC count in the CSF when RBCs are also present.

51. Define erythrophagocytosis and discuss its meaning.
52. State the three most common causes of CSF xanthochromia and describe how to distinguish them.
53. Enumerate the widely available laboratory tests on the CSF and give normal values for the constituents of the CSF routinely tested (Fig. 13-7).
54. Give the normal cell count in the CSF for young infants and mature Pts and state the type of cells normally present.
55. List some of the types of neoplastic cells that invade the CSF and state in principle how they are identified.
56. Describe in principle the methods for identifying the various common bacteria and viruses that cause meningitis and encephalitis.
57. Explain why the vast array of laboratory tests available for the identification of microorganisms places even more value on the clinical findings than ever before.
58. State the normal value for the CSF glucose concentration and how it relates to the blood glucose level.
59. State the normal value for the CSF protein and describe in principle the importance of fractionating the immunoglobulins.
60. State how to correct the CSF protein value to compensate for blood in the CSF.
61. State in principle the differences in the CSF pressure, cell count, and protein content from early infancy to maturity.
62. State the typical CSF profiles found in encephalitis, meningitis, pre-existing bleeding, multiple sclerosis, and neoplasm (Table 13-2).

III. Neuroradiology

1. Enumerate, in principle, the features of bone anatomy displayed by plain skull radiographs.
2. Discuss, in principle, the clinical indications for ordering skull radiographs.
3. Discuss, in principle, the indications for ordering plain spine films.
4. Enumerate the major pathologic categories of CNS lesions disclosed by MRI scan (Fig. 13-9).
5. Explain which procedure, an MRI or CT scan, is usually the procedure of choice to visualize most CNS lesions.
6. Recite the common indications for ordering an MRI scan.
7. State what additional information an MRI scan enhanced with gadolinium would provide.
8. State a special circumstance that would contraindicate an MRI scan because of physical danger to the Pt.
9. Describe what must be done to obtain an MRI scan on a Pt unable to cooperate by holding still for several minutes.
10. State the one tissue shown by CT that MRI scan does not visualize.
11. Describe some clinical circumstances when a CT substitutes for, or is superior to, an MRI scan.

****12. State some clinical circumstances when direct arteriography by arterial catheter may be needed to supplement visualization of the vessels on routine MRI scan.
13. State two clinical circumstances that would preclude use of contrast material for angiography.
14. Describe the use of ultrasound in neuroimaging and neurovascular imaging.
**15. State the indications for radionuclide brain scans.

IV. Electroencephalography (EEG) and evoked potentials

1. State, in principle, what the EEG records.
2. Define a seizure and epilepsy.
3. Describe, in principle, the kinds of abnormal EEG waves seen with seizures (Fig. 13-9).
4. State in principle the difference in the EEG waves in diffuse cerebral disease versus focal destructive lesions (Fig. 13-9).
5. Describe how to use EEG to differentiate seizures and pseudoseizures.
6. Describe the routine activating procedures used during EEG and explain why they are used.
7. State why an EEG cannot "rule out" epilepsy.
8. Describe how the EEG may aid in differentiating the causes of changes in mental state, particularly disorientation and coma.
9. State three conditions in which the EEG displays no recordable cerebral activity.
10. State the major clinical indications for ordering an EEG (Table 13-5).
11. Describe in principle the criteria that identify a capable electroencephalographer and explain why reading EEGs by long distance telephone is worse than useless.
12. Recite the three sensory pathways ordinarily utilized for evoked potentials.
13. Describe in principle some typical clinical indications for use of evoked potentials.

V. Electronystagmography (ENG)

1. State the clinical indications for ENG.
2. Distinguish operationally between what is recorded in the ENG and in the EEG and evoked potential tests.

**VI. Magnetic stimulation

State which motor pathway can be readily studied by magnetic stimulation.

VII. Electromyography (EMG) nerve conduction velocity

1. Describe, in principle, what the EMG records.
2. State, in principle, the clinical indications for an EMG.
3. Describe the EMG changes typical of denervation and of myopathies (Fig. 7-22).
4. Describe how EMG aids in the diagnosis of myasthenia gravis.

5. Enumerate some of the major clinical indications for measurement of motor or sensory nerve conduction velocities.

VIII. Muscle, nerve and brain biopsy

1. State the major classes of diseases diagnosed by a muscle biopsy.

**2. State the clinical indications for a nerve biopsy and state which type of nerve, motor or sensory, is biopsied.

**3. State the indications for a brain biopsy.

IX. A perspective on the use of laboratory procedures
(from Robert Wartenberg)
Discuss in principle the pitfalls in laboratory tests.

Chapter Fourteen

Clinical and Laboratory Tests to Distinguish Hysteria from Neurologic Disease

Much will be gained if we succeed in transforming hysterical misery into common unhappiness.   **Sigmund Freud** (1856–1939)

Note: I have not programmed this chapter. Try programming it yourself to reach the emancipation stage in self-instruction. Learn it one way or another, since you face two distinct tests: the Learning Objectives at the end of the chapter and your first hysterical Pt.

I. The general clinical features of hysteria

A. *Definition of hysteria (conversion reaction, DSM-III)*
Hysteria means transient motor or sensory dysfunctions mimicking neurologic disease but arising from unconscious determinants, not from neuroanatomic lesions in the sites that should produce the dysfunctions (Table 14-1).

B. *Primary and secondary gain in hysteria:* Classical psychoanalytic theory holds that a hysterical symptom represents an *unconscious* mental mechanism that relieves overwhelming anxiety by converting it into symptoms (Weintraub, 1983). The symptom provides both *primary* and *secondary* gains for the Pt.
1. The *primary* gain consists of the relief of anxiety.
2. The *secondary* gains consist of manipulative control over the emotional responses and actions of other persons and relief from responsibilities. Overall, the gains make the symptom more acceptable to the Pt than the anxiety that the symptom relieves.
3. Walker et al (1989) suggest that operant conditioning, with its theory of reinforcement of behavior by reward, provides an alternative paradigm to analytic theory. "Simply put, those behaviors that obtain reward are those that are expressed."

C. *Distinction between hysteria and malingering*
1. The origins of the dysfunction and the purposes it serves seem to operate at a subconscious level in hysteria. The Pt experiences the illness as genuine.

TABLE 14-1 Pseudoneurologic manifestations of conversion hysteria and other non-organic disorders

A. *Mental*
1. Pseudoepileptic seizures
2. Amnestic and fugue states

B. *Motor*
1. Paralysis (monoplegia, paraplegia, or hemiplegia)
2. Hyperkinesia: tremors, flailing, and spasms
2. Astasia-abasia
3. Aphonia-dysphagia
4. Hyperventilation, often with dizziness and syncope; weak, shallow respiration; or grunting, demonstrative respiration
5. Blepharospasm, convergence spasm, pseudo-VIth nerve palsy, and ptosis
6. Vomiting

C. *Sensory*
1. Anesthesia, paresthesia, hyperesthesia, or pain
2. Dimness of vision, tunnel vision and spiral fields, blindness, double vision, and photophobia
3. Deafness and dizziness
4. Globus hystericus

At the opposite nosologic pole stands the malingerer, who consciously fakes an illness to achieve some tangible goal, such as getting money in a lawsuit, or avoiding criminal prosecution, or other responsibilities.
2. A spectrum of illnesses, such as Munchausen's syndrome, pseudoepileptic seizures, and many chronic pain syndromes, fall somewhere in between hysteria and malingering on the scale of conscious awareness. Instead of debating the degree of conscious awareness, let us just focus on the salient fact that the same examination techniques effectively separate organic diseases from the entire spectrum of psychogenic or functional diseases.

    D. *Criteria for the diagnosis of hysteria*
        1. *Explicit criteria for the diagnosis of hysteria* (Table 14-2)
        2. *History in conversion hsyteria*
            a. Females, usually between 10 and 35 years of age, predominate about 3:1. The quoted ratio may reflect a diagnostic bias. Hysteria unequivocally affects males. The history discloses long-standing personality problems, with some immediate emotional stress that triggers the hysterical episodes. For example, a neurotic Pt, after getting engaged, may display hysterical paraplegia as an unconscious defense against the sexual performance or the duties implied by marriage. The history of predisposing emotional problems and of the precipitating event is essential to the diagnosis of hysteria. Don't diagnose hysteria in a previously well-

---

TABLE 14-2 Criteria for the diagnosis of conversion hysteria

1. Presence of symptoms and signs that imitate neurological disease but do not match organic patterns of illness. The symptoms reflect the Pt's mental image of the body and the way it functions rather than the wiring diagram of the nervous system.
2. Absence of signs of organic illness. Symptoms abound, but signs can't be found.
3. History of pre-existing psychiatric problems and of a precipitating or triggering incident.
4. Full remission of the symptom with time.

adjusted, 60-year-old Pt who suddenly has neurologic symptoms. *Always assume that such a Pt has organic disease until proven otherwise.*

    b. During the interview, or NE, when the Ex focuses on the hysterical dysfunction, such as a tremor, it worsens. The dysfunction also worsens in the presence of family members or significant acquaintances. In other words, the symptom varies with the attention directed to it, or with the presence of emotionally significant people. It is socially dependent. Remember, however, that emotional stress may similarly enhance organic tremors and involuntary movements.

  3. *The diagnosis of hysteria rests on two pillars*

    a. Pillar one. The negative pillar is the absence of neurologic signs that would have to be present if an organic lesion caused the disability.

    b. Pillar two. The positive pillar is the history of overt psychiatric stress and the complete disappearance of the symptoms with time, as the psychiatric problems resolve.

 E. Affective status in hysteria

  1. No single affect or personality pattern accompanies hysteria (Woolsey, 1976). Some hysterical Pts appear blandly indifferent (la belle indifférence) to the disability, accepting it stoically or good-naturedly, as it were. They do not ask about nor seem concerned about the cause or prognosis.

  2. In contrast to the passive acceptance by some hysterical Pts, others with hysterical symptoms, particularly sensory ones, such as pain, overreact with much wailing or dramatic prostration. They literally "go into hysterics" over it. The art of diagnosis—the art—is to recognize the *disproportionate* overreaction or underreaction in either case.

  3. *Caveats for the history*

    a. In searching for psychiatric predispositions, the naive Ex may overlook the *high achiever syndrome,* or even misinterpret it as evidence against hysteria. Consider the "all-American child syndrome." The child, a straight A student, runs cross-country in the fall, plays varsity basketball in the winter, plays Little League baseball and swims competitively in the summers, and receives the yearly citizenship award at school. After school hours, the child goes to dance lessons, choir practice, and baby-sits for the mother on weekends. The over-scheduling denies the child a childhood. In desperation, the child becomes paraplegic. In such a Pt, the unremitting excellence of function, maintained at too high a cost in psychic energy, constitutes the psychiatric predisposition.

    b. Some Pts with multiple sclerosis or frontal lobe damage may seem blandly unconcerned about their disability and its implications.

II. Hysterical disorders of motor function

 A. Range of motor disorders

  1. Hysteria may cause paralysis or hyperkinesias. The hyperkinesias usually take the form of tremors, spasms, or flailing about. The paralysis may affect cranial nerve muscles, causing aphonia or dysphagia, or it may affect the rest of the body in monoplegic, hemiplegic, or paraplegic distributions. Hysterical quadriplegia virtually never occurs.

  2. Impotence, the most common form of psychogenic or functional paralysis, does not qualify as hysteria, because it represents failure of autonomic function, rather than willfully directed muscular activity.

B. *Oculomotor manifestations of hysteria*

1. *Common oculomotor manifestations.* Eyelid tics, blepharospasm, convergence spasm, pseudo-VIth-nerve palsy, and pseudoptosis.

2. *Blepharospasm.* The eyelids remain tonically closed and strongly resist any attempt by the Pt or Ex to open them. The spasm affects only the orbicularis oculi muscles, but their action also pulls the eyebrows down.

3. *Convergence spasm.* The pupils constrict along with the forceful adduction of the eyes, indicating an overactive accommodation mechanism (Griffin et al, 1976). Review accommodation in Table 4-3.

4. *Pseudo-VIth-nerve palsy.* The Pt, on attempting to look to one side, say the right, will move the eyes conjugately to, or a little past, the midline. Then as the *ad*ducting eye continues to progress to the right, the *ab*ducting eye deviates inward, as if the lateral rectus muscle had failed to act. Careful inspection will show that the Pt has learned to utilize convergence. As the errant eye breaks off of conjugate movement to adduct, the pupil simultaneously constricts. Thus, a volitional convergence stimulus has arrested the abduction of the eye, not failure of action of the lateral rectus muscle (Troost and Troost, 1979). In organic VIth-nerve palsy, the pupil of the eye that fails to abduct does not change in size.

5. *Pseudoptosis.* The Pt will lower the eyebrow on the side of the ptosis, rather than automatically lifting it by using the frontalis muscle in compensation. The malingerer may also use mydriatic drops to dilate the pupil, further simulating a IIId nerve palsy (Keane, 1982).

6. *Caveats.* Blepharospasm occurs as an involuntary movement disorder and idiopathically (Cavenar et al, 1978). Organic diseases can cause convergence spasm, but usually neighborhood signs of midbrain-pretectal region lesions are present. Gilles de la Tourette's syndrome may cause a variety of tics affecting the eyelids and ocular movements.

C. *Hysterical dysfunctions of voice production, swallowing, and breathing*

1. *Range of dysfunction.* Mutism or low voice volume, spasmodic dysphonia, dysphagia, and respiratory dysrhythmias.

2. *Hysterical mutism.* The hysteric may exhibit complete mutism, or speak with a low voice volume. Although aphonic, the hysteric has normal vocal cord action during laryngoscopy, or shows pure adductor palsy. Yet, the Pt can produce a Valsalva maneuver, or a normal, strong cough, proving that the adductor muscles of the vocal cords can, in fact, act forcefully. The Pt has no palatal palsy, and may breathe, and swallow normally, and may whisper with perfect articulation. The Pt may talk or phonate during sleep, establishing the integrity of the vocal apparatus.

3. *Spasmodic dysphonia.* When the Pt attempts to speak, the vocal cords go into spasm, causing a tight, hoarse, or strained voice (Aminoff et al, 1978).

4. *Hysterical dysphagia.* The Pt chokes, or cannot swallow, but may have no accompanying signs of palatal, laryngeal, or pharyngeal dysfunction. The Pt swallows normally when asleep. The Pt may also experience *globus hystericus,* a distressing sensation of a lump lodged in the throat.

5. *Respiratory dysrhythmias.* Disturbances include apnea, often in association with a Valsalva maneuver; weak, shallow, or "asthenic" breathing in a Pt who avoids eye contact; or theatrical gagging, with guttural noises, stridor, rolling of the head and trunk, and demonstrative, expressive eyes (Walker et al, 1989). The authors liken the latter state of respiratory gymnastics to astasia-abasia: In both the Pt totters on the brink but escapes

disaster. Hyperventilation may accompany or precede many hysterical symptoms such as syncope. Most Pts with psychogenic breathing disorders show no cyanosis and have a normal arterial O_2, but if misdiagnosed may be treated by endotracheal intubation (Walker et al, 1989).
6. *Caveat.* Dystonia may cause spasmodic dysphonia, and early stages of several organic diseases—such as amyotrophic lateral sclerosis and myasthenia gravis—may cause dysphonia and dysphagia.

D. *Hysterical vomiting.* The vomiting occurs mainly in the presence of emotionally significant people. The malingering Pt can, on one occasion or another, be observed to induce the vomiting by gagging themselves, or malingerers may simulate GI bleeding by secretly adding blood to their vomitus or stool.

E. *Hysterical disturbances of station and gait (astasia-abasia)*
1. *Astasia* means the inability to stand, and *abasia* the inability to walk. The astasia-abasia Pt typically shows wild gyrations when standing or walking. The Pt rarely falls, or falls into the Ex's arms (or a chair) without suffering bodily injury. The flamboyant gyrations without falling testify eloquently to the competency of the Pt's motor system and balance. When in bed, or sitting, the Pt may show no disability or only minor disturbances of movement.
2. On the Romberg test, the Pt will usually sway much more with the eyes closed. Review section V, F, 4 of Chap. 10 for the methods by which the Ex can divert the functional Pt into a normal performance on this test.
3. *Caveats.* Recall that Pts with the rostral or caudal vermis syndromes may show little dysfunction when reclining, but display dystaxia when walking, particularly when tandem walking. Pts with involuntary movement syndromes, particularly dystonia musculorum deformans, frequently get diagnosed as having a hysteric gait in the early stages of their illness. See the gait essay, at the end of Chap. 8.

F. *Hysterical paresis or paralysis of trunk and limbs*
1. *Demeanor of the Pt.* The Pt's demeanor during testing of strength often provides a clue to hysteria. Usually the Pt with hysterical paralysis makes a great show of effort to move the afflicted part. Thus, the Pt may grimace, grunt, or squirm, and show obvious strain. It is a dramatic performance meant to communicate sincerity of effort, rather than a simple attempt to move the part, as in organic paralysis. The hysteric with partial paralysis usually moves the part very slowly. Often the Ex can see and feel that the putatively weak muscles in such a movement, in fact, contract very strongly. Thus, in grip testing, the Pt contracts the flexors very strongly, demonstrating intact innervation, which the Ex can see and palpate, but the Pt's fingers only encircle the Ex's fingers very lightly, not actually closing tightly on them. When the Ex tugs against a muscle to test strength, the hysteric may offer considerable resistance and then yield suddenly, or may show a series of jactitating, cogwheel-like releases. Objective recording of strength by myometry shows different patterns of contractions in hysterics, normals, and organically paralyzed Pts (van der Ploeg and Oosterhuis, 1991).
2. *Distribution of hysterical paralysis.* While the paralysis of hysteria may follow monoplegic, hemiplegic, or paraplegic distributions, it seldom affects individual muscles, or groups of muscles, innervated by a single peripheral

nerve or root. The limbs do not assume organic postures, as in organic hemiplegia, and the overall lack of signs establishes the functional nature of the paralysis (Table 14-3).

3. *Eliciting inadvertent or automatic movements of the paralyzed parts in hysteria*

a. *Sleep.* Several observations or maneuvers establish the integrity of the putatively paralyzed part by inadvertent or automatic mechanisms. The Pt with hysterical monoplegia, hemiplegia, or paraplegia moves the parts in the normal manner during sleep. When dressing, the Pt may inadvertently reach out with the affected part or use it automatically for postural support. *This is a key principle: The Ex finds some way to activate the putatively paralyzed muscles automatically or inadvertently, as it were.*

b. *Monrad-Krohn's cough test (1922).* To identify functional paralysis of the arm, the Ex stands behind the Pt and grasps the two latissimus dorsi muscles between the thumb and fingers of the right and left hands. Ask the Pt to cough forcefully. Both latissimus dorsi muscles should contract automatically, establishing the integrity of the motor pathway through the brachial plexus.

c. *Make a fist test.* To test for a functional wrist drop, ask the Pt to make a strong fist. Watch for action of the wrist extensors. If intact, the putatively paralyzed wrist extensors automatically cock the hand up into the

TABLE 14-3 Differentiation of non-organic and organic paraplegia		
	Non-organic paraplegia	Organic paraplegia
Onset	Usually arises suddenly after stress or discord in a person with a psychiatric predisposition	May evolve slowly or suddenly in a patient who may have a predisposing organic cause
Attitude to illness	May seem indifferent or histrionic	Appropriate concern
MSRs	Present and normal	May be absent in spinal shock or very brisk
Clonus	Absent or unsustained	Sustained
Muscle tone	Normal	Flaccid acutely, then spastic
Plantar response	Normal plantar flexion of great toe	Dorsiflexion of great toe unless spinal shock is present
Abdominal-cremasteric reflexes	Present	Absent, depending on level
Umbilical migration	Absent	Upward migration if lesion affects T_{10} (Beevor's sign)
Sphincter control	Present	Lost
Anal wink reflex	Present	May be absent
Sensory level	Extends around waist in horizontal plane. Varies from exam to exam. May not match motor loss.	Slants obliquely downward; constant border if lesion static.
Inadvertent use of legs	May move legs inadvertently for postural support, in sleep, or with Hoover's test	Does not move legs if the paraplegia is complete, but may show flexor spasms
MRI, SSEV, and cystometrogram	Normal but usually not needed if neurologic exam done carefully.	Abnormal

"anatomic position" when the Pt makes a fist. Make a strong fist to notice this action on yourself and palpate your forearm muscles with your other hand while they spring into action.

d. *Displacement test.* To test for a functional foot drop, ask the Pt to stand with the eyes closed. Place one hand on the Pt's chest and suddenly displace the Pt backwards, using the other hand on the Pt's back to prevent a fall. The Ex will see the dorsiflexor tendons of the feet spring into action as the Pt automatically reacts to the displacement.

e. *Hoover test.* To test for functional leg paralysis, ask the Pt to lie supine on the bed. The Ex stands at the foot with one hand under each of the Pt's heels. The Ex then asks the Pt to lift the *normal* leg to a right angle briskly in one motion. Hysterics usually automatically brace the putatively paralyzed limb, which the Ex can see and feel. The same principle of causing inadvertent bracing of the putatively paralyzed part works in testing adduction and abduction of the legs. When the Ex squeezes both knees together or tries to pull them both apart, the Pt often automatically braces the putatively paralyzed limb against the action of the intact limb.

f. *Reversed hands test.* To identify hysterical hand paralysis, the Ex has the Pt reverse and invert the hands (Fig. 14-1). Then the Ex asks the Pt to look at the fingers, and the Ex points to, but does not touch, a finger and asks the Pt to move that finger. Usually the Pt moves the finger of the hand opposite to the one pointed to by the Ex. Try this test on a partner. Notice that after a few trials, the subject learns to respond accurately. Thus, it serves best during the first trials. The test also works to confuse a malingerer who claims anesthesia for one arm.

g. Try all of the foregoing tests on a companion.

4. Magnetic stimulation of the motor cortex can prove that the pyramidal pathways are intact (Pilai et al, 1992).

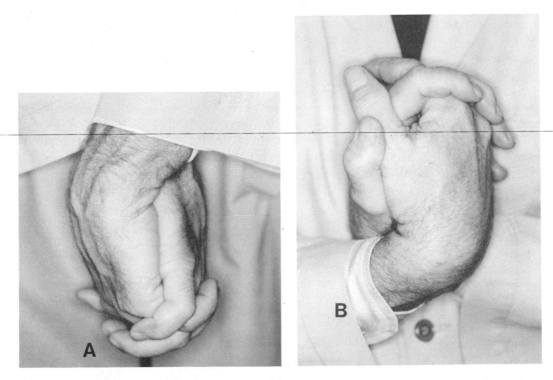

FIG. 14-1. Method of inverting hands to test for hysterical loss of sensation or motor function. The final posture in *B* reverses right for left. (*A*) Clasp fingers as shown. (*B*) Invert the hands.

> **TABLE 14-4 Clinical features of psychogenic tremor**
>
> 1. Abrupt onset
> 2. Static course
> 3. Spontaneous remissions
> 4. Unclassifiable tremors (complex tremors)
> 5. Clinical inconsistencies (selective disabilities)
> 6. Changing tremor characteristics
> 7. Unresponsiveness to anti-tremor drugs
> 8. Tremor increases with attention
> 9. Tremor lessens with distractibility
> 10. Responsiveness to placebo
> 11. Absence of other neurologic signs
> 12. Remission with psychotherapy

Source: From Koller et al, 1989.

G. *Psychogenic tremors.* The tremor varies greatly in intensity, and frequently is present at rest, during a sustained posture, and during movement, in contrast to most organic tremors (Koller et al, 1989), midbrain or so-called rubral tremor excepted (Reza Samie et al, 1990). See Chap. 7 and Table 14-4.

III. Hysterical disorders of vision

A. *Range of symptoms.* Hysterical visual symptoms usually consist of diminished vision or blindness, nonanatomic visual field defects, diplopia, and photophobia.

B. *Hysterical blindness*
   1. *Establishing the integrity of the visual pathways.* The eyes of the hysterically blind Pt often will fixate upon moving objects that appear unexpectedly. Placing a mirror directly in front of the Pt and moving it may cause the Pt's eyes to pursue their reflection. The Pt retains pupillary light reactions, and the fundi appear normal. The hysterical Pt may show optokinetic nystagmus (railroad nystagmus) when exposed to a rotating drum, or moving stripes. However, Pts can inhibit optokinetic nystagmus. Its presence thus establishes the integrity of the retino-geniculocalcarine pathway and the efferent optomotor pathway to the brainstem from the occipital cortex, but the absence of nystagmus does not prove that the Pt has a lesion. The electroretinogram in hysterics remains normal, the EEG shows a photic driving response, and more refined visual evoked potential studies prove that impulses reach the visual cortex (see Chap. 13). Even evoked responses are not beyond manipulation, since the Pt's thought processes can change the pattern evoked (Baumgartner and Epstein, 1982; Tan et al, 1984). If the Pt has monocular hysterical blindness, the Ex may induce the Pt to have double vision by applying canthal compression (Fig. 4-4), or the ophthalmologist can do so by use of prisms, proving that the putatively blind eye sees.
   2. *Caveats*
      a. Acute retrobulbar neuritis can cause acute, complete blindness in an eye with a normal-appearing fundus, before optic atrophy sets in. The diseased eye will show a diminished or absent direct pupillary light reflex, and the opposite pupil will fail to show a consensual reflex. Try the swinging flashlight test (Chap. 4, section VI, A, 5).

b. In Anton's syndrome, a bilateral, occipital lobe lesion causes bilateral cortical blindness, yet the pupillary responses remain intact. Although obviously blind, the Pt confabulates vision, describing nonexistent scenes around him, qualifying this syndrome as an anosognosia for blindness. During the stage of diaschisis that may follow an acute, severe unilateral occipital lobe lesion, Anton's syndrome may occur temporarily.

C. *Hysterical visual field defects:* The typical hysterical visual field defect consists of constriction of the diameter of the field, producing tunnel or tubular vision, as if the person were looking through a tunnel. In a closely allied phenomenon, the *spiral visual field,* the size of the field diminishes on successive trials. In tunnel vision, the visual field remains the same diameter for near and far objects (Fig. 14-2).

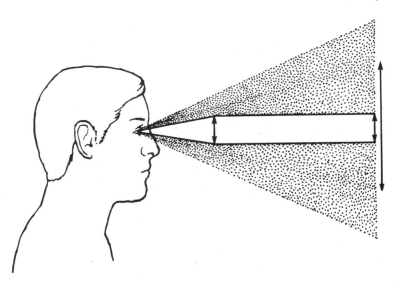

FIG. 14-2. Illustration of tunnel vision in a Pt with hysteria. The normal visual field expands. In tunnel vision, the field remains the same size for targets of different distances.

D. *Monocular diplopia*
1. Hysterics may report monocular diplopia. The diplopia will not follow any of the laws of diplopia (Chap. 4), the corneal light reflections remain aligned, and the cover-uncover test remains normal.
2. *Caveat.* A dislocated lens; a fold, detachment, or elevation of the retina; or a hole in the iris may cause organic monocular diplopia, but the ocular examination and opthalmoscopy differentiate these conditions easily.

E. *Photophobia:* Pain in the eyes on exposure to light may occur with hysteria or with organic illnesses—e.g., iritis. Careful slit-lamp examination and ophthalmologic investigation must rule out definable organic disease.

IV. Hysterical deafness

A. *Clinical and laboratory tests to establish the integrity of the auditory pathways:* The hysterically deaf Pt may turn when addressed unexpectedly from the side or may show a startle response to sudden sound when awake or asleep. The presence of a response indicates an intact auditory pathway, but absence of a response does not establish organic disease. The tuning fork tests of Weber and Rinne described in Chap. 9 may give bizarre results. Audiologists have several methods of manipulating sound to recognize hysterical deafness, which, combined with the BAER test (Chap. 13) showing evoked potentials recorded over the auditory cortex, document the integrity of the auditory pathways.

B. *Caveat:* Acute viral illness can cause sudden deafness, with no other evidence of neurologic disease.

V. Hysterical disorders of somatic sensation

A. *Range of disorders:* Pts with hysterical somatosensory disorders usually complain of anesthesia, paresthesia, hyperesthesia, or pain in the body or extremities. The anesthesia usually affects all sensory modalities. If the Pt loses only one modality, it is usually touch or pain, not vibration or position sense.

B. *Non-anatomical distribution of hysterical sensory loss*

1. Hysterical sensory losses follow non-anatomical distributional patterns and often have variable but very sharp borders from exam to exam. Hysterical sensory losses conform to the Pt's mental image of the body, not the actual anatomic pattern of innervation by peripheral nerves, nerve roots, or central pathways (Fig. 10-3). Chap. 10 has explained how organic facial anesthesia from a Vth nerve lesion spares the angle of the mandible, which receives its sensory innervation from C_2. See Figs. 10-2, 14-3*A*.

2. In hysterical anesthesia of an extremity, the loss usually includes the hand or foot and extends proximally to stop abruptly at a line transverse to the long axis of the limb, as if the extremity were amputated. Often the transverse line crosses the wrist or elbow. In hysterical anesthesia of the whole arm, the loss often stops at the shoulder joint, conforming to the Pt's mental image of an arm, but not to the actual innervation by dermatomes, peripheral nerves, or central pathways. See Fig. 14-3*C* and *D*. In hysterical lower-extremity anesthesia, the proximal border often falls at the waist or the gluteal fold posteriorly or the inguinal line anteriorly (Fig. 14-3*E* and *F*). As the hysterical anesthesia improves, the border moves distally along the limb, stopping at successive transverse levels until it disappears.

3. In hysterical paraplegia with a sensory level, the line circles the body horizontally, while in organic paraplegia the dermatomes slant downwards in the lower abdomen (Fig. 2-10, Table 14-3).

4. A striking example of the body image loss of sensation occurs in hysterical hemianesthesia. The Pt not only loses all somatic sensation from one half of the body but may also lose sight, hearing, taste, and smell on the affected side, an obvious anatomic impossibility. In hysterical hemianesthesia, the sensory loss stops sharply at the midline and may run up the entire body and head as in the mental image of one half of the body. Pts with organic

FIG. 14-3. Contrast between functional and organic sensory losses. (*A*) Functional facial anesthesia usually includes the angle of the mandible and may stop at the hairline. (*B*) Organic facial anesthesia from a Vth nerve lesion spares the angle of the mandible (innervated by C_2). The border follows the distribution of the entire Vth nerve or one of its three branches. See also Fig. 10-2. (*C*) Functional loss of upper limb sensation usually cuts off transversely at the wrist, elbow, or shoulder. (*D*) Organic sensory loss when limited to a region of an upper extremity follows an anatomic distribution, either dermatomal (D_1, C_6 dermatome) or peripheral nerve (D_2, ulnar nerve). See also Figs. 2-10 and 2-11. (*E*) Functional loss of lower-extremity sensation usually cuts off at a joint or the gluteal fold dorsally, or the inguinal line ventrally, or it may cut off transversely at any lower level. (*F*) Organic sensory loss, when limited to a region of a lower extremity, follows an anatomic distribution, either dermatomal (F_1, L_5 dermatome) or peripheral nerve (F_2, lateral femoral cutaneous nerve). See also Figs. 2-10 and 2-11.

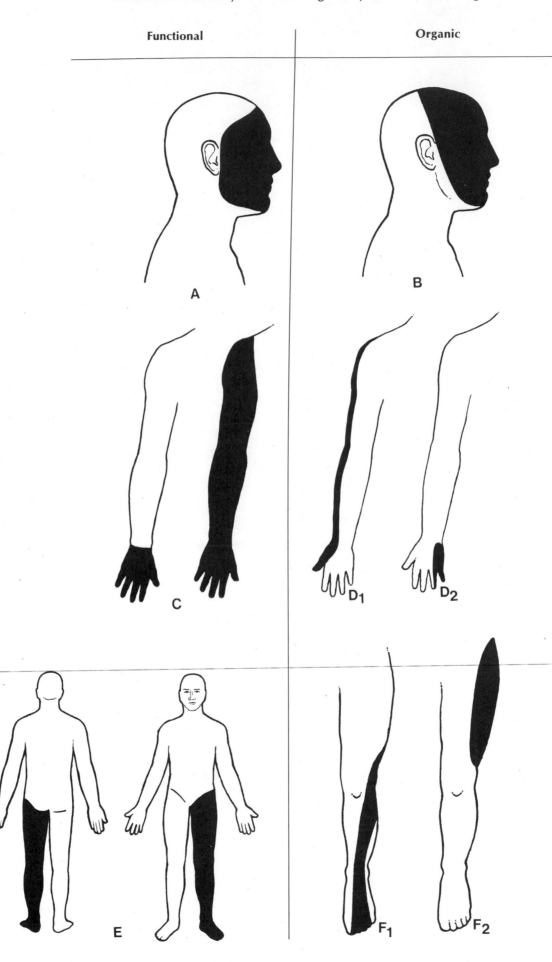

hemisensory loss usually have an indistinct midline border. The hysteric, for example, will report complete absence of vibratory sensation when a tuning fork, applied to the sternum or forehead, just reaches the midline. In fact, the vibration travels some distance through the bone and its perception cannot be cut off sharply at the midline (Fig. 14-4A and B).

5. Figures 14-3 to 14-5 show the differences in the borders of organic and hysterical sensory losses. The border between the anesthetic and the normal zone, although usually sharp, may change from time to time.

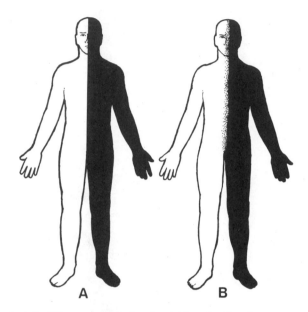

FIG. 14-4. Some characteristic differences in the borders of functional and organic sensory losses functional and organic hemianesthesia. (*A*) In functional hemianesthesia, the sensory loss usually stops abruptly at the midline for all modalities. (*B*) In organic hemianesthesia, the sensory loss usually fades gradually at the midline, particularly for vibration.

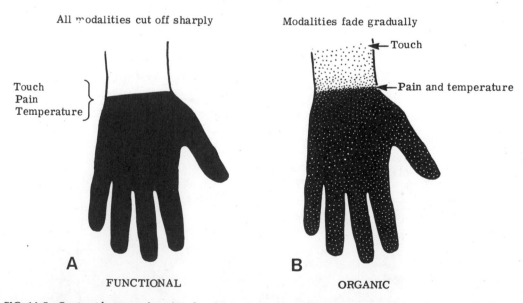

FIG. 14-5. Contrast between functional and organic stocking-glove sensory loss. (*A*) In functional stocking-glove sensory loss, the proximal border usually stops sharply at a joint line or skin crevice for all modalities. (*B*) In organic stocking-glove sensory loss, the proximal border usually fades gradually and differs for the various modalities.

6. Some inversions of the body parts can provide a quick answer to a hysterical hemisensory loss. In males with hemianesthesia, the penis can be twisted to reverse right and left. Then touching the previously anesthetic half, now reversed, will produce a sensory response, whereas the previously normal side becomes anesthetic, a striking proof of the "body" image loss of sensation in hysteria. Similarly, reversal of the hands may reverse or confuse the sensory responses. See Fig. 14-1.

C. *Inadvertent proof that a sensory deficit is non-organic*
   1. *Normal motor function.* If the hysteric has anesthesia for all modalities, not anesthesia plus paralysis, the Pt may use the part completely normally, which is impossible without proprioception. This fact plus the *preservation* of stretch reflexes and *absence* of hypotonia, atrophy, and dystaxia proves that the Pt cannot have anesthesia. Complete sensory loss must produce areflexia, hypotonia, and sensory dystaxia. (Review Table 10-2, for the features of sensory dystaxia). Testing the Pt during sleep will disclose withdrawal of the putatively anesthetic extremity from pain.
   2. *Rhythmic responses.* In testing touch or pain responses, the Ex may elicit a rhythm of answering that inadvertently discloses the integrity of the sensation in the putatively anesthetic or analgesic area. Ordinarily, in order to maintain the Pt's attention, the Ex avoids such a rhythm in organic Pts. Starting with areas of intact sensation, get the Pt to respond by saying "yes" when you apply the stimulus or "no" when you withhold it. Then unexpectedly, out of rhythm, incorporate the anesthetic region in the testing. Often the hysteric says "no" each time just after the Ex unexpectedly touches the anesthetic zone, indicating that, at some level of consciousness, the Pt has perceived the stimulus.
   3. *Pattern of exactly opposite responses.* In responding to position sense testing, the functional Pt may display a pattern of exactly opposite answers, saying, for example, "down" each time for "up." The fact that the Pt gives exactly the reverse response each time means that position sense has to be intact. Even with total absence of position sense, the Pt should guess the right answer about one-half of the time.
   4. *Histrionic underreaction or exaggerated overreaction.* Hysterics sometimes respond very slowly and deliberately to sensory stimuli during the examination. The Pt conveys the impression of trying very hard to feel the stimulus and report it correctly, a pseudocooperation. Other Pts give a studied response of feeling it "just a little bit," even after strong stimulation. In hysterical analgesia, the Ex should not continue to make increasingly strong pain stimuli to prove a point (or express frustration with a puzzling sensory examination). In contrast to these underreacting Pts, others manifestly overreact to sensory stimuli. The Ex learns to recognize the histrionic overreaction or studied underreaction as inadvertent evidence of the non-organic nature of the sensory deficit.
   5. *Forced-choice testing.* Hysterics show a very different response to forced-choice testing of sensation than organic Pts (Tegner, 1988).

D. *Caveats:* In deciding whether a sensory loss is functional or not, review the *Steps in the Analysis of a Sensory Complaint* (Chap. 10, section VII). Recall also that organic pain may be referred to or radiate beyond the confines of an anatomic territory. Some Pts with organic disease have true hyperesthesia, sometimes of excruciating type, as in causalgia, or trigger zones where the slightest stimulus elicits unbearable pain, as in trigeminal neuralgia. On some occasions Pts with thalamic or parietal lesions will show hemisensory losses that suggest hysteria (Yarnell et al, 1978). See Fig. 14-4. Recall also that the Pt may have an organic lesion but with a functional overlay.

VI. Pseudoepileptic seizures

A. *Range of expression:* Hysteria frequently manifests by dizziness, blackout spells, fainting, or pseudoepileptic seizures. Hysterical lapses of consciousness occur after some identifiable, precipitating event. Most commonly, they occur in the presence of someone emotionally significant to the Pt, such as a parent or lover, or to avoid some unpleasant obligation. *No pathognomonic clinical features separate true from pseudoepileptic seizures.* Pseudoepileptic seizures may manifest as pure unresponsiveness without motor activity—in other words, a swoon (Leis et al, 1992). When present, the motor activity shows bizarre patterns that usually differ from the in-phase, bilaterally symmetrical tonic-clonic jerks of grand mal epilepsy. Pseudoseizure Pts show more random, out-of-phase movements, with the extremities on the two sides doing different things. In addition to extremity movements, the Pts make pelvic thrusts and side-to-side head movements, rarely seen in true epilepsy, and the posturing and jerking vary in intensity during the seizure (Meierkord et al, 1991; Rowan and Gates, 1993). Epileptic Pts may injure themselves by biting their tongue or falling, and they often become incontinent. Pseudoseizure Pts may do the same, although much less frequently. Usually, in pseudoepileptic seizures, the blood pressure, pulse rate, and pupillary size do not change, whereas in organic seizures they often change dramatically.

B. *Caveats*
   1. *Range of epileptic seizures.* Almost every conceivable neurologic symptom or sign has occurred in some Pt at some time as an epileptic seizure. No matter how bizarre, the attack may be organic, including fugue states or confusional attacks (Ellis and Lee, 1978; Kanner et al, 1990; Manford and Shorvon, 1992; Markand et al, 1978). *In many instances, even the most experienced neurologist observing an attack cannot distinguish psychogenic attacks from organic ones.* Pseudoseizures occur in adolescents and children (Finlayson and Lucas, 1979). Hyperventilation can precipitate pseudoseizures and organic seizures, particularly petit mal. The resolution requires combined video and EEG monitoring in a laboratory or ambulatory monitoring until the attacks can be recorded (Rowan and Gates, 1993). Normal records during an attack virtually exclude epilepsy, but even then, the EEG, which depends on surface electrical activity, may appear normal even during some epileptic attacks. The most difficult problem is the not-rare combination of seizures and pseudoseizures. Many Pts with unrecognized pseudoseizures erroneously receive intravenous medication for status epilepticus (Leis et al, 1992; Pakalnis et al, 1991).
   2. *Rule out hypoglycemia.* Whenever a Pt exhibits any undiagnosed attack that alters or obtunds consciousness, or results in a frank seizure, always measure the blood glucose level and, if indicated, other blood constituents and blood gases.

VII. Factitious fevers

Malingerers may produce false temperature readings by manipulating a thermometer. If a Pt has a puzzling fever or hypothermia of unknown origin, measure a fresh sample of urine with your own thermometer. The urine specimen will reflect the true body temperature, by passing any manipulation the Pt manages with the thermometer (Murray et al, 1977). The Ex always has to consider doing a lumbar puncture, and culturing the blood and urine, in Pts with true fever of unknown origin.

VIII. Some final caveats on the diagnosis of hysteria

A. *Remain patient:* The Ex should avoid confrontation and tricks, such as hypnosis or electric shocks, to "speed up" recovery. Avoid the impression of trying to unmask, expose, or trick functional Pts. The Ex can hint that the findings suggest a disorder that may end in recovery; but beyond that, let the Pt retain the dignity of patienthood until the symptoms resolve.

B. *Consider a functional overlay:* Some Pts with undiagnosed illnesses, in shopping from physician to physician, elaborate on or exaggerate their organic symptoms in desperation as they try to convince the physician of the reality of their illness. The many physicians will have asked the same questions over and over in the review of systems, inadvertently suggesting new symptoms for the Pt to worry about or to imagine. Such Pts may be neither malingering nor frankly hysterical, but legitimately worried about their health. The Ex has to recognize the possibility that an organic disease underlies the functional complaints (Benson and Blumer, 1975; DePaulo and Folstein, 1978).

C. *Maintain professionalism to avoid diagnostic errors:* Those puzzling and troublesome Pts whose illnesses consist of organic. functional, and factitious factors often provoke anger. Neophyte physicians may refer to these Pts by such inexcusable names as "crocks," "gomers," or "gorks." Remember yet another aphorism: *If the physician deprecates the Pt, the physician has failed to understand the Pt's problem.* By remaining curious about what it is in the brain, body chemistry, or life experiences that caused the Pt's condition, the physician remains receptive and potentially helpful, rather than dismissing the Pt as a cheat, liar, and fraud. Regard every event in the consulting room, whether an extensor plantar response or a factitious fever, neutrally as a clinical phenomenon. React to it objectively, as reflecting the state of the Pt's nervous system, as deriving from nerve impulses shuttling through neuroanatomic circuits (Chap. 1, Sections A and B). Emotional responses, particularly hostility, will degrade the quality of your examination and greatly increase the possibility of an error in diagnosis or management. Retain the grace of professionalism and the humility to recognize the fallibility of your own judgments.

D. *Avoid the Pt's trap:* The intimacy of the medical interview and the physical examination provides a prime opportunity for Pts to indulge in pathologic manipulation. Such Pts may act seductively, try to exploit their illness for pity or favors, or consciously or subconsciously try to provoke hostility. The physician duped by these manipulations loses any possibility of helping the Pt. For this and many other reasons, the medical model forbids the physician to react emotionally to the Pt, whether with love, pity, or hostility.

E. *The Pt may have some disease you have not thought of, nor even heard of:* Lastly, never diagnose a functional illness by exclusion because you cannot think of another diagnosis. Call in a consultant who just may recognize the

---

TABLE 14-5 Organic disorders with bizarre or subtle neurologic manifestations often mistaken for hysteria

1. Early multiple sclerosis: fleeting sensory loss, retrobulbar neuritis, transient paraplegia
2. Porphyria: abdominal pain, peripheral neuropathy, seizures, and mental changes
3. Endocrinopathies: fatigue, weakness, nervousness, and tremors
4. Involuntary movement syndromes with bizarre gait disturbances, particularly dystonia with tortipelvis and camptocormia, and early degenerative diseases such as spinocerebellar degenerations
5. Seizures with bizarre auras affecting vision, somatic sensation, and visceral auras with crawling sensations, abdominal auras of something like fluid running through the chest or abdomen, odd smells or odors, sexual feelings such as orgasm, forced thoughts, and forced laughter
6. Myasthenia gravis with transient cranial nerve dysfunction, fatigability, and weakness
7. Neuropathies, particularly carpal tunnel syndrome, causalgia, and autonomic neuropathies
8. Early Tourette's syndrome with multiple tics, throaty sounds, and urgent, obsessive personality patterns with poor interpersonal relations
9. Midline neoplasms or butterfly gliomas with personality changes but no objective signs
10. Collagen-vascular disease with neuropathy, fleeting CNS symptoms, fatigue, and fever
11. Syringomyelia with dissociated pain and temperature loss
12. Foramen magnum meningioma with slight dysarthria and spastic ataxic gait.

---

porphyria, smoldering collagen disease, occult carcinoma, parasitic infestation, chronic liver abscess, multiple sclerosis, or masked depression that you didn't even consider. Remember this:

> *There are more things in heaven and earth, Horatio,*
> *than are dreamt of in your philosophy.*
> **William Shakespeare** (1564–1616), *Hamlet*

See Table 14-5.

BIBLIOGRAPHY FOR HYSTERIA

Aminoff MJ, Dedo HH, Izdebski K: Clinical aspects of spasmodic dysphoria. *J Neurol Neurosurg Psychiatr* 1978;41:361–365

Benson DF, Blumer D: *Psychiatric Aspects of Neurological Disease.* New York, Grune & Stratton, 1975

Breuer J, Freud S: Studies on hysteria, in Strachey J (ed): *The Standard Edition of the Complete Psychological Words of Sigmund Freud* (vol II). London, Hogarth Press, 1955

Bumgartner J, Epstein CM: Voluntary alteration of visual evoked potentials. *Ann Neurol* 1982;12:475–478

Cavenar JO Jr, Brantley IJ, Braasch E: Blepharospasm: Organic or functional? *Psychosomatics* 1978;19:623–628

DePaulo JR, Folstein MF: Psychiatric disturbances in neurological patients: Detection, recognition, and hospital course. *Ann Neurol* 1978;4:225–289

Ellis JM, Lee SI: Acute prolonged confusion in later life as an ictal state. *Epilepsia* 1978;19:119–128

Finlayson RE, Lucas AR: Pseudo-epileptic seizures in children and adolescents. *Mayo Clin Proc* 1979;54:83–87

Griffin JR, Wray SH, Anderson DP: Misdiagnosis of spasm of the near reflex. *Neurology* 1976;26:1018–1020

Keane JR: Neuro-ophthalmic, signs and symptoms of hysteria. *Neurology* 1982;32:757–762

Kanner AM, Morris HH, Luders H, et al: Supplementary motor seizures mimicking pseudoseizures: Some clinical differences. *Neurology* 1990;40:1404–1407

Koller W, Lang A, Vetere-Overfield B, et al: Psychogenic tremors. *Neurology* 1989;39:1094–1099

Leis AA, Ross MA, Summers AK: Psychogenic seizures: Ictal characteristics and diagnostic pitfalls. *Neurology* 1992;42:95–99

Manford M, Shorvon SD: Prolonged sensory or visceral symptoms: An under-diagnosed form of non-convulsive focal (simple partial) status epilepticus. *J Neurol Neurosurg Psychiatr* 1992;55:714–716

Markand ON, Wheeler GL, Pollack SL: Complex partial status epilepticus. *Neurology* 1978;28:189–196

Meierkord H, Will B, Fish D, et al: The clinical features and prognosis of pseudo-seizures diagnosed using video-EEG telemetry. *Neurology* 1991;41:1643–1646

Monrad-Krohn GH: On the function of the latissimus dorsi muscle and a sign of functional dissociation in simulated and "functional" paralysis of the arm. *Acta Medica Scand* 1922;56:9–11

Morris HH III, Dinner DS, Luders H, et al: Supplementary motor seizures: Clinical and electroencephalographic findings. *Neurology* 1988;38:1075–1082

Murray HW, Tuazon CU, Guerrero IC, et al: Urinary temperature: a clue to early diagnosis of factitious fever. *N Engl J Med,* 1977;296:23.

Pillai JJ, Markind S, Streletz LJ, et al: Motor evoked potentials in psychogenic paralysis. *Neurology* 1991;42:935–936

Reza Samie M, Selhorst JB, Koller WC: Post-traumatic midbrain tremors. *Neurology* 1990;40:62–66

Rowan AJ, Gates JR: *Non-epileptic Seizures.* Stoneham, MA, Butterworth-Heinemann, 1993

Tan CT, Murray NMF, Sawyers D, et al: Deliberate alteration of the visual evoked potential. *J Neurol Neurosurg Psychiatr* 1984;47:518–523

Tegner R: A technique to detect psychogenic sensory loss. *J Neurol Neurosurg Psychiatr* 1988;51:1455–1456

Troost BT, Troost EG: Functional paralysis of horizontal gaze. *Neurology* 1979;29:82–85

van der Ploeg RJO, Oosterhuis HJGH: The "make/break test" as a diagnostic tool in functional weakness. *J Neurol Neurosurg Psychiatr* 1991;54:248–251

Walker FO, Alessi AG, Digre KB, et al: Psychogenic respiratory distress. *Arch Neurol* 1989;46:196–200

Weintraub MI: *Hysterical Conversion Reactions. A Clinical Guide to Diagnosis and Treatment.* Jamaica, NY, SP Medical & Scientific Books, 1983

Woolsey RM: Hysteria: 1875–1975. *Dis Nerv Syst* 1976;37:379–386

Yarnell P, Melamed E, Silverberg R: Global hemianesthesia: A parietal perceptual distortion suggesting non-organic illness. *J Neurol Neurosurg Psychiatr* 1978;41:843–846

Learning Objectives for Chapter Fourteen

I. The general clinical features of hysteria

1. Define hysteria.
2. Describe the concepts of *primary* and *secondary gain* in hysteria.
3. Describe the most important distinction between hysteria and malingering.
4. State the usual goals or purposes of the malingerer.

5. Recite the explicit criteria for the diagnosis of hysteria (Table 14-2).
6. Describe the usual age range and sex of Pts presenting with hysteria, and state, in principle, the psychiatric background of the hysterical Pt.
7. Describe what happens to the magnitude of the hysterical symptom in the presence of emotionally significant persons, or when the Ex focuses attention on it.
8. Discuss whether exacerbation of a symptom or sign by emotional stress establishes a hysterical origin.
9. State the major negative and positive findings required to support the diagnosis of hysteria.
10. Describe some of the attitudes or reactions of hysterical Pts toward their symptoms.
11. Explain in principle why some hysterical Pts may show a seemingly stoic or bland attitude (la belle indifférence).
12. Describe a pervasive lifestyle that may appear to argue against hysteria but, in fact, provides evidence for it.
13. Describe two organic neurologic conditions in which the Pts may appear to be indifferent to their symptoms.

II. Hysterical disorders of motor function

1. Describe some of the common hysterical disorders of the eye-associated muscles, or EOM.
2. Describe the pseudo-VIth nerve palsy syndrome and state how to prove that the arrest of abduction is not due to a VIth nerve palsy.
3. Describe the difference in the action of the frontalis muscle, and the corresponding height of the eyebrow, in hysteria and organic ptosis.
4. Describe some of the ways hysteria affects the oropharyngeal muscles and breathing.
5. Define *astasia-abasia* and explain how it proves that the Pt has a very competent motor system.
6. Describe the difference in the amount of effort overtly displayed by functional and organic Pts when they try to move a paralyzed part.
7. Describe how to divert the hysterical Pt who sways excessively on the Romberg test into performing well.
8. Describe the demeanor of many hysterical Pts during strength testing.
9. State what observations, during grip testing, show that the functionally paralyzed Pt actually has intact forearm muscles.
10. Describe the major differences in the NE in functional and organic paraplegia with a sensory level at the umbilicus (T_{10}).
11. Explain the value of observing a hysterically paralyzed Pt during sleep.
12. Describe how to produce inadvertent movement of the putatively paralyzed parts in the following circumstances in hysteria: arm paralysis, wrist drop, foot drop, and leg paralysis.

**13. Describe the use of the inverted hands test to detect functional paralysis of the hand (Fig. 14-1).
**14. Describe a laboratory test that can prove that the pyramidal tract is intact.
15. Describe some major differences in psychogenic and organic tremors.

III. Hysterical disorders of vision

1. List some of the ways in which hysteria affects vision.
2. Describe some bedside methods of establishing the integrity of the retino-geniculo-calcarine pathway in hysterical blindness.
3. Describe some laboratory tests that will establish the integrity of the visual pathways.
4. Name a lesion of sudden onset that may cause complete blindness in an eye without ophthalmoscopic changes early in the course.
5. Describe the differences in the NE that would distinguish functional monocular blindness from retrobulbar neuritis.
6. Explain whether the presence of the pupillary light reflexes would exclude cortical blindness.
7. Describe the typical non-organic visual field defects in hysterical Pts (Fig. 14-2).
**8. Name some organic causes for monocular diplopia.

IV. Hysterical deafness

Describe some clinical and laboratory methods for establishing that a functionally deaf Pt has intact auditory pathways.

V. Hysterical disorders of somatic sensation

1. Describe the common kinds of functional somatic sensory disturbances (exclusive of special senses).
2. Explain this aphorism: Hysterical Pts lose sensation according to their mental image of the body rather than the anatomy and physiology of the nervous system. Give some examples of this principle (Fig. 14-3).
3. Describe how to use vibration sense to help distinguish organic from non-organic hemianesthesia (Fig. 14-4).
4. Describe the difference in the stocking-glove distribution of sensory loss in organic and non-organic Pts (Fig. 14-5).
5. Describe objective findings on the NE that prove that a functional Pt cannot have an organic basis for total anesthesia of a limb.
**6. Describe some bedside techniques to reverse body orientation or awareness of the side of the stimulus to disclose non-organic sensory losses (Fig. 14-1).
7. Describe some of the characteristic ways that functional Pts respond to sensory stimuli that may provide clues to the non-organic nature of the disorder.
8. Explain how to interpret it when the Pt gives exactly

opposite answers to the up or down position of the digit when the Ex tests position sense.

9. Describe some of the demeanors or patterns of reaction of the hysterical Pt to sensory testing that suggest non-organic sensory loss.

10. List some organic sensory disorders that may be mistaken for hysteria.

VI. Pseudoepileptic seizures

1. Describe some circumstances which may elicit or trigger pseudoepileptic seizures.

2. Describe several of the ways that pseudoepileptic seizures differ from typical, generalized epileptic seizures.

3. Discuss the difficulty of distinguishing pseudoepileptic seizures from true seizures at the bedside.

4. Discuss, in principle, the use of the EEG to distinguish pseudoepileptic seizures from epileptic seizures.

5. State what blood chemistry determinations the Ex should consider when observing any undiagnosed attack that alters consciousness or, causes a frank loss of consciousness, or that could be an epileptic seizure.

VII. Factitious fevers

Describe a simple, foolproof method of measuring the true body temperature without the Pt's having any knowledge of what you are doing.

VII. Some final caveats on hysteria and other non-organic, pseudoneurologic disorders

1. Discuss whether the physician should focus on early elimination of symptoms when the findings suggest a non-organic illness.

2. Discuss the concept of functional overlay and some reasons why it arises.

3. Discuss why the medical model calls for the physician to respond neutrally to all events in the Pt-physician transaction, whether organic or factitial, as clinical phenomena and to forgo moral judgments and emotional responses.

4. Discuss the difficulty in trying to decide whether a Pt is hysterical or malingering, and explain why the physician should avoid a pejorative attitude to either type of Pt.

5. Discuss the danger of the common practice of applying pejorative names to Pts with puzzling and troublesome neuropsychiatric syndromes.

6. Explain how adherence to the medical model keeps the manipulative, seductive, or hostility-provoking Pt from gaining control over the physician and maintains the possibility for effective management.

7. List several organic disorders that may present with puzzling symptoms that may suggest a non-organic illness.

Chapter Fifteen

A Synopsis of the Neurologic Investigation and a Formulary of Neurodiagnosis

I. The routine screening neurologic examination (NE) when the Pt has no symptoms suggesting neurologic disease

A. *What is the minimum allowable NE?* Every new Pt and every routine physical checkup requires the Ex to complete a minimum screening examination of all body systems. To this requirement students often respond fretfully, "But it takes too long to do an NE on everyone." In fact, with sufficient practice, you can learn to do a basic screening NE in about 6 min in the mentally normal, cooperative Pt who has no neurologic symptoms. This statement presupposes a thorough history. The better the history, the briefer the examination required. The Ex need not and should not do every test on every Pt. The Ex contracts and expands the NE to fit the history. If a Pt presents only with a sore throat and has no neurologic symptoms whatsoever, the Ex squanders time in testing smell and taste, doing caloric irrigation and a detailed aphasia examination, and in tugging against every muscle. The expanded examination required to explore neurologic symptoms, of course, takes much, much longer. But recall that the history and clinical examination constitute the most efficient method known for the detection of disease.

B. *Format for the mandatory 6-min neurologic examination for every Pt*
1. *Appraisal during the history.* During the history, the Ex appraises the Pt's mental status, notes the facial features, the eyes and ears, ocular movements, speech and swallowing, and observes the posture, gait, and movement patterns.
2. *Examination of the head.* Inspect the head shape, and palpate the head. Record the OFC of every infant.
3. *Visual system.* Test visual acuity (central fields), peripheral fields, and ocular movements, and do ophthalmoscopy.
4. *Do the 45-sec motor examination of cranial nerves III, IV, V, VI, VII, IX, X, XI, and XII* (Table 6-8).
5. *Hearing.* Test by conversational voice, by finger rustling, and by tuning fork, if necessary.

6. *Somatic motor examination*
   a. Undress the Pt, note the somatotype, and inspect for muscle atrophy, fasciculations, tremors, involuntary movements, and neurocutaneous stigmata.
   b. Test gait by free walking; toe, heel, and tandem walking; and deep-knee bend.
   c. Test strength of abduction of arms, wrist dorsiflexion, grip, hip flexion, and foot dorsiflexion.
   d. Test cerebellar function by finger-to-nose and heel-to-knee tests, in addition to the gait.
   e. Elicit MSRs of biceps, triceps, quadriceps femoris, and triceps surae.
   f. Elicit plantar reflexes.
7. *Sensory examination*
   a. Test *superficial* sensation by light, touch, and temperature discrimination on the face, hands, and feet (Fig. 10-4*A* and *B*).
   b. Test *deep* sensation by the directional scratch test (Chap. 10, section V, I), or position sense in fingers and toes, and vibration sense at ankles. Test for astereognosis with coins or paper clip.

C. *Recording the routine NE:* In reading someone's NE, I personally want to find out the mental status and whether the Pt can see, hear, talk, swallow, breathe, stand, walk, and feel normally. Surprisingly, many write-ups fail to include that information. Hurriedly scribbling that the "Neuro exam is physiological" or "WNL" just won't do. When a Pt has neurologic findings, no forms or checkoff lists record the NE as well as a series of statements, best dictated and typed. If the Pt has no neurologic findings, you still may prefer to write out the screening NE, but a checkoff sheet can save time, and you may expand it as needed to record positive findings. See Table 15-1.

II. Closing the neurologic investigation when the Pt has signs or symptoms suggesting neurologic diseases

A. *Hypothesis testing and reaching a provisional diagnosis:* When the history suggests neurologic disease, the NE must include every clinical test for the integrity of neural structures that the lesion or disease could affect. The goal is to achieve the best provisional diagnosis. To reach a provisional diagnosis, the Ex poses and tests numerous diagnostic hypotheses during the history, physical examination, and later the laboratory work-up. The thinking process is one of posing *if*s: "If the Pt has such and such a disease or sign, then I should also find so and so. Very well, I will look for that next."

B. *The concept of closure:* After the history and after the examination and the hypothesizing, the next event in the medical process is the *closure,* or *cloture.* The term *closure* is, in fact, a technical term meaning *now that the arguments have been heard and the data presented, now is the time to pose the critical question(s) for decision and action.* The decision is the provisional diagnosis and the differential diagnosis derived from it, and the action is the management (Fig. 15-1).

C. *The diagnostic catechism:* The closure requires, in fact, five fundamental questions, the first three primary and the second two derivative, which form the *diagnostic catechism* (Table 15-2).

TABLE 15-1 The screening neurological examination

Name: _____ #: _____ Date: _____

Normal   Abnormal

_____   _____   1. *General appearance and mental status:* well-developed & well-nourished ____-____-old,
                       __ W/ B/ O __ male/ female, oriented, cooperative, affectively appropriate, and gives
                       an apparently reliable history. Occupation: _____.

_____   _____   2. *Head:* normocephalic—no bruits, bumps, tenderness, or depressions. OFC _____cm.

_____   _____   3. *Visual system:*
                       a. Acuity and visual fields
                       b. PERLA; _____ mm in size
                       c. EOM full. No nystagmus
                       d. Fundi (describe)

_____   _____   4. *Nonocular motor cranial nerves:*
                       a. Facial movements symmetrical
                       b. Tongue, jaw, and palate midline
                       c. Word articulation
                       d. Swallowing
                       e. Breathing

_____   _____   5. *Motor system:*
                       a. Gait/station: free walking, toe, heel, & tandem walking, & deep-knee bend
                       b. Atrophy or fasciculations
                       c. Tremor/involuntary mvmts
                       d. Dystaxia/dysdiadochokinesia
                       e. Strength: shoulder girdle, dorsiflexors of hands, & feet, grip, & hip flexors
                       f. Muscle tone

_____   _____   6. *Sensory system:*
                       a. Hearing: voice, finger rustling, tuning fork tests
                       b. Touch and temperature discrimination over the face, hands, and feet
                       c. Directional scratch test, position & vibratory sensation, & coin recognition

_____   _____   7. *Skin:*

                    8. *Case summary (no more than three lines):*

                    9. *Provisional diagnosis/differential diagnosis:*

                    10. *Recommendations:*

                                                              Signature: _____

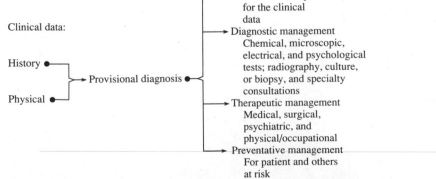

FIG. 15-1. Summary of the operational steps of the closure process. The clinical encounter leads to a provisional diagnosis. That determines the differential diagnosis and all of the future choices in the management of the Pt.

TABLE 15-2 The diagnostic catechism
1. Is there a lesion or disease?
2. If so, where is the lesion or the disease?
3. What is the lesion or the disease (the provisional diagnosis)?
4. What laboratory tests (if any) will confirm or reject the provisional diagnosis or establish a final diagnosis?
5. What is the optimum therapeutic and preventive management?

D. *What the questions of the diagnostic catechism encompass: Is there a lesion or a disease?* The Ex initially tries to discover neurologic signs that identify an anatomic lesion. Then the Ex considers organic disorders with biochemical lesions, such as some types of epilepsy or migraine, that exhibit no signs in the interictal examination. Next, the Ex considers emotional disorders with no lesion. The Ex must try to separate psychogenic from organic disorders, because the provisional diagnosis thus achieved determines the extent and type of clinical and laboratory tests required to establish the final diagnosis. To answer "Yes" to the question, "Is there a lesion?" the Ex hopes to find at least one sign. One firm sign may mean more than a multitude of symptoms. In answering the question, think through Fig. 15-2 to start generating the possibilities in your mind.

E. *Where is the lesion or the disease?* If the clinical evidence suggests a lesion or disease, ask these further questions:
   1. Is the lesion or disease in the structure or biochemistry of the Pt?
   2. Is it at the level of gene, chromosome, or cell? Is it at the level of blending of cells into tissues or of tissues into organs, or of organs into systems, or of systems into the general somatotype of the patient? In other words, do the findings constitute a neuroanatomic, morphologic, biochemical, or genetic syndrome?
   3. Can a decision be made as to the organ or organs, system or systems, involved by the lesion? If it affects the nervous system, is the lesion:
      a. In the PNS or CNS?
      b. If in the CNS, is the lesion intra-axial or extra-axial?
      c. If intra-axial, is it *focal;* in cerebrum, ventricular cavities or passageways, basal ganglia, brainstem, cerebellum, or spinal cord; or is it *multifocal* or *diffuse?*
      d. If it could be extra-axial, is it:
         (1) In a meningeal or bony covering?
         (2) In a meningeal space: epidural, subdural, or subarachnoid?
         (3) In a nerve root, plexus, peripheral nerve, neuromyal junction, or muscle?
   4. When the Pt's symptoms and signs suggest a neurologic disease, try to classify it as motor, sensory, sensorimotor, headache, or organic mental syndrome.
      a. If motor, see Fig. 15-3 to locate the neuronal system affected, or if an involuntary movement syndrome, see Fig. 15-4.
      b. If sensory, see Fig. 15-5.
      c. If a headache, see Fig. 15-6.
      d. If an organic mental syndrome, see Fig. 15-7.

F. *What is the lesion or the disease?*
Having hypothesized the neuronal system, or systems, involved, and the lesion site, the Ex next has to hypothesize *what* the lesion is. For this purpose, system-

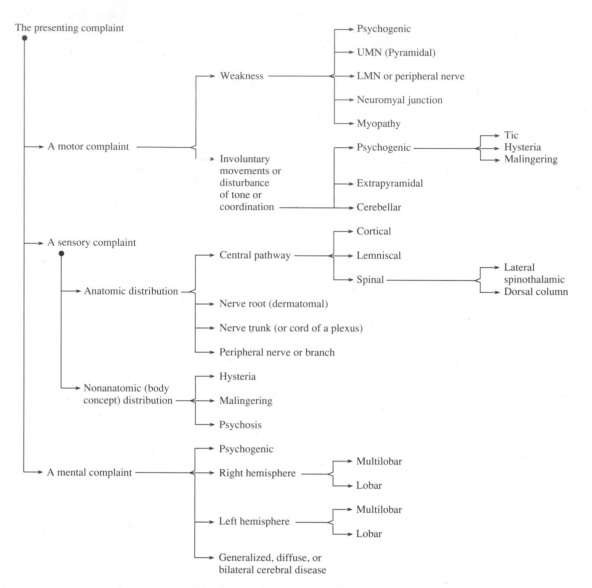

FIG. 15-2. Consider these preliminary possibilities when the Pt's complaint suggests neurologic disease.

atically think through the entities in Fig. 15-8. Then state a provisional diagnosis. State the provisional diagnosis according to the principle of parsimony: The simplest diagnosis that will explain the signs and symptoms.

G. *What tests, clinical or laboratory, will confirm or reject the provisional diagnosis and establish the final diagnosis?*
1. The explicitly stated provisional diagnosis then serves as a basis to generate a differential diagnosis list. The Ex selects any further clinical tests that will best affirm or deny the provisional diagnosis or point to another diagnosis. Having exhausted all clinical tests, the Ex selects laboratory tests according to these principles:
   a. Select the one or two *best* tests to support or reject the provisional diagnosis.
   b. Given tests of approximately equal value, select the simplest, safest, and cheapest ones, but never curtail the investigation in the sole interest of "cost containment." Failure to diagnose a diagnosable disease is the costliest mistake of all.

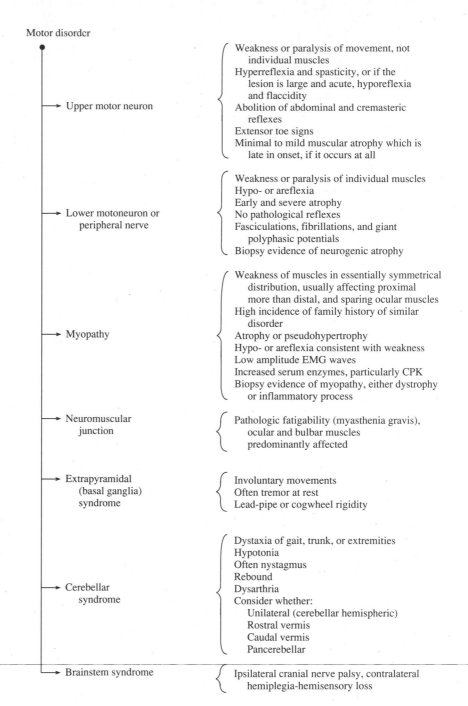

Motor disorder

Upper motor neuron
- Weakness or paralysis of movement, not individual muscles
- Hyperreflexia and spasticity, or if the lesion is large and acute, hyporeflexia and flaccidity
- Abolition of abdominal and cremasteric reflexes
- Extensor toe signs
- Minimal to mild muscular atrophy which is late in onset, if it occurs at all

Lower motoneuron or peripheral nerve
- Weakness or paralysis of individual muscles
- Hypo- or areflexia
- Early and severe atrophy
- No pathological reflexes
- Fasciculations, fibrillations, and giant polyphasic potentials
- Biopsy evidence of neurogenic atrophy

Myopathy
- Weakness of muscles in essentially symmetrical distribution, usually affecting proximal more than distal, and sparing ocular muscles
- High incidence of family history of similar disorder
- Atrophy or pseudohypertrophy
- Hypo- or areflexia consistent with weakness
- Low amplitude EMG waves
- Increased serum enzymes, particularly CPK
- Biopsy evidence of myopathy, either dystrophy or inflammatory process

Neuromuscular junction
- Pathologic fatigability (myasthenia gravis), ocular and bulbar muscles predominantly affected

Extrapyramidal (basal ganglia) syndrome
- Involuntary movements
- Often tremor at rest
- Lead-pipe or cogwheel rigidity

Cerebellar syndrome
- Dystaxia of gait, trunk, or extremities
- Hypotonia
- Often nystagmus
- Rebound
- Dysarthria
- Consider whether:
  - Unilateral (cerebellar hemispheric)
  - Rostral vermis
  - Caudal vermis
  - Pancerebellar

Brainstem syndrome
- Ipsilateral cranial nerve palsy, contralateral hemiplegia-hemisensory loss

FIG. 15-3. Consider these loci as the possible site for the lesion if the Pt has symptoms and signs suggesting an organic disorder of the motor system.

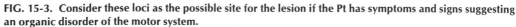

    c. When faced with a hopeless or untreatable disorder, take all reasonable steps to exclude a treatable disorder.

  2. To select the most appropriate laboratory tests, review the possible ones listed in Table 13-1.

H. *What is the optimum therapeutic and preventive management?*

  1. State the therapeutic goals and how to meet them. Just what can you hope to do for the Pt?

  2. What emotional, educational, or socioeconomic perils does the Pt face

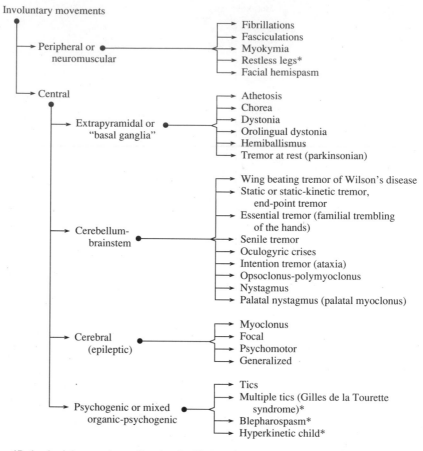

*Pathophysiology unclear—disorder classified more or less arbitrarily

FIG. 15-4. Consider these loci as the possible site for the lesion if the Pt has an involuntary movement disorder.

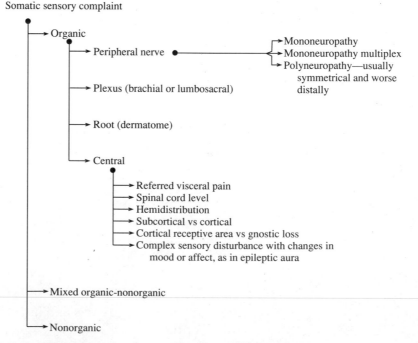

FIG. 15-5. Consider these loci as the possible site for the lesion if the Pt has a sensory complaint.

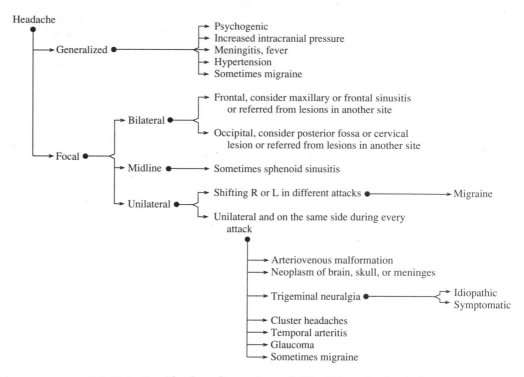

FIG. 15-6. Consider these diagnostic possibilities if the Pt has headaches.

because of the illness? What agencies—lay, rehabilitative, vocational, or governmental—might help?

3. Having identified the Pt's illness, the Ex has to identify other persons at risk. How can they be reached and offered prophylaxis? Consider for Pts with environmentally induced, contagious-infectious, or hereditary diseases.

4. Follow the Pt to insure that your final diagnosis is indeed final and that the Pt's subsequent course continues to confirm its finality.

III. A precis for success in the NE; or, common errors to be avoided

Note: I wanted to end the text by reviewing the common errors made in the performance of the NE, but then I decided to phrase them as a list of *dos,* not *don'ts.*

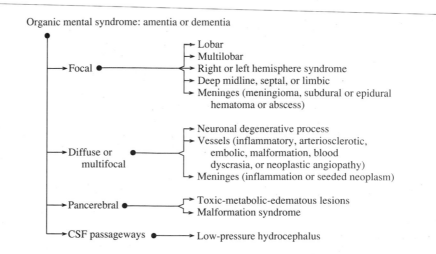

FIG. 15-7. Consider these diagnostic possibilities if the Pt has mental, emotional, or intellectual deficits that suggest an organic neurologic disorder.

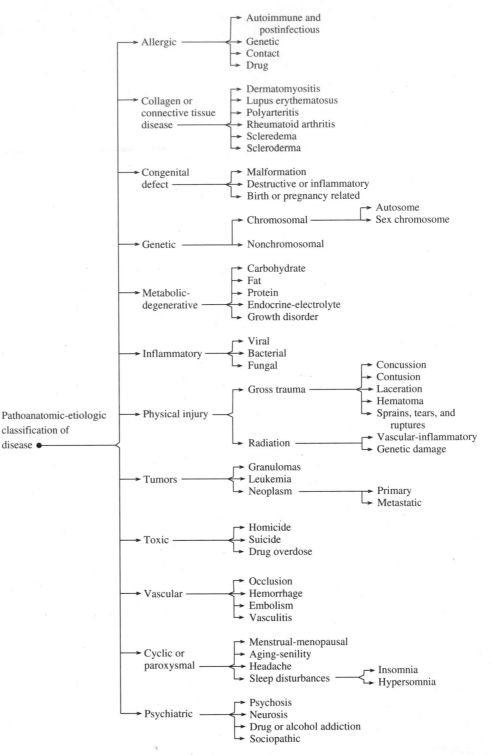

FIG. 15-8. Pathoanatomic-etiologic classification of disease. Review this dendrogram systematically for each patient to generate the gamut of etiologic possibilities that may cause the clinical findings. The branching of the dendrogram to the right can be continued almost endlessly.

Interpret them either way, but if you heed what they say, you will avoid the mistakes that they convey.

A. *Attitudes for success in the NE*
   1. *Maintain professionalism.* Accept every revelation by the Pt and every behavior neutrally, as purely clinical phenomena. If you react emotionally

to the Pt, either by love or hate, you lose the objective judgment required to make correct clinical decisions.

2. *Expect the abnormal.* By expecting every finding to be abnormal, you will do a much more vigilant examination than if you expect normality.

3. *Enjoy the NE.* Make the NE a game of friendly challenges in order to maintain the interest of both the Ex and Pt in the outcome of each test. "Let's see how light a touch you can feel?" Or ". . . how soft a sound you can hear." "Hold your hands out in front and let's see how still you can keep them." In testing strength, "Do your best, don't let me win," etc.

B. *Overall principles of performance*
   1. *Do an organized NE.* A disorganized examination is the most common error of all. Correct it by laying out your instruments in order of use and proceeding rostrocaudally, doing the head and cranial nerve examination, motor examination, and sensory examination in order (see the summarized NE at the start of the text).
   2. *Insure the Pt's comfort and safety during each test.*
   3. *Understand each test and each definition operationally.* Separate observation and description from interpretation. If you understand the operation and the purpose of each test of the NE, you will interpret the findings correctly.
   4. *Titrate, or match, the Pt's sensory or motor functions against yours wherever possible.* Titrate or match visual fields, visual acuity, vibration and hearing thresholds, and strength.
   5. *Quantify or scale the test results whenever possible.* Measure circumferences of the head and extremities. Scale dysfunctions as minimal, mild, moderate, or severe, or enumerate 0 to 4+.
   6. *Think circuitry.* Visualize the connections of each circuit as you test it. Unless you review circuitry daily, you forget it. If you find a neurological abnormality, postulate the neighborhood signs that should accompany it by visualizing the conjunction of the circuits of the nervous system and test for these neighborhood signs. Actually drawing the circuits helps.
   7. *Consider whether any finding is a normal variation or reflects the genetic background of the Pt.* Commonly, the Ex fails to call in and examine the whole family to decide about pseudopapilledema, the OFC, height of the arch of the foot, facial features, overall somatotype, etc.
   8. *Consider whether any finding pre-existed:* Ptosis, VIth nerve palsy, anisocoria, hemiplegia, and atrophy. This is especially important in examining the comatose Pt when a pre-existing finding, such as anisocoria, may mislead the Ex. Get old photographs or family videos.
   9. *Extend the basic NE when required.* Reproduce triggering factors: hyperventilation, fatigability during exercise, dizziness on change of position, or trouble in swallowing. Have the Pt return when symptomatic and repeat the tests.

C. *The mental status examination*
   1. *Weave in the questions that test the sensorium skillfully, as ordinary conversation, not as an inquisition.* Do not ask the *who, where, when,* and *what* questions in machine-gun style, except in an acute head injury.
   2. *Complete the Halstead-Reitan battery if the history raises the question of a cerebral lesion.*
   3. *Estimate intelligence.* Severely, moderately, or mildly retarded or demented, or normal.

D. *Examination of the cranial nerves and head*
1. *Measure the OFC of every infant.*
2. *Test the visual fields on the diagonals, not the meridians.* Testing on the vertical or horizontal meridians may entirely miss a quadrantic defect (Fig. 3-10).
3. *Test pupilloconstriction correctly.* Darken the room, ask the Pt to fixate on a distant point to eliminate pupilloconstriction from accommodation, and flash the light into each eye separately from the side. Then do the swinging flashlight test.
4. *Test the corneal reflex from the side.* Bring the cotton wisp in from the side out of sight of the Pt's vision to avoid a visually induced blink response. Don't use the cotton tip of an applicator stick (no sticks around the eyes).
5. *Press on the zygomatic arch (cheekbone), not the jaw, to test the strength of the sternocleidomastoid muscle and other rotators of the head.* Direct pressure on the cheekbone tests the head rotators without working through the lateral pterygoid muscles. If the pterygoids are weak, strong lateral pressure on the jaw may dislocate the temporomandibular joint, especially in elderly and edentulous Pts.

E. *Motor examination*
1. *Recognize that each positive behavior produced by the unconscious Pt establishes the integrity of some neuroanatomic circuit.* By observing and correctly interpreting all of the spontaneous and elicited behaviors of the unconscious Pt, the Ex can test most of the sensory and motor circuits that can be tested in the conscious Pt.
2. *Apply the concept of deficit and release phenomena and of neural shock (diaschisis) to the Pt with an acute neurologic lesion.* Neural shock means that UMN lesions manifest only by deficit signs, not the classical release signs as with acute lesions, and that signs and symptoms temporarily extend beyond those suggested by the actual anatomic boundaries of acute lesions.
3. *Test every Pt's gait, where possible.* Nothing tests the integrity of the Pt's nervous system so quickly (Chap. 8, section VI), yet Exs often fail to test it.
4. *Test strength by use of principles.* The length-strength law, the law of predominant strength of the antigravity muscles, and the law of matching the Pt and Ex muscle to muscle, particularly in testing finger strength (Fig. 7-3).
5. *Elicit the MSRs by a whiplash swing, not a peck.* Be a swinger of hammers, not a pecker (Fig. 7-5). If no reflexes are elicited, try re-positioning and relaxing the part, altering the pressure or tension on the tendon, and use Jendrassik's reinforcement.
6. *Try first to elicit the extensor toe sign from the lateral side of the foot, not the sole.* Demented, psychotic, or retarded Pts, the elderly and often the ticklish young, or those with painful peripheral neuropathies resist the discomfort of plantar stimulation but may tolerate pressure on the lateral side of the foot.

F. *Sensory examination*
1. *Establish good communication.* Inform the Pt of the nature of the stimulus and the response to make. "Which is the sharpest, number one or number two?" "Is the toe up or down?" etc.

2. *Isolate the modality to be tested.* Conceal the test object from sight or perception by any modality other than the one tested.
3. *Monitor the Pt's attention and reliability.* The Ex sometimes withholds a stimulus when the Pt expects it, and forewarns the Pt of that possibility.
4. *Test temperature discrimination rather than pain around the face and in children.* (Fig. 10-4). Both pain and temperature sensations test the same pathways. Testing temperature discrimination is more comfortable for every Pt. Children as young as three years will accept it, but often will not accept pain testing at all. In this time of AIDS, the fewer the pinpricks, the better.

F. *Closure of the NE*
   1. *Write a three-line summary.* If you have come to grips with the clinical problem, you can write it out in no more than three lines, no matter how complicated. *Your ability to summarize the findings is the best single test of your ability to function as a physician.* "This is a 64-yr-old hypertensive WM salesman who had the acute onset of coma, eyes deviated to the left, complete flaccid right hemiplegia, and nuchal rigidity." From that summary, the probable diagnosis leaps out at you: intracranial hemorrhage in the left middle cerebral artery distribution, probably extending into the ventricle and subarachnoid space.
   2. *Always recite the diagnostic catechism:* (Table 15-2).
   3. *If tempted to make a nonorganic diagnosis, review the list of organic diseases commonly misdiagnosed* (Table 14-5).
   4. *Write out the NE informatively, or use a checkoff list to state what you have actually tested and found to be negative or positive (Table 15-1).* Your notes should, at least, enable the reader to find out about the Pt's mental state and whether the Pt can sit, stand, walk, talk, breathe, see, hear, and feel normally. I'd rather you simply said that than write out every negative finding, but negatives are also important as exclusionary evidence.

IV. Beneficence: the ultimate objective of every Pt-physician contact

For hundreds, even thousands, of years, physicians have understood the goals of the medical model and have expressed them in aphorisms. The two given here apparently arose in the Middle Ages; their exact authorship is lost in obscurity. Here is the first:

> A painless examination
> A complete cure
> Leaving no blemish behind

And here is the other:

> The physician can only rarely cure,
> Can sometimes palliate,
> But can always give comfort.

At the end of every Pt-physician contact, the Pt should at least feel benefited and comforted, although the physician cannot cure or even palliate. Comfort comes not from false optimism, pity, patronizing pap, nor condescending platitudes, but through honest compassion and competence. Each Pt-physician contact remains incomplete, the ring remains open and the physician remains but a technocrat, until the Pt feels this beneficence.

Learning Objectives for Chapter Fifteen

I. The routine screening neurological examination

1. Enumerate what the Ex may elect to omit from the complete NE when screening a Pt who has no symptoms of neurologic disease.

2. Describe what you should record in your notes after completing the screening NE (Table 15-1).

II. The neurologic examination when the Pt has symptoms or signs suggesting neurologic disease

1. State the five questions of the diagnostic catechism (Table 15-2).

2. Explain the meaning of each of the five questions of the diagnostic catechism.

3. Discuss the importance of posing diagnostic hypotheses during the history and examination.

4. Describe how and why to use differential diagnostic dendrograms to analyze the Pt's presenting complaint (Figs. 15-2 through 15-7).

5. Enumerate the major pathologic categories of disease to consider in differential diagnosis. (If you wish, make a dendrogram and extend it as far to the right as you can.) (Fig. 15-8).

6. State the principles involved in selecting laboratory tests.

III. A precis of the NE (see text)

IV. Beneficence

Describe the one feeling that the physician attempts to provide or convey at every encounter with every Pt.

Index